Handbook of Pediatric Nephrology

Handbook of Pediatric Nephrology

Editor: Jasper Dempsey

AMERICAN
MEDICAL PUBLISHERS
www.americanmedicalpublishers.com

AMERICAN
MEDICAL PUBLISHERS
www.americanmedicalpublishers.com

Cataloging-in-Publication Data

Handbook of pediatric nephrology / edited by Jasper Dempsey.
p. cm.
Includes bibliographical references and index.
ISBN 979-8-88740-369-4
1. Pediatric nephrology. 2. Nephrology. 3. Children--Diseases. 4. Kidneys--Diseases. I. Dempsey, Jasper.
RJ476.K5 H36 2023
618.926 1--dc23

American Medical Publishers,
41 Flatbush Avenue,
1st Floor, New York,
NY 11217, USA

ISBN 979-8-88740-369-4 (Hardback)

Contents

Preface

This book has been an outcome of determined endeavour from a group of educationists in the field. The primary objective was to involve a broad spectrum of professionals from diverse cultural background involved in the field for developing new researches. The book not only targets students but also scholars pursuing higher research for further enhancement of the theoretical and practical applications of the subject.

Pediatric nephrology refers to a sub-specialty of pediatrics. It is responsible for managing infants, children and young people having acute and chronic kidney disease. It also includes treating kidney diseases through kidney transplantation and dialysis. Pediatric nephrology involves the detailed study of renal physiology, fluid management, and disturbances in acid-base balance and electrolytes. It is involved in the management of various diseases such as acute glomerulonephritis, acute kidney failure, nephritis and inherited cystic kidney disease. Pediatric nephrology investigates and treats children in a manner that helps them to cooperate and relax. Moreover, medical equipment specifically designed for children is used within this field. This book aims to understand the clinical perspectives of pediatric nephrology. It presents researches and studies performed by experts across the globe. Researchers and students in this field will be assisted by this book.

It was an honour to edit such a profound book and also a challenging task to compile and examine all the relevant data for accuracy and originality. I wish to acknowledge the efforts of the contributors for submitting such brilliant and diverse chapters in the field and for endlessly working for the completion of the book. Last, but not the least; I thank my family for being a constant source of support in all my research endeavours.

Editor

1

Meckel–Gruber Syndrome: An Update on Diagnosis, Clinical Management and Research Advances

*Verity Hartill[1,2], Katarzyna Szymanska[2], Saghira Malik Sharif[1], Gabrielle Wheway[3] and Colin A. Johnson[2]**

[1] *Department of Clinical Genetics, Yorkshire Regional Genetics Service, Leeds Teaching Hospitals NHS Trust, Leeds, United Kingdom,* [2] *Leeds Institute of Biomedical and Clinical Sciences, University of Leeds, Leeds, United Kingdom,* [3] *Faculty of Health and Applied Sciences, Department of Applied Sciences, UWE Bristol, Bristol, United Kingdom*

Correspondence:
Colin A. Johnson
c.johnson@leeds.ac.uk

Meckel–Gruber syndrome (MKS) is a lethal autosomal recessive congenital anomaly syndrome caused by mutations in genes encoding proteins that are structural or functional components of the primary cilium. Conditions that are caused by mutations in ciliary genes are collectively termed the ciliopathies, and MKS represents the most severe condition in this group of disorders. The primary cilium is a microtubule-based organelle, projecting from the apical surface of vertebrate cells. It acts as an "antenna" that receives and transduces chemosensory and mechanosensory signals, but also regulates diverse signaling pathways, such as Wnt and Shh, that have important roles during embryonic development. Most MKS proteins localize to a distinct ciliary compartment called the transition zone (TZ) that regulates the trafficking of cargo proteins or lipids. In this review, we provide an up-to-date summary of MKS clinical features, molecular genetics, and clinical diagnosis. MKS has a highly variable phenotype, extreme genetic heterogeneity, and displays allelism with other related ciliopathies such as Joubert syndrome, presenting significant challenges to diagnosis. Recent advances in genetic technology, with the widespread use of multi-gene panels for molecular testing, have significantly improved diagnosis, genetic counseling, and the clinical management of MKS families. These include the description of some limited genotype–phenotype correlations. We discuss recent insights into the molecular basis of disease in MKS, since the functions of some of the relevant ciliary proteins have now been determined. A common molecular etiology appears to be disruption of ciliary TZ structure and function, affecting essential developmental signaling and the regulation of secondary messengers.

Keywords: Meckel–Gruber syndrome, renal cystic dysplasia, oligohydramnios, primary cilium, transition zone, Shh signaling

CLINICAL FEATURES

Meckel–Gruber syndrome (MKS, OMIM number #249000), sometimes simply termed Meckel syndrome, was first described by Johann Friedrich Meckel in 1822. Meckel noted two siblings who died soon after birth with typical features that included occipital encephalocele, polycystic kidneys, and polydactyly (1). Gruber described the same condition later, naming it dysencephalia splanchnocystica (2). In the 1960s, the condition was further delineated by Opitz and Howe (3) with subsequent refinement of the diagnostic criteria (4–7).

Meckel–Gruber syndrome is a lethal developmental syndrome characterized by posterior fossa abnormalities (most frequently occipital encephalocele) (**Figures 1A,B**), bilateral enlarged cystic kidneys (**Figures 1C–E**), and hepatic developmental defects that include ductal plate malformation associated with hepatic fibrosis and cysts (**Figure 1F**) (8). A common additional feature is postaxial polydactyly, usually affecting both hands and feet (**Figure 1A**), which is seen in 70–80% of cases (5–7, 9). Other occasional features, seen in 25–40% of fetuses include bowing and shortening of the long bones, abnormalities of the male genitalia, microcephaly or anencephaly, cleft lip and palate, and other craniofacial abnormalities, congenital heart defects, and pulmonary hypoplasia (5, 6, 8, 9). Rare features (seen in less than 20% of cases) include cystic dysplasia of the lungs or thyroid, retinal colobomata, and *situs* defects (8–14). Central nervous system (CNS) defects are considered to be obligate features of MKS but appear to have a variable presentation, varying between total craniorachischisis, partial defects of the corpus callosum, Dandy–Walker malformation, and most frequently occipital encephalocele (15).

Renal cystic dysplasia is the most characteristic feature of MKS, but differs from those typical of polycystic kidney disease. The degree of cyst formation varies between individuals with MKS, but the kidneys will often be grossly enlarged, causing massive swelling of the abdomen (**Figures 1A,D**). Large, fluid-filled cysts are visible by eye in most affected individuals. However, in other small cysts, cystic changes of the proximal tubules and the absence of normal renal parenchyma are visible by microscopic investigation (**Figure 1E**). Cysts develop first in the glomeruli in the cortex, and cystogenesis progresses along the tubules and collecting ducts in the medulla. Abnormal fetal renal function is a frequent cause of oligohydramnios or anhydramnios, a common complication of an MKS pregnancy (7, 9). Potter's sequence is frequent (pulmonary hypoplasia, growth restriction, club feet, and contractures) with a distinctive facies (comprising slanting forehead, flattened nose, and low-set ears) (**Figure 1A**), and is secondary to oligohydramnios or anhydramnios during pregnancy. In addition to cystic kidney dysplasia, hepatic involvement is an obligate feature of MKS (6). The typical histology shows bile duct proliferation and dilation (**Figure 1F**), associated with excess collagenous connective tissues (8), which are thought to arise from the incomplete development of the hepatic biliary system (16, 17).

GENETICS AND ALLELISM

Autosomal recessive (AR) inheritance for MKS is confirmed by equal occurrence in males and females, concordance in monozygotic twins, examples of affected siblings, and, in some cases, parental consanguinity. If the condition has occurred in previous pregnancies then the recurrence risk is 25%. The worldwide incidence of MKS has been estimated at 1 in 135,000 live births (18), but higher incidences of MKS are observed in endogamous populations, such as Gujarati Indians (19), Tatars (20), Hutterites (21), and in Finland (22) where 1 in every 9,000 live births is affected. MKS incidence is also higher in consanguineous populations, such as Kuwaiti Bedouin tribes (1 in 3,530 births) (23) and populations in Saudi Arabia (1 in 3,500 births) (24).

Meckel–Gruber syndrome has extreme genetic heterogeneity and displays allelism with other ciliopathies such as Joubert syndrome (JBTS), COACH syndrome (cerebellar vermis hypo/aplasia, oligophrenia, congenital ataxia, ocular coloboma, and hepatic fibrosis), oro-facio-digital syndrome (OFD), nephronophthisis (NPHP), and Bardet–Biedl syndrome (BBS). To date, mutations in 14 genes (including *TXNDC15*) are identified as causative for MKS (**Table 1**). Mutations in a further three genes, specifically *C5orf42* (25), *CSPP1* (26), and *CEP55* (27), are implicated on the basis of pathogenic private mutations in individual families with either MKS or MKS-like phenotypes (**Table 1**). Two other genes, comprising *SEC8* (also known as *EXOC4*) (25) and *EXOC3L2* (28), have private mutations as a cause of probable MKS phenotypes. In total, mutations in these genes appear to explain only 50–60% of MKS cases (28, 29).

Mutations in *TMEM67*, *RPGRIP1L*, and *TMEM216* can cause both JBTS and MKS, demonstrating allelism between these conditions (31, 35, 36, 46) (**Table 1**). Biallelic mutations in the known MKS genes can also cause other related and allelic ciliopathies. Most notably, mutations in *CEP290* (*MKS4*) can also occur in patients with NPHP (47), Senior-Løken syndrome (SLSN), JBTS (34), BBS (48), COACH syndrome (49), and Leber congenital amaurosis (50). The variable expressivity of the MKS phenotype can complicate the diagnosis of the condition, since this can extend to intra-familial variation for individuals that carry the same pathogenic mutation within families (31), even between monozygotic twins (7). The effect of non-Mendelian inheritance modes or the influence of genetic modifier alleles has frequently been proposed to explain some of this variation. However, in a cohort of JBTS patients who shared causal alleles but had discordant phenotypic features, digenic, or oligogenic inheritance modes were largely excluded as disease mechanisms (51). A second recent study suggests that ciliopathy phenotypes, including those for MKS, are allele-specific and that stochastic effects have a more important role on phenotypic variability than modifier alleles (28).

GENOTYPE–PHENOTYPE CORRELATIONS

In recent years, the identification of pathogenic alleles specific to MKS, limited genotype–phenotype correlations and founder mutations for particular ethnic groups (**Table 1**) have facilitated the rapid and accurate genetic diagnosis of this condition. Mutations in *MKS1* cause ca. 7% of all MKS cases and ca. 70% cases in Finland. Most Finnish MKS patients share the common "Finn major" mutation (*MKS1* IVS15-7_35del; **Table 1**), which is thought to have arisen in a founder of the Finnish population (52). Skeletal involvement including shortening and bowing of the long bones, polydactyly, and occipital encephalocele are frequently seen in patients with the Finn major mutation (18). More generally, *MKS1* mutations are associated with higher rates of polydactyly and occipital encephalocele, bone dysplasia, cleft palate, and *situs* defects (52). All *MKS1* mutations reported in MKS patients are null mutations, but a hypomorphic mutation has been reported in an individual with BBS (48), and recently in individuals with JBTS (53, 54).

TMEM67 mutations are estimated to cause 16% of MKS cases (55), making them the most frequent cause of MKS. Both CNS malformations and polydactyly are less frequent in *TMEM67*-mutated individuals than those with *MKS1* mutations (56).

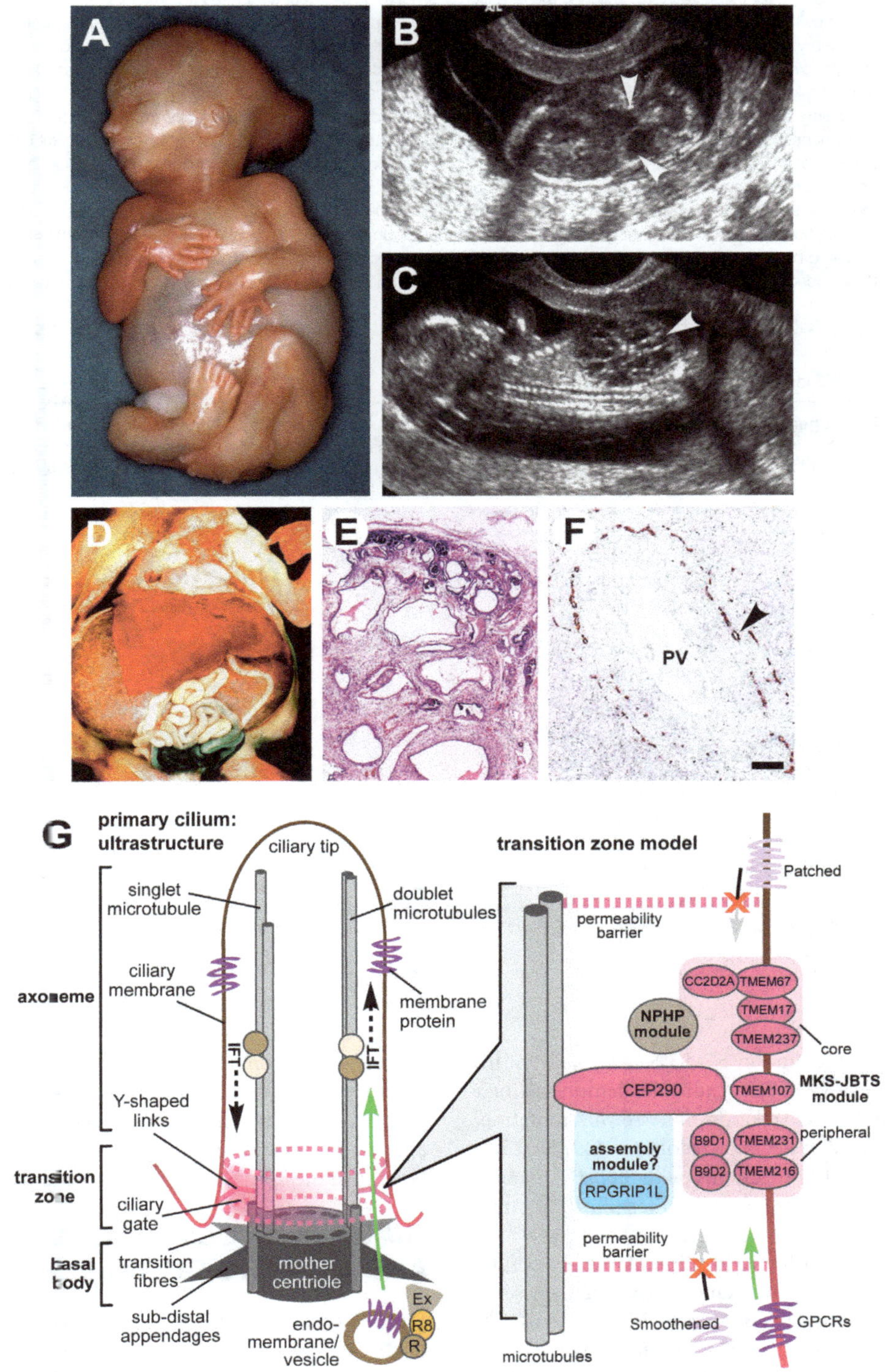

FIGURE 1 | Continued

FIGURE 1 | Continued
Clinical features of Meckel–Gruber syndrome (MKS) and schematic of primary cilia structure. **(A)** Typical external features for a fetus with MKS at gestation age 16/40, showing typical clinical features comprising occipital encephalocele, massive flank masses due to bilateral renal cystic dysplasia, postaxial hexadactyly of all limbs, and a typical Potter's sequence facies with a slanting forehead and flattened nose. **(B,C)** Ultrasound findings at 14+/40 weeks of gestation for MKS showing **(B)** encephalocele (arrowheads), and **(C)** large cystic kidneys (arrowhead). **(D)** Massive swelling of the abdomen of a fetus at gestation age 18+/40 with MKS due to grossly enlarged, cystic kidneys. **(E)** Hematoxylin-eosin staining of MKS fetal kidney at gestation age 18+/40 showing cystic dysplasia, comprising large, fluid-filled cysts, small cysts, and cystic swelling of the proximal tubules and glomeruli, with the absence of normal renal parenchyma. **(F)** Immunohistochemical staining of MKS fetal liver at gestation age 18+/40 for cytokeratin-19, showing the retention of embryonic bile duct structures (the ductal plate malformation) without the formation of patent bile ducts (arrowhead). PV, hepatic portal vein. **(G)** Left: simplified schematic of cilium ultrastructure (individual components are not to scale). For the purposes of clarity, the ciliary axoneme is represented by two doublets of microtubules (the A- and B-tubules; gray rods), and the nine-fold symmetry in the structure is indicated by dark gray ovals in the mother centriole. The axoneme is bound by ciliary membrane (red/brown line and shading). The ciliary transition zone (TZ) is characterized by Y-shaped links (pink) that mediate interactions with the ciliary membrane. The permeability barrier called the "ciliary gate" is indicated by the dashed pink ovals and pink shading, and is thought to consist of transition fibers and TZ proteins. Ciliary cargo proteins (purple) are trafficking by vesicular transport mediated by coordinated interactions between the Rab family of small GTPases (RAB11 and RAB8; R8), the RAB8 activator protein Rabin8 (R), and the exocyst protein complex (Ex) at the ciliary base. The exocyst tethers vesicles to the periciliary membrane, facilitating transport through the ciliary gate (green arrow), followed by transport within the cilium mediated by intraflagellar transport (IFT; dashed black arrows). Right: schematic of a TZ model, showing the possible location of TZ proteins mutated in MKS and related ciliopathies (pink ovals) forming the "MKS-JBTS module," RPGRIP1L (blue oval) which is thought to be a component of a ciliary assembly module, and a third functional module (brown) that is associated with nephronophthisis (NPHP) proteins. The selective transport of cargo transmembrane proteins (lilac or purple) is indicated by arrows. The proteins include G-protein-coupled receptors (GPCRs), and effectors of the Shh signaling pathway (Smoothened and Patched). Images **(A–C)** are used by kind permission of Dr. Riitta Salonen (Rinnekoti Foundation, Helsinki, Finland) from the Robert J. Gorlin Slide Collection. JBTS, Joubert syndrome.

TABLE 1 | Summary of known MKS loci and identified genes.

Locus	Gene	Entrez gene ID	Aliases	Location	Founder mutation(s)	Reference
MKS1	*MKS1*	54903	MKS, BBS13, JBTS28	17q22	Finnish c.1408-35_1408-7del29	(30)
MKS2	*TMEM216*	51259	JBTS2, CORS2	11q12.2	Ashkenazi c.218G > T (p.R73L)	(31, 32)
MKS3	*TMEM67*	91147	JBTS6, NPHP11, MECKELIN	8q22.1	Pakistani c.1575 + 1G > A	(33)
MKS4	*CEP290*	80184	KIAA0373, 3H11AG, JBTS5, SLSN6, LCA10, BBS14, NPHP6	12q21.32		(34)
MKS5	*RPGRIP1L*	23322	KIAA1005, JBTS7, CORS3, FTM, NPHP8	16q12.2	European c.1843A > C (p.T625P)	(35, 36)
MKS6	*CC2D2A*	57545	KIAA1345, JBTS9	4p15.32	Finnish c.1762C > T (p.?)	(37)
MKS7	*NPHP3*	27031	SLSN3, NPHP3, NPH3, RHPD1	3q22.1		(38)
MKS8	*TCTN2*	79867	C12orf38, TECT2, JBTS24	12q24.31		(39)
MKS9	*B9D1*	27077	MKSR1, JBTS27	17p11.2		(40)
MKS10	*B9D2*	80776	MKSR2	19q13.2		(41)
MKS11	*TMEM231*	79583	JBTS20	16q23.1		(42)
NA	*C5orf42*	65250	OFD6, JBTS17	5p13.2		(25)
NA	*CSPP1*	79848	JBTS21, CSPP	8q13.1-q13.2		(26)
MKS12	*KIF14*	9928	KIAA0042	1q32.1		(43)
MKS13	*TMEM107*	84314	JBTS29, PRO1268	17p13.1		(44, 45)
NA	*TXNDC15*	79770	C5orf14, UNQ335	5q31.1		(28)
NA	*CEP55*	55165	CT111, URCC6, C10orf3	10q23.33		(27)

Assigned locus names are listed, with unassigned ones indicated by NA. Alias names of genes or loci summarize the alternative gene symbols, names, and any reported allelism with other ciliopathies (indicated by the gene symbol or locus name). Any reported founder mutations in specific populations are also listed, in addition to the original gene discovery paper or papers.
CORS, cerebellar–ocular–renal syndrome; JBTS, Joubert syndrome; MKS, Meckel–Gruber syndrome; NPHP, nephronophthisis; OFD, oro-facio-digital syndrome; SLSN, Senior-Løken syndrome.

TMEM67 mutations also account for 57–83% (49, 55, 57) of the JBTS variant phenotype of COACH syndrome, demonstrating a strong genotype–phenotype correlation of *TMEM67* mutations with hepatic developmental defects or coloboma (49, 58). This correlation indicates that JBTS patients with hepatic involvement are prioritized for *TMEM67* mutation testing (57). Other genotype–phenotype correlations for MKS or JBTS have been identified by mutation type, or by the location of missense mutations within protein domains. For example, *CC2D2A* missense mutations are associated with JBTS whereas MKS is caused by null alleles (59). Missense mutations in exons 8–15 of *TMEM67*, particularly in combination with a second truncating mutation, are also associated with MKS (29, 55). Homozygous truncating mutations in *RPGRIP1L* are associated with MKS, whereas missense mutations (either in the homozygous state or compound heterozygous with a truncating mutation) are prevalent for JBTS patients. MKS phenotypes associated with *RPGRIP1L* mutations tend to be severe, including anencephaly and shortening and bowing of the long bones, in addition to the classic triad (36).

DIAGNOSIS, CLINICAL MANAGEMENT, AND GENETIC COUNSELING

Meckel–Gruber syndrome is lethal *in utero* or immediately after birth, often due to pulmonary hypoplasia, although an unusual survivor has been described aged 28 months (60). MKS has a broad, multi-organ phenotype with considerable variation, but it is generally diagnosed by the presence of cystic kidney dysplasia (**Figure 1C**), in addition to at least one other hallmark feature of the disease. These comprise occipital encephalocele (**Figure 1B**), polydactyly (**Figure 1A**), or hepatic developmental abnormalities such as the ductal plate malformation (**Figure 1F**) (6, 7). The presence of abnormal intrahepatic bile ducts and cystic kidneys has been proposed to be invariant features of MKS and appears to be pathognomonic for the condition (6, 17). Salonen (6) has proposed that the minimal diagnostic criteria for MKS are CNS malformation, bilateral multicystic kidneys, and hepatic fibrotic changes.

Transabdominal ultrasonography, performed at 10–14 weeks gestation, has been shown to successfully detect several of the fetal anomalies associated with MKS, including polycystic kidneys (from 9 weeks gestation), occipital encephalocele (from 13 weeks), and polydactyly (from 11 weeks), in both high-risk and low-risk pregnancies (**Figure 1B**) (60–64). Visualization can be compromised by oligohydramnios (65), but this is less problematic when performed in the first trimester of pregnancy (62). Further investigation of anomalies is possible by transvaginal scanning. Enlargement of the fetal trunk can give an early indication of multicystic renal dysplasia (66), in addition to unusually heterogeneous corticomedullary differentiation, reduced echogenicity of the medulla, increased echogenicity of the cortex, and the visualization of small medullary cysts (**Figure 1C**) (67). The fetal bladder can also be visualized by ultrasonography from 11 weeks, and the absence of a visible fetal bladder is often indicative of renal dysfunction.

Fetal MRI is an alternative if ultrasonography findings are inconclusive or lack of amniotic fluid prevents clear imaging. MRI offers better soft-tissue resolution than ultrasonography, and can provide clearer images of intracranial structures to enable an accurate diagnosis of CNS malformations, but is rarely performed before 18 weeks gestation. Fetal movement and maternal aortic pulsation do not preclude a successful diagnosis of MKS using MRI (68), since imaging artifacts caused by fetal movement can be minimized by a fetal neuromuscular blockade (69) or general anesthesia of the mother. Transabdominal or vaginal endoscopy in the first trimester of pregnancy allows diagnosis of MKS by visualization of the surface anatomy of the embryo. Fetoscopy enables the direct observation of polydactyly and occipital encephalocele from 11 weeks gestational age (70). Prenatal diagnosis is also possible by using a combination of these imaging techniques, α-fetoprotein testing of amniotic fluid, and DNA testing of fetus and parents. For example, elevated levels of maternal α-fetoprotein during antenatal screening may be associated with MKS (61).

Definitive diagnosis is often possible by using DNA testing to screen for mutations in the known MKS genes. Molecular diagnostic strategies include mutation screening of individual genes or targeted clonal sequencing of multi-gene panels. Single gene testing has low diagnostic sensitivity because of the absence of clear genotype–phenotype correlations for MKS. However, once a pathogenic variant in a family has been identified, then prenatal genetic diagnosis by chorionic villus sampling can be prioritized for at-risk pregnancies. Multi-gene panels can include MKS genes, and other ciliopathy genes of interest, that can be tested by sequence analysis and deletion/duplication analysis (71). However, their diagnostic sensitivity can vary between laboratories because panels can include genes that are unrelated to MKS. Referring clinicians should therefore decide which multi-gene panel has the best balance of sensitivity and affordability. If testing by a multi-gene panel does not confirm a clinical diagnosis of MKS, then more comprehensive testing by either whole-exome sequencing or whole-genome sequencing (WES or WGS) should be considered for obligate carriers. However, these tests may support or suggest unexpected diagnoses, in view of the broad range of possible differential diagnoses for MKS. These are extensive and include Smith–Lemli–Opitz syndrome, trisomy 13, hydrolethalus syndrome, and other related ciliopathies that include AR polycystic kidney disease, BBS, JBTS, and OFD. In particular, the prenatal features of BBS (polydactyly, renal defects, hepatic anomalies, genital hypoplasia, and heart malformations) can lead to a misdiagnosis of MKS (72). The extensive range of differential diagnoses and the broad allelism between different ciliopathies highlights the clinical need for accurate molecular diagnosis and the refinement of genotype–phenotype correlations (71, 73).

Since MKS has an AR inheritance pattern, couples with a previously affected child should have the opportunity for genetic counseling with a medical professional in order to discuss the nature, inheritance, and implications of an MKS diagnosis. The possibility of prenatal testing needs appropriate counseling of parents if it is being considered for the purpose of pregnancy termination in addition to early diagnosis. Individual opinions regarding prenatal testing and pregnancy termination may depend on a number of factors such as religious and cultural beliefs, and previous experiences of the medical condition (74, 75). An accurate perception of their genetic risk, a clear impact of genetic disorder and previous experience of having an affected child can help parents to make an informed decision (76). It is therefore appropriate to discuss these issues at an early stage to ensure that families can make informed medical and personal decisions.

With consanguineous MKS families, geneticists will encourage disclosure to at-risk relatives. The fact that these individuals often do not seek carrier testing suggests that many families are not sharing this information. In families with an AR disorder who practice consanguinity, the concern that their children's carrier status would affect their marriage prospects can contribute to non-disclosure of this important information to their wider family (76–78). Furthermore, there is a widespread assumption among healthcare professionals that Muslim patients will not accept termination of pregnancy (79). However, under a *fatwā* (an Islamic legal pronouncement), termination of pregnancy is permitted before "ensoulment" at 120 days in cases of severe disability such as MKS, or where there is a risk to the mother's life (75, 80), but knowledge of the *fatwā* is limited among Muslim populations (75, 81).

INSIGHTS INTO MOLECULAR PATHOMECHANISMS

The primary cilium is a microtubule-based organelle, projecting from the apical surface of vertebrate cells. It acts as an "antenna" that receives and transduces chemosensory and mechanosensory signals (**Figure 1G**). Primary cilia are thought to be hubs of developmental signaling that regulate diverse pathways such as Wnt and Shh that have essential roles during embryonic development. In particular, mutations MKS genes cause defective Shh signaling in several mouse models of ciliopathies (82–85). Primary cilia have a complex architecture that defines the compartmentalization of ciliary proteins, and many genes that are mutated in MKS encode proteins that localize to the ciliary TZ. This is a distinct molecular compartment located at proximal regions of cilia (86, 87) that has been defined by genetic and biochemical approaches to consist of protein complexes forming the so-called "MKS-JBTS module" (**Figure 1G**). The TZ connects the microtubules of the ciliary axoneme to the plasma and ciliary membranes, and it has been suggested to both limit and assist the regulated trafficking of cargo proteins and lipids into and out of the cilium (88). The TZ is therefore thought to modulate the composition of essential ciliary compartments such as the ciliary membrane, axoneme, and associated proteins (88). A recent study demonstrated that the disruption of ciliary TZ architecture causes JBTS (89), but how this affects ciliary trafficking and causes the MKS or other ciliopathy phenotypes remains a research question of paramount importance.

Genetic, biochemical, and proteomic approaches have delineated the networks of protein-protein interactions that underlie the functional "MKS-JBTS module" at the TZ, as well providing insights into the structural basis of selective permeability at this ciliary compartment (90, 91). For example, several small tetraspanin-like transmembrane proteins (TMEMs) that are mutated as a cause of MKS and other ciliopathies (TMEM216, TMEM231, and TMEM107) appear to localize to the specialized ciliary membrane at the TZ. Other transmembrane proteins at this compartment include the Tectonic proteins (TCTN1, TCTN2, and TCTN3) and the Frizzled-like receptor TMEM67. In turn, the TMEM and Tectonic transmembrane proteins are likely to mediate interactions with and modulate the function of membrane-targeting proteins such as RPGRIP1L and CC2D2A that contain C2 domains (90, 91). TCTN1, for example, forms a biochemical complex at the TZ with CC2D2A, other ciliary transmembrane proteins (TCTN2, TMEM216, and TMEM67), and other known ciliopathy proteins (MKS1, CEP290, and B9D1) (92). The role of CEP290 and the B9 domain-containing proteins B9D1 (MKS9) and B9D2 (MKS10) at the TZ is undefined, but by analogy with the C2 domain-containing proteins, they are likely to mediate protein–protein interactions through their coiled-coil or B9 domains. One plausible model suggests that these proteins link TMEMs with either vesicular cargo at the TZ during the process of ciliogenesis, or then subsequently during the ciliary trafficking of cargo proteins through the TZ (**Figure 1G**). However, functional work on AHI1/jouberin, a ciliary TZ protein that contains WD40 and Src Homology 3 protein interaction domains, tends to support a general role for TZ proteins during vesicular trafficking because AHI1/jouberin interacts with RAB8A (93). RAB8A is an important small GTP/GDP-binding protein that is essential for vesicular protein trafficking from the endoplasmic reticulum to the Golgi apparatus and plasma membrane (93). Interestingly, AHI/jouberin also directly interacts and sequestrates β-catenin (a downstream effector of canonical Wnt signaling) at the cilium (94, 95) and it therefore has functions that are additional and distinct to those of CEP290.

Several recent studies have provided mechanistic insights into how the disruption of selective permeability at the TZ results in the incorrect trafficking of proteins at the cilium, with a focus on the trafficking of enzymes, receptors, and other transmembrane proteins involved in intracellular signaling. Although two TMEMs, TMEM17 and TMEM231, localize to the ciliary TZ, other TZ proteins (CC2D2A and B9D1) are required for TMEM231 localization to the TZ (82). In turn, these functional interactions in the TZ regulated the trafficking of ciliary G-protein-coupled receptors (GPCRs; somatostatin and serotonin receptors SSTR3 and HTR6) into the ciliary membrane, and both B9D2 and TMEM231 mutations caused defective ciliogenesis and Shh signaling in mice (82). In a separate study, loss of TCTN1 did not affect ciliogenesis, but nevertheless caused defective ciliary localizations of the transmembrane signaling proteins Smoothened and PKD2/polycystin-2, adenylyl cyclase 3 (ACIII; forming the secondary messenger cAMP), and ARL13B (a small Arf-family GTPase that localizes to the ciliary membrane) (92). Furthermore, the normal trafficking and localization of Smoothened at both the TZ and cilium is lost as a consequence of JBTS-associated mutations in RPGRIP1L that disrupt ciliary TZ architecture (89). In turn, the disruption of ciliary structure and function prevent Smoothened from mediating correct developmental Shh signaling (89). Disrupted compartmentalization could also prevent the correct ciliary transport of KIF7, a kinesin motor-protein that controls Shh signaling by regulating the amounts of activator and repressor isoforms of GLI transcription factors (96, 97). GLI proteins mediate gene expression changes as a consequence of Shh signaling, and the regulatory roles of KIF7 appear to be both negative, by preventing the incorrect activation of GLI2 in the absence of Shh ligand, and positive, by preventing the processing of GLI3 into the repressor isoform.

FUTURE PERSPECTIVES

At the present time, the molecular cause for only 60% of cases can be explained by mutations in the known MKS genes (28, 29, 71). The entire series of causative genes for MKS, MKS-like, and related ciliopathy phenotypes are therefore incomplete, but the remaining genes will be either uncommon or carry private mutations that are likely to be represented by single families. However, the widespread use of targeted clonal sequencing techniques such as multi-gene panels and WGS now allows the affordable re-investigation of molecular causes in the known MKS genes for individuals that have previously been mutation negative. These studies are likely to identify potential pathogenic causes that include intronic mutations, copy number variations, and other genic variants in promoter sequences or *cis*-regulatory elements. Although this will improve diagnostic rates for MKS families, these efforts are complicated by both allelism and extreme phenotypic variability for MKS and related ciliopathies. The mechanistic basis of phenotypic variability in MKS still remains largely unclear, and it is undefined what the relative contributions are made by modifier alleles in other genes, in contrast to the general stochastic effects of variability in developmental signaling during embryogenesis. A future research challenge is to delineate the complex relationships between ciliary architecture and organization, and how these relate to and regulate ciliary function.

AUTHOR CONTRIBUTIONS

VH, KS, SS, GW, and CJ made substantial contributions to the writing, drafting, and revision of this manuscript. All authors approved the final published version of the manuscript.

ACKNOWLEDGMENTS

We thank Dr. Riitta Salonen (Rinnekoti Foundation, Helsinki, Finland) for permission to use clinical images.

FUNDING

This work was supported by funding from the Medical Research Council (grant numbers MR/K011154/1 and MR/M000532/1) and the European Community's Seventh Framework Programme FP7/2009 under grant agreement no. 241955 SYSCILIA (to CJ). VH was supported by a British Heart Foundation clinical training fellowship (grant number FS/13/32/30069). GW was supported by National Eye Research Centre Small Grant SAC019 and Wellcome Trust Seed Award in Science 204378/Z/16/Z.

REFERENCES

1. Meckel J. Beschreibung zweier, durch sehr ähnliche Bildungsabweichungen entstellter Geschwister. *Dtsch Arch Physiol* (1882) 7:99–172.
2. Gruber G. Beitrage zur frage "gekoppelter" Miszbildungen (Akrocephalo-syndactylie und dysencephalia splanchnocystica). *Beitr Pathol Anat* (1934) 93:459–76.
3. Opitz JM, Howe JJ. The Meckel syndrome (dysencephalia splanchnocystica, the Grüber syndrome). *Birth Defects Orig Art Ser* (1969) 2:167–79.
4. Mecke S, Passarge E. Encephalocele, polycystic kidneys and polydactyly as an autosomal recessive trait simulating certain other disorders – Meckel syndrome. *Ann Genet* (1971) 14:97–103.
5. Fraser FC, Lytwyn A. Spectrum of anomalies in the Meckel syndrome, or maybe there is a malformation syndrome with at least one constant anomaly. *Am J Med Genet* (1981) 9:67–73. doi:10.1002/ajmg.1320090112
6. Salonen R. The Meckel syndrome – clinicopathological findings in 67 patients. *Am J Med Genet* (1984) 18:671–89. doi:10.1002/ajmg.1320180414
7. Hsia YE, Bratu M, Herbordt A. Genetics of Meckel syndrome (dysencephalia-splanchnocystica). *Pediatrics* (1971) 48:237–47.
8. Salonen R, Paavola P. Meckel syndrome. *J Med Genet* (1998) 35:497–501. doi:10.1136/jmg.35.6.497
9. Majewski F, Stoss H, Goecke T, Kemperdick H. Are bowing of long tubular bones and preaxial polydactyly signs of the Meckel syndrome? *Hum Genet* (1983) 65:125–33. doi:10.1007/BF00286648
10. Lowry RB, Hill RH, Tischler B. Survival and spectrum of anomalies in the Meckel syndrome. *Am J Med Genet* (1983) 14:417–21. doi:10.1002/ajmg.1320140303
11. Moerman P, Verbeken E, Fryns JP, Goddeeris P, Lauweryns JM. The Meckel syndrome. Pathological and cytogenetic observations in eight cases. *Hum Genet* (1982) 62:240–5. doi:10.1007/BF00333528
12. Seppanen U, Herva R. Roentgenologic features of the Meckel syndrome. *Pediatr Radiol* (1983) 13:329–31. doi:10.1007/BF01625959
13. Rapola J, Salonen R. Visceral anomalies in the Meckel syndrome. *Teratology* (1985) 31:193–201. doi:10.1002/tera.1420310204
14. Paavola P, Salonen R, Weissenbach J, Peltonen L. The locus for Meckel syndrome with multiple congenital anomalies maps to chromosome 17q21-q24. *Nat Genet* (1995) 11:213–5. doi:10.1038/ng1095-213
15. Ahdab-Barmada M, Claassen D. A distinctive triad of malformations of the central nervous system in the Meckel-Gruber syndrome. *J Neuropathol Exp Neurol* (1990) 49:610–20. doi:10.1097/00005072-199011000-00007
16. Blankenberg TA, Ruebner BH, Ellis WG, Bernstein J, Dimmick JE. Pathology of renal and hepatic anomalies in Meckel syndrome. *Am J Med Genet Suppl* (1987) 3:395–410. doi:10.1002/ajmg.1320280546
17. Sergi C, Adam S, Kahl P, Otto HF. Study of the malformation of ductal plate of the liver in Meckel syndrome and review of other syndromes presenting with this anomaly. *Pediatr Dev Pathol* (2000) 3:568–83. doi:10.1007/s100240010104
18. Auber B, Burfeind P, Herold S, Schoner K, Simson G, Rauskolb R, et al. A disease causing deletion of 29 base pairs in intron 15 in the *MKS1* gene is highly associated with the campomelic variant of the Meckel-Gruber syndrome. *Clin Genet* (2007) 72:454–9. doi:10.1111/j.1399-0004.2007.00880.x
19. Young ID, Rickett AB, Clarke M. High-incidence of Meckels syndrome in Gujarati Indians. *J Med Genet* (1985) 22:301–4. doi:10.1136/jmg.22.4.301
20. Lurie IW, Prytkov AN, Meldere LV. Meckel syndrome in different populations. *Am J Med Genet* (1984) 18:661–9. doi:10.1002/ajmg.1320180413
21. Schurig V, Bowen P, Harley F, Schiff D. The Meckel syndrome in the Hutterites. *Am J Med Genet* (1980) 5:373–81. doi:10.1002/ajmg.1320050408
22. Salonen R, Norio R. The Meckel syndrome in Finland: epidemiologic and genetic aspects. *Am J Med Genet* (1984) 18:691–8. doi:10.1002/ajmg.1320180415
23. Teebi AS, Alsaleh QA, Odeh H. Meckel syndrome and neural-tube defects in Kuwait. *J Med Genet* (1992) 29:140. doi:10.1136/jmg.29.2.140-a
24. Teebi AS, Teebi SA. Genetic diversity among the Arabs. *Community Genet* (2005) 8:21–6. doi:10.1159/000083333
25. Shaheen R, Faqeih E, Alshammari MJ, Swaid A, Al-Gazali L, Mardawi E, et al. Genomic analysis of Meckel-Gruber syndrome in Arabs reveals marked genetic heterogeneity and novel candidate genes. *Eur J Hum Genet* (2013) 21:762–8. doi:10.1038/ejhg.2012.254
26. Shaheen R, Shamseldin HE, Loucks CM, Seidahmed MZ, Ansari S, Ibrahim Khalil M, et al. Mutations in CSPP1, encoding a core centrosomal protein, cause a range of ciliopathy phenotypes in humans. *Am J Hum Genet* (2014) 94:73–9. doi:10.1016/j.ajhg.2013.11.010
27. Bondeson ML, Ericson K, Gudmundsson S, Ameur A, Pontén F, Wesström J, et al. A nonsense mutation in CEP55 defines a new locus for a Meckel-like syndrome, an autosomal recessive lethal fetal ciliopathy. *Clin Genet* (2017) 92(5):510–6. doi:10.1111/cge.13012
28. Shaheen R, Szymanska K, Basu B, Patel N, Ewida N, Faqeih E, et al. Characterizing the morbid genome of ciliopathies. *Genome Biol* (2016) 17:242. doi:10.1186/s13059-016-1099-5
29. Szymanska K, Berry I, Logan CV, Cousins SR, Lindsay H, Jafri H, et al. Founder mutations and genotype-phenotype correlations in Meckel-Gruber syndrome and associated ciliopathies. *Cilia* (2012) 1:18. doi:10.1186/2046-2530-1-18
30. Kyttälä M, Tallila J, Salonen R, Kopra O, Kohlschmidt N, Paavola-Sakki P, et al. MKS1, encoding a component of the flagellar apparatus basal body proteome, is mutated in Meckel syndrome. *Nat Genet* (2006) 38:155–7. doi:10.1038/ng1714
31. Valente EM, Logan CV, Mougou-Zerelli S, Lee JH, Silhavy JL, Brancati F, et al. Mutations in TMEM216 perturb ciliogenesis and cause Joubert, Meckel and related syndromes. *Nat Genet* (2010) 42:619–25. doi:10.1038/ng.594
32. Edvardson S, Shaag A, Zenvirt S, Erlich Y, Hannon GJ, Shanske AL, et al. Joubert syndrome 2 (JBTS2) in Ashkenazi Jews is associated with a TMEM216 mutation. *Am J Hum Genet* (2010) 86:93–7. doi:10.1016/j.ajhg.2009.12.007

33. Smith UM, Consugar M, Tee LJ, McKee BM, Maina EN, Whelan S, et al. The transmembrane protein meckelin (MKS3) is mutated in Meckel-Gruber syndrome and the *wpk* rat. *Nat Genet* (2006) 38:191–6. doi:10.1038/ng1713
34. Sayer J, Otto EA, O'Toole JF, Nurnberg G, Kennedy MA, Becker C, et al. The centrosomal protein nephrocystin-6 is mutated in Joubert syndrome and activates transcription factor ATF4. *Nat Genet* (2006) 38:674–81. doi:10.1038/ng1786
35. Arts HH, Doherty D, van Beersum SE, Parisi MA, Letteboer SJ, Gorden NT, et al. Mutations in the gene encoding the basal body protein RPGRIP1L, a nephrocystin-4 interactor, cause Joubert syndrome. *Nat Genet* (2007) 39:882–8. doi:10.1038/ng2069
36. Delous M, Baala L, Salomon R, Laclef C, Vierkotten J, Tory K, et al. The ciliary gene RPGRIP1L is mutated in cerebello-oculo-renal syndrome (Joubert syndrome type B) and Meckel syndrome. *Nat Genet* (2007) 39:875–81. doi:10.1038/ng2039
37. Tallila J, Jakkula E, Peltonen L, Salonen R, Kestilä M. Identification of CC2D2A as a Meckel syndrome gene adds an important piece to the ciliopathy puzzle. *Am J Hum Genet* (2008) 82:1361–7. doi:10.1016/j.ajhg.2008.05.004
38. Bergmann C, Fliegauf M, Brüchle NO, Frank V, Olbrich H, Kirschner J, et al. Loss of nephrocystin-3 function can cause embryonic lethality, Meckel-Gruber-like syndrome, situs inversus, and renal-hepatic-pancreatic dysplasia. *Am J Hum Genet* (2008) 82:959–70. doi:10.1016/j.ajhg.2008.02.017
39. Shaheen R, Faqeih E, Seidahmed MZ, Sunker A, Alali FE, AlQahtani K, et al. A TCTN2 mutation defines a novel Meckel Gruber syndrome locus. *Hum Mutat* (2011) 32:573–8. doi:10.1002/humu.21507
40. Hopp K, Heyer CM, Hommerding CJ, Henke SA, Sundsbak JL, Patel S, et al. B9D1 is revealed as a novel Meckel syndrome (MKS) gene by targeted exon-enriched next-generation sequencing and deletion analysis. *Hum Mol Genet* (2011) 20:2524–34. doi:10.1093/hmg/ddr151
41. Dowdle WE, Robinson JF, Kneist A, Sirerol-Piquer MS, Frints SG, Corbit KC, et al. Disruption of a ciliary B9 protein complex causes Meckel syndrome. *Am J Hum Genet* (2011) 89:94–110. doi:10.1016/j.ajhg.2011.06.003
42. Shaheen R, Ansari S, Mardawi EA, Alshammari MJ, Alkuraya FS. Mutations in TMEM231 cause Meckel-Gruber syndrome. *J Med Genet* (2013) 50:160–2. doi:10.1136/jmedgenet-2012-101431
43. Filges I, Nosova E, Bruder E, Tercanli S, Townsend K, Gibson WT, et al. Exome sequencing identifies mutations in KIF14 as a novel cause of an autosomal recessive lethal fetal ciliopathy phenotype. *Clin Genet* (2014) 86:220–8. doi:10.1111/cge.12301
44. Shaheen R, Almoisheer A, Faqeih E, Babay Z, Monies D, Tassan N, et al. Identification of a novel MKS locus defined by TMEM107 mutation. *Hum Mol Genet* (2015) 24:5211–8. doi:10.1093/hmg/ddv242
45. Lambacher NJ, Bruel AL, van Dam TJ, Szymańska K, Slaats GG, Kuhns S, et al. TMEM107 recruits ciliopathy proteins to subdomains of the ciliary transition zone and causes Joubert syndrome. *Nat Cell Biol* (2016) 18:122–31. doi:10.1038/ncb3273
46. Baala L, Romano S, Khaddour R, Saunier S, Smith UM, Audollent S, et al. The Meckel-Gruber syndrome gene, MKS3, is mutated in Joubert syndrome. *Am J Hum Genet* (2007) 80:186–94. doi:10.1086/510499
47. Chang B, Khanna H, Hawes N, Jimeno D, He S, Lillo C, et al. In-frame deletion in a novel centrosomal/ciliary protein CEP290/NPHP6 perturbs its interaction with RPGR and results in early-onset retinal degeneration in the rd16 mouse. *Hum Mol Genet* (2006) 15:1847–57. doi:10.1093/hmg/ddl107
48. Leitch CC, Zaghloul NA, Davis EE, Stoetzel C, Diaz-Font A, Rix S, et al. Hypomorphic mutations in syndromic encephalocele genes are associated with Bardet-Biedl syndrome. *Nat Genet* (2008) 40:443–8. doi:10.1038/ng.97
49. Brancati F, Iannicelli M, Travaglini L, Mazzotta A, Bertini E, Boltshauser E, et al. MKS3/TMEM67 mutations are a major cause of COACH syndrome, a Joubert syndrome related disorder with liver involvement. *Hum Mutat* (2009) 30:E432–42. doi:10.1002/humu.20924
50. Den Hollander AI, Koenekoop RK, Yzer S, Lopez I, Arends ML, Voesenek KEJ, et al. Mutations in the CEP290 (NPHP6) gene are a frequent cause of Leber congenital amaurosis. *Am J Hum Genet* (2006) 79:556–61. doi:10.1086/507318
51. Phelps IG, Dempsey JC, Grout ME, Isabella CR, Tully HM, Doherty D, et al. Interpreting the clinical significance of combined variants in multiple recessive disease genes: systematic investigation of Joubert syndrome yields little support for oligogenicity. *Genet Med* (2017). doi:10.1038/gim.2017.94
52. Khaddour R, Smith U, Baala L, Martinovic J, Clavering D, Shaffiq R, et al. Spectrum of MKS1 and MKS3 mutations in Meckel syndrome: a genotype-phenotype correlation. Mutation in brief #960. Online. *Hum Mutat* (2007) 28:523–4. doi:10.1002/humu.9489
53. Bader I, Decker E, Mayr JA, Lunzer V, Koch J, Boltshauser E, et al. MKS1 mutations cause Joubert syndrome with agenesis of the corpus callosum. *Eur J Med Genet* (2016) 59:386–91. doi:10.1016/j.ejmg.2016.06.007
54. Irfanullah F, Khan S, Ullah I, Nasir A, Meijer CA, Laurense-Bik M, et al. Hypomorphic MKS1 mutation in a Pakistani family with mild Joubert syndrome and atypical features: expanding the phenotypic spectrum of MKS1-related ciliopathies. *Am J Med Genet A* (2016) 170:3289–93. doi:10.1002/ajmg.a.37934
55. Iannicelli M, Brancati F, Mougou-Zerelli S, Mazzotta A, Thomas S, Elkhartoufi N, et al. Novel TMEM67 mutations and genotype-phenotype correlates in meckelin-related ciliopathies. *Hum Mutat* (2010) 31:E1319–31. doi:10.1002/humu.21239
56. Consugar M, Kubly V, Lager D, Hommerding C, Wong W, Bakker E, et al. Molecular diagnostics of Meckel-Gruber syndrome highlights phenotypic differences between MKS1 and MKS3. *Hum Genet* (2007) 121:591–9. doi:10.1007/s00439-007-0341-3
57. Doherty D, Parisi MA, Finn LS, Gunay-Aygun M, Al-Mateen M, Bates D, et al. Mutations in 3 genes (MKS3, CC2D2A and RPGRIP1L) cause COACH syndrome (Joubert syndrome with congenital hepatic fibrosis). *J Med Genet* (2010) 47:8–21. doi:10.1136/jmg.2009.067249
58. Otto EA, Tory K, Attanasio M, Zhou W, Chaki M, Paruchuri Y, et al. Hypomorphic mutations in meckelin (MKS3/TMEM67) cause nephronophthisis with liver fibrosis (NPHP11). *J Med Genet* (2009) 46:663–70. doi:10.1136/jmg.2009.066613
59. Mougou-Zerelli S, Thomas S, Szenker E, Audollent S, Elkhartoufi N, Babarit C, et al. CC2D2A mutations in Meckel and Joubert syndromes indicate a genotype-phenotype correlation. *Hum Mutat* (2009) 30:1574–82. doi:10.1002/humu.21116
60. Ramadani HM, Nasrat HA. Prenatal diagnosis of recurrent Meckel syndrome. *Int J Gynaecol Obstet* (1992) 39:327–32. doi:10.1016/0020-7292(92)90265-K
61. Sepulveda W, Sebire NJ, Souka A, Snijders RJM, Nicolaides KH. Diagnosis of the Meckel-Gruber syndrome at eleven to fourteen weeks' gestation. *Am J Obstet Gynecol* (1997) 176:316–9. doi:10.1016/S0002-9378(97)70491-5
62. Braithwaite JM, Economides DL. First-trimester diagnosis of Meckel-Gruber syndrome by transabdominal sonography in a low-risk case. *Prenat Diagn* (1995) 15:1168–70. doi:10.1002/pd.1970151215
63. Pachi A, Giancotti A, Torcia F, Deprosperi V, Maggi E. Meckel-Gruber syndrome – ultrasonographic diagnosis at 13 weeks gestational age in an at-risk case. *Prenat Diagn* (1989) 9:187–90. doi:10.1002/pd.1970090307
64. Nizard J, Bernard JP, Ville Y. Fetal cystic malformations of the posterior fossa in the first trimester of pregnancy. *Fetal Diagn Ther* (2005) 20:146–51. doi:10.1159/000082440
65. Verjaal M, Meyer AH, Beckerbloemkolk MJ, Leschot NJ, Weduwen JJD, Gras J. Oligohydramnios hampering prenatal-diagnosis of Meckel syndrome. *Am J Med Genet* (1980) 7:85–6. doi:10.1002/ajmg.1320070112
66. Kaffe S, Rose JS, Godmilow L, Walker BA, Kerenyi T, Beratis N, et al. Prenatal diagnosis of renal anomalies. *Am J Med Genet* (1977) 1:241–51. doi:10.1002/ajmg.1320010210
67. Ickowicz V, Eurin D, Maugey-Laulom B, Didier F, Garel C, Gubler MC, et al. Meckel-Gruber syndrome: sonography and pathology. *Ultrasound Obstet Gynecol* (2006) 27:296–300. doi:10.1002/uog.2708
68. Chao A, Wong AM, Hsueh C, Chang YL, Wang TH. Integration of imaging and pathological studies in Meckel-Gruber syndrome. *Prenat Diagn* (2005) 25:267–8. doi:10.1002/pd.1111
69. Williamson RA, Weiner CP, Yuh WTC, Abuyousef MM. Magnetic-resonance imaging of anomalous fetuses. *Obstet Gynecol* (1989) 73:952–6.

70. Quintero RA, Abuhamad A, Hobbins JC, Mahoney MJ. Transabdominal thin-gauge embryofetoscopy – a technique for early prenatal diagnosis and its use in the diagnosis of a case of Meckel-Gruber syndrome. *Am J Obstet Gynecol* (1993) 168:1552–7. doi:10.1016/S0002-9378(11)90797-2
71. Watson CM, Crinnion LA, Berry IR, Harrison SM, Lascelles C, Antanaviciute A, et al. Enhanced diagnostic yield in Meckel-Gruber and Joubert syndrome through exome sequencing supplemented with split-read mapping. *BMC Med Genet* (2016) 17:1. doi:10.1186/s12881-015-0265-z
72. Karmous-Benailly H, Martinovic J, Gubler MC, Sirot Y, Clech L, Ozilou C, et al. Antenatal presentation of Bardet-Biedl syndrome may mimic Meckel syndrome. *Am J Hum Genet* (2005) 76:493–504. doi:10.1086/428679
73. Chen CP. Meckel syndrome: genetics, perinatal findings, and differential diagnosis. *Taiwan J Obstet Gynecol* (2007) 46:9–14. doi:10.1016/S1028-4559(08)60100-X
74. Ahmed S, Green JM, Hewison J. Attitudes towards prenatal diagnosis and termination of pregnancy for thalassaemia in pregnant Pakistani women in the North of England. *Prenat Diagn* (2006) 26:248–57. doi:10.1002/pd.1391
75. Ahmed S, Ahmed M, Sharif SM, Sheridan E, Taylor GR. Attitudes towards prenatal testing and termination of pregnancy in British Pakistani parents and relatives of children with recessive conditions in the UK. *Prenat Diagn* (2012) 32:954–9. doi:10.1002/pd.3940
76. Ahmed S, Bryant LD, Cole P. Midwives' perceptions of their role as facilitators of informed choice in antenatal screening. *Midwifery* (2013) 29:745–50. doi:10.1016/j.midw.2012.07.006
77. Middleton A, Robson F, Burnell L, Ahmed M. Providing a transcultural genetic counseling service in the UK. *J Genet Couns* (2007) 16:567–82. doi:10.1007/s10897-007-9089-0
78. Ali TS, Gunilla K, Gul R, Asad N, Johansson E, Mogren I. Gender roles and their influence on life prospects for women in urban Karachi, Pakistan: a qualitative study. *Glob Health Action* (2011) 4:7448. doi:10.3402/gha.v4i0.7448
79. Modell B, Harris R, Lane B, Khan M, Darlison M, Petrou M, et al. Informed choice in genetic screening for thalassaemia during pregnancy: audit from a national confidential inquiry. *BMJ* (2000) 320:337–41. doi:10.1136/bmj.320.7231.337
80. Al-Matary A, Ali J. Controversies and considerations regarding the termination of pregnancy for foetal anomalies in Islam. *BMC Med Ethics* (2014) 15:10. doi:10.1186/1472-6939-15-10
81. Jafri H, Ahmed S, Ahmed M, Hewison J, Raashid Y, Sheridan E. Islam and termination of pregnancy for genetic conditions in Pakistan: implications for Pakistani health care providers. *Prenat Diagn* (2012) 32:1218–20. doi:10.1002/pd.3987
82. Chih B, Liu P, Chinn Y, Chalouni C, Komuves LG, Hass PE, et al. A ciliopathy complex at the transition zone protects the cilia as a privileged membrane domain. *Nat Cell Biol* (2011) 14:61–72. doi:10.1038/ncb2410
83. Cui C, Chatterjee B, Francis D, Yu Q, SanAgustin JT, Francis R, et al. Disruption of Mks1 localization to the mother centriole causes cilia defects and developmental malformations in Meckel-Gruber syndrome. *Dis Model Mech* (2011) 4:43–56. doi:10.1242/dmm.006262
84. Weatherbee SD, Niswander LA, Anderson KV. A mouse model for Meckel syndrome reveals Mks1 is required for ciliogenesis and Hedgehog signaling. *Hum Mol Genet* (2009) 18:4565–75. doi:10.1093/hmg/ddp422
85. Abdelhamed ZA, Wheway G, Szymanska K, Natarajan S, Toomes C, Inglehearn C, et al. Variable expressivity of ciliopathy neurological phenotypes that encompass Meckel-Gruber syndrome and Joubert syndrome is caused by complex de-regulated ciliogenesis, Shh and Wnt signalling defects. *Hum Mol Genet* (2013) 22:1358–72. doi:10.1093/hmg/dds546
86. Szymanska K, Johnson CA. The transition zone: an essential functional compartment of cilia. *Cilia* (2012) 1:10. doi:10.1186/2046-2530-1-10
87. Reiter JF, Blacque OE, Leroux MR. The base of the cilium: roles for transition fibres and the transition zone in ciliary formation, maintenance and compartmentalization. *EMBO Rep* (2012) 13:608–18. doi:10.1038/embor.2012.73
88. Williams CL, Li C, Kida K, Inglis PN, Mohan S, Semenec L, et al. MKS and NPHP modules cooperate to establish basal body/transition zone membrane associations and ciliary gate function during ciliogenesis. *J Cell Biol* (2011) 192:1023–41. doi:10.1083/jcb.201012116
89. Shi X, Garcia G III, Van De Weghe JC, McGorty R, Pazour GJ, Doherty D, et al. Super-resolution microscopy reveals that disruption of ciliary transition-zone architecture causes Joubert syndrome. *Nat Cell Biol* (2017) 19(10): 1178–88. doi:10.1038/ncb3599
90. Garcia-Gonzalo FR, Reiter JF. Scoring a backstage pass: mechanisms of ciliogenesis and ciliary access. *J Cell Biol* (2012) 197:697–709. doi:10.1083/jcb.201111146
91. Blacque OE, Sanders AA. Compartments within a compartment: what *C. elegans* can tell us about ciliary subdomain composition, biogenesis, function, and disease. *Organogenesis* (2014) 10:126–37. doi:10.4161/org.28830
92. Garcia-Gonzalo FR, Corbit KC, Sirerol-Piquer MS, Ramaswami G, Otto EA, Noriega TR, et al. A transition zone complex regulates mammalian ciliogenesis and ciliary membrane composition. *Nat Genet* (2011) 43:776–84. doi:10.1038/ng.891
93. Hsiao YC, Tong ZJ, Westfall JE, Ault JG, Page-McCaw PS, Ferland RJ. AHI1, whose human ortholog is mutated in Joubert syndrome, is required for Rab8a localization, ciliogenesis and vesicle trafficking. *Hum Mol Genet* (2009) 18:3926–41. doi:10.1093/hmg/ddp335
94. Lancaster MA, Louie CM, Silhavy JL, Sintasath L, Decambre M, Nigam SK, et al. Impaired Wnt-beta-catenin signaling disrupts adult renal homeostasis and leads to cystic kidney ciliopathy. *Nat Med* (2009) 15:1046–54. doi:10.1038/nm.2010
95. Lancaster MA, Schroth J, Gleeson JG. Subcellular spatial regulation of canonical Wnt signalling at the primary cilium. *Nat Cell Biol* (2011) 13:700–7. doi:10.1038/ncb2259
96. Dafinger C, Liebau MC, Elsayed SM, Hellenbroich Y, Boltshauser E, Korenke GC, et al. Mutations in KIF7 link Joubert syndrome with Sonic Hedgehog signaling and microtubule dynamics. *J Clin Invest* (2011) 121:2662–7. doi:10.1172/JCI43639
97. Putoux A, Thomas S, Coene KL, Davis EE, Alanay Y, Ogur G, et al. KIF7 mutations cause fetal hydrolethalus and acrocallosal syndromes. *Nat Genet* (2011) 43:601–6. doi:10.1038/ng.826

2

Is Autosomal Dominant Polycystic Kidney Disease Becoming a Pediatric Disorder?

Stéphanie De Rechter[1,2], Luc Breysem[3] and Djalila Mekahli[1,2]*

[1] PKD Lab, Department of Development and Regeneration, KU Leuven, Leuven, Belgium, [2] Department of Pediatric Nephrology, University Hospitals Leuven, Leuven, Belgium, [3] Department of Radiology, University Hospitals Leuven, Leuven, Belgium

***Correspondence:**
Stéphanie De Rechter
stephanie.derechter@uzleuven.be

Autosomal dominant polycystic kidney disease (ADPKD) affects 1 in 400 to 1,000 live births, making it the most common monogenic cause of renal failure. Although no definite cure is available yet, it is important to affect disease progression by influencing modifiable factors such as hypertension and proteinuria. Besides this symptomatic management, the only drug currently recommended in Europe for selected adult patients with rapid disease progression, is the vasopressin receptor antagonist tolvaptan. However, the question remains whether these preventive interventions should be initiated before extensive renal damage has occurred. As renal cyst formation and expansion begins early in life, frequently *in utero*, ADPKD should no longer be considered an adult-onset disease. Moreover, the presence of hypertension and proteinuria in affected children has been reported to correlate well with disease severity. Until now, it is controversial whether children at-risk for ADPKD should be tested for the presence of the disease, and if so, how this should be done. Herein, we review the spectrum of pediatric ADPKD and discuss the pro and contra of testing at-risk children and the challenges and unmet needs in pediatric ADPKD care.

Keywords: autosomal dominant polycystic kidney disease, children, testing, prevention, treatment

AUTOSOMAL DOMINANT POLYCYSTIC KIDNEY DISEASE (ADPKD) AND ITS SPECTRUM IN PEDIATRIC PATIENTS

Autosomal dominant polycystic kidney disease affects 1 in 400 to 1,000 live births, making it the most common monogenic cause of renal failure and representing a major socio-economic medical problem in the world (1). The disorder arises as a consequence of *PKD1* or *PKD2* gene mutations, encoding polycystin-1 (PC1) and -2 (PC2), and accounting for 85 and 15% of patients with a *PKD* gene mutation, respectively. Recently, a third gene has been identified to cause ADPKD when mutated, namely *GANAB* (Glucosidase, Alpha, Neutral AB form), encoding the glucosidase IIa subunit (2). Although most cases are familial, in 10–25% of patients, a positive family history is absent, posing a diagnostic challenge. These cases are explained by *de novo* disease in up to 10–15% (3), missing parental medical records, germline or somatic mosaicism, or mild disease from hypomorphic *PKD1* and *PKD2* mutations (4).

Abbreviations: ACEi, angiotensin converting enzyme inhibitor; ADPKD, autosomal dominant polycystic kidney disease; ARB, angiotensin receptor blocker; CKD, chronic kidney disease; (e)GFR, (estimated) glomerular filtration rate; LVH, left ventricular hypertrophy; MRI, magnetic resonance imaging; RAAS, renin-angiotensin-aldosterone system; TKV, total kidney volume; VEO, very early onset; US, ultrasound.

Autosomal dominant polycystic kidney disease is characterized by a progressive growth of cysts in all nephron segments, ultimately leading to end-stage renal disease (ESRD) in 50% of patients in the sixth decade. ADPKD patients with a *PKD2* mutation have a milder phenotype and reach ESRD approximately 20 years later than *PKD1* patients. Within the *PKD1* population, patients with a truncating mutation are more severely affected than those with a non-truncating. Therefore, *PKD* gene mutation analysis is one of the elements forming the PROPKD scoring system, an algorithm to predict renal survival in adult ADPKD patients (5). Moreover, ADPKD as a bona fide ciliopathy is a systemic disorder, comprising extrarenal symptoms such as cyst formation in other organs, mostly in the liver, hypertension, intracranial arterial aneurysms, cardiac valvular defects, inguinal and abdominal herniation, etc. (6). Recently, there is also evidence of bone and mineral metabolism anomalies, from both studies in different animal ADPKD models (7–9) as from clinical studies in adult and pediatric patients (7, 10–14).

As the majority of patients remain *a-* or *pauci*-symptomatic until adulthood, ADPKD is still often considered as a late-onset disease (15). Historically, ADPKD was termed "adult" polycystic kidney disease due to this classic presentation (16). However, comorbidities might be underdiagnosed in childhood if not actively looked for by caregivers as not all cause complaints. Moreover, the glomerular filtration rate (GFR) masks the underlying renal damage for several decades, due to hyperfiltration and hypertrophy of unaffected residual nephrons (17). The parameter proven to be a strong and independent predictor for ESRD development in ADPDK patients was the factual anatomic damage, indirectly assessed as the height-adjusted total kidney volume (TKV) on magnetic resonance imaging (MRI) (18, 19). Although evidence is growing that renal injury starts with the formation of the first renal cysts *in utero* (20), a consensus for the management of children at-risk for or diagnosed with ADPKD is lacking. Indeed, of all ADPKD patients, 2–5% present in childhood with a broad phenotypic spectrum, ranging from severe neonatal presentations mimicking autosomal recessive polycystic kidney disease (21) to the incidental sonographic finding of renal cysts (22). Here, we aimed to summarize the most important manifestations of ADPKD in childhood.

Renal Manifestations in Childhood

Possible presenting symptoms of renal disease in children with ADPKD are frequency, nocturia and/or, hematuria, urinary tract infection(s) and back, flank or abdominal pain (23). Often, the earliest biological renal manifestation of childhood ADPKD is a decreased urinary concentrating ability, resulting in polyuria and polydipsia (15). 58% of children ($N = 53$) showed a decreased renal concentrating capacity when performing a standardized renal concentrating capacity test after nasal drop application of desmopressin (24). In several study cohorts, children were included having a decreased estimated GFR (eGFR): 12 (25) to 39% (26) of the ADPKD children had eGFR levels < 90 mL/min/1.73 m^2, and ESRD was seldom observed. Indeed, cases of ESRD in childhood due to ADPKD are rare and in these cases, coexisting reasons for renal function decline should be ruled out. Other reasons might be the coinheritance of a hypomorphic *PKD1* allele in trans with an inactivating *PKD1* allele or the inheritance of two incompletely penetrant *PKD1* alleles—most likely leading to very early onset (VEO) ADPKD (27, 28). Children with ADPKD display glomerular hyperfiltration in 18 (29) to 21% (25). Importantly, the occurrence of hyperfiltration was associated with a significantly faster renal function impairment and a higher renal growth rate over time (29). Also, proteinuria and microalbuminuria are seen in ADPKD, and more frequently in children and adolescents than in adults. In different pediatric cohorts, the prevalence of micro-albuminuria and proteinuria ranges from 30 to 48% and 10 to 23%, respectively (25, 26, 30). From studies performed in both pediatric (30) and adult (31) patient cohorts, it was shown that patients with established proteinuria have a more aggressive course of renal disease. Indeed, adult proteinuric patients had higher mean arterial pressures, larger renal volumes and lower creatinine clearances compared to the non-proteinuric subjects (31). Similarly, proteinuric children had a more severe renal disease -defined as having more than 10 renal cysts—then those without proteinuria. However, unlike in adults, no correlation between proteinuria and hypertension, one of the most prevalent extrarenal manifestations, was seen in children (30). Last, hematuria, both possible after an antecedent of abdominal trauma, for instance in patients playing contact sports, as spontaneously (32), and nephrolithiasis are rather uncommon in children (15). A prevalence of the latter is lacking, as information comes from case reports (33). Moreover, nephrolithiasis is seen in up to 28% of ADPKD patients, which is 5–10 times the rate in the general population, due to both anatomic and metabolic abnormalities; but none in the patients below 20 years of age (34). Different from the general population is that nephrolithiasis in ADPKD patients should only be made after ruling out a superimposed urinary tract infection, cyst infection or hemorrhage and that screening for underlying urinary metabolic abnormalities should be performed from the first presentation (35).

The anatomic renal damage can often already be seen from a young age as renal cysts and/or uni- or bilateral nephromegaly. In a cohort of 47 ADPKD children, all had accelerated renal growth relative to the normal population, and half had nephromegaly (26). Affected individuals who do not yet have cysts detectable by ultrasound (US) were shown to have larger age-adjusted kidneys, suggesting ongoing microscopic cyst development and growth (36). Importantly, mathematical models computing volume changes of solitary and multiple cysts in function of time show that cysts formed early in life, are the main contributors to the final total cyst volume (37).

Another major symptom of childhood ADPKD, explained by anomalies in both the renal and cardiovascular system, namely hypertension, will be discussed in Section "Extrarenal Manifestations in Childhood: Cardiovascular Symptoms."

Extrarenal Manifestations in Childhood: Cardiovascular Symptoms

Cardiovascular manifestations are the most prominent extrarenal manifestation in ADPKD, also in childhood, of which hypertension occurs in a majority of patients, prior to renal function decline. The reported incidence in childhood varies widely in different cohorts, namely from 5 to 44% (15): 6% (25), 15% (26), 21% (30), 33% (38), and 37% (29). The most reliable assessment probably is a recently published meta-analysis covering 14 studies, estimating 20% of ADPKD children having hypertension (39).

The pathogenesis of hypertension in ADPKD includes a complex and multifactorial process, involving the renin–angiotensin–aldosterone system (RAAS), the sympathetic nervous system, sodium retention, and endothelial dysfunction. First, the presence of growing renal cysts was shown to attenuate intrarenal blood vessels, suggesting the presence of local renal ischemia and hypoxia. This in turn suggests stimulation of the RAAS in ADPKD. Both increased circulating (40) as intrarenal (41) RAAS activity was demonstrated in patients with ADPKD. Second, it is known that RAAS activation stimulates the sympathetic nervous system and *vice versa*. Indeed, adult hypertensive ADPKD patients have significantly higher plasma catecholamine concentrations compared to patients with essential hypertension (42). Third, sodium retention plays a role. Interestingly, adult patients with normotension were shown to exhibit an increased total body sodium as compared with their unaffected siblings, suggesting an early role of RAAS (43). Last, expression of Pkd1 and Pkd2 was shown in the major vessels and in the cilia of endothelial and vascular smooth muscle cells. Decreased or absent PC1 or -2 levels are associated with abnormal vascular structure and function, *via* reduced nitric oxide (NO) levels due to diminished Ca^{2+}-dependent endothelial NO syntheses activity, resulting in an altered endothelial response to shear stress with attenuation in vascular relaxation. Moreover, decreased NO production leads to the activation of the RAAS, next to its triggering by cyst enlargement and intra-renal ischemia (44). However, it is still unclear which factor hypertension in ADPKD is mainly due to. The early onset of hypertension in ADPKD, probably still underdetected and therefore left untreated, is associated with left ventricular hypertrophy (LVH) in half of the patients in their 40s (45). Importantly, cardiovascular complications appear to be the leading cause of death in patients with ADPKD. Therefore, LVH should be prevented in patients with ADPKD, as it is known to be associated with coronary heart disease, cardiac failure, arrhythmias, and sudden death (46).

A correlation between TKV and cyst volume, and hypertension was observed in a longitudinal MRI study in ADPKD children: the hypertensive subgroup had a larger increase in both cyst volume and number than the normotensive (47). Also, the prevalence of hypertension was found to be significantly higher in children with a decreased urinary concentrating capacity compared to those with a normal concentrating capacity. Significant negative correlations were shown between urinary concentrating capacity, blood pressure and the number of renal cysts (24).

Vascular dysfunction begins early in the course of ADPKD. In normotensive patients with preserved renal function, the endothelium-dependent dilatation and arterial stiffness were evaluated and compared to age and sex matched healthy controls, by measuring the brachial artery flow-mediated dilation (FMD_{BA}) and the carotid-femoral pulse wave velocity (CFPWV), respectively. FMD_{BA} was lower in 25% of patients, indicating an impaired endothelium-dependent dilatation, while CFPWV was higher in 14% of patients, designating increased arterial stiffness. Both are well-known independent predictors of future cardiovascular comorbidity and mortality (48).

Another possible cardiovascular feature in ADPKD, is mitral valve prolapse, occurring in 12% of children (15). Next, the association of ADPKD with intracranial aneurysm formation is well known (49). Almost all cases of ruptured intracranial aneurysms occur in adult patients with a median age at rupture of 40 years. In a study screening ADPKD patients, aged 7–87 years, the prevalence of intracranial aneurysm was 12.4%, reaching a peak in the 60–69 years age group; and higher in patients with a positive family history of hemorrhagic stroke or intracranial aneurysm. Only 1 patient had an aneurysm before the age of 29 years, but the authors do not state the exact age of this patient (49). However, case reports describe rupture at very young ages, even neonatal (50, 51). Although rare, this complication might be lethal in young patients.

Extrarenal Manifestations in Childhood: Others

Recently, evidence has emerged showing bone involvement in ADPKD (7–14). Indeed, PC1 is highly expressed in both osteoblasts and osteocytes and a homozygous *PKD1* null mutation in mice was shown to cause polyhydramnios, hydrops fetalis, spina bifida, and osteochondrodysplasia (52, 53). Moreover, the PC1 C terminal tail regulates TAZ expression, an enhancer of RUNX2-mediated osteoblast differentiation and suppressor of PPARγ-stimulated adipocyte differentiation. A causal relationship between mutant PC1, decreased Runx2 levels, and impaired osteoblast differentiation leading to a defect skeletogenesis was described (9, 54).

It has been demonstrated that fibroblast growth factor 23 (FGF23), a phosphaturic hormone secreted by osteocytes, was studied in different ADPKD rodent models. FGF23 levels were raised, but a peripheral biologic resistance to FGF23 was hypothesized to account for the absence of a renal phosphate leak or hypophosphatemia. Importantly, FGF23 was detected in cells lining renal cysts, from a rodent model (7). In ADPKD adults in chronic kidney disease (CKD) stages 1–2, FGF23 levels were highly increased compared to both healthy controls and CKD matched controls. However, the majority of the ADPKD population displayed FGF23 resistance, given the absence of a phosphaturic phenotype, confirming the observations from the animal models. This was hypothesized to be due to the deficiency of the FGF coreceptor, namely serum Klotho (sKlotho) (13). FGF23 has also been studied in ADPKD children with preserved renal function. Compared to healthy controls, patients had significantly lower serum phosphate SDS. In a quarter of the patient population, this was accompanied by low TmP/GFR levels for age, based on the reference values (55). Although FGF23 levels were similar in both groups, it is inappropriately normal for the ADPKD cohort, given the hypophosphatemia in the latter. Also sKlotho levels were similar between both groups. Apart from the phenotypic differences in adulthood vs. childhood concerning FGF23 and phosphate metabolism, these anomalies seem to be ADPDK specific, as markedly FGF23 elevation is only found in non-ADPKD patients with advanced CKD stage, where it is thought to counteract phosphate retention and is classically accompanied by an increased parathyroid hormone and decreased 1,25-dihydroxyvitamin D levels (14). Moreover, given the observations in the pediatric cohort, it is an early disease phenomenon.

In the same pediatric ADPKD cohort, significantly lower values of bone alkaline phosphatase were seen compared to healthy controls (10). Based on these data and the findings from a bone biopsy study in which a low bone turnover was observed in young adult ADPKD patients with preserved kidney function (56), bone formation suppression is hypothesized in ADPKD.

Also sclerostin, known to inhibit the osteo-anabolic Wnt/β-catenin pathway, is an emerging player in the mineral metabolism phenotype of ADPKD. Higher osseous sclerostin expression has been reported in *jck* mouse model (57) and in a small cohort of adult ADPKD patients in ESRD (11). However, it could not be confirmed in a pediatric ADPKD cohort (10). This discrepancy remains to be elucidated, next to the clinical relevance of sclerostin overactivity in ADPKD, if confirmed in future studies.

In general, one of the main extrarenal manifestations of ADPKD is polycystic liver disease (PLD). In contrast to renal cyst formation, liver cyst formation does not affect liver function, although it can cause symptoms related to its mass effect when significant liver enlargement has occurred, or due to cyst bleeding or infection (58). In children, liver cyst formation is very rare (59). PLD is the result of ductal plate—the primitive biliary structure—malformations. Normally, ductal plate remodeling takes place from 12 weeks gestational age, up to term, but with a slowing down between the 20th and the 32nd week of gestation (60). Ductal plate malformation leads to a partial to complete arrest of ductal plate remodeling, and therefore a persistent excess of embryonic biliary structures (61). Typically, these structures are present from a very early disease stage, but remain asymptomatic until cyst growth initiates in adulthood (62).

DIAGNOSING ADPKD IN CHILDREN

The diagnosis of ADPKD in children can be made either unintentionally or actively, *via* screening. First, children at-risk for ADPKD might present with symptoms such as urinary tract infection(s), hematuria, enuresis etcetera, leading to their diagnosis when further investigated. Children might be diagnosed unintentionally as well, starting from the routinely performed prenatal US during pregnancy. Prenatally, the typical—although not specific for ADPKD—sonographic characteristics are moderately enlarged hyperechogenic kidneys with an increased corticomedullary differentiation (CMD). Other prenatal sonographic features such as an absent or decreased CMD and cortical cysts are less frequently seen (21). Although a prenatal presentation of ADPKD is rare, this form is recurrent within families, suggesting a common genetic modifying background with low levels of PC1 function (63) or the association with other modifying genes such as *HNF1B* or *PKHD1* (64). In other cases, children might be diagnosed unintentionally postnatally, after the coincidental detection of renal cysts on an abdominal US performed for other reasons, most frequently abdominal pain. Second, active presymptomatic testing might be requested by the parents and/or the adolescents themselves. However, the diagnosis of ADPKD, especially its timing, represents controversies that we will discuss later in this review.

We first aim to demonstrate the challenges and limitations in the methods for the diagnosis of ADPKD in children and the lack of definite criteria for individuals under the age of 15 years. Indeed, presymptomatic testing in children at-risk for ADPKD, due to their positive familial history, can be executed by clinical evaluation and/or imaging. However, genetic evaluation is needed to resolve some cases. Most diagnoses of ADPKD are established on a positive family history combined with imaging [sonographic (65, 66) or MRI (67)] findings. However, for individuals under the age of 15 years, there are no validated diagnostic imaging criteria available (36, 68). As simple renal cysts occur rarely in childhood (69), a child with a positive family history for ADPKD, having a single cyst, preferably > 1 cm in diameter, is generally assumed to have the diagnosis of ADPKD, although this was never fully evaluated and validated. Moreover, based on renal US findings, one can only exclude disease presence in at-risk individuals aged 30–40 years or older (65–67). Based on MRI, this will probably be possible at an earlier age, but a cutoff age for a definite exclusion is not set yet. In case of a negative US and the patient and their family are willing to have a more definitive evaluation, gene sequencing of the *PKD* genes can be performed. However, this is not yet routinely used in clinical practice yet due to its high cost and challenging analysis. These are explained by the presence of six *PKD1* pseudogenes and the remarkable allelic heterogeneity. While the diagnostic accuracy of *PKD1* and *PKD2* gene mutation testing was found to be lower than the accuracy of US examination in adults above the age of 30 years, the relative accuracy of genetic vs. sonographic testing was comparable for children younger than 15 years in *PKD1* and superior in *PKD2* individuals (65). Also, in case the familial mutation has been identified, it is more cost effective to sequence the exon with the known mutation in at-risk individuals of this specific family. However, in that case, there is still a chance of a non-familial *de novo* mutation, not completely excluding the disease. Also, in case of a non *PKD1* non *PKD2* family, in which there is a clear ADPKD family history, but the *PKD* gene mutational analysis remains negative, exclusion of the disease in at-risk individuals will be possible only by means of a negative renal US at the age of 30–40 years or older (70).

Importantly, children who were diagnosed *in utero* or within their first 18 months of life, the so-called VEO group, represent a particularly high-risk group of ADPKD patients and should be managed accordingly. Indeed, this group was shown to have more hypertension and progression of eGFR < 90 mL/min/1.73 m^2 by the last follow-up at the median age of 16 years; although they had similar rates of glomerular hyperfiltration compared to a non-VEO ADPKD control group (27).

THE CONTROVERSY OF TESTING AT-RISK CHILDREN FOR THE PRESENCE OF ADPKD

Currently, apart from the Kidney Disease: Improving Global Outcomes (KDIGO) Controversies Conference Report (71) and the European ADPKD Forum (EAF) Report (72), no guidelines are available for the clinical care of ADPKD families.

In the KDIGO consensus, it is recommended to have at-risk children screened for hypertension, starting at the age of 5 years, and repeated every 3 years in case of normotension. Presymptomatic screening of ADPKD by means of US or genetic analysis is not currently recommended for at-risk children, while it is accepted for at-risk adults, in whom the potential benefits of presymptomatic diagnosis usually outweigh the risks. However, on the other hand, this consensus suggests the following three options for at-risk children to be discussed thoroughly with their parents, so the parents can decide which approach will be taken. First, to screen the children and to disclose the results to the whole family; second to screen the children and disclose the results only to their parents, or last, not to screen the children. Moreover, according to the consensus, molecular genetic testing should be considered in cases of atypical renal imaging, discordant disease within a family; very mild PKD; in a patient without a family history for PKD; early and severe forms of PKD or PKD associated with syndromic features; and reproductive counseling (71).

In the EAF report, it is not discussed whether at risk children should be tested, although it is stated that genetic testing is vital for diagnosing ADPKD in children and that genetic counseling including informing the patients on the possibility of preimplantation genetic diagnosis for ADPKD should be offered at initial diagnosis (72).

Taken together, it is still a matter of controversy whether asymptomatic individuals at-risk for ADPKD, especially minors, should be tested for the presence of the disease or not (73). However, they and their family should be informed about the possibility of testing, and reasons why (not) to test. An important contra to testing, is the current absence of a cure (6). Although over the last decade, several drug targets based on the cellular mechanisms were tested in *in vitro* and *in vivo* models to slow down cystogenesis, only one drug demonstrated a moderate effect on disease progression in adult ADPKD patients, namely the vasopressin V2 receptor antagonist tolvaptan (74), as also concluded by a recent Cochrane review on interventional studies in adult patients (75). Despite its adverse effects of polydipsia and polyuria, it is currently the only drug available in Europe, indicated in selected adult patients with CKD stages 1–3, having evidence of rapidly progressing disease (76). Important to take into account are the methodological issues, limiting the interpretation of results of the published trials up till now. Though these are often encouraging, they are frequently restricted because of inadequate power, short study duration, patients' heterogeneity (large differences in TKV and/or underlying mutation class for instance), doses with inadequate pharmacological effects and uncertain target organ concentration (77). Moreover, the question remains whether it would be more efficacious to start treatment before extensive renal damage has occurred. A second contra is the potential induction of psychological stress in an at-risk individual and his/her family, possibly causing feelings of (survival) guilt; although not only the certainty of having a diagnosis might be experienced as unbearable, but also the uncertainty when not testing (78, 79). A recently published mono-center survey performed in adults diagnosed with ADPKD, prior to the start of renal replacement therapy, showed that 22% had a clinically significant depression and 62% felt guilty about passing the disease on to their children. The latter represented one of the major psychological challenges confronting patients with ADPKD (80). A third argument against presymptomatic testing is the negative financial consequences a diagnosis with ADPKD might cause, such as difficulties obtaining insurances (81).

On the other hand however, presymptomatic testing not only has a prognostic value, by means of TKV measurement and *PKD* genotyping; it may also give caregivers the opportunity to target modifiable risk factors for disease progression from an early disease stage (82), thereby improving long-term renal outcome (71). This is supported by the observation of similar outcomes in a study comparing the presence of nephromegaly, hypertension, microalbuminuria and decreased eGFR between a cohort in which diagnosis was based on postnatal US screening vs. after presenting symptoms (26). This emphasizes the importance of regular screening for hypertension and proteinuria in at-risk children, but could also be seen as supporting argument for presymptomatic testing. Indeed, the significance of early treatment of disease symptoms should not be neglected. In children, this was demonstrated by slower cyst growth in ADPKD children with normotension compared to those with hypertension (47). Moreover, effective blood pressure control from childhood on may ameliorate the cardiovascular outcomes in these patients, known to be at high risk for early cardiovascular events (83, 84). Although glomerular hyperfiltration was shown to correlate with a more severe renal phenotype (29), there is no evidence (yet) for regular screening and/or treatment of it. Also, for some identified disease progression markers in adults, it remains to be determined to what extent their modification may influence the clinical course of ADPKD, such as for higher urinary sodium excretion and lower serum HDL cholesterol (85). A benefit accruing to all tested individuals, is their empowerment, namely the process through which people gain greater control over decisions and actions affecting their health and life, an important aspect is informed reproductive decision making (79).

A survey performed among European pediatric and adult nephrologist and geneticists before the KDIGO publication and the EMA approval of tolvaptan, demonstrated that their clinical practice and beliefs are very heterogeneous regarding testing of asymptomatic offspring and other ethical issues in the management of ADPKD families (86). In this study, agreement between respondents was observed regarding clinical testing of at-risk minors, although pediatric nephrologists supported this significantly stronger compared to geneticists. Also, the three groups of caregivers showed a moderate disagreement on the performance of genetic testing for ADPKD in at-risk minors. However, the differences observed in their counseling attitude were only attributable to their professional discipline. Therefore, ADPKD patients and their family tend to receive conflicting and/or incomplete information from their caregivers. As suggested in the article, a reevaluation in a few years from now, to evaluate how the KDIGO consensus statement and the availability of tolvaptan and probably other upcoming treatment options influence both professionals and patients beliefs on these issues, would be interesting to perform (86).

CHILDHOOD AS A CRITICAL THERAPEUTIC WINDOW FOR (FUTURE) THERAPIES

As suggested earlier, we should ask ourselves whether the best chance for preserving long term renal function in ADPKD is to take an early start. Starting prevention before extensive renal damage has occurred, thus at a young(er) age, might indeed improve the long term renal survival. Moreover, as suggested by Grantham et al., based on the assumption that decline in GFR is linked to the progressive increase in TKV, early treatment has the potential to delay renal dysfunction progression by more than a decade. When therapy is started at 18 years of age, reduction in the rate of TKV growth is predicted to shift from 5 to 2.5%, or 1.25% per year—a change that yields a vastly different effect on GFR decline than that induced by starting therapy later in life (87).

However, before heading toward cystogenesis inhibiting treatment options in children, disease manifestations requiring symptomatic treatment should be identified and managed adequately (16).

In both children and adults with ADPKD, hypertension is a predictor of worse renal outcome. Moreover, it is associated with increased cardiovascular morbidity and mortality (15).

In adults with ADPKD, LVH, a major cardiovascular risk factor, was significantly further decreased by rigorous (<120/80 mmHg) than standard blood pressure control (<140/90 mmHg), although this was not associated with a statistically significant difference in renal function between the two treatment arms (88). Moreover, from the HALT/PKD study, it was shown in an early ADPKD cohort that as compared with standard blood pressure control (120/70 to 130/80 mmHg), rigorous blood-pressure control (95/60 to 110/75 mmHg) was associated with a slower increase in TKV, no overall change in the eGFR, a greater decline in left ventricular mass index, and a greater reduction in albuminuria levels (89). These data may be particularly applicable to children as the study cohort represented early stages of ADPKD. However, a study using angiotensin converting enzyme inhibitors (ACEi) in children and young adolescents with ADPKD, over a period of 5 years, failed to demonstrate a significant effect on renal growth in the total cohort. Importantly, ACEi treatment was associated with stable renal function and left ventricular mass index in the (borderline) hypertensive children, who are at particular risk for increases in renal volume and left ventricular mass index and decreased renal function as compared with the other study groups (90).

KDIGO states that treatment of hypertension in pediatric ADPKD patients should follow prevailing pediatric guidelines; meaning a goal blood pressure below the 90th percentile for age, sex, and height; with the only exception that RAAS blockade is preferred as first-line treatment (71). However, given these findings, it was recommended recently to use an ACEi with a target blood pressure of <110/75 in young adults older than 18 years; and in adolescents and children with borderline hypertension (75–95th percentile) or hypertension (≥95th percentile), to use an ACEi to achieve a goal blood pressure ≤50th percentile. Angiotensin receptor blockers (ARBs) can be used in patients who do not tolerate ACEi (15). Combination of both RAAS blockers should be avoided as no benefit was demonstrated by adding an ARB (telmisartin) to an ACEi (lisinopril) on ADPKD progression in adult patients with early or moderately advanced kidney disease (89). Moreover, girls of childbearing potential and their families should be informed on fetal toxicity of ACEi and ARBs (15).

Next, in a 3-year, phase III clinical trial of pravastatin on TKV and left ventricular mass index, pravastatin was effective in slowing the progression of structural kidney disease in older children and young adults with ADPKD. There was no beneficial effect on the left ventricular mass index, nor on their urinary micro albumin excretion (91). However, a recently published *post hoc* analysis of the HALT PKD trials, comparing the outcomes of participants who never used statins with those who used statin for at least 3 years, failed to demonstrate a benefit of statin therapy in both subjects with a preserved renal function (Study A) as a reduced renal function (Study B) (92). Conclusions remain preliminary, as the first study consisted of a relatively small cohort, and the *post hoc* analysis of the HALT PKD is limited given the small number of statin users in Study A, different statin drugs and doses used, non-randomized allocation and advanced disease stage in Study B. Also, as with ACEi, potential risks to the fetus with statin exposure during pregnancy should be reviewed prior to treatment to females of appropriate pubertal development.

As mentioned before, currently, the only drug available for selected (<50 years, CKD stages 1-3a, rapidly progressing disease) adult patients in Europe (76) is the vasopressin V2 receptor antagonist tolvaptan. Tested in the TEMPO clinical trials, including adult patients with a relatively advanced disease stage (TKV > 750 mL), tolvaptan use was demonstrated to induce both a slower annual increase in TKV and a slower annual decline in kidney function in treated patients vs. controls (74). Despite its possible adverse effects—polydipsia, polyuria and significant liver enzyme elevation—tolvaptan is currently studied in a phase III double-blind placebo controlled clinical trial in a pediatric ADPKD cohort within Europe (NCT02442674) (93). Apart from this, there is one case report, describing the off-label use of tolvaptan in a severely affected neonate with ADPKD (94). Other coming exciting therapies, such as the AMPK activator metformin, are currently tested in adult patients, and will be tested in pediatric ADPKD depending on the results in adults (95). A general remark on (future) studies including children with ADPKD is that the subjects often are performed in tertiary and specialist centers. This might reflect highly selected populations, likely to contain a higher proportion of symptomatic children and "fast-progressors," influencing the results.

CHALLENGES AND UNMET NEEDS IN PEDIATRIC ADPKD CARE

In the care of pediatric ADPKD and their families, there is a clear need of a more standardized management. Few initiatives have been taken so far, namely the KDIGO consensus and EAF report, however, conflicting recommendations still need standardization and completion such as testing of at-risk minors and the target blood pressure when treating hypertension (50th vs. 90th percentile) as discussed earlier. Moreover, there are no details provided on how blood pressure should be monitored, namely *via* an office blood pressure measurement or a 24-h ambulatory blood pressure monitoring. There is evidence that the latter should be performed routinely from a large pediatric cohort, in which 51.9% of patients lacked a physiological nocturnal blood pressure dipping and 18.2% had isolated nocturnal hypertension (Massella L et al. High prevalence of hypertension in a European cohort of children with ADPKD: results of the ADPKiDs study. IPNA; 2016; Iguacu, Brazil) (96).

Others recommendations are absent, such as on screening for intracranial aneurysms, both in adults and in children, a topic in which many areas of uncertainty remain, as observed in a recent survey among European French speaking nephrologists (97). However, there is recent evidence that systematic screening in all ADPKD patients, regardless of the family history for intracranial aneurysms, is cost-effective (98). Moreover, despite the recommendations, it will take time to implement these. Till now, many at risk children with ADPKD are not under regular follow-up and remain undiagnosed (39). Thus, leaving the important issue who should be responsible for informing them in adulthood: only the family, both the family and the caregivers or only the caregivers? From the caregivers' point of view, this is a shared responsibility for professionals with the family (86), although it would be interesting to know the opinion of ADPKD patients on this.

Next, there is a need of diagnostic imaging criteria under the age of 15 years apart from the currently used eminence-based guidelines. The most important is the need for clear prognostic criteria from childhood, as a validated method to identify slow vs. rapid progressors does not exist in the pediatric population, except in case of VEO ADPKD (27). However, this is necessary for the stratification of young patients in clinical trials, and possibly as new and better outcome measures. Indeed, TKV as a prognostic marker is well-assessed and accepted, but only in studies starting to include patients from the age of 15 years (87). Moreover, TKV measurements *via* MRI were shown to be more accurate and reproducible compared to US in adults (99), however, unfeasible in many young children due to the need of sedation or general anesthesia. Therefore, new modalities should be tested for TKV measurement in ADPKD children. One promising option is a three dimensional US technique, which was shown a valuable alternative to MRI to measure, although underestimating MRI TKV (96, 100).

Untill now, most studies published were performed on small pediatric cohorts, while we need to build large cohorts before we will be able to define evidence-based recommendation for children with ADPKD. Therefore, we recently have launched our initiative of the "ADPedKD" international registry to collect retrospective and prospective longitudinal clinical, imaging, and genetic data of children until the age of 19 years.

CONCLUSION

In conclusion, children and young adults with ADPKD may represent a critical therapeutic window to reduce future renal and cardiovascular risk. However, we are still far from standardized care for this population. Moreover, the ultimate goal should be to empower patients to make their own informed decisions.

According to the KDIGO consensus, the advised follow-up of at-risk children should encompass regular monitoring for disease manifestations such as hypertension and proteinuria, so treatment of these disease modifying factors is initiated as early as possible.

AUTHOR CONTRIBUTIONS

The authors confirm being the sole contributors of this work and approved it for publication.

FUNDING

DM is supported by the Clinical Research Fund of UZ Leuven, by the Fund for Scientific Research, Flanders G0B1313N and by a research grant from the European Society for Pediatric Nephrology. SR is supported by the Fund for Scientific Research, Flanders 11M5214N.

REFERENCES

1. Gabow PA. Autosomal dominant polycystic kidney disease. *N Engl J Med* (1993) 329:332–42. doi:10.1056/NEJM199307293290508
2. Porath B, Gainullin VG, Cornec-Le Gall E, Dillinger EK, Heyer CM, Hopp K, et al. Mutations in GANAB, encoding the glucosidase IIalpha subunit, cause autosomal-dominant polycystic kidney and liver disease. *Am J Hum Genet* (2016) 98:1193–207. doi:10.1016/j.ajhg.2016.05.004
3. Reed B, McFann K, Kimberling WJ, Pei Y, Gabow PA, Christopher K, et al. Presence of de novo mutations in autosomal dominant polycystic kidney disease patients without family history. *Am J Kidney Dis* (2008) 52:1042–50. doi:10.1053/j.ajkd.2008.05.015
4. Iliuta IA, Kalatharan V, Wang K, Cornec-Le Gall E, Conklin J, Pourafkari M, et al. Polycystic kidney disease without an apparent family history. *J Am Soc Nephrol* (2017) 28:2768–76. doi:10.1681/ASN.2016090938
5. Cornec-Le Gall E, Audrezet MP, Rousseau A, Hourmant M, Renaudineau E, Charasse C, et al. The PROPKD score: a new algorithm to predict renal survival in autosomal dominant polycystic kidney disease. *J Am Soc Nephrol* (2015) 27:942–51. doi:10.1681/ASN.2015010016
6. Grantham JJ. Clinical practice. Autosomal dominant polycystic kidney disease. *N Engl J Med* (2008) 359:1477–85. doi:10.1056/NEJMcp0804458
7. Spichtig D, Zhang H, Mohebbi N, Pavik I, Petzold K, Stange G, et al. Renal expression of FGF23 and peripheral resistance to elevated FGF23 in rodent models of polycystic kidney disease. *Kidney Int* (2014) 85:1340–50. doi:10.1038/ki.2013.526
8. Xiao Z, Zhang S, Cao L, Qiu N, David V, Quarles LD. Conditional disruption of Pkd1 in osteoblasts results in osteopenia due to direct impairment of bone formation. *J Biol Chem* (2010) 285:1177–87. doi:10.1074/jbc.M109.050906
9. Xiao Z, Zhang S, Magenheimer BS, Luo J, Quarles LD. Polycystin-1 regulates skeletogenesis through stimulation of the osteoblast-specific transcription factor RUNX2-II. *J Biol Chem* (2008) 283:12624–34. doi:10.1074/jbc.M710407200
10. De Rechter S, Bacchetta J, Godefroid N, Dubourg L, Cochat P, Maquet J, et al. Evidence for bone and mineral metabolism alterations in children with

autosomal dominant polycystic kidney disease. *J Clin Endocrinol Metab* (2017) 102:4210–7. doi:10.1210/jc.2017-01157
11. Jankowska M, Haarhaus M, Qureshi AR, Lindholm B, Stenvinkel P, Evenepoel P. Sclerostin – a debutant on the autosomal dominant polycystic kidney disease scene? *Kidney Int Rep* (2017) 2:481–5. doi:10.1016/j.ekir.2017.01.001
12. Mekahli D, Bacchetta J. From bone abnormalities to mineral metabolism dysregulation in autosomal dominant polycystic kidney disease. *Pediatr Nephrol* (2013) 28:2089–96. doi:10.1007/s00467-012-2384-5
13. Pavik I, Jaeger P, Ebner L, Poster D, Krauer F, Kistler AD, et al. Soluble klotho and autosomal dominant polycystic kidney disease. *Clin J Am Soc Nephrol* (2012) 7:248–57. doi:10.2215/CJN.09020911
14. Pavik I, Jaeger P, Kistler AD, Poster D, Krauer F, Cavelti-Weder C, et al. Patients with autosomal dominant polycystic kidney disease have elevated fibroblast growth factor 23 levels and a renal leak of phosphate. *Kidney Int* (2011) 79:234–40. doi:10.1038/ki.2010.375
15. Reddy BV, Chapman AB. The spectrum of autosomal dominant polycystic kidney disease in children and adolescents. *Pediatr Nephrol* (2016) 32:31–42. doi:10.1007/s00467-016-3364-y
16. Patil A, Sweeney WE Jr, Avner ED, Pan C. Childhood polycystic kidney disease. In: Li X, editor. *Polycystic Kidney Disease*, Chapter 2. Brisbane, Australia: Codon Publications (2015).
17. Grantham JJ. Rationale for early treatment of polycystic kidney disease. *Pediatr Nephrol* (2014) 30:1053–62. doi:10.1007/s00467-014-2882-8
18. Chapman AB, Bost JE, Torres VE, Guay-Woodford L, Bae KT, Landsittel D, et al. Kidney volume and functional outcomes in autosomal dominant polycystic kidney disease. *Clin J Am Soc Nephrol* (2012) 7:479–86. doi:10.2215/CJN.09500911
19. Chapman AB, Guay-Woodford LM, Grantham JJ, Torres VE, Bae KT, Baumgarten DA, et al. Renal structure in early autosomal-dominant polycystic kidney disease (ADPKD): the Consortium for Radiologic Imaging Studies of Polycystic Kidney Disease (CRISP) cohort. *Kidney Int* (2003) 64:1035–45. doi:10.1046/j.1523-1755.2003.00185.x
20. Grantham JJ, Cook LT, Wetzel LH, Cadnapaphornchai MA, Bae KT. Evidence of extraordinary growth in the progressive enlargement of renal cysts. *Clin J Am Soc Nephrol* (2010) 5:889–96. doi:10.2215/CJN.00550110
21. Brun M, Maugey-Laulom B, Eurin D, Didier F, Avni EF. Prenatal sonographic patterns in autosomal dominant polycystic kidney disease: a multicenter study. *Ultrasound Obstet Gynecol* (2004) 24:55–61. doi:10.1002/uog.1098
22. Fick-Brosnahan G, Johnson AM, Strain JD, Gabow PA. Renal asymmetry in children with autosomal dominant polycystic kidney disease. *Am J Kidney Dis* (1999) 34:639–45. doi:10.1016/S0272-6386(99)70387-2
23. Fick GM, Duley IT, Johnson AM, Strain JD, Manco-Johnson ML, Gabow PA. The spectrum of autosomal dominant polycystic kidney disease in children. *J Am Soc Nephrol* (1994) 4:1654–60.
24. Seeman T, Dusek J, Vondrák K, Bláhová K, Simková E, Kreisinger J, et al. Renal concentrating capacity is linked to blood pressure in children with autosomal dominant polycystic kidney disease. *Physiol Res* (2004) 53:629–34.
25. Selistre L, de Souza V, Ranchin B, Hadj-Aissa A, Cochat P, Dubourg L. Early renal abnormalities in children with postnatally diagnosed autosomal dominant polycystic kidney disease. *Pediatr Nephrol* (2012) 27:1589–93. doi:10.1007/s00467-012-2192-y
26. Mekahli D, Woolf AS, Bockenhauer D. Similar renal outcomes in children with ADPKD diagnosed by screening or presenting with symptoms. *Pediatr Nephrol* (2010) 25:2275–82. doi:10.1007/s00467-010-1617-8
27. Nowak KL, Cadnapaphornchai MA, Chonchol MB, Schrier RW, Gitomer B. Long-term outcomes in patients with very-early onset autosomal dominant polycystic kidney disease. *Am J Nephrol* (2016) 44:171–8. doi:10.1159/000448695
28. Shamshirsaz AA, Reza Bekheirnia M, Kamgar M, Johnson AM, McFann K, Cadnapaphornchai M, et al. Autosomal-dominant polycystic kidney disease in infancy and childhood: progression and outcome. *Kidney Int* (2005) 68:2218–24. doi:10.1111/j.1523-1755.2005.00678.x
29. Helal I, Reed B, McFann K, Yan XD, Fick-Brosnahan GM, Cadnapaphornchai M, et al. Glomerular hyperfiltration and renal progression in children with autosomal dominant polycystic kidney disease. *Clin J Am Soc Nephrol* (2011) 6:2439–43. doi:10.2215/CJN.01010211
30. Sharp C, Johnson A, Gabow P. Factors relating to urinary protein excretion in children with autosomal dominant polycystic kidney disease. *J Am Soc Nephrol* (1998) 9:1908–14.
31. Chapman AB, Johnson AM, Gabow PA, Schrier RW. Overt proteinuria and microalbuminuria in autosomal dominant polycystic kidney disease. *J Am Soc Nephrol* (1994) 5:1349–54.
32. Gabow PA, Duley I, Johnson AM. Clinical profiles of gross hematuria in autosomal dominant polycystic kidney disease. *Am J Kidney Dis* (1992) 20:140–3. doi:10.1016/S0272-6386(12)80541-5
33. Firinci F, Soylu A, Kasap Demir B, Turkmen M, Kavukcu S. An 11-year-old child with autosomal dominant polycystic kidney disease who presented with nephrolithiasis. *Case Report Med* (2012) 2012:428749. doi:10.1155/2012/428749
34. Dimitrakov D, Simeonov S. Studies on nephrolithiasis in patients with autosomal dominant polycystic kidney disease. *Folia Med* (1994) 36:27–30.
35. Mallett A, Patel M, Tunnicliffe DJ, Rangan GK. KHA-CARI autosomal dominant polycystic kidney disease guideline: management of renal stone disease. *Semin Nephrol* (2015) 35:603–6.e3. doi:10.1016/j.semnephrol.2015.10.009
36. Gabow PA, Kimberling WJ, Strain JD, Manco-Johnson ML, Johnson AM. Utility of ultrasonography in the diagnosis of autosomal dominant polycystic kidney disease in children. *J Am Soc Nephrol* (1997) 8:105–10.
37. Grantham JJ, Cook LT, Torres VE, Bost JE, Chapman AB, Harris PC, et al. Determinants of renal volume in autosomal-dominant polycystic kidney disease. *Kidney Int* (2008) 73:108–16. doi:10.1038/sj.ki.5002624
38. Cadnapaphornchai MA, McFann K, Strain JD, Masoumi A, Schrier RW. Increased left ventricular mass in children with autosomal dominant polycystic kidney disease and borderline hypertension. *Kidney Int* (2008) 74:1192–6. doi:10.1038/ki.2008.397
39. Marlais M, Cuthell O, Langan D, Dudley J, Sinha MD, Winyard PJ. Hypertension in autosomal dominant polycystic kidney disease: a meta-analysis. *Arch Dis Child* (2016) 101:1142–7. doi:10.1136/archdischild-2015-310221
40. Chapman AB, Johnson A, Gabow PA, Schrier RW. The renin-angiotensin-aldosterone system and autosomal dominant polycystic kidney disease. *N Engl J Med* (1990) 323:1091–6. doi:10.1056/NEJM199010183231602
41. Loghman-Adham M, Soto CE, Inagami T, Cassis L. The intrarenal renin-angiotensin system in autosomal dominant polycystic kidney disease. *Am J Physiol Renal Physiol* (2004) 287:F775–88. doi:10.1152/ajprenal.00370.2003
42. Cerasola G, Vecchi M, Mulè G, Cottone S, Mangano MT, Andronico G, et al. Sympathetic activity and blood pressure pattern in autosomal dominant polycystic kidney disease hypertensives. *Am J Nephrol* (1998) 18:391–8. doi:10.1159/000013382
43. Harrap SB, Davies DL, Macnicol AM, Dominiczak AF, Fraser R, Wright AF, et al. Renal, cardiovascular and hormonal characteristics of young adults with autosomal dominant polycystic kidney disease. *Kidney Int* (1991) 40:501–8. doi:10.1038/ki.1991.238
44. Arlene B, Chapman KS, Rahbari-Oskoui F. Hypertension in autosomal dominant polycystic kidney disease. *Adv Chronic Kidney Dis* (2010) 17:153–63. doi:10.1053/j.ackd.2010.01.001
45. Chapman AB, Johnson AM, Rainguet S, Hossack K, Gabow P, Schrier RW. Left ventricular hypertrophy in autosomal dominant polycystic kidney disease. *J Am Soc Nephrol* (1997) 8:1292–7.
46. Schrier RW. Renal volume, renin-angiotensin-aldosterone system, hypertension, and left ventricular hypertrophy in patients with autosomal dominant polycystic kidney disease. *J Am Soc Nephrol* (2009) 20:1888–93. doi:10.1681/ASN.2008080882
47. Cadnapaphornchai MA, Masoumi A, Strain JD, McFann K, Schrier RW. Magnetic resonance imaging of kidney and cyst volume in children with ADPKD. *Clin J Am Soc Nephrol* (2011) 6:369–76. doi:10.2215/CJN.03780410
48. Nowak KL, Farmer H, Cadnapaphornchai MA, Gitomer B, Chonchol M. Vascular dysfunction in children and young adults with autosomal dominant polycystic kidney disease. *Nephrol Dial Transplant* (2017) 32:342–7. doi:10.1093/ndt/gfw013
49. Xu HW, Yu SQ, Mei CL, Li MH. Screening for intracranial aneurysm in 355 patients with autosomal-dominant polycystic kidney disease. *Stroke* (2011) 42:204–6. doi:10.1161/STROKEAHA.110.578740
50. Kubo S, Nakajima M, Fukuda K, Nobayashi M, Sakaki T, Aoki K, et al. A 4-year-old girl with autosomal dominant polycystic kidney disease complicated by a ruptured intracranial aneurysm. *Eur J Pediatr* (2004) 163:675–7.
51. Thong KM, Ong AC. Sudden death due to subarachnoid haemorrhage in an infant with autosomal dominant polycystic kidney disease. *Nephrol Dial Transplant* (2014) 29(Suppl 4):iv121–3. doi:10.1093/ndt/gfu014

52. Lu W, Shen X, Pavlova A, Lakkis M, Ward CJ, Pritchard L, et al. Comparison of Pkd1-targeted mutants reveals that loss of polycystin-1 causes cystogenesis and bone defects. *Hum Mol Genet* (2001) 10:2385–96. doi:10.1093/hmg/10.21.2385
53. Qiu N, Cao L, David V, Quarles LD, Xiao Z. Kif3a deficiency reverses the skeletal abnormalities in Pkd1 deficient mice by restoring the balance between osteogenesis and adipogenesis. *PLoS One* (2010) 5:e15240. doi:10.1371/journal.pone.0015240
54. Byun MR, Jeong H, Bae SJ, Kim AR, Hwang ES, Hong JH. TAZ is required for the osteogenic and anti-adipogenic activities of kaempferol. *Bone* (2012) 50:364–72. doi:10.1016/j.bone.2011.10.035
55. Payne RB. Renal tubular reabsorption of phosphate (TmP/GFR): indications and interpretation. *Ann Clin Biochem* (1998) 35(Pt 2):201–6. doi:10.1177/000456329803500203
56. Gitomer BY, Pereira RC, Malaczewski MR, Wolf MS, Salusky IB, Stoneback JW, et al. Identification of a Bone Defect in ADPKD. *ANS Kidney Week* Philadelphia (2014).
57. Sabbagh Y, Graciolli FG, O'Brien S, Tang W, dos Reis LM, Ryan S, et al. Repression of osteocyte Wnt/beta-catenin signaling is an early event in the progression of renal osteodystrophy. *J Bone Miner Res* (2012) 27:1757–72. doi:10.1002/jbmr.1630
58. Cornec-Le Gall E, Torres VE, Harris PC. Genetic complexity of autosomal dominant polycystic kidney and liver diseases. *J Am Soc Nephrol* (2017). doi:10.1681/ASN.2017050483
59. Dell KM. The spectrum of polycystic kidney disease in children. *Adv Chronic Kidney Dis* (2011) 18:339–47. doi:10.1053/j.ackd.2011.05.001
60. Sergi C, Adam S, Kahl P, Otto HF. The remodeling of the primitive human biliary system. *Early Hum Dev* (2000) 58:167–78. doi:10.1016/S0378-3782(00)00065-7
61. Desmet VJ. [Cystic diseases of the liver. From embryology to malformations]. *Gastroenterol Clin Biol* (2005) 29:858–60. doi:10.1016/S0399-8320(05)86360-2
62. de Miranda Henriques MS, de Morais Villar E. *The Liver and Polycystic Kidney Disease*. Brisbane, Australia: Codon Publications (2015).
63. Audrézet MP, Corbiere C, Lebbah S, Morinière V, Broux F, Louillet F, et al. Comprehensive PKD1 and PKD2 mutation analysis in prenatal autosomal dominant polycystic kidney disease. *J Am Soc Nephrol* (2016) 27:722–9. doi:10.1681/ASN.2014101051
64. Bergmann C, von Bothmer J, Ortiz Brüchle N, Venghaus A, Frank V, Fehrenbach H, et al. Mutations in multiple PKD genes may explain early and severe polycystic kidney disease. *J Am Soc Nephrol* (2011) 22:2047–56. doi:10.1681/ASN.2010101080
65. Chapman AB, Wei W. Imaging approaches to patients with polycystic kidney disease. *Semin Nephrol* (2011) 31:237–44. doi:10.1016/j.semnephrol.2011.05.003
66. Pei Y, Obaji J, Dupuis A, Paterson AD, Magistroni R, Dicks E, et al. Unified criteria for ultrasonographic diagnosis of ADPKD. *J Am Soc Nephrol* (2009) 20:205–12. doi:10.1681/ASN.2008050507
67. Pei Y, Hwang YH, Conklin J, Sundsbak JL, Heyer CM, Chan W, et al. Imaging-based diagnosis of autosomal dominant polycystic kidney disease. *J Am Soc Nephrol* (2015) 26:746–53. doi:10.1681/ASN.2014030297
68. Reed B, Nobakht E, Dadgar S, Bekheirnia MR, Masoumi A, Belibi F, et al. Renal ultrasonographic evaluation in children at risk of autosomal dominant polycystic kidney disease. *Am J Kidney Dis* (2010) 56:50–6. doi:10.1053/j.ajkd.2010.02.349
69. Ravine D, Gibson RN, Donlan J, Sheffield LJ. An ultrasound renal cyst prevalence survey: specificity data for inherited renal cystic diseases. *Am J Kidney Dis* (1993) 22:803–7. doi:10.1016/S0272-6386(12)70338-4
70. Paul BM, Consugar MB, Ryan Lee M, Sundsbak JL, Heyer CM, Rossetti S, et al. Evidence of a third ADPKD locus is not supported by re-analysis of designated PKD3 families. *Kidney Int* (2014) 85:383–92. doi:10.1038/ki.2013.227
71. Chapman AB, Devuyst O, Eckardt KU, Gansevoort RT, Harris T, Horie S, et al. Autosomal-dominant polycystic kidney disease (ADPKD): executive summary from a kidney disease: Improving Global Outcomes (KDIGO) Controversies Conference. *Kidney Int* (2015) 88:17–27. doi:10.1038/ki.2015.59
72. Forum EA. *Translating Science into Policy to Improve ADPKD Care*. (2015). Available from: https://www.nvn.nl/files/nvn_nl/EAF%20Report_Jan2015_eng.pdf
73. European Society of Human Genetics. Genetic testing in asymptomatic minors: Recommendations of the European Society of Human Genetics. *Eur J Hum Genet* (2009) 17:720–1. doi:10.1038/ejhg.2009.26
74. Torres VE, Chapman AB, Devuyst O, Gansevoort RT, Grantham JJ, Higashihara E, et al. Tolvaptan in patients with autosomal dominant polycystic kidney disease. *N Engl J Med* (2012) 367:2407–18. doi:10.1056/NEJMoa1205511
75. Bolignano D, Palmer SC, Ruospo M, Zoccali C, Craig JC, Strippoli GF. Interventions for preventing the progression of autosomal dominant polycystic kidney disease. *Cochrane Database Syst Rev* (2015) (7):CD010294. doi:10.1002/14651858.CD010294.pub2
76. Gansevoort RT, Arici M, Benzing T, Birn H, Capasso G, Covic A, et al. Recommendations for the use of tolvaptan in autosomal dominant polycystic kidney disease: a position statement on behalf of the ERA-EDTA Working Groups on Inherited Kidney Disorders and European Renal Best Practice. *Nephrol Dial Transplant* (2016) 31:337–48. doi:10.1093/ndt/gfv456
77. Iliuta IA, Kitchlu A, Pei Y. Methodological issues in clinical trials of polycystic kidney disease: a focused review. *J Nephrol* (2017) 30:363–71. doi:10.1007/s40620-016-0358-6
78. Borry P, Goffin T, Nys H, Dierickx K. Predictive genetic testing in minors for adult-onset genetic diseases. *Mt Sinai J Med* (2008) 75:287–96. doi:10.1002/msj.20038
79. Marsick R, Limwongse C, Kodish E. Genetic testing for renal diseases: medical and ethical considerations. *Am J Kidney Dis* (1998) 32:934–45. doi:10.1016/S0272-6386(98)70087-3
80. Simms RJ, Thong KM, Dworschak GC, Ong AC. Increased psychosocial risk, depression and reduced quality of life living with autosomal dominant polycystic kidney disease. *Nephrol Dial Transplant* (2016) 31:1130–40. doi:10.1093/ndt/gfv299
81. Golin CO, Johnson AM, Fick G, Gabow PA. Insurance for autosomal dominant polycystic kidney disease patients prior to end-stage renal disease. *Am J Kidney Dis* (1996) 27:220–3. doi:10.1016/S0272-6386(96)90544-2
82. Gabow PA, Johnson AM, Kaehny WD, Kimberling WJ, Lezotte DC, Duley IT, et al. Factors affecting the progression of renal disease in autosomal-dominant polycystic kidney disease. *Kidney Int* (1992) 41:1311–9. doi:10.1038/ki.1992.195
83. Wuthrich RP, Kistler AD, Rodriguez D, Kapoor S, Mei C. Blood pressure control for polycystic kidney disease. In: Li X, editor. *Polycystic Kidney Disease*, Chapter 5. Brisbane, Australia: Codon Publications (2015).
84. Sans L, Pascual J, Radosevic A, Quintian C, Ble M, Molina L, et al. Renal volume and cardiovascular risk assessment in normotensive autosomal dominant polycystic kidney disease patients. *Medicine* (2016) 95:e5595. doi:10.1097/MD.0000000000005595
85. Torres VE, Grantham JJ, Chapman AB, Mrug M, Bae KT, King BF Jr, et al. Potentially modifiable factors affecting the progression of autosomal dominant polycystic kidney disease. *Clin J Am Soc Nephrol* (2011) 6:640–7. doi:10.2215/CJN.03250410
86. De Rechter S, Kringen J, Janssens P, Liebau MC, Devriendt K, Levtchenko E, et al. Clinicians' attitude towards family planning and timing of diagnosis in autosomal dominant polycystic kidney disease. *PLoS One* (2017) 12:e0185779. doi:10.1371/journal.pone.0185779
87. Grantham JJ, Torres VE. The importance of total kidney volume in evaluating progression of polycystic kidney disease. *Nat Rev Nephrol* (2016) 12:667–77. doi:10.1038/nrneph.2016.135
88. Schrier R, McFann K, Johnson A, Chapman A, Edelstein C, Brosnahan G, et al. Cardiac and renal effects of standard versus rigorous blood pressure control in autosomal-dominant polycystic kidney disease: results of a seven-year prospective randomized study. *J Am Soc Nephrol* (2002) 13:1733–9. doi:10.1097/01.ASN.0000018407.60002.B9
89. Schrier RW, Abebe KZ, Perrone RD, Torres VE, Braun WE, Steinman TI, et al. Blood pressure in early autosomal dominant polycystic kidney disease. *N Engl J Med* (2014) 371:2255–66. doi:10.1056/NEJMoa1402685
90. Cadnapaphornchai MA, McFann K, Strain JD, Masoumi A, Schrier RW. Prospective change in renal volume and function in children with ADPKD. *Clin J Am Soc Nephrol* (2009) 4:820–9. doi:10.2215/CJN.02810608
91. Cadnapaphornchai MA, George DM, McFann K, Wang W, Gitomer B, Strain JD, et al. Effect of pravastatin on total kidney volume, left ventricular mass index, and microalbuminuria in pediatric autosomal dominant polycystic kidney disease. *Clin J Am Soc Nephrol* (2014) 9:889–96. doi:10.2215/CJN.08350813

92. Brosnahan G, Abebe KZ, Rahbari-Oskoui FF, Patterson CG, Bae KT, Schrier RW, et al. Effect of statin therapy on the progression of autosomal dominant polycystic kidney disease. A secondary analysis of the HALT PKD trials. *Curr Hypertens Rev* (2017). doi:10.2174/1573402113666170427142815
93. Janssens P, Weydert C, De Rechter S, Wissing KM, Liebau MC, Mekahli D. Expanding the role of vasopressin antagonism in polycystic kidney diseases: from adults to children? *Pediatr Nephrol* (2017). doi:10.1007/s00467-017-3672-x
94. Olalekan K, Fox A, Gilbert R. Tolvaptan use in severe neonatal autosomal dominant polycystic kidney disease (Adpkd): the pharmaceutical challenge. *Arch Dis Child* (2016) 101:e2. doi:10.1136/archdischild-2016-311535.61
95. Cadnapaphornchai MA. Clinical trials in pediatric autosomal dominant polycystic kidney disease. *Front Pediatr* (2017) 5:53. doi:10.3389/fped.2017.00053
96. Abstracts for the 17th IPNA Congress, Iguacu, Brazil, September 2016: oral presentations. *Pediatr Nephrol* (2016) 31:1723–64.
97. Flahault A, Trystram D, Fouchard M, Knebelmann B, Nataf F, Joly D. Screening for unruptured intracranial aneurysms in autosomal dominant polycystic kidney disease: a survey of 420 nephrologists. *PLoS One* (2016) 11:e0153176. doi:10.1371/journal.pone.0153176
98. Flahault A, Trystram D, Nataf F, Fouchard M, Knebelmann B, Grünfeld JP, et al. Screening for intracranial aneurysms in autosomal dominant polycystic kidney disease is cost-effective. *Kidney Int* (2017). doi:10.1016/j.kint.2017.08.016
99. O'Neill WC, Robbin ML, Bae KT, Grantham JJ, Chapman AB, Guay-Woodford LM, et al. Sonographic assessment of the severity and progression of autosomal dominant polycystic kidney disease: the Consortium of Renal Imaging Studies in Polycystic Kidney Disease (CRISP). *Am J Kidney Dis* (2005) 46:1058–64. doi:10.1053/j.ajkd.2005.08.026
100. Breysem L, De Rechter S, De Keyzer F, Smet MH, Bammens B, Van Dyck M, et al. 3D US as an alternative to MR for measuring renal volume in children with Autosomal Dominant Polycystic Kidney Disease. *Pediatric Nephrology* (2017).

3

The KOUNCIL Consortium: From Genetic Defects to Therapeutic Development for Nephronophthisis

Kirsten Y. Renkema[1]*, *Rachel H. Giles*[2], *Marc R. Lilien*[3], *Philip L. Beales*[4], *Ronald Roepman*[5], *Machteld M. Oud*[5], *Heleen H. Arts*[6] *and Nine V. A. M. Knoers*[1]

[1] Department of Genetics, Center for Molecular Medicine, University Medical Center Utrecht, Utrecht University, Utrecht, Netherlands, [2] Department of Nephrology and Hypertension, University Medical Center Utrecht, Utrecht University, Utrecht, Netherlands, [3] Department of Pediatric Nephrology, Wilhelmina Children's Hospital, University Medical Center Utrecht, Utrecht University, Utrecht, Netherlands, [4] UCL Great Ormond Street Institute of Child Health, London, United Kingdom, [5] Department of Genetics, Radboud University Medical Center, Nijmegen, Netherlands, [6] Department of Pathology and Molecular Medicine, McMaster University, Hamilton, ON, Canada

***Correspondence:**
Kirsten Y. Renkema
k.renkema@umcutrecht.nl

Nephronophthisis (NPH) is the most common monogenic cause of renal failure in children. Treatment options are limited to dialysis and transplantation. Therapeutics to significantly delay or prevent end-stage renal disease (ESRD) in children are currently not available. In the Dutch-Anglo KOUNCIL (**K**idney-**O**riented **UN**derstanding of correcting **CIL**iopathies) consortium, several groups and specialties united to perform scientific groundwork with the aim to develop genetic and therapeutic personalized care for NPH patients. At the start of this consortium, a genetic diagnosis for NPH was available for only 30–40% of patients, which improved to 50–60% during the course of the 4-year KOUNCIL project. Other major accomplishments of the consortium were (1) the establishment of a Dutch renal ciliopathy patient database with genotype and phenotype data; (2) composition of a proteomics-based integrated network of protein modules disrupted in NPH; (3) the development of non-invasive, urine-based assays that allow functional assessment of genomic variants in NPH and of therapeutic efficiency of drugs; and (4) chemical screening toward the identification of compounds that delay or prevent disease progression in NPH, which resulted in four potential medical interventions for NPH. In conclusion, the KOUNCIL consortium effectively channeled complementary approaches to broaden our understanding of NPH pathogenesis, resulted in 54 publications, improvement of genome diagnostics for NPH patients, awareness in the nephrology and clinical genetics communities for NPH, and new avenues for patient management.

Keywords: cilia, pediatric kidney disease, nephronophthisis, renal ciliopathy, genetics

INTRODUCTION

Nephronophthisis (NPH; OMIM Phenotypic Series PS256100) is an autosomal recessive, genetically heterogeneous disorder that results in chronic renal disease in children and young adults (1). NPH is initially characterized by polydipsia and polyuria. Progression of the disease is characterized by renal interstitial fibrosis, tubular basement membrane disruption, and—in a subset of cases—renal cyst formation, eventually leading to renal failure.

NPH can occur as an isolated disorder but is also often accompanied by a variety of extrarenal manifestations such as in Senior-Løken-, Joubert-, Bardet-Biedl-, Meckel-Gruber-, Jeune-, Short-Rib-Polydactyly-, and Sensenbrenner syndromes. These disorders overlap phenotypically, as well as genetically and functionally. All are thought to result from defective ciliary signaling, and are classified as renal ciliopathies or nephronophthisis-related ciliopathies (NPH-RCs). Although NPH patients are usually diagnosed when renal failure has developed, NPH patients typically experience a 5–10-year period between diagnosis and renal replacement therapy, which offers a therapeutic window of opportunity. Currently, no medical interventions are available for NPH patients. We anticipate that the identified molecular defect in each patient will ultimately steer the development and use of personalized therapies (2).

Gene identification is essential for development of personalized therapies. However, genetic causes of NPH are unknown in ~50% of cases (3, 4). Twenty genes are known to date to be mutated in NPH. The vast majority of gene mutations results in loss-of-function of proteins that are important for ciliary architecture or regulation of signaling cascades. Cilia are the tail-like microtubule-based protrusions from the plasma membrane that reside on the apical surface of virtually every vertebrate cell, including renal tubular cells. Cilia act as the cell's antenna by sensing the extracellular environment through an array of specific receptors and transmitting a signal response to the cell that reacts upon the signal. Ciliary gene disruption can disrupt cilia-dependent signaling cascades, which may lead to apoptosis and misaligned cell division (5). This results in heterogeneous phenotypes that affect multiple organs, including kidneys (6).

Despite steady progress in gene discovery over the past decade, a significant number of genes mutated in NPH still await identification because a significant proportion of NPH cases remains unexplained. To address this issue and advance NPH research and diagnostics collectively, our research groups united in a Dutch-Anglo consortium, funded by the Dutch Kidney Foundation. In this review, we aim to demonstrate the value of synergistic consortia in obtaining the critical mass required for patient cohort recruitment, while combining complementary expertise to work toward gene identification and targeted therapies for NPH.

THE KOUNCIL CONSORTIUM

The KOUNCIL (**K**idney-**O**riented **UN**derstanding of correcting **CIL**iopathies) consortium was founded to perform scientific groundwork for the improvement of personalized care for NPH patients. Our consortium augmented the individual expertise of the collaborating workgroups toward reaching the challenging goals. The consortium included research groups with established expertise in renal ciliopathy research and diagnostics, including clinical geneticists, pediatric nephrologists, molecular biologists, cell biologists, and bioinformaticians (**Figure 1**). The international scientific advisory board of the Dutch Kidney Foundation reviewed and supported the consortium, and a tailored internal scientific advisory board reviewed our progress and suggested solutions to problems encountered.

We designed and conducted an integrated work plan aimed to (1) identify novel genes associated with NPH and related disorders by using next generation sequencing (NGS) approaches, (2) gain insights in genotype-phenotype relations through the setup and analysis of a renal ciliopathy database, (3) increase our understanding of the composition and function NPH-related protein modules in the ciliary proteome and explore mutational effects by state-of-the-art proteomics, and (4) initiate the development of targeted therapies to delay or prevent renal failure in NPH patients by drug screening in zebrafish and 3D culturing of cells derived from patients' urine samples.

By bringing together the three university medical centers in our project we maximized patient inclusion. This was an important aspect of our study as NPH and -related disorders are individually rare. Combining our efforts has led to significant conclusions and high impact findings. The interactions within and between the different groups and work packages have been very open and effective, and by connecting different disciplines in the KOUNCIL project, a robust workflow could be implemented in the clinic that results from this synergy. We believe that without the close and successful collaboration within the consortium, the results would have been less optimal.

RESULTS OF KOUNCIL

Patient Recruitment, Database Generation, and Diagnostics

The success of research consortia relies heavily on patient numbers, diagnostic accuracy, and deep-phenotyping of patients. In KOUNCIL, we used the AGORA data- and biobank protocols to systematically recruit and include patients (http://www.agoraproject.nl) (7). Furthermore, we involved the professional Society for Dutch Pediatric Nephrologists and requested participation of pediatric nephrologists in recruiting patients for the renal ciliopathy database. Patients were also directly informed via the Dutch Kidney Patient Association and the KOUNCIL website (http://www.kouncil.nl). Clinical data including renal and extrarenal phenotypic information was obtained and manually curated for inclusion in the renal ciliopathy database (**Figure 2**). So far, 88 patients with NPH and -related disorders have been included in our coded database. Inclusion is ongoing and the database will be maintained as a resource during the following years. The database is a valuable source of clinical and genetic information, and is currently being assessed for investigations on genotype-phenotype correlations to improve early diagnosis, prognosis, and genetic counseling. Furthermore, the database offers opportunities to match with other renal ciliopathy databases such as the German language cohort Nephreg (http://www.nephreg.de), and we hope to follow up on that initiative.

We applied NGS approaches to identify causative genetic defects in 50 patients with unexplained renal ciliopathies. These methods include targeted gene panel sequencing and whole exome sequencing that facilitate the parallel analysis of multiple

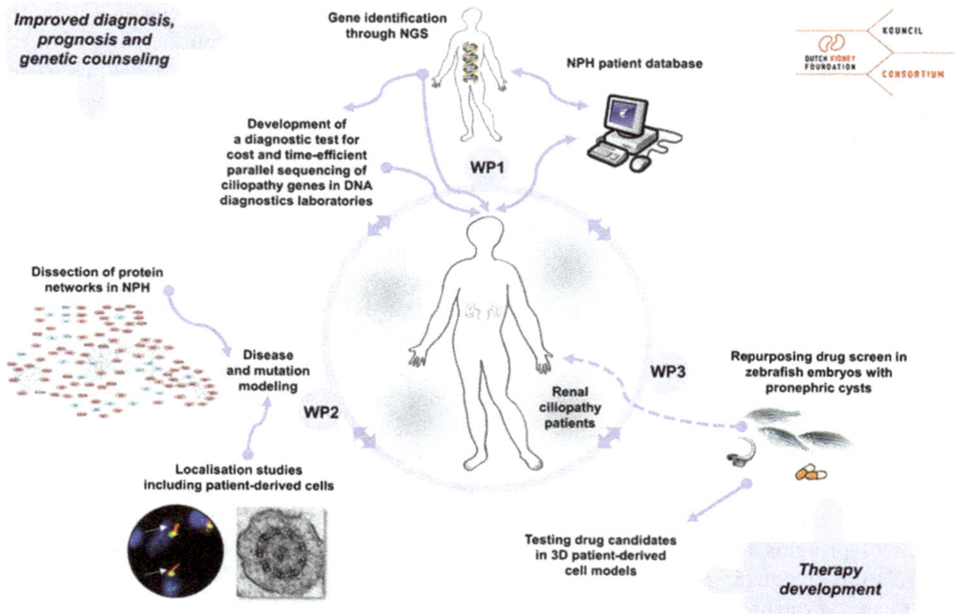

FIGURE 1 | Overview of the KOUNCIL consortium work plan that aims to improve personalized diagnostics, counseling, and treatment for nephronophthisis (NPH) patients. In work package 1 (WP1), genotypes and phenotypes were extensively studied and recorded in the nephronophthisis (NPH) database. In work package 2 (WP2), NPH protein modules were identified and NPH-related genes and gene variants were functionally characterized *in vitro* and *in vivo*. Work package 3 (WP3) focused on therapy development by drug screening in zebrafish that displayed nephric cysts. NGS; next generation sequencing.

genes in one sequencing run in a cost- and time-efficient manner. This has led to the identification and confirmation of multiple genes for renal ciliopathy-related diseases: *WDR60* (8), *WDR34* (9), *IFT172* (10), *DCDC2* (11), *CEP120* (12), *ICK* (13), *EXTL3* (14), and *TCTEX1D2* (15). Causal variant identification in new and known genes resulted in a genetic diagnosis for 31 patients from our cohort, who had not received a prior molecular diagnosis. We have implemented renal ciliopathy-specific gene screening in our genome diagnostic divisions and ensure high sensitivity and optimal diagnostic yield by periodically updating available tests.

Understanding Functional Defects Underlying Renal Ciliopathies

Cilia are regulated by defined protein complexes, some of which act as molecular machines (16). It is estimated that 1,000–2,000 proteins contribute to ciliary architecture or signaling. Through large-scale interaction assays, many of these proteins have been delineated in functional modules that are interconnected. Disrupting ciliary protein-protein interactions interferes with modules regulating cilia function. Because different ciliopathies are characterized by multiple and overlapping phenotypes, we hypothesized that there is also overlap in the molecular defects and protein modules that are disrupted in the different ciliopathies, including eye, brain, and kidney abnormalities (**Figure 3**) (17). Work that was performed prior to KOUNCIL suggested that proteomics-based dissection of molecular modules can relate biological mechanisms to specific genotypes in ciliopathy patients (18). Proof of principle ignited our interest to expand this approach to renal ciliopathies. Although our approach involving state-of-the art quantitative proteomics such as Stable Isotope Labeling with Amino acids in Cell culture (SILAC) combined with mass spectrometry proved technically challenging and involved multiple rounds of troubleshooting and adaptation, we were eventually successful in increasing our understanding of the ciliary protein complexes that are disturbed in NPH and allied ciliopathies (**Figure 4** and unpublished data), which is indispensable for the development of targeted therapies (17, 18). Another lesson learned was that patients remain their own best model of disease, since patient cells such as urine-derived renal epithelial cells (URECs) and fibroblasts delivered the most relevant information about possible pathogenic effects of detected genomic variation and more generally, mechanisms of disease (**Figure 4**) (20). Thus, implementation of the developed non-invasive methods for patient-derived cell investigations has proven to be tremendously useful in diagnostics for renal diseases and therapy development.

Advancing Therapeutics for NPH

Since there is no targeted cure for NPH, research toward the development of therapies that slow renal disease progression in NPH patients is warranted. We aimed to identify drugs that delay or prevent renal cyst formation, and used zebrafish embryos with pronephric cysts for a high-throughput drug screen to achieve this goal. We first developed a robust zebrafish model for NPH, using both morpholinos and CRISPR/Cas9 gene editing

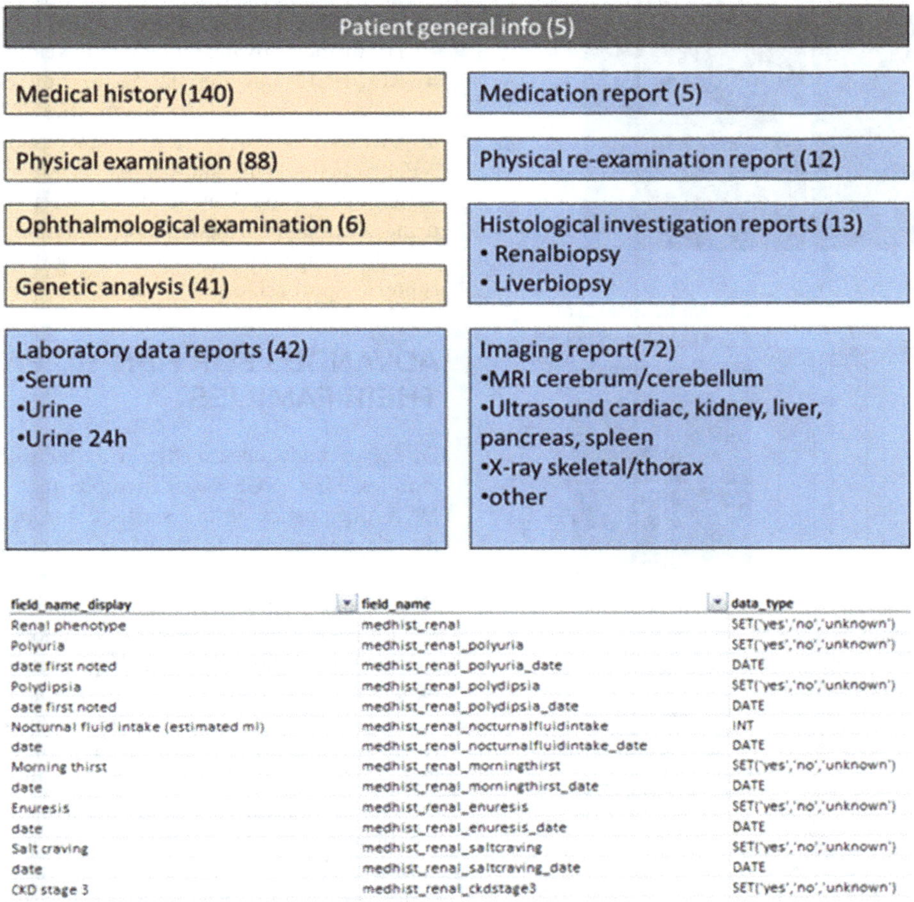

field_name_display	field_name	data_type
Renal phenotype	medhist_renal	SET('yes','no','unknown')
Polyuria	medhist_renal_polyuria	SET('yes','no','unknown')
date first noted	medhist_renal_polyuria_date	DATE
Polydipsia	medhist_renal_polydipsia	SET('yes','no','unknown')
date first noted	medhist_renal_polydipsia_date	DATE
Nocturnal fluid intake (estimated ml)	medhist_renal_nocturnalfluidintake	INT
date	medhist_renal_nocturnalfluidintake_date	DATE
Morning thirst	medhist_renal_morningthirst	SET('yes','no','unknown')
date	medhist_renal_morningthirst_date	DATE
Enuresis	medhist_renal_enuresis	SET('yes','no','unknown')
date	medhist_renal_enuresis_date	DATE
Salt craving	medhist_renal_saltcraving	SET('yes','no','unknown')
date	medhist_renal_saltcraving_date	DATE
CKD stage 3	medhist_renal_ckdstage3	SET('yes','no','unknown')

FIGURE 2 | Screenshots from parts of the nephronophthisis database. Numbers indicate the number of fields attributed to a specific theme.

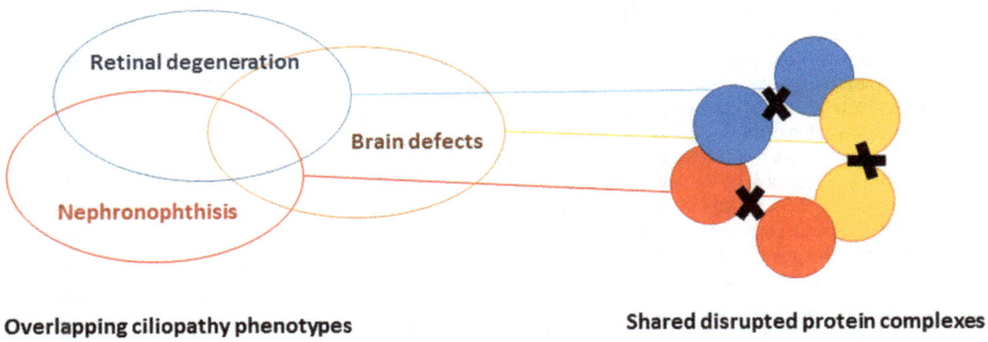

FIGURE 3 | Schematic representation of understanding proteomic modules underlying ciliopathies. By performing systematic agnostic proteomic profiling of protein complexes, it is possible to distinguish and find overlap in the disrupted protein modules in ciliopathies, featuring retinal degeneration, brain malformation, and/or renal ciliopathies.

technologies. A popular drug screening strategy is repurposing, whereby already FDA-approved drugs are investigated for new uses. We hypothesized that such a strategy is likely effective toward the identification of drugs that slow renal failure in NPH as it would allow a fast conversion from drug identification to actual clinical use. As such, we tested a library of FDA-approved compounds for inhibitory effects on renal cystogenesis. Two approaches were taken to screen for effective compounds. First, we performed a screen of 640 drugs in zebrafish embryos with NPH, which was a non-hypothesis driven approach. Secondly,

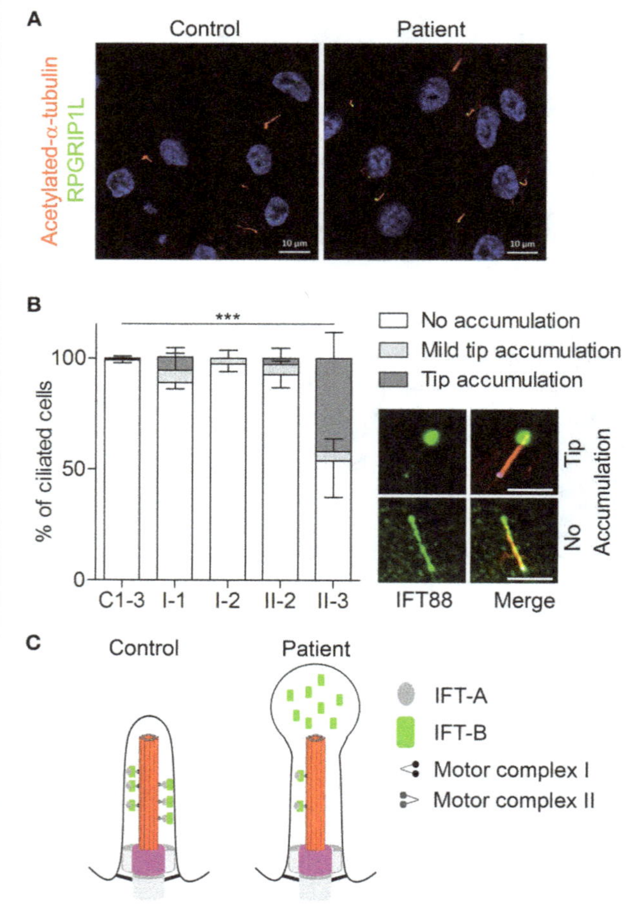

FIGURE 4 | Defective retrograde transport in urine-derived cells from a Mainzer-Saldino syndrome patient. URECs derived from a patient (referred to as "patient" or "II-3") with compound heterozygous variants in *IFT140* (one pathogenic frameshift and one missense variant of uncertain significance), were compared to URECs from three control individuals (C1-3). **(A)** URECs stained for ciliary marker acetylated-α-tubulin (red) and RPGRIP1L (green). **(B)** Analysis of retrograde transport in controls, healthy family members (I-1, I-2, and II-2) and patient (II-3) URECs. Cilia were visualized with acetylated-α-tubulin (red) and RPGRIP1L (pink). The cells were analyzed for the presence of IFT88 (green) accumulation at the ciliary tip. Patient II-3 showed a significant tip accumulation of IFT88 in 41% of the cells (Fisher's exact two-tailed test showed a $p < 0.0001$ when comparing the cells of the patient to those of the controls). Scale bar represents 5μm. **(C)** A schematic overview of the cilium in controls and in the patient with pathogenic variants in *IFT140*. The control shows normal intraflagellar transport with the IFT-B complex transporting proteins from the base of the cilium to the tip (axoneme is shown in red and the transition zone marks the base of the cilium in pink) and the IFT-A complex transporting proteins back down to the base. The image shows defective retrograde transport leading to an abnormal bulge at the ciliary tip, which is filled with IFT-B proteins. This image was adapted from Oud et al. (19). https://ciliajournal.biomedcentral.com/articles/10.1186/s13630-018-0055-2.

we extensively examined 14 therapies based on known beneficial effects in polycystic kidney disease (PKD), as a candidate-selected approach. From the second approach, four individual drugs and one drug combination significantly rescued the NPH phenotype in zebrafish embryos with acceptable toxicity profiles. These drugs warrant further *in vivo* investigations for their potential in modulating NPH-progression.

To further advance therapy development, a major effort in KOUNCIL was the standardization of the use of URECs in molecular and cellular diagnostics (20). The 3D culturing of URECs resulted in clear characteristic growth patterns in NPH patients. This allowed us to adapt a non-invasive drug screening methodology in patient-derived 3D spheroids from urine. Although expansion and validation of the URECs and 3D models is ongoing, we are excited by the potential this patient-centered approach offers.

ADVANCES FOR NPH-RC PATIENTS AND THEIR FAMILIES

Our project advanced medical care for kidney patients and their families. First, NGS-based methods that were implemented in DNA diagnostics at the start of our project almost doubled the diagnostic yield for NPH-RC. Secondly, NGS-based DNA diagnostics for renal ciliopathies allow clinicians to make the NPH diagnosis at a much earlier stage, which resolves the need for invasive renal biopsies for diagnostic purposes. Third, a solidified work flow has been implemented for renal ciliopathy patients in our dedicated multidisciplinary outpatient clinics for kidney diseases in the Radboud university medical center, Nijmegen, The Netherlands and the University Medical Center Utrecht, Utrecht, The Netherlands. In London, UK, multi-disciplinary clinics for Bardet-Biedl Syndrome (BBS) patients are provided. NPH-RC patients are seen by a nephrologist, ophthalmologist, geneticist, dietician, general pediatricians, endocrinologist (diabetes type II), and a clinical psychologist. The aim is to provide a "one stop" visit to ensure that patients receive specialized and expert attention and management. This should result in a major change in how NPH and BBS is managed, with a focus on diagnosis, early intervention and appropriate health management. These multidisciplinary clinics form a role model for other hospitals worldwide and will hopefully be more widely implemented in the near future.

The fourth improvement in patient care results from the setup of a renal ciliopathy database, which increased our insight into the relation between genotypes and phenotypes of NPH-RC patients. In the future, the database can be connected to other databases and converted to an interactive, international online registry. This will in turn allow for more refined insights in genotype-phenotype correlations and prognosis (6). Finally, we have developed a non-invasive protocol for research on renal cells that does not require patients (and their parents) to visit the hospital. In conclusion, KOUNCIL improved opportunities for patient management, led to advancements in the diagnostic trajectory and resulted in optimal genetic counseling for patients and their families.

SCIENTIFIC IMPACT

KOUNCIL and KOUNCIL collaborations revealed several new renal ciliopathy genes and molecular mechanisms of disease, which significantly improved the diagnostic yield for NPH and related disorders as well as advanced knowledge of ciliopathy pathophysiology. In combination with the phenotypic characteristics sampled in our coded renal ciliopathy database, the power of genotype-phenotype correlations for NPH is just emerging and will require further prospective validation. Continued genetic screening and ongoing deep phenotyping of NPH-RC patients will further dissect these correlations, ultimately improving patient counseling. Understanding the impact of allelic variants from patients on disease manifestations demands understanding of the extensive molecular connectivity of cilium-directed pathways; to this end, we have developed a proteomics-based approach to evaluate the assembly defects of the ciliary transport particles (IFT) in a subset of ciliopathy patients. Although ciliopathies represent a class of rare pediatric diseases, through the work of KOUNCIL, we have found novel insights into the molecular mechanisms of chronic renal disease progression widespread in the general population. Preliminary work suggesting that cilia are key repressors of cellular fibrosis in the kidney, will direct and further streamline future efforts to develop therapeutic intervention with a focus on fibrosis treatment.

It should be noted that development of methodologies independent of animal experimentation are a priority for most scientific bodies today. We have generated a robust protocol growing renal cells from urine that is non-invasive to patients, yet is patient-specific, and is amenable to screening (20). We showed that functional tests in URECs and CRISPR/Cas9-derived knockdown cells can more widely clarify the pathogenicity of genetic variants of unknown significance identified in NPH-RC patients. Growing 3D spheroids from urine ("urinoids") may also be appropriate for variant interpretation and with appropriate quality assurance measures, are potentially adaptable for diagnostic support (21).

CONCLUSIONS

The KOUNCIL consortium, consisting of pediatric nephrologists, clinical geneticists, molecular biologists and bioinformaticians, provided a unique, coherent inter- and transdisciplinary team to combat juvenile kidney failure. The resulting five PhD theses from three centers in two countries implicated the relevance of our consortium for the next generation of renal clinicians and scientists, and will continue to have a high impact on the renal field.

This consortium aimed to improve the understanding of genetics and biology of renal ciliopathies with innovative NGS and biochemical techniques, and set the first important steps toward therapeutic approaches to delay the progressive degenerative defects in the kidney. The results of this consortium project have already significantly impacted the clinical management of NPH-RC by improvements in diagnosis, prognosis, and accuracy of genetic risk assessment. Our project has provided us with optimal preparations for the development and refinement of future personalized therapies, and is a message of hope for NPH patients for whom there is currently no satisfactory treatment.

AUTHOR CONTRIBUTIONS

KR, RG, and HA performed the writing of the manuscript; ML, MO, and RR provided figures; RG, PB, RR, HA, and NK were work package leaders in the KOUNCIL consortium. All authors provided feedback on the revised manuscript.

ACKNOWLEDGMENTS

We thank the patients and parents who participated in the research performed within the KOUNCIL consortium. We also thank the scientific advisory board of the KOUNCIL consortium: Dr. Richard Sandford, Prof. Dr. Christine Mummery, and Prof. Dr. Irene van Langen; and the international scientific advisory board of Dutch Kidney Foundation chaired by Prof. Dr. Jo Berden. The KOUNCIL consortium was financially supported by the Dutch Kidney Foundation under grant agreement number CP11.18. The authors thank Simone Dusseljee for project management and Dr. Arjen Rienks and Dr. Eveline Martens of the Dutch Kidney Foundation for program management. PB is an NIHR Senior Investigator.

REFERENCES

1. Stokman M, Lilien M, Knoers N. *GeneReviews®*. Adam, MP, Ardinger, HH, Pagon, RA, Wallace, SE, Bean, LJH, Mefford, HC, et al. editors. (Seattle, WA: University of Washington). (1993).
2. Arts HH, Knoers NV. Current insights into renal ciliopathies: what can genetics teach us? *Pediatr Nephrol.* (2013) **28**:863–74. doi: 10.1007/s00467-012-2259-9
3. Schueler M, Halbritter J, Phelps IG, Braun DA, Otto EA, Porath JD, et al. Large-scale targeted sequencing comparison highlights extreme genetic heterogeneity in nephronophthisis-related ciliopathies. *J Med Genet.* (2016) **53**:208–14. doi: 10.1136/jmedgenet-2015-103304
4. Kang HG, Lee HK, Ahn YH, Joung JG, Nam J, Kim NK, et al. Targeted exome sequencing resolves allelic and the genetic heterogeneity in the genetic diagnosis of nephronophthisis-related ciliopathy. *Exp Mol Med.* (2016) **48**:e251. doi: 10.1038/emm.2016.63
5. Reiter JF, Leroux MR. Genes and molecular pathways underpinning ciliopathies. *Nat Rev Mol Cell Biol.* (2017) **18**:533–47. doi: 10.1038/nrm.2017.60
6. Konig J, Kranz B, Konig S, Schlingmann KP, Titieni A, Tonshoff B, et al. Phenotypic Spectrum of Children with Nephronophthisis and Related Ciliopathies. *Clin J Am Soc Nephrol.* (2017) **12**:1974–83. doi: 10.2215/CJN.01280217
7. van Rooij IA, van der Zanden LF, Bongers EM, Renkema KY, Wijers CH, Thonissen M, et al. AGORA a data- and biobank for birth defects and childhood cancer. *Birth Defects Res A Clin Mol Teratol.* (2016) **106**:675–84. doi: 10.1002/bdra.23512

8. McInerney-Leo AM, Schmidts M, Cortes CR, Leo PJ, Gener B, Courtney AD, et al. Short-rib polydactyly and Jeune syndromes are caused by mutations in WDR60. *Am J Hum Genet.* (2013) **93**:515–23. doi: 10.1016/j.ajhg.2013.06.022
9. Schmidts M, Vodopiutz J, Christou-Savina S, Cortes CR, McInerney-Leo AM, Emes RD, et al. Mutations in the gene encoding IFT dynein complex component WDR34 cause Jeune asphyxiating thoracic dystrophy. *Am J Hum Genet.* (2013) **93**:932–44. doi: 10.1016/j.ajhg.2013.10.003
10. Halbritter J, Bizet AA, Schmidts M, Porath JD, Braun DA, Gee HY, et al. Defects in the IFT-B component IFT172 cause jeune and mainzer-saldino syndromes in humans. *Am J Hum Genet.* (2013) **93**:915–25. doi: 10.1016/j.ajhg.2013.09.012
11. Schueler M, Braun DA, Chandrasekar G, Gee HY, Klasson TD, Halbritter J, et al. DCDC2 mutations cause a renal-hepatic ciliopathy by disrupting Wnt signaling. *Am J Hum Genet.* (2015) **96**:81–92. doi: 10.1016/j.ajhg.2014.12.002
12. Shaheen R, Schmidts M, Faqeih E, Hashem A, Lausch E, Holder I, et al. A founder CEP120 mutation in Jeune asphyxiating thoracic dystrophy expands the role of centriolar proteins in skeletal ciliopathies. *Hum Mol Genet.* (2015) **24**:1410–19. doi: 10.1093/hmg/ddu555
13. Roosing S, Romani M, Isrie M, Rosti RO, Micalizzi A, Musaev D, et al. Mutations in CEP120 cause Joubert syndrome as well as complex ciliopathy phenotypes. *J Med Genet.* (2016) **53**:608–15. doi: 10.1136/jmedgenet-2016-103832
14. Oud MM, Tuijnenburg P, Hempel M, van Vlies N, Ren Z, Ferdinandusse S, et al. Mutations in EXTL3 cause neuro-immuno-skeletal dysplasia syndrome. *Am J Hum Genet* (2017) **100**:281–96. doi: 10.1016/j.ajhg.2017.01.013
15. Schmidts M, Hou Y, Cortes CR, Mans DA, Huber C, Boldt K, et al. TCTEX1D2 mutations underlie Jeune asphyxiating thoracic dystrophy with impaired retrograde intraflagellar transport. *Nat Commun.* (2015) **6**:7074. doi: 10.1038/ncomms8074
16. Lechtreck KF, Van De Weghe JC, Harris JA, Liu P. Protein transport in growing and steady-state cilia. *Traffic* (2017) **18**:277–86. doi: 10.1111/tra.12474
17. Boldt K, van Reeuwijk J, Lu Q, Koutroumpas K, Nguyen TM, Texier Y, et al. An organelle-specific protein landscape identifies novel diseases and molecular mechanisms. *Nat Commun.* (2016) **7**:11491. doi: 10.1038/ncomms11491
18. Boldt K, Mans DA, Won J, van Reeuwijk J, Vogt A, Kinkl N, et al. Disruption of intraflagellar protein transport in photoreceptor cilia causes Leber congenital amaurosis in humans and mice. *J Clin Invest.* (2011) **21**:2169–80. doi: 10.1172/JCI45627
19. Oud MM, Latour BL, Bakey Z, Letteboer SJ, Lugtenberg D, Wu KM, et al. Cellular ciliary phenotyping indicates pathogenecity of novel variants in IFT140 and confirms a Mainzer-Saldino syndrome diagnosis. *Cilia* (2018) **7**:1. doi: 10.1186/s13630-018-0055-2
20. Ajzenberg H, Slaats GG, Stokman MF, Arts HH, Logister I, Kroes HY, et al. Non-invasive sources of cells with primary cilia from pediatric and adult patients. *Cilia* (2015) **4**:8. doi: 10.1186/s13630-015-0017-x
21. Srivastava S, Ramsbottom SA, Molinari E, Alkanderi S, Filby A, White K, et al. A human patient-derived cellular model of Joubert syndrome reveals ciliary defects which can be rescued with targeted therapies. *Hum Mol Genet.* (2017) **26**:4657–67. doi: 10.1093/hmg/ddx347

4

Cystic Kidney Diseases from the Adult Nephrologist's Point of View

Roman-Ulrich Müller and Thomas Benzing*

Department II of Internal Medicine and Center for Molecular Medicine Cologne, University of Cologne, Cologne, Germany

***Correspondence:**
Roman-Ulrich Müller
roman-ulrich.mueller@uk-koeln.de

Cystic kidney diseases affect patients of all age groups with the onset spanning from prenatal disease to late adulthood. Autosomal-dominant polycystic kidney disease (ADPKD) is by far the most common renal cystic disease. However, there are various cystic kidney diseases, the onset of which occurs at different times in life and depends on the type of the disease and the causative genes involved. When genetic kidney diseases are discussed in the adult setting this view is usually limited on autosomal-dominant kidney disease, the most frequent genetic disorder causing adult onset ESRD. Other diseases—such as autosomal-recessive polycystic kidney disease—are often being viewed as a disorder only important in pediatric nephrology. However, more recent data has revealed that, despite clear age peaks of onset for each disorder, all of them can also show highly variable phenotypes with classical adult onset genetic diseases being of importance in pediatrics and *vice versa*. Furthermore, the affected children need to be seen by adult nephrologists in the long term after transition, requiring knowledge on the underlying pediatric disease, potential extrarenal manifestations, and genetic counseling. Consequently, the view on these diseases should be widened on both ends. Close interaction between pediatric and adult nephrology is key to appropriate care of patients suffering from genetic kidney disease to profit from each other's experience.

Keywords: polycystic kidney diseases, autosomal dominant polycystic kidney disease, autosomal-recessive polycystic kidney disease, tuberous sclerosis complex, von Hippel–Lindau disease, nephronophthisis, genetic kidney disease, Birt–Hogg–Dubé syndrome

INTRODUCTION

While pediatric nephrologists are rather experienced in managing patients with genetic kidney diseases, most adult nephrologists are faced with congenital disease less frequently (1, 2). This is mainly due to the reason that genetic disorders are the minority of causes of end-stage renal disease in the adult population whereas in children they are common. Autosomal-dominant polycystic kidney disease (ADPKD) reveals most of its burden in adulthood and has long been considered to be the only cystic kidney disease in adults. Other cystic kidney diseases—primarily nephronophthisis (NPH) and autosomal-recessive polycystic kidney disease (ARPKD)—start much earlier and are entities that have primarily been studied and treated by pediatric nephrologists. However, with the advent of the first targeted treatment strategies—such as tolvaptan in ADPKD patients—the question arises whether early detection of disease and an early commencement of a potential therapy may be beneficial.

Genetic causes of kidney disease are on the brink to become much more of a visible problem in adult nephrology. This is not limited to cystic kidney diseases, but also true for other disorders, such as the MCD-FSGS spectrum. On the one hand, an increasing number of children suffering from kidney disease reach adulthood raising the question of transition and continued care in the adult nephrology setting. On the other hand, the advent of novel sequencing technologies has paved the way for elucidating more complex genetic factors in kidney disease and will allow for novel associations between the genetic background and pathogenic aspects. Clearly, chronic kidney disease in general in adulthood has an important genetic component. However, many of the genetic alterations are not simply monogenetic causes, but must rather be considered as complex genetic diseases. Consequently, knowledge on genetic diseases of the kidney will play an increasingly important role in adult nephrology and profit from a close interaction with colleagues from pediatric nephrology. Here, we will use the example of cystic kidney diseases—and ADPKD specifically—to point out the most important aspects and advances in the care of adult patients.

CYSTIC KIDNEY DISEASE—A CILIOPATHY

The introduction of next-generation sequencing techniques in the last decade—starting in basic research and being currently introduced in clinical diagnostics—made the large-scale analysis of potential disease-causing mutations in patients with cystic kidney diseases feasible (3–6). This has led to the identification of numerous novel disease-causing genes enabling the discovery of more than 100 genes to be involved in cystic kidney diseases (7). Nonetheless, a significant proportion of cases remains unsolved which will require further research in well-characterized families and cohorts (3, 5). Despite this enormous genetic complexity of cystic kidney diseases, they are unified by a single pathophysiological concept. Nearly all protein products of disease-causing genes identified so far have been linked to the generation or function of the primary cilium—a membranous protrusion of the apical cell membrane of close to all cell types that is supported by a microtubular skeleton (7). Primary cilia may function as chemo- and mechanoreceptors and ciliary dysfunction which initiates numerous signaling aberrations in epithelial kidney cells—like increased cAMP generation or mTOR-signaling—that are crucial to cyst formation (8). This has led to the definition of the cystic disease complex as a ciliopathy. The fact that pretty much all tissues in the human body contain ciliated cells explains why ciliary defects can be the basis to complex syndromes affecting different organs—e.g., the combination of cystic kidneys with *situs inversus* and retinitis pigmentosa observed in several NPH-associated syndromes (9).

ADPKD—EPIDEMIOLOGY

Autosomal-dominant polycystic kidney disease is the most common entity among cystic kidney diseases (10). Its lifetime morbid risk is estimated to be around 1:1,000 while point prevalence—which rather reflects clinically relevant disease—has recently been shown to be approximately 1:2,500 (11–14). The frequency of ADPKD is thus comparable to much more commonly known disorders, such as cystic fibrosis or multiple sclerosis. Consequently, it is also the most frequent genetic cause of end-stage renal disease in adults with a prevalence of 5–10% in the dialysis population (15). However, a decline in renal function is rarely observed in childhood leading to ADPKD being primarily viewed as a disease of adult patients. Nonetheless, with the advent of novel targeted therapeutic strategies—e.g., tolvaptan and somatostatin-analogs—and seeing that a subpopulation of children with ADPKD suffer from clinically meaningful hypertension (16), ADPKD has gained increasing attention among pediatric nephrologists—a fact that is reflected by the initiation of a pediatric ADPKD registry in 2017 (www.adpedkd.org) that has successfully started recruiting patients. Nonetheless, the predominant time at which ADPKD gets manifest is above the age of 30 years and ESRD is reached at an average age of 50–60 years (17). Consequently, while there is no clear consensus of how to care for children of affected parents, the period in life during which interventions are necessary is primarily adulthood for now. Obviously, this may change in the future, e.g., with upcoming clinical trials on drugs such as the V2 receptor antagonist tolvaptan in pediatric cohorts (18).

DIFFERENTIAL DIAGNOSIS OF ADPKD

Due to its typical clinical manifestation, the diagnosis of ADPKD can be made solely on clinical grounds in the vast majority of affected patients. This is primarily based on three considerations: (1) morphology of the kidneys, (2) extrarenal manifestations, and (3) mode of inheritance.

Using these criteria ADPKD can—in most cases—clearly be separated from the rarer causes of cystic kidney diseases in adulthood. This is very important, since—even though ADPKD is by far the most common diagnosis—distinguishing other disorders, including autosomal-dominant tubulointerstitial disease (ADTKD), NPH, and ARPKD and a clear separation from simple renal cysts is crucial to make the correct diagnosis. This has become even more important with targeted therapies getting available for particular disorders.

Kidney Morphology

With the morphology of the kidneys being the key to diagnosing or excluding ADPKD in individuals at risk, imaging modalities are highly important screening tools. As to this point, several different key factors have to be taken into consideration: (1) kidney size, (2) number of cysts, (3) unilateral/bilateral disease, and (4) distribution of the cysts.

(1) Autosomal-dominant polycystic kidney disease generally goes along with enlarged kidneys. Since the disease is gradually progressing during lifetime, size has to be considered in an age-dependent fashion. The correlation of age-adjusted kidney size with disease progression allows for using the information obtained by imaging to—beyond making a diagnosis—help guiding treatment decisions using, e.g., MRI volumetry (19) (**Figure 1**). Large polycystic kidneys are also found in ARPKD as well as the much less common tumor-associated syndromes (tuberous sclerosis, Von Hippel–Lindau disease, Birt–Hogg–Dubé syndrome) and *HNF1b*-associated kidney disease (20–22). In contrast to this, diseases of the NPH complex are characterized by small (to normal) sized kidneys. (2) Ravine et al. were the first to come up with a classification based on cyst numbers that allowed for diagnosing ADPKD in individuals with a positive family history using ultrasonography more than 20 years ago (23). Since then this approach has been revised twice in order to account for the advances in imaging technologies that strongly increased sensitivity of cyst detection accompanied with decreasing positive predictive values (24, 25). York Pei and colleagues validated novel criteria in a well-designed

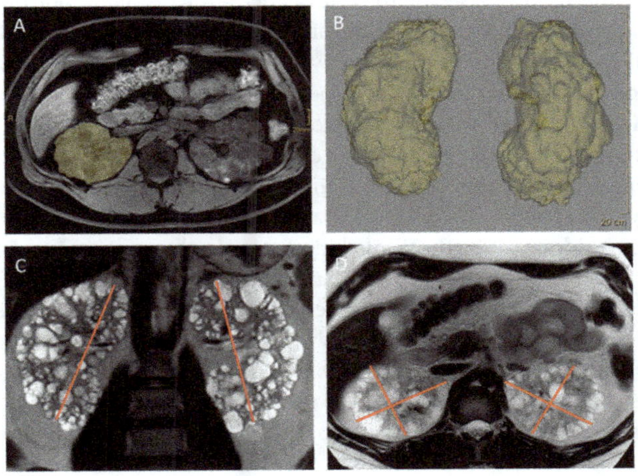

FIGURE 1 | MRI imaging and volumetry of kidneys in autosomal-dominant polycystic kidney disease (ADPKD). These images reveal the classical features of ADPKD: strongly enlarged kidneys showing a ubiquitous distribution of cysts throughout the parenchyma. Kidney volume—an important prognostic feature now used in algorithm for making treatment decisions—can be obtained by planimetry **(A,B)** as done in the clinical trials. However, for everyday clinical decisions volumetry based on measuring the axes and using the ellipsoid formula has been shown to be sufficient (19) **(C,D)**. From Müller et al. (27) (images kindly provided by Dr. Thorsten Persigehl, Institute of Radiology, University of Cologne).

study in 2015 that now allows for clear detection of ADPKD by ultrasound from the age of 30 onwards. Interestingly, all affected individuals showed more than ten cysts when measured by MRI clearly distinguishing them from unaffected individuals. This held true already from the age of 16 years providing data that imaging-based exclusion of disease may be possible starting in adolescence (25). One caveat regarding the diagnosis of ADPKD based on cyst number is the fact that these approaches have only been validated in patients showing a positive family history. (3) However, there is still more conclusions that can be drawn from kidney morphology in cystic kidney diseases. First, based on the fact that these are genetic diseases that go along with the same genetic alteration in all kidney cells, bilateral disease is to be expected. There is few and very rare exceptions to this rule due to potential genetic somatic mosaicism (26). (4) In ADPKD, the bilateral cysts are generally distributed ubiquitously throughout the parenchyma, since cyst formation occurs along the entire nephron (**Figure 1**). This leads to an entirely different pattern compared to NPH, where the cysts are strictly localized at the corticomedullary junction. In ARPKD, cyst formation occurs primarily in the collecting duct, however, the imaging findings can be similar to ADPKD. The same holds true for the tumor syndromes mentioned above and *HNF1b*-associated disease that can all phenocopy ADPKD as to kidney morphology. Here, apart from the fact that—due to its frequency—ADPKD is clearly the most likely diagnosis, extrarenal findings help to distinguish the different entities.

Renal Manifestations Beyond Cysts

As to the kidneys themselves, ADPKD is not only characterized by renal cysts but also includes kidney stones, flank pain, cyst infections, and macrohematuria. While these manifestations are common in adult patients and may lead to the diagnosis—especially in cases with a negative family history—they are rare in childhood. Importantly, early onset of these symptoms may indicate rapid progression of disease as pointed out by the data from the French GENKYST cohort (PROPKD score, see section on "Targeted therapies") (28).

Extrarenal Manifestations

As explained above cystic kidney diseases are one of the best characterized ciliopathies. Knowing that cilia are present on nearly all cells of the human body and are expected to play important roles in cellular polarity signaling and cell proliferation it is not surprising that the clinical manifestation of a ciliopathy is normally not limited to one organ, but causes a multitude of syndromic clinical pictures. Knowledge of the extrarenal manifestations is crucial to patient care, since they do not only explain symptoms but may also require specific interventions/diagnostic strategies—e.g., in the case of intracranial aneurysms in ADPKD. As to diagnosing a specific cystic kidney disease these manifestations are very helpful, especially in cases where the decision is not clear based on kidney morphology. Hence, a complete workup of these aspects by patient history and clinical examination is essential when seeing PKD patients.

Extrarenal Manifestations in ADPKD

The most common extrarenal finding in ADPKD patients is extrarenal cysts with the majority of patients also showing liver cysts (and less frequently in other organs, such as the seminal vesicles, pancreas, or spleen). Furthermore, diverticulosis is a common manifestation. As to cardiac manifestations cardiac valve abnormalities—primarily mitral valve prolaps and insufficiency—are the most common findings, a fact that makes echocardiography a useful tool in the workup of these patients. Abdominal and inguinal hernias are also associated with ADPKD and are probably a consequence of both an altered strength of the abdominal wall and the increased intra-abdominal pressure due to enlarged kidneys and liver. An aspect that may be especially worrisome for ADPKD patients is the increased occurrence of intracranial aneurysms. Here, a tailored screening strategy in high-risk patients (e.g., those with a positive family history) as well as an interdisciplinary workup (neurosurgeons, neuroradiologists, nephrologists) are crucial—especially when taking into account that interventions to close these aneurysms can also lead to significant morbidity and mortality (29, 30). A more complete workup of potential extrarenal associations with ADPKD and their management can be found in the recent literature (10, 31, 32).

Extrarenal Manifestations of Tumor Syndromes Associated With Polycystic Kidneys

In contrast to ADPKD, the tumor syndromes—associated with polycystic kidneys that often resemble ADPKD—tuberous sclerosis, BHD syndrome, and VHL syndrome—all go along with a significantly increased risk of kidney cancer (clear-cell renal cell carcinoma in VHL and TSC; chromophobe renal cell carcinoma in BHD). Furthermore, all of these syndromes have characteristic extrarenal manifestations—TSC: e.g., giant-cell astrocytomas and other CNS tumors, renal angiomyolipomas, pulmonary lymphangioleiomyomatosis, cardiac rhabdomyomas, and multiple dermatological signs (facial angiofibromas, periungual fibromas, ash leaf spots, Shagreen patches, etc.); BHD: recurrent pneumothoraces and fibrofolliculomas; VHL: e.g., CNS/retinal hemangioblastomas, pancreatic neuroendocrine tumors, and pheochromocytoma (33). All of these can and should be used for differential diagnosis. While VHL and BHD patients often do not show any symptoms before late adolescence or adulthood, TSC—especially due to the CNS and cardiac manifestations—is frequently already highly symptomatic in early childhood. Nonetheless, there are a considerable proportion of TSC patients that are not diagnosed before adulthood and present with an oligosymptomatic course that, e.g., is mainly characterized by multiple renal angiomyolipomas.

Extrarenal Manifestations in ARPKD and HNF1B-Associated Kidney Disease

Another disease that can phenocopy the renal phenotype of ADPKD patients is ARPKD. However, the spectrum of extrarenal manifestations differs between these two entities. While in childhood pulmonary hypoplasia is one of the most dramatic findings, patients reaching adulthood without having been diagnosed do generally not show pulmonary symptoms. However, ARPKD has an obligatory association with liver fibrosis (in combination with dilated bile ducts—Caroli syndrome). Consequently, these patients need a workup, including liver imaging (sonography, fibroscan) and gastroscopy (screening for varices). Combined kidney-liver transplantation always needs to be considered when reaching end-stage renal disease (34).

HNF1b is a key transcription factor influencing numerous renal and extrarenal disease genes. Consequently, its mutation can lead to a range of symptoms. As to extrarenal manifestation-associated disorders, which include elevated liver enzymes, MODY diabetes mellitus, pancreatic insufficiency, hypomagnesemia, hyperparathyroidism, gout, and mental retardation (22).

Extrarenal Manifestations in Diseases of the NPH Complex

Even though diseases of the NPH complex are much less common in the adult population knowledge about their characteristics is important for identifying individuals affected by non-ADPKD cystic kidney diseases. Due to the nature of these disorders as a ciliopathy a wide range of affected tissues and symptoms are possible. In the following, we will summarize the most common examples that may sometimes not be diagnosed before reaching adulthood (9). Importantly, the attribution of a disorder to the NPH complex is—due to genetic complexity—not primarily guided by genetic diagnostics, but by the clinical characterization of the syndromic pattern of manifestations. The most frequent extrarenal finding in NPH patients is retinitis pigmentosa, which is characterized by night blindness followed by tunnel vision and eventually blindness. The combination of NPH and retinitis pigmentosa is classified as Senior–Løken syndrome. Furthermore—based on the role of cilia at the primary node during embryonal determination of laterality—many patients with NPH-associated syndromes show *situs inversus* as a characteristic finding. Another entity to be specifically named here is Bardet–Biedl syndrome which is characterized by polydactyly, juvenile obesity (often accompanied by diabetes mellitus), mental retardation of different degrees, retinitis pigmentosa, anosmia, and hypogonadism. Interestingly, Bardet–Biedl patients often show large kidneys at birth. While kidney size in the majority returns to normal by the age of 1–2 years, renal phenotypes that resemble ADPKD have been described in adult patients. Most other diseases of the NPH complex are nearly exclusively diagnosed in early childhood, such as Joubert syndrome (characterized by cerebellar vermis hypoplasia) or result in perinatal lethality as for Meckel–Gruber syndrome (20).

The Role of Genetic Diagnostics

Using the clinical criteria mentioned above, the diagnosis can be made correctly in the vast majority of patients without requiring a molecular genetics workup (20, 25, 35). In NPH, there is only very limited phenotype–genotype correlation which makes targeted genetics difficult. However, since *NPHP1* is the most commonly affected gene, testing for alterations in *NPHP1* may be of diagnostic utility (36, 37). This may change in the future with always cheaper and easier access to next-generation sequencing panels. ADPKD is—in patients with a positive family history—diagnosed almost exclusively on clinical grounds. However, molecular genetics may play a major important role in these patients for predicting disease progression (which may be a piece of the puzzle for making therapeutic decisions) in the future (28). The tumor syndromes on the other hand require different considerations when discussing molecular genetics. Here, a clear diagnosis based on the mutation is essential to distinguish these entities from ADPKD which then allows for the design of screening strategies for individual patients and prognostic testing in family members. An overview of a diagnostic strategy in cystic kidney diseases including clinical and genetic considerations is illustrated in (**Figure 2**). Importantly, current clinical diagnostic algorithms may require adaptation in the future due to novel culprit genes and associated disease entities identified—e.g., *GANAB* recently described as a new gene in ADPKD (5). Obviously, diseases not expected in adulthood—e.g., ARPKD and rare disorders that go along with variable clinical manifestations like HNF1b-associated kidney disease—may also require a molecular genetic diagnosis.

CLINICAL TRIALS TO PREVENT DISEASE PROGRESSION OF CYSTIC KIDNEY DISEASE

Supportive Measures

Knowledge of the various manifestations is key to the therapy of cystic kidney diseases in general. ESRD can obviously be addressed by renal transplantation in all entities (with a combined liver transplantation to be considered in ARPKD patients). Yet, data from randomized trials as well as a targeted therapy are only available for ADPKD. Until the year 2015 merely

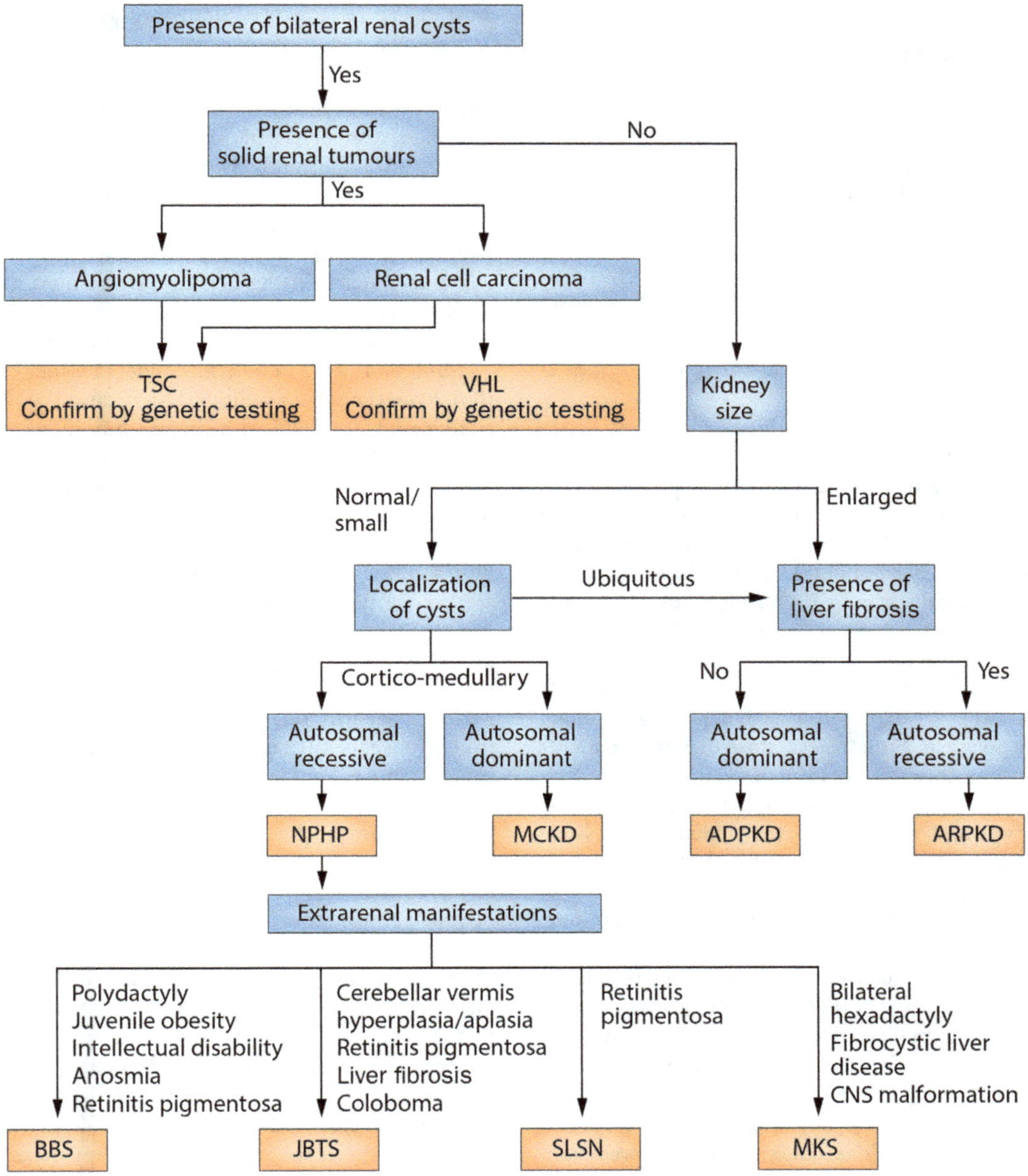

FIGURE 2 | Scheme of the diagnostic algorithm for polycystic kidney diseases combining clinical judgment with imaging modalities and molecular genetics. From Kurschat et al. (20). NPHP, nephronophthisis; MCKD, medullary cystic kidney disease (better to be termed now: autosomal-dominant tubulointerstitial disease); BBS, Bardet–Biedl syndrome; JBTS, Joubert syndrome; SLSN, Senior–Loken syndrome; MKS, Meckel–Gruber syndrome.

supportive measures were available. The most important recommendations to all of the affected individuals are summarized in **Table 1**, however, the degree of evidence is limited for some of these recommendations. As an example, sufficient fluid intake is mainly based on pathophysiological considerations regarding ADH-suppression (38–40). Here, a recently initiated randomized trial will hopefully clarify the impact of fluid intake (41). On the contrary, there is solid data regarding blood pressure control which was recently emphasized again by the randomized HALT-PKD trials (42). Study arm A showed that lowering blood pressure to 95/60–110/70 mmHg compared to 120/70–130/80 mmHg using an ACE-inhibitor or an AT1-blocker leads to a significant decrease in the kidney growth rate (42) in young patients with preserved kidney function (15–49 years of age, CKD stages G1 and 2). Dual RAAS-blockade once again did not show any additional benefit (43). Interestingly, a *post hoc* analysis of the same trial confirmed that salt restriction should be part of the general management of ADPKD patients (44).

Targeted Therapies—Tolvaptan

The TEMPO 3:4 trial which was published in 2012 entirely changed the approach to ADPKD, since it led to the approval of

TABLE 1 | Supportive measures in autosomal-dominant polycystic kidney disease (ADPKD).

Supportive measures in ADPKD
Blood pressure control (42)
Limiting NaCl intake to <5–7 g/day (44)
Sufficient fluid intake (>3 L/day) (38–41)
Avoid estrogen intake (which stimulates liver growth) (45–47)
Healthy diet (e.g., Mediterranean diet) (48, 49)

While strict blood pressure control is based upon the results from an RCT (HALT-PKD study arm A), the strongest data regarding limiting salt intake specifically in ADPKD relies on a post hoc analysis of HALT-PKD. The effect of estrogens was observed both in pregnant women and more specifically in a small cohort regarding postmenopausal substitution. As to healthy diets, trial results regarding cardiovascular endpoints—the risk of which is increased in ADPKD—can be extrapolated to this cohort. Sufficient fluid intake inhibits ADH secretion, however, its impact on disease progression still needs to be confirmed.

the very first targeted therapy in Europe. TEMPO 3:4 showed—in a double-blind randomized design—that vasopressin receptor (V2R) inhibition could significantly slow down the rate of kidney growth by close to 50% (50). Even more importantly, eGFR loss was decreased by about 26%, an effect size that is comparable to the large trials on RAAS-blockade in diabetic nephropathy. This effect has recently been confirmed by the REPRISE trial that showed tolvaptan to be effective not only in early-stage ADPKD but also in patients having reached early CKD stage G4 (51). As expected V2R-blockade goes along with significant polyuria. Nonetheless, close to 80% of patients enrolled did continue through 3 years of the trial; a finding that is confirmed by recent real-world experiences (52). Furthermore, even though rare and reversible, liver toxicity is possible and requires regular screening of liver enzymes. In order for ADPKD patients to benefit from this therapy, careful selection of patients in whom the treatment is started is of utmost importance. Individuals that will not reach ESRD during lifetime are not suitable candidates for such an approach making only rapid progressors candidates for this therapy. Consequently, several publications have been published in the past 2 years trying to give guidance to nephrologists as to patient selection (27, 53). Past data on eGFR loss is the best indicator of rapid disease progression, yet, these data are not always available and do not help in CKD stage G1. Consequently, a row of predictors of disease progression in ADPKD—including models using total kidney volume ("Mayo classification") (19), mutation status, and clinical symptoms ("PROPKD Score") (28)—have been validated that can help in treatment decisions and patient counseling. While ultrasonography is usually sufficient to make a diagnosis of ADPKD, MRI volumetry has proven very helpful to obtain more precise kidney volumes as the basis to treatment decisions (**Figure 1**). A more detailed summary of these criteria can be found in the recent literature (27, 53).

Targeted Therapies Beyond Tolvaptan

Even though tolvaptan is a major step forward in the care of ADPKD patients it only slows down disease progression and will not prevent reaching ESRD in the vast majority of patients. Consequently, additional strategies targeting others of the multiple dysregulated cellular signal transduction pathways are necessary (54). One promising target was the mTOR-signaling pathway based on data from mouse models (55, 56). However, two clinical trials did unfortunately not show any benefit in the patient setting (57, 58). The use of somatostatin-analogs targets the same intracellular secondary messenger—cAMP—as tolvaptan. A small trial has shown a potential benefit in ADPKD patients (59). Currently, two phase 3 trials—the LIPS trial in France and the DIPAK1 trial in the Netherlands—are examining this approach in larger cohorts. Somatostatin-analogs would have the advantage to also influence liver disease in ADPKD, while an impact on the hepatic involvement has by now not been shown in the case of tolvaptan. Interestingly, with the use of pravastatin in ADPKD, a double-blind randomized trial in children and young adults has added another potential target (60). Even though a recent *post hoc* analysis of the HALT-PKD trials could not confirm a disease-modifying effect of statin therapy in ADPKD, final clarification of the potential of these drugs will need a larger prospective clinical trial (61). With the overactivation of several kinases in ADPKD, re-purposing of kinase inhibitors has gained interest in the past years. In this line, a phase 2 trial examining the potential of bosutinib—a src/bcr-abl tyrosine kinase inhibitor—has recently been published. In this 2-year trial, bosutinib was able to slow down kidney growth. However, there was no effect on eGFR loss and close to 50% of the patients discontinued the initial treatment period, primarily due to treatment-associated adverse events (62). Consequently, more efforts are necessary to continue translating basic research in ADPKD to clinically meaningful therapies. Apart from the identification of novel treatment targets and their translation into clinical trials—e.g., as for CDC25 inhibition using vitamin K3, treatment with niacinamide, re-purposing of metformin, dietary interventions, or reversal of the Warburg effect (63–67)—combination therapies could also help in improving the effects and reducing side effects of pharmacological therapies in ADPKD in the future (68, 69). Furthermore, as to tolvaptan, a trial that started recruitment in the past year is currently examining V2R-inhibition as a therapeutic principle in a pediatric cohort. Even though clinical disease onset in ADPKD does primarily occur in adulthood, patients with clear indicators of very rapid disease progression could profit from an early start of therapy making this trial an interesting endeavor.

CONCLUSION

There has been an enormous breakthrough in the understanding of polycystic kidney diseases both in the adult as well as in the pediatric population. A large number of underlying gene defects have been identified and pathogenic pathways characterized. In ADPKD this resulted in the development of the first available treatment strategies and the approval of tolvaptan to prevent progression of the disorder. Even though ADPKD is primarily a disease of adulthood and ADPKD patients are thus mainly seen by adult nephrologists, a close interaction between pediatric and adult nephrology will be of benefit to patients and their families. Not only do genetic diseases always involve more than one individual. Unusual courses can also lead to onset of classical diseases of adulthood (e.g., ADPKD) in children and of classical pediatric diseases (e.g., ARPKD and NPH complex) in adult patients. Adult nephrologists can benefit from the wide experience of pediatric disciplines regarding genetic diseases on the one hand. On the other hand, this interaction helps in combining the knowledge on childhood interventions with outcome in adulthood and allows to learn from each other's experiences in the treatment of polycystic kidney diseases.

AUTHOR CONTRIBUTIONS

R-UM and TB wrote the manuscript. R-UM designed the figures.

FUNDING

Ministerium für Kultur und Wissenschaft des Landes NRW (Nachwuchsgruppen.NRW 2015-2021) Deutsche Nierenstiftung Marga und Walter Boll Stiftung.

REFERENCES

1. Atkins RC. The epidemiology of chronic kidney disease. *Kidney Int Suppl* (2005) 67:S14–8. doi:10.1111/j.1523-1755.2005.09403.x
2. Becherucci F, Roperto RM, Materassi M, Romagnani P. Chronic kidney disease in children. *Clin Kidney J* (2016) 9:583–91. doi:10.1093/ckj/sfw047
3. Schueler M, Munschauer M, Gregersen LH, Finzel A, Loewer A, Chen W, et al. Differential protein occupancy profiling of the mRNA transcriptome. *Genome Biol* (2014) 15:R15. doi:10.1186/gb-2014-15-1-r15
4. Hildebrandt F, Benzing T, Katsanis N. Ciliopathies. *N Engl J Med* (2011) 364:1533–43. doi:10.1056/NEJMra1010172
5. Cornec-Le Gall E, Torres VE, Harris PC. Genetic complexity of autosomal dominant polycystic kidney and liver diseases. *J Am Soc Nephrol* (2017) 29(1):13–23. doi:10.1681/ASN.2017050483
6. Lu H, Galeano MCR, Ott E, Kaeslin G, Kausalya PJ, Kramer C, et al. Mutations in DZIP1L, which encodes a ciliary-transition-zone protein, cause autosomal recessive polycystic kidney disease. *Nat Genet* (2017) 49:1025–34. doi:10.1038/ng.3871
7. Braun DA, Hildebrandt F. Ciliopathies. *Cold Spring Harb Perspect Biol* (2017) 9(3):a028191. doi:10.1101/cshperspect.a028191
8. Vivante A, Hildebrandt F. Exploring the genetic basis of early-onset chronic kidney disease. *Nat Rev Nephrol* (2016) 12:133–46. doi:10.1038/nrneph.2015.205
9. Benzing T, Schermer B. Clinical spectrum and pathogenesis of nephronophthisis. *Curr Opin Nephrol Hypertens* (2012) 21:272–8. doi:10.1097/MNH.0b013e3283520f17
10. Torres VE, Harris PC. Autosomal dominant polycystic kidney disease: the last 3 years. *Kidney Int* (2009) 76:149–68. doi:10.1038/ki.2009.128
11. Neumann HP, Jilg C, Bacher J, Nabulsi Z, Malinoc A, Hummel B, et al. Epidemiology of autosomal-dominant polycystic kidney disease: an in-depth clinical study for south-western Germany. *Nephrol Dial Transplant* (2013) 28:1472–87. doi:10.1093/ndt/gfs551
12. McGovern AP, Jones S, van Vlymen J, Saggar AK, Sandford R, de Lusignan S. Identification of people with autosomal dominant polycystic kidney disease using routine data: a cross sectional study. *BMC Nephrol* (2014) 15:182. doi:10.1186/1471-2369-15-182
13. Dalgaard OZ. Bilateral polycystic disease of the kidneys; a follow-up of 284 patients and their families. *Dan Med Bull* (1957) 4:128–33.
14. Willey CJ, Blais JD, Hall AK, Krasa HB, Makin AJ, Czerwiec FS. Prevalence of autosomal dominant polycystic kidney disease in the European Union. *Nephrol Dial Transplant* (2017) 32:1356–63. doi:10.1093/ndt/gfw240
15. Hildebrandt F. Genetic kidney diseases. *Lancet* (2010) 375:1287–95. doi:10.1016/S0140-6736(10)60236-X
16. Marlais M, Cuthell O, Langan D, Dudley J, Sinha MD, Winyard PJ. Hypertension in autosomal dominant polycystic kidney disease: a meta-analysis. *Arch Dis Child* (2016) 101:1142–7. doi:10.1136/archdischild-2015-310221
17. Spithoven EM, Kramer A, Meijer E, Orskov B, Wanner C, Abad JM, et al. Renal replacement therapy for autosomal dominant polycystic kidney disease (ADPKD) in Europe: prevalence and survival – an analysis of data from the ERA-EDTA registry. *Nephrol Dial Transplant* (2014) 29(Suppl 4):iv15–25. doi:10.1093/ndt/gfu017
18. *Safety, Pharmacokinetics, Tolerability and Efficacy of Tolvaptan in Children and Adolescents with ADPKD (Autosomal Dominant Polycystic Kidney Disease)*. ClinicalTrials.gov (2017). Available from: https://clinicaltrials.gov/ct2/show/NCT02964273. (accessed October 23, 2017).
19. Irazabal MV, Rangel LJ, Bergstralh EJ, Osborn SL, Harmon AJ, Sundsbak JL, et al. Imaging classification of autosomal dominant polycystic kidney disease: a simple model for selecting patients for clinical trials. *J Am Soc Nephrol* (2015) 26:160–72. doi:10.1681/ASN.2013101138
20. Kurschat CE, Müller RU, Franke M, Maintz D, Schermer B, Benzing T. An approach to cystic kidney diseases: the clinician's view. *Nat Rev Nephrol* (2014) 10:687–99. doi:10.1038/nrneph.2014.173
21. Schmidt LS, Linehan WM. Molecular genetics and clinical features of Birt-Hogg-Dubé syndrome. *Nat Rev Urol* (2015) 12:558–69. doi:10.1038/nrurol.2015.206
22. Verhave JC, Bech AP, Wetzels JFM, Nijenhuis T. Hepatocyte nuclear factor 1β-associated kidney disease: more than renal cysts and diabetes. *J Am Soc Nephrol* (2016) 27:345–53. doi:10.1681/ASN.2015050544
23. Ravine D, Gibson RN, Donlan J, Sheffield LJ. An ultrasound renal cyst prevalence survey: specificity data for inherited renal cystic diseases. *Am J Kidney Dis* (1993) 22:803–7. doi:10.1016/S0272-6386(12)70338-4
24. Pei Y, Obaji J, Dupuis A, Paterson AD, Magistroni R, Dicks E, et al. Unified criteria for ultrasonographic diagnosis of ADPKD. *J Am Soc Nephrol* (2009) 20:205–12. doi:10.1681/ASN.2008050507
25. Pei Y, Hwang YH, Conklin J, Sundsbak JL, Heyer CM, Chan W, et al. Imaging-based diagnosis of autosomal dominant polycystic kidney disease. *J Am Soc Nephrol* (2015) 26:746–53. doi:10.1681/ASN.2014030297
26. Iliuta IA, Kalatharan V, Wang K, Cornec-Le Gall E, Conklin J, Pourafkari M, et al. Polycystic kidney disease without an apparent family history. *J Am Soc Nephrol* (2017) 28:2768–76. doi:10.1681/ASN.2016090938
27. Müller R-U, Haas CS, Sayer JA. Practical approaches to the management of autosomal dominant polycystic kidney disease patients in the era of tolvaptan. *Clin Kidney J* (2018) 11(1):62–9. doi:10.1093/ckj/sfx071
28. Cornec-Le Gall E, Audrézet MP, Rousseau A, Hourmant M, Renaudineau E, Charasse C, et al. The PROPKD score: a new algorithm to predict renal survival in autosomal dominant polycystic kidney disease. *J Am Soc Nephrol* (2016) 27:942–51. doi:10.1681/ASN.2015010016
29. Wiebers DO, Whisnant JP, Huston J 3rd, Meissner I, Brown RD Jr, Piepgras DG, et al. Unruptured intracranial aneurysms: natural history, clinical outcome, and risks of surgical and endovascular treatment. *Lancet* (2003) 362:103–10. doi:10.1016/S0140-6736(03)13860-3
30. Pirson Y, Chauveau D, Torres V. Management of cerebral aneurysms in autosomal dominant polycystic kidney disease. *J Am Soc Nephrol* (2002) 13:269–76.
31. Halvorson CR, Bremmer MS, Jacobs SC. Polycystic kidney disease: inheritance, pathophysiology, prognosis, and treatment. *Int J Nephrol Renovasc Dis* (2010) 3:69–83.
32. Luciano RL, Dahl NK. Extra-renal manifestations of ADPKD: considerations for routine screening and management. *Nephrol Dial Transplant* (2014) 29(2):247–54. doi:10.1093/ndt/gft437
33. Schmidt LS, Linehan WM. Genetic predisposition to kidney cancer. *Semin Oncol* (2016) 43:566–74. doi:10.1053/j.seminoncol.2016.09.001
34. Wehrman A, Kriegermeier A, Wen J. Diagnosis and management of hepatobiliary complications in autosomal recessive polycystic kidney disease. *Front Pediatr* (2017) 5:124. doi:10.3389/fped.2017.00124
35. Hildebrandt F, Zhou W. Nephronophthisis-associated ciliopathies. *J Am Soc Nephrol* (2007) 18:1855–71. doi:10.1681/ASN.2006121344

36. Salomon R, Saunier S, Niaudet P. Nephronophthisis. *Pediatr Nephrol* (2009) 24:2333–44. doi:10.1007/s00467-008-0840-z
37. Schueler M, Halbritter J, Phelps IG, Braun DA, Otto EA, Porath JD, et al. Large-scale targeted sequencing comparison highlights extreme genetic heterogeneity in nephronophthisis-related ciliopathies. *J Med Genet* (2016) 53:208–14. doi:10.1136/jmedgenet-2015-103304
38. Barash I, Ponda MP, Goldfarb DS, Skolnik EY. A pilot clinical study to evaluate changes in urine osmolality and urine cAMP in response to acute and chronic water loading in autosomal dominant polycystic kidney disease. *Clin J Am Soc Nephrol* (2010) 5:693–7. doi:10.2215/CJN.04180609
39. van Gastel MDA, Torres VE. Polycystic kidney disease and the vasopressin pathway. *Ann Nutr Metab* (2017) 70:43–50. doi:10.1159/000463063
40. Wang CJ, Creed C, Winklhofer FT, Grantham JJ. Water prescription in autosomal dominant polycystic kidney disease: a pilot study. *Clin J Am Soc Nephrol* (2011) 6:192–7. doi:10.2215/CJN.03950510
41. Wong ATY, Mannix C, Grantham JJ, Allman-Farinelli M, Badve SV, Boudville N, et al. Randomised controlled trial to determine the efficacy and safety of prescribed water intake to prevent kidney failure due to autosomal dominant polycystic kidney disease (PREVENT-ADPKD). *BMJ Open* (2018) 8:e018794. doi:10.1136/bmjopen-2017-018794
42. Schrier RW, Abebe KZ, Perrone RD, Torres VE, Braun WE, Steinman TI, et al. Blood pressure in early autosomal dominant polycystic kidney disease. *N Engl J Med* (2014) 371:2255–66. doi:10.1056/NEJMoa1402685
43. Torres VE, Abebe KZ, Chapman AB, Schrier RW, Braun WE, Steinman TI, et al. Angiotensin blockade in late autosomal dominant polycystic kidney disease. *N Engl J Med* (2014) 371:2267–76. doi:10.1056/NEJMoa1402686
44. Torres VE, Abebe KZ, Schrier RW, Perrone RD, Chapman AB, Yu AS, et al. Dietary salt restriction is beneficial to the management of autosomal dominant polycystic kidney disease. *Kidney Int* (2017) 91:493–500. doi:10.1016/j.kint.2016.10.018
45. Eckardt KU, Alper SL, Antignac C, Bleyer AJ, Chauveau D, Dahan K, et al. Autosomal dominant tubulointerstitial kidney disease: diagnosis, classification, and management – a KDIGO consensus report. *Kidney Int* (2015) 88:676–83. doi:10.1038/ki.2015.28
46. Sherstha R, McKinley C, Russ P, Scherzinger A, Bronner T, Showalter R, et al. Postmenopausal estrogen therapy selectively stimulates hepatic enlargement in women with autosomal dominant polycystic kidney disease. *Hepatology* (1997) 26:1282–6. doi:10.1053/jhep.1997.v26.pm0009362373
47. Savige J, Mallett A, Tunnicliffe DJ, Rangan GK. KHA-CARI autosomal dominant polycystic kidney disease guideline: management of polycystic liver disease. *Semin Nephrol* (2015) 35:618–22.e5. doi:10.1016/j.semnephrol.2015.10.015
48. Estruch R, Ros E, Salas-Salvadó J, Covas MI, Corella D, Arós F, et al. Primary prevention of cardiovascular disease with a mediterranean diet. *N Engl J Med* (2013) 368:1279–90. doi:10.1056/NEJMoa1200303
49. Di Iorio BR, Cupisti A, D'Alessandro C, Bellasi A, Barbera V, Di Lullo L. Nutritional therapy in autosomal dominant polycystic kidney disease. *J Nephrol* (2018). doi:10.1007/s40620-018-0470-x
50. Torres VE, Chapman AB, Devuyst O, Gansevoort RT, Grantham JJ, Higashihara E, et al. Tolvaptan in patients with autosomal dominant polycystic kidney disease. *N Engl J Med* (2012) 367:2407–18. doi:10.1056/NEJMoa1205511
51. Torres VE, Chapman AB, Devuyst O, Gansevoort RT, Perrone RD, Koch G, et al. Tolvaptan in later-stage autosomal dominant polycystic kidney disease. *N Engl J Med* (2017) 377:1930–42. doi:10.1056/NEJMoa1710030
52. *The German ADPKD Tolvaptan Treatment Registry*. ClinicalTrials.gov (2017). Available from: https://clinicaltrials.gov/ct2/show/NCT02497521 (accessed October 23, 2017)
53. Gansevoort RT, Arici M, Benzing T, Birn H, Capasso G, Covic A, et al. Recommendations for the use of tolvaptan in autosomal dominant polycystic kidney disease: a position statement on behalf of the ERA-EDTA working groups on inherited kidney disorders and European renal best practice. *Nephrol Dial Transplant* (2016) 31:337–48. doi:10.1093/ndt/gfv456
54. Harris PC, Torres VE. Polycystic kidney disease. *Annu Rev Med* (2009) 60:321–37. doi:10.1146/annurev.med.60.101707.125712
55. Shillingford JM, Murcia NS, Larson CH, Low SH, Hedgepeth R, Brown N, et al. The mTOR pathway is regulated by polycystin-1, and its inhibition reverses renal cystogenesis in polycystic kidney disease. *Proc Natl Acad Sci U S A* (2006) 103:5466–71. doi:10.1073/pnas.0509694103
56. Shillingford JM, Piontek KB, Germino GG, Weimbs T. Rapamycin ameliorates PKD resulting from conditional inactivation of Pkd1. *J Am Soc Nephrol* (2010) 21:489–97. doi:10.1681/ASN.2009040421
57. Serra AL, Poster D, Kistler AD, Krauer F, Raina S, Young J, et al. Sirolimus and kidney growth in autosomal dominant polycystic kidney disease. *N Engl J Med* (2010) 363:820–9. doi:10.1056/NEJMoa0907419
58. Walz G, Budde K, Mannaa M, Nürnberger J, Wanner C, Sommerer C, et al. Everolimus in patients with autosomal dominant polycystic kidney disease. *N Engl J Med* (2010) 363:830–40. doi:10.1056/NEJMoa1003491
59. Caroli A, Perico N, Perna A, Antiga L, Brambilla P, Pisani A, et al. Effect of longacting somatostatin analogue on kidney and cyst growth in autosomal dominant polycystic kidney disease (ALADIN): a randomised, placebo-controlled, multicentre trial. *Lancet* (2013) 382:1485–95. doi:10.1016/S0140-6736(13)61407-5
60. Cadnapaphornchai MA, George DM, McFann K, Wang W, Gitomer B, Strain JD, et al. Effect of pravastatin on total kidney volume, left ventricular mass index, and microalbuminuria in pediatric autosomal dominant polycystic kidney disease. *Clin J Am Soc Nephrol* (2014) 9:889–96. doi:10.2215/CJN.08350813
61. Brosnahan GM, Abebe KZ, Rahbari-Oskoui FF, Patterson CG, Bae KT, Schrier RW, et al. Effect of statin therapy on the progression of autosomal dominant polycystic kidney disease. A secondary analysis of the HALT PKD trials. *Curr Hypertens Rev* (2017) 13(2):109–20. doi:10.2174/1573402113666170427142815
62. Tesar V, Ciechanowski K, Pei Y, Barash I, Shannon M, Li R, et al. Bosutinib versus placebo for autosomal dominant polycystic kidney disease. *J Am Soc Nephrol* (2017) 28(11):3404–13. doi:10.1681/ASN.2016111232
63. Masyuk TV, Masyuk AI, LaRusso NF. Therapeutic targets in polycystic liver disease. *Curr Drug Targets* (2017) 18:950–7. doi:10.2174/1389450116666150427161743
64. Masyuk TV, Radtke BN, Stroope AJ, Banales JM, Masyuk AI, Gradilone SA, et al. Inhibition of Cdc25A suppresses hepato-renal cystogenesis in rodent models of polycystic kidney and liver disease. *Gastroenterology* (2012) 142:622–33.e4. doi:10.1053/j.gastro.2011.11.036
65. Magistroni R, Boletta A. Defective glycolysis and the use of 2-deoxy-D-glucose in polycystic kidney disease: from animal models to humans. *J Nephrol* (2017) 30:511–9. doi:10.1007/s40620-017-0395-9
66. Chang MY, Ma TL, Hung CC, Tian YC, Chen YC, Yang CW, et al. Metformin inhibits cyst formation in a zebrafish model of polycystin-2 deficiency. *Sci Rep* (2017) 7:7161. doi:10.1038/s41598-017-07300-x
67. Zhou X, Fan LX, Sweeney WE Jr, Denu JM, Avner ED, Li X. Sirtuin 1 inhibition delays cyst formation in autosomal-dominant polycystic kidney disease. *J Clin Invest* (2013) 123:3084–98. doi:10.1172/JCI64401
68. Hopp K, Hommerding CJ, Wang X, Ye H, Harris PC, Torres VE. Tolvaptan plus pasireotide shows enhanced efficacy in a PKD1 model. *J Am Soc Nephrol* (2015) 26:39–47. doi:10.1681/ASN.2013121312
69. Zhu P, Sieben CJ, Xu X, Harris PC, Lin X. Autophagy activators suppress cystogenesis in an autosomal dominant polycystic kidney disease model. *Hum Mol Genet* (2017) 26:158–72. doi:10.1093/hmg/ddw376

5

The Genetic and Cellular Basis of Autosomal Dominant Polycystic Kidney Disease—A Primer for Clinicians

Adrián Cordido[†], Lara Besada-Cerecedo[†] and Miguel A. García-González[*]

Grupo de Genética y Biología del Desarrollo de las Enfermedades Renales, Laboratorio de Nefrología (n.° 11), Instituto de Investigación Sanitaria (IDIS), Complexo Hospitalario de Santiago de Compostela (CHUS), Santiago de Compostela, Spain

Correspondence:
Miguel A. García-González
miguel.garcia.gonzalez@sergas.es

Autosomal dominant polycystic kidney disease (ADPKD) is one of the most common genetic disorders worldwide. In recent decades, the field has undergone a revolution, starting with the identification of causal ADPKD genes, including *PKD1*, *PKD2*, and the recently identified *GANAB*. In addition, advances defining the genetic mechanisms, protein localization and function, and the identification of numerous pathways involved in the disease process, have contributed to a better understanding of this illness. Together, this has led to a better prognosis, diagnosis, and treatment in clinical practice. In this mini review, we summarize and discuss new insights about the molecular mechanisms underlying ADPKD, including its genetics, protein function, and cellular pathways.

Keywords: autosomal dominant polycystic kidney disease, genetics, molecular biology, diagnosis, therapy

INTRODUCTION

Polycystic kidney disease (PKD) is a heterogeneous group of monogenic disorders characterized by the bilateral formation and progressive expansion of renal cyst that lead to end stage renal disease (ESRD) (1). Several Mendelian diseases including autosomal dominant polycystic kidney disease (ADPKD), autosomal recessive polycystic kidney disease (ARPKD), and atypical forms of PKD can be grouped under this pathological entity.

Autosomal dominant polycystic kidney disease is the most common inherited kidney disease affecting ~1/400–1/1,000 individuals (2). The hallmark characteristic of ADPKD is the progressive development and expansion of cysts in the kidney leading to ESRD. It can be associated with several extrarenal manifestations including hypertension, symptomatic extrarenal cysts, and subarachnoid hemorrhage from intracranial aneurysms (3–5). The vast majority of the patients develop the disease between the ages of 20–40 s, but there have been sporadic cases that range in onset from late to childhood ("early onset," before 15 years old) or even *in utero* ("very early onset") (6).

GENETICS OF THE ADPKD

Autosomal dominant polycystic kidney disease is genetically heterogeneous and associated with mutations in *PKD1* (responsible of ADPKD-Type I), *PKD2* (-Type II), and *GANAB*. *PKD1* is a complex gene mapping to chromosome 16 (16p13.3) (**Figure 1A**). Its genomic structure has a number of features that complicate its evaluation (7, 8): (a) it is highly GC-rich with a large number of

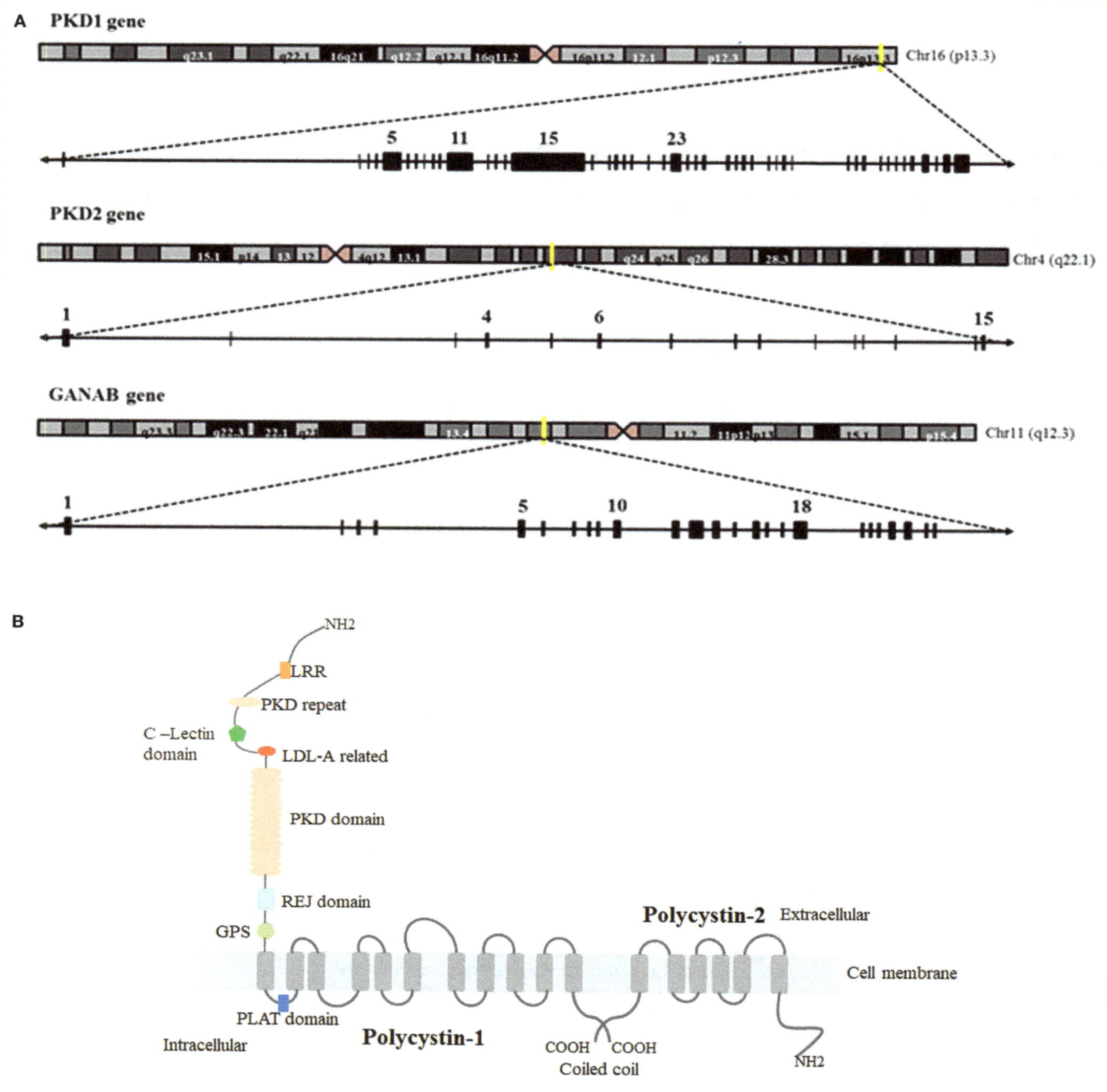

FIGURE 1 | Chromosome localization and genomic structure of *PKD1*, *PKD2*, and *GANAβ* genes and structure of polycystin-1 (PC1) and polycystin-2 (PC2). **(A)** Schematic representation of chromosomes and genomic structure for the genes. **(B)** Representation of *PKD1* and *PKD2* protein products: PC1 and PC2. *GIIα (encoded by GANAβ) is not included because the tertiary structure of the protein is not available in the bibliography or protein date bases.

CpG dinucleotides, (b) 70% of *PKD1* is duplicated multiple times throughout chromosome 16 with high sequence fidelity (95% identity) (9), and (c) it contains a 2.5 kb polypyrimidine tract in intron 21 (the largest in the human genome) (10). In contrast to *PKD1*, the *PKD2* gene is located on chromosome 4 (4q21) and has simpler features and structure (11) (**Figure 1A**). Approximately, 80–85% of ADPKD families were associated with *PKD1* mutations, and 15–20% to *PKD2* mutations in the literature (12). Recently, Porath and colleagues identified causal mutations in *GANAB*, a gene on chromosome 11q12.3 (**Figure 1A**), in ADPKD patients that are negative for *PKD1* and *PKD2* mutations. They report that *GANAB* accounts for ~0.3% of total ADPKD and it is associated with a milder manifestation of PKD and autosomal dominant polycystic liver disease (ADPLD) (5).

DIAGNOSIS OF ADPKD

The diagnosis of ADPKD is dependent on the stage of the disease. When the disease is fully established, the diagnosis is clinically based on patient's history and physical examination (13, 14). However, definitive diagnosis can be difficult due to other disorders having overlapping symptoms. Therefore, complementary approaches such as diagnostic imaging or genetic tests are necessary to confirm the diagnosis. Imaging techniques, including ultrasound, computed axial tomography, or nuclear magnetic resonance, allow for the detection of cysts in the kidney, liver, or pancreas (15). The magnetic resonance technique has proven to be more sensitive than ultrasound, allowing measurements of height-adjusted total kidney volume (htTKV) and better definition of the cysts without the use of contrast agents. However, these imaging tests are expensive (16) and are often not performed on a subset of the ADPKD population including those who are young individuals at risk or patients with atypical or *de novo* renal cystic disease (13) for whom complementary genetic tests is the method for definitive diagnosis. Direct DNA sequencing (DS) could offer a molecular diagnosis; however, the genetic analysis of the *PKD1* (responsible for most ADPKD cases) is complicated. The 5′-region of the gene (exon 1–34) is replicated in at least six highly homologous copies on chromosome 16 (7, 9, 17). To date, direct sequencing based on a Long-Rage PCR strategy with specific primers has been the accepted strategy by the ADPKD community (18). Isolated gene by gene sequencing is laborious and expensive, and provides limited amount of information to provide a better diagnosis and prognosis for the patients. Moreover, it has been described that the main mutation responsible of the disease may interact with other PKD or ciliopathy loci modifying the phenotype and extending the genetic complexity of the disease (18–20). For this reason, ADPKD experts are highlighting the necessity to screen all cystic genes in a common strategy to allow for a more accurate diagnosis, including those genes responsible of atypical forms of PKD. Under this context, next-generation sequencing strategies followed by the validation of variants by DS have become the recommended methodology allowing for faster, more cost-effective, and more reliable genetic diagnosis of large ADPKD cohorts (21).

GENOTYPE–PHENOTYPE CORRELATIONS

It has been described that patients with mutations in *PKD1* gene have larger kidneys and earlier onset (mean age at ESRD, 53.4 versus 72.7 years old, respectively) with lower eGFR and higher htTKV than *PKD2* patients (22, 23). In addition, *GANAB* mutations seem to be associated with a mild renal phenotype, closer to a *PKD2* than a *PKD1* phenotype, revealing the importance of molecular diagnosis (5). Moreover, a strong correlation between the type of the mutation and the severity of the disease was observed, illustrating the importance of quantifying genetic heterogeneity in ADPKD. Truncating *PKD1* mutations (frameshift, splicing, and nonsense) have a more severe disease prognosis with lower eGFR; however. the type of mutation does not correlate with htTKV (23, 24). Non-truncating *PKD1* mutations (missense, inframe deletion/insertion) or mutations in *PKD2* are associated with a milder form of the disease. In addition, males with truncating *PKD1* are associated with larger kidneys and increased risk for ESRD, while women with truncating *PKD1* have a more severe liver phenotype (23, 24). In addition, disease manifestation in ADPKD patients from the same family, or patients with the same mutation, can have varying severity and differential disease progression, which may be due to the presence of variation in a modifying gene. This phenomenon is known as genetic interaction and epistasis, and usually aggravates or attenuates the phenotype cause by the primary mutation (17, 25).

Based on genetic and clinical data, Cornec-Le Gall and colleagues (26) developed a robust prognostic model, the PROPKD score (with a range from 0 to 9), to predict survival in ADPKD patients. They described critical variables associated with ESRD including age of onset (median age reported to be 70.6 years for low risk, 56.9 years for intermediate risk, and 49 years for high risk) and a scoring system to predict disease progression: sex (being male 1 point), need for antihypertensive therapy before 35 years old (2 points), occurrence of the first urologic event before 35 years old (2 points), and genetic status (having PKD2 mutations: 0 points, non-truncating PKD1 mutation: 2 points and truncating PKD1 mutations: 4 points). Three risk categories were then defined to describe the putative risk for progression to ESRD: low risk (0–3 points), intermediate risk (4–6 points), and high risk (7–9 points) (26).

PKD PROTEINS: STRUCTURE AND FUNCTION

PKD1 and *PKD2* encode the proteins PC1/Polycystin-1 and PC2/Polycystin-2 or TRPP2, respectively. PC1 is a putative receptor for an unidentified ligand which contains a long extracellular N-terminal domain, 11 transmembrane domains and a short intracellular C-terminal domain (27). PC2/TRPP2 has similar characteristics to TRP channel, having six transmembrane segments, a pore loop domain (separating the first two transmembrane segments), and an N- and C-terminal domains (28) (**Figure 1B**). PC2 is a Ca^{2+}-permeable non-selective ion cation channel and together with PC1 forms a receptor–channel complex implicated in the Ca^{2+} pathway called PC complex (29).

In contrast to *PKD1* and *PKD2*, *GANAB* encodes the alpha subunit of glucosidase II (GIIα) which is the catalytic subunit of GII. GIIα together with the regulatory subunit of GII, GIIβ (also called hepatocystin) (5) form a functional holoenzyme in the endoplasmic reticulum (ER). This holoenzyme is implicated in the proper folding and translocation of glycoproteins into the ER, and its dysfunction has been reported to be associated with maturation and localization defects of PC1 (30).

DISEASE MECHANISM

Two-Hit Model for ADPKD

The human kidney has approximately one million nephrons, and an ADPKD patient will develop around a 1,000 cysts (31). ADPKD disease progression is highly variable and depends directly from the nature of the mutated gene. The "Two-Hit Model," in which two different mutations affect proper genetic/cellular interactions, has been the proposed theory to explain the kidney phenotype observed in ADPKD patients. While an individual has inherited a germ line mutation ("first hit"), the development of cysts does not occur until another mutation (somatic mutations) in either *PKD1* or *PKD2* occurs ("second hit") (32, 33).

Localization of PKD Proteins: The Role of Primary Cilia

There have been a number of different localizations proposed for the PC1/PC2, including the ER, apical and basolateral cell membranes, or secreted exosomes (31). However, there is evidence supporting their presence in primary cilia based on their central role in ADPKD pathogenesis. Cilia are microtubule-based, non-motile organelles on the apical surface of the cells and play an essential role in cellular detection and regulation of external signals. Dysfunction of this organelle result in a group of disorders called the ciliopathies (34). Data from animal models (*C. elegans*, *Drosophila*, and *Mus musculus*) support the idea that defects in function or structure of primary cilia contribute to the pathomechanisms of PKD (35). PKD proteins such as PC1, PC2, and polyductin/FPC (encoded from the ARPKD gene, *PKHD1*) localized to the primary cilium (36–38). These PKD proteins interact with each other (17, 29, 36, 39, 40) and form a functional complex with common downstream signaling pathways (41). In addition, deleted in azoospermia interacting protein 1-like, the protein encoded from the recently identified ARPKD gene (*DZIP1L*), was reported to localize to the centrioles and basal bodies of cilia and are also associated with ciliary trafficking defects (19).

There has also been additional evidence to support the functional role of PKD proteins within the cilium. Urine flow has been linked to an increase in intracellular calcium (42), likely driven by the mechanical response of the primary cilium (43). The large extracellular domain of PC1 has been proposed to be the flow mechanosensor that opens the PC2-channel, allowing calcium entry leading to mechanotransduction activation (44). A different model proposes that the primary cilia's role in flow sensing is required for proper centrosomal localization that results in oriented cell division (OCD). In addition, defects in cilia drive the loss of planar cell polarity and consequently abnormal OCD (45); however, this model is controversial and remains unclear (46, 47). Several observations support the idea of the mechanosensory role of polycystins in the primary cilium (48, 49). PC2 directly interacts with KIF3A and KIF3B, two essential proteins for ciliary assembly and function (37, 50). In addition, PC2 is required for the flow-mediated increase of cytosolic Ca^{2+} (51, 52), and mechanical stimuli can induce proteolytic cleavage of the intracellular C-terminal domain of PC1 (53). Interestingly, there have been controversial results reporting that mechanosensation does not occur *via* Ca^{2+} signaling within cilia (54). In spite of this, there are some unanswered questions as while Delling and colleagues do not exclude the presence of others mechanosensitive elements in primary cilia (55) and the cilia seems to increase cytoplasmic Ca^{2+} concentration by diffusion (56).

A very interesting and unexpected finding by Ma and colleagues showed that loss of cilia results in a significant reduction of PKD severity (57). Authors reported that a simultaneous inactivation of polycystins and cilia assembly resulted in the reduction of the cystic phenotype associated with polycystins inactivation. These findings suggest that the polycystins modulate a pathway involved in the cilia signaling, but require intact cilia function (58).

Threshold or Dosage Model

Genetic background influences the phenotypic variability of ADPKD. As we previously mentioned, patients with mutations in *PKD1* have worse prognosis than those with mutations in *PKD2* (59), and those with truncating *PKD1* mutations were associated with more severe polycystic renal pathology than those with non-truncating mutations (60). In addition, unaffected patients who carry a missense variant in *PKD1* indicate that some alleles are incompletely dominant in the disease (61). Similarly, other studies suggest that incomplete, penetrant alleles can influences disease severity in ADPKD (62).

These data support that a threshold or dosage model could explain cystogenesis in ADPKD (63). According to this model, cyst initiation and cystic expansion depends on PKD gene dosage, starting when the level of functional PC falls below the cystogenic threshold (58, 63). Defects in that threshold may occur by a combination of one or more factors: the nature of germline mutation ("first-hit"), somatic mutations ("second hit"), modifier genes or environmental factors such as renal injury or inflammation (58, 64). Several studies support this: (1) García-González and colleagues reported genetic interaction between ADPKD and ARPKD genes in a common pathway (17), (2) it has been reported that ADPLD genes (*Prkcsh* and *Sec63*), ARPKD gene (*Pkhd1*) and ADPKD gene (*Pkd1*) interact with each other suggesting a central role of PC1 in cystogenesis (65), and (3) a developmental window for cystogenesis has been identified, suggesting that timing of secondary events may influence the severity of ADPKD (66).

A crucial step in the protein maturation of functional PCs is also related to the *dosage model*. Autoproteolytic cleavage of PC1 at the GPS domain, mediated by larger GAIN [G protein-coupled receptor (GPCR)-autoproteolysis inducing] domain which includes a GPCR proteolysis site (GPF) motif, is crucial for PC1 maturation (67, 68). Besse and colleagues have described that specific isolated-PLD proteins (encoded by SEC61β, ALG8, and GANAβ), from the ER protein biogenesis pathway, are directly related to PC1 biogenesis (30). Furthermore, PC1 maturation requires PC2 in a dose-dependent manner (69). It is also known that mature PC assembles at the PC complex-bearing vesicles in the Golgi before trafficking to the ciliary/plasmatic membrane (70) (**Figure 2**). In addition, Cai and colleagues described the effect of several mutations in *Pkd1* and *Pkd2* in the importance of PCs trafficking to cilia using *in vitro* and *in vivo* models, concluding that altered trafficking and dysfunctional maturation of PC complex underlie PKD pathology (71) These facts suggest a central role for PC1 in the cystogenesis process and in regulating the severity of ADPKD, ARPKD, and ADPLD (72).

Signaling Pathways and Targeted Therapies in ADPKD

Several signaling pathways and transcription factors control the progression and development of cystogenesis (64, 73). Calcium signaling is one of the most studied pathways in the PKD field.

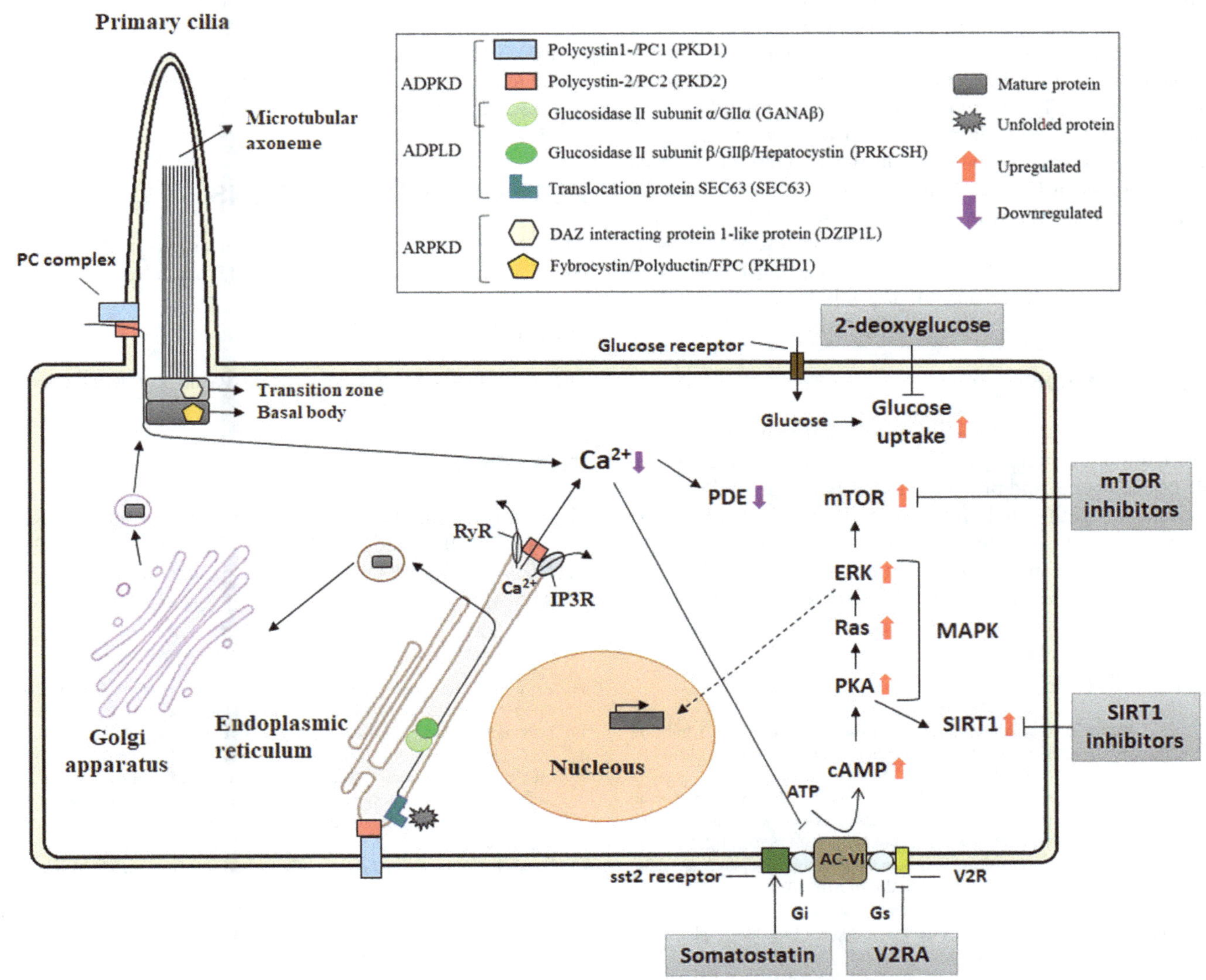

FIGURE 2 | Diagram of the localization of the polycystic kidney disease (PKD) proteins, the pathways implicated in its pathogenesis, and putative therapeutic targets. The polycystin-1 (PC1) and polycystin-2 (PC2), associated with autosomal dominant polycystic kidney disease (ADPKD), and FPC and DIZP1L, associated with autosomal recessive polycystic kidney disease (ARPKD), are ciliary proteins and have functions in relation with the primary cilia. GANAβ [associated with ADPKD and autosomal dominant polycystic liver disease (ADPLD)], together with the classical genes of the ADPLD, PRKCSH, and Sec63, is localized in the endoplasmic reticulum (ER) and plays a role in the translocation and folding of the protein maturation. PC1 and PC2 form a receptor–channel complex in the cilium and is implicated in the Ca^{2+} pathway. PC2 also regulates intracellular calcium in the ER. PC mutations result in deregulation of Ca^{2+} leading an increase in cAMP and upregulation of the PKA and MAPK pathways. Abbreviations: RyR, ryanodine receptor; IP3R, IP3 receptor; PDE, phosphodiesterase; AC-VI, adenylyl cyclase 6; Gs and Gi, guanosine nucleotide-binding proteins; V2R, V2 receptor; cAMP, cyclic AMP; PKA, protein kinase A; MAPK, MAP kinases; SIRT1, sirtuin 1.

PC2 is a calcium permeable non-selective cation channel that is abundantly expressed in the ER and interacts with others calcium channel proteins (51). It binds to the inositol 1,4,5-trisphosphate receptor (IP_3R) regulating Ca^{2+} homeostasis and the activity of ryanodine receptors (74, 75). In contrast to PC2, PC1 accelerates the decay of the intracellular calcium response to ATP by increasing ER calcium uptake. All of this suggests a major role of polycystins in intracellular calcium hometostasis (76, 77). Cystic epithelial cells have an aberrant cross talk between intracellular calcium and cAMP signaling as elevated levels of cAMP stimulate cyst fluid secretion, enhancing protein kinase A activity (78–80). Furthermore, V2 receptor antagonists (Tolvaptan) ameliorate the progression of PKD by the inhibition of cAMP signaling pathway in both animal models (81, 82) and in clinical trials (83) (**Figure 2**). Importantly, adverse secondary effects could appear with Tolvaptan treatment such as polyuria, nocturia, and elevation of liver enzymes (84). Taking this into account, Tolvaptan is the first therapy approved for indication of ADPKD in several countries.

Alterations to other pathways have been reported to affect cystic volume or cystic progression, but to date; attempts to completely inhibit cystogenesis have been unsuccessful. The mTOR pathway is highly activated in cystic tissues independent of the PKD gene mutation (85). Preclinical trials with sirolimus and everolimus blocked cystic progression in a rodent model of ADPKD (86, 87). In addition, somatostatin analogs, as octreotide and lanreotide reduced hepatic and renal volume expansion in ADPKD (88–90). Treatment of PKD animal models, which have defective glucose metabolism associated with cystic expansion, with 2-deoxyglucose, an analog of glucose, also result in reduced cystic progression (91, 92) (**Figure 2**). Adding to the hunt for therapeutics, other alternate mechanisms also exist, such as sirtuin 1, microRNAs, and MCP1 which have been postulated as possible therapies for PKD (93–95) and recently, ongoing Phase-II and Phase-I clinical trials of a multi-kinase inhibitor, tesevatinib, are ongoing for ADPKD and children with ARPKD (96, 97).

CONCLUSION

In the last two decades, there have been significant contributions toward our understanding of the genetic, cellular, and functional role of PKD genes and proteins, as well as, the identification of a number of pathways implicated in the pathogenesis of the disease. Nevertheless, several questions remain unresolved and controversial in the PKD community. The complexity of this disease is reflected along all scientific levels, starting at the genetic level with critical refinement of the mutations, followed by the study of protein function and dosage to understand the spectrum of clinical manifestations in PKD, and finally the study of related pathways and modifier mechanisms that all should be taken into account for future clinical trials and personalized medicine.

AUTHOR CONTRIBUTIONS

All authors listed have made a substantial, direct, and intellectual contribution to the work and approved it for publication.

ACKNOWLEDGMENTS

The authors would like to thank María Pardo and Perciliz Tan for their comments.

FUNDING

This work was supported by grants from the Instituto de Salud Carlos III FEDER funds ISCIII RETIC REDINREN RD12/0016, PI11/00690, PI15/001467, Sociedad Española de Nefrología, and Xunta de Galicia.

REFERENCES

1. Lee K, Battini L, Gusella GL. Cilium, centrosome and cell cycle regulation in polycystic kidney disease. *Biochim Biophys Acta* (2001) 1812(10):1263–71. doi:10.1016/j.bbadis.2011.02.008
2. Reiterová J, Štekrová J, Merta M, Kotlas J, Elišáková V, Lněnička P, et al. Autosomal dominant polycystic kidney disease in a family with mosaicism and hypomorphic allele. *BMC Nephrol* (2013) 14:59. doi:10.1186/1471-2369-14-59
3. Torres VE, Harris PC, Pearson Y. Autosomal dominant polycystic kidney disease. *Lancet* (2007) 369(9569):1287–301. doi:10.1016/S0140-6736(07)60601-1
4. Harris PC, Rossetti S. Molecular diagnostics for autosomal dominant polycystic kidney disease. *Nat Rev Nephrol* (2010) 6(4):197–206. doi:10.1038/nrneph.2010.18
5. Porath B, Gainullon VG, Cornec-Le Gall E, Dillinger EK, Heyer CM, Hopp K, et al. Mutations in *GANAB*, encoding glucosidase IIα subunit, cause autosomal dominant polycystic kidney disease and liver disease. *Am J Hum Genet* (2016) 98(6):1193–207. doi:10.1016/j.ajhg.2016.05.004
6. Loftus H, Ong AC. Cystic kidney diseases: many ways to form a cyst. *Pediatr Nephrol* (2013) 28(1):33–49. doi:10.1007/s00467-012-2221-x
7. Hughes J, Ward CJ, Peral B, Aspinwall R, Clark K, San Millán JL, et al. The polycystic kidney disease 1 (*PKD1*) gene encodes a novel protein with multiple cell recognition domains. *Nat Genet* (1995) 10(2):151–60. doi:10.1038/ng0695-151
8. Burn TC, Connors TD, Dackowski WR, Petry LR, Van Raay TJ, Millholland JM, et al. Analysis of the genomic sequence for the autosomal dominant polycystic kidney disease (PKD1) gene predicts the presence of a leucine-rich repeat. *Hum Mol Genet* (1995) 4(4):575–82. doi:10.1093/hmg/4.4.575
9. Bogdanova N, Markoff A, Gerke V, McCluskey M, Horst J, Dworniczak B. Homologues to the first gene for autosomal dominant polycystic kidney disease are pseudogenes. *Genomics* (2001) 74(3):333–41. doi:10.1006/geno.2001.6568
10. Van Raay TJ, Burn TC, Connors TD, Petry LR, Germino GG, Klinger KW, et al. A 2.5kb polypyrimidine tract in the PKD1 gene contains at least 23 H-DNA-forming sequences. *Microb Comp Genomics* (1996) 1(4):317–27. doi:10.1089/mcg.1996.1.317
11. Harris PC, Torres VE. Polycysic kidney disease. *Annu Rev Med* (2009) 60:321–37. doi:10.1146/annurev.med.60.101707.125712
12. Cornec-Le Gall E, Audrézet MP, Renaudineau E, Hourmant M, Charasse C, Michez E, et al. *PKD2*-related autosomal dominant polycystic kidney disease: prevalence, clinical presentation, mutation spectrum and prognosis. *Am J Kidney Dis* (2017) 6386(17):30537–30531. doi:10.1053/j.ajkd.2017.01.046
13. Pei Y. Diagnostic approach in autosomal dominant polycystic kidney disease. *Clin J Am Soc Nephrol* (2006) 1(5):1108–14. doi:10.2215/CJN.02190606
14. Igarashi P, Somlo S. Genetics and pathogenesis of polycystic kidney disease. *J Am Soc Nephrol* (2002) 13(9):2384–98. doi:10.1097/01.ASN.0000028643.17901.42
15. Mosetti MA, Leonardou P, Motohara T, Kanematsu M, Armao D, Semelka RC. Autosomal dominant polycystic kidney disease: MR imaging evaluation using current techniques. *J Magn Reson Imaging* (2003) 18(2):210–5. doi:10.1002/jmri.10347
16. Irazabal MV, Rangel LJ, Bergstralh EJ, Osborn SL, Harmon AJ, Sundsbak JL, et al. Imaging classification of autosomal dominant polycystic kidney disease: a simple model for selecting patients for clinical trials. *J Am Soc Nephrol* (2015) 26(1):160–72. doi:10.1681/ASN.2013101138
17. Garcia-Gonzalez M, Menezes L, Piontek K, Kaimori J, Huso D, Watnick T, et al. Genetic interaction studies link autosomal dominant and recessive polycystic kidney disease in a common pathway. *Hum Mol Genet* (2007) 16(16):1940–50. doi:10.1093/hmg/ddm141
18. Garcia-Gonzalez MA, Jones JG, Allen SK, Palatucci CM, Batish SD, Seltzer WK, et al. Evaluating the clinical utility of a molecular genetic test for polycystic kidney disease. *Mol Genet Metab* (2007) 92(1–2):160–7. doi:10.1016/j.ymgme.2007.05.004
19. Lu H, Rondón-Galeano M, Ott E, Kaeslin G, Kausalya P, Kramer C, et al. Mutations in DZIP1L, which encodes a ciliary-transition-zone protein, cause autosomal recessive polycystic kidney disease. *Nat Genet* (2017) 49(7):1025–34. doi:10.1038/ng.3871
20. Hartung E, Guay-Woodford L. DZIP1L defines a new functional zip code for autosomal recessive PKD. *Nat Rev Nephrol* (2017) 13(9):519–20. doi:10.1038/nrneph.2017.102
21. Renkema KY, Stokman MF, Giles RH, Knoers NV. Next-generation sequencing for research and diagnostics in kidney disease. *Nat Rev Nephrol* (2014) 10(8):433–44. doi:10.1038/nrneph.2014.95
22. Harris PC, Bae KT, Rossetti S, Torres VE, Grantham JJ, Chapman AB, et al. Cyst number but not the rate of cystic growth is associated with the mutated gene in autosomal dominant polycystic kidney disease. *J Am Soc Nephrol* (2006) 17(11):3013–9. doi:10.1681/ASN.2006080835
23. Heyer CM, Sundsbak JL, Abebe KZ, Chapman AB, Torres VE, Grantham JJ, et al. Predicted mutation strength of nontruncating PKD1 mutations aids genotype-phenotype correlations in autosomal dominant polycystic kidney disease. *J Am Soc Nephrol* (2016) 27(9):2872–84. doi:10.1681/ASN.2015050583

24. Hwang YH, Conklin J, Chan W, Roslin NM, Liu J, He N, et al. Refining genotype-phenotype correlation in autosomal dominant polycystic kidney disease. *J Am Soc Nephrol* (2016) 27(6):1861–8. doi:10.1681/ASN.2015060648
25. Bergmann C, von Bothmer J, Ortiz Brüchle N, Venghaus A, Frank V, Fehrenbach H, et al. Mutations in multiple PKD genes may explain early and severe polycystic kidney disease. *J Am Soc Nephrol* (2011) 22(11):2047–56. doi:10.1681/ASN.2010101080
26. Cornec-Le Gall E, Audrézet MP, Rousseau A, Hourmant M, Renaudineau E, Charasse C, et al. The PROPKD Score: a new algorithm to predict renal survival in autosomal dominant polycystic kidney disease. *J Am Soc Nephrol* (2016) 27(3):942–51. doi:10.1681/ASN.2015010016
27. Wilson P. Polycystic kidney disease. *N Engl J Med* (2004) 350(2):151–64. doi:10.1056/NEJMra022161
28. Hofherr A, Köttgen M. TRPP channels and polycystins. *Adv Exp Med Biol* (2011) 704:287–313. doi:10.1007/978-94-007-0265-3_16
29. Hanaok K, Qian F, Boletta A, Bhunia A, Piontek K, Tsiokas L, et al. Co-assembly of polycystin-1 and -2 produces unique cation-permeable current. *Nature* (2000) 408(6815):990–4. doi:10.1038/35050128
30. Besse W, Dong K, Choi J, Punia S, Fedeles SV, Choi M, et al. Isolated polycystic liver disease genes define effectors of polycystin-1 function. *J Clin Invest* (2017) 127(9):3558–3558. doi:10.1172/JCI96729
31. Grantham J. Clinical practice: autosomal dominant polycystic kidney disease. *N Engl J Med* (2008) 359(14):1477–85. doi:10.1056/NEJMcp0804458
32. Qian F, Watnick T, Onuchic L, Germino G. The molecular basis of focal cyst formation in human autosomal dominant polycystic kidney disease type I. *Cell* (1996) 87(6):979–87. doi:10.1016/S0092-8674(00)81793-6
33. Watnick T, Torres VE, Gandolph MA, Qian F, Onuchic LF, Klinger KW, et al. Somatic mutation in individual liver cysts supports a two-hit model of cystogenesis in autosomal dominant polycystic kidney disease. *Mol Cell* (1998) 2(2):247–51. doi:10.1016/S1097-2765(00)80135-5
34. Hildebrandt F, Benzing T, Katsanis N. Ciliopathies. *N Engl J Med* (2011) 364(16):1533–43. doi:10.1056/NEJMra1010172
35. Gerdes J, Davis E, Katsanis N. The vertebrate primary cilium in development, homeostasis and disease. *Cell* (2009) 137(1):32–45. doi:10.1016/j.cell.2009.03.023
36. Yorder B, Hou X, Guay-Woodford L. The polycystic kidney disease proteins, polycystin-1, polycystin-2, polaris, and cystin, are co-localized in renal cilia. *J Am Soc Nephrol* (2002) 13(10):2508–16. doi:10.1097/01.ASN.0000029587.47950.25
37. Wu Y, Dai X, Li Q, Chen C, Mai W, Hussain Z, et al. Kinesin-2 mediates physical and functional interactions between polycystin-2 and fibrocystin. *Hum Mol Genet* (2006) 15(22):3280–92. doi:10.1093/hmg/ddl404
38. Watnick T, Germino G. From cilia to cyst. *Nat Genet* (2003) 34(4):355–6. doi:10.1038/ng0803-355
39. Wang S, Zhang J, Nauli S, Li X, Starremans P, Luo Y, et al. Fibrocystin/polyductin, found in the same protein complex with polycystin-2, regulates calcium responses in kidney epithelia. *Mol Cell Biol* (2007) 27(8):3241–52. doi:10.1128/MCB.00072-07
40. Kim I, Fu Y, Hui K, Moeckel G, Mai W, Li C, et al. Fibrocystin/polyductin modulates renal tubular formation by regulating polycystin-2 expression and function. *J Am Soc Nephrol* (2008) 19(3):455–68. doi:10.1681/ASN.2007070770
41. Kaimori J, Germino G. ARPKD and ADPKD: first cousins or more distant relatives? *J Am Soc Nephrol* (2008) 19(3):416–23. doi:10.1681/ASN.2008010033
42. Praetorius H, Frokiaer J, Nielsen S, Spring K. Bending the primary cilium opens Ca2+-sensitive intermediate-conductance K+ channels in MDCK cells. *J Membr Biol* (2003) 191(3):193–200. doi:10.1007/s00232-002-1055-z
43. Goetz S, Anderson K. The primary cilium: a signalling centre during vertebrate development. *Nat Rev Gen* (2010) 11(5):331–44. doi:10.1038/nrg2774
44. Nauli S, Alenghat F, Luo Y, Williams E, Vassilev P, Li X, et al. Polycystins 1 and 2 mediate mechanosensation in the primary cilium of kidney cells. *Nat Genet* (2003) 33(2):129–37. doi:10.1038/ng1076
45. Fischer E, Legue E, Doyen A, Nato F, Nicolas J, Torres V, et al. Defective planar cell polarity in polycystic kidney disease. *Nat Genet* (2006) 38(1):21–3. doi:10.1038/ng1701
46. Nishio S, Tian X, Gallagher AR, Yu Z, Patel V, Igarashi P, et al. Loss of oriented cell division does not initiate cyst formation. *J Am Soc Nephrol* (2010) 21(2):295–302. doi:10.1681/ASN.2009060603
47. Kunimoto K, Bayly RD, Vladar EK, Vonderfecht T, Gallagher AR, Axelrod JD. Disruption of core planar cell polarity signaling regulates renal tubule morphogenesis but is not cystogenic. *Curr Biol* (2017) 27(20):3120–31. doi:10.1016/j.cub.2017.09.011
48. Retailleau K, Duprat F. Polycystins and partners: proposed role in mechanosensitivity. *J Physiol* (2014) 592(12):2453–71. doi:10.1113/jphysiol.2014.271346
49. Ma M, Gallagher A, Somlo S. Ciliary mechanisms of cyst formation in polycystic kidney disease. *Cold Spring Harb Perspect Biol* (2017) 9:a028209. doi:10.1101/cshperspect.a028209
50. Li Q, Montalbetti N, Wu Y, Ramos A, Raychowdhurry M, Cheng X, et al. Polycystin-2 cation channel function is under the control of microtubular structures in primary cilia of renal epithelial cells. *J Biol Cem* (2006) 281(49):37566–75. doi:10.1074/jbc.M603643200
51. Köttgen M, Buchholz B, Garcia-Gonzalez MA, Kotsis F, Fu X, Doerken M, et al. TRPP2 and TRPV4 form a polymodal sensory channel complex. *J Cell Biol* (2008) 182(3):437–47. doi:10.1083/jcb.200805124
52. Boehlke C, Kotsis F, Patel V, Braeg S, Voelker H, Beyer T, et al. Primary cilia regulate mTORC1 activity and cell size through Lkb1. *Nat Cell Biol* (2010) 12(11):1115–22. doi:10.1038/ncb2117
53. Chauvet V, Tian X, Husson H, Grimm D, Wang T, Hiesberger T, et al. Mechanical stimuli induce cleavage and nuclear translocation of the polycystin-1 C terminus. *J Clin Invest* (2004) 114(10):1433–43. doi:10.1172/JCI21753
54. Delling M, Indzhykulian A, Liu X, Li Y, Xie T, Corey D, et al. Primary cilia are not calcium-responsive mechanosensors. *Nature* (2016) 531(7596):656–60. doi:10.1038/nature17426
55. Hofherr A, Köttgen M. Polycystic kidney disease: cilia and mechanosensation revisited. *Nat Rev Nephrol* (2016) 12(6):318–9. doi:10.1038/nrneph.2016.61
56. Delling M, DeCaen P, Doerner J, Febvay S, Clapham D. Primary cilia are specialized calcium signalling organelles. *Nature* (2013) 504(7479):311–4. doi:10.1038/nature12833
57. Ma M, Tian X, Igarashi P, Pazour GJ, Somlo S. Loss cilia suppresses cyst growth in genetic models of autosomal polycystic kidney disease. *Nat Genet* (2013) 45(9):1004–12. doi:10.1038/ng.2715
58. Antignac C, Calvet JP, Germino GG, Grantham JJ, Guay-Woodford LM, Harris PC, et al. The future of polycystic kidney disease research – as seen by the 12 Kaplan awardees. *J Am Soc Nephrol* (2015) 26(9):2081–95. doi:10.1681/ASN.2014121192
59. Harris PC, Hopp K. The mutation, a key determinant of phenotype in ADPKD. *J Am Soc Nephrol* (2013) 24(6):868–70. doi:10.1681/ASN.2013040417
60. Cornec-Le Gall E, Audrézet MP, Chen JM, Hourmant M, Morin MP, Perrichot R, et al. Type of PKD1 mutation influences renal outcome in ADPKD. *J Am Soc Nephrol* (2013) 24(6):1006–13. doi:10.1681/ASN.2012070650
61. Rossetti S, Kubly VJ, Consugar MB, Hopp K, Roy S, Horsley SW, et al. Incompletely penetrant PKD1 alleles suggest a role for gene dosage in cyst initiation in polycystic kidney disease. *Kidney Int* (2009) 75(8):848–55. doi:10.1038/ki.2008.686
62. Hopp K, Ward CJ, Hommerding CJ, Nasr SH, Tuan HF, Gainullin VG, et al. Functional polycystin-1 dosage governs autosomal dominant polycystic kidney disease severity. *J Clin Invest* (2012) 122(11):4257–73. doi:10.1172/JCI64313
63. Ong AC, Harris PC. A polycystin-centric view of cyst formation and disease: the polycystins revisited. *Kidney Int* (2015) 88(4):699–710. doi:10.1038/ki.2015.207
64. Harris PC, Torres VE. Genetic mechanisms and signaling pathways in autosomal dominant polycystic kidney disease. *J Clin Invest* (2014) 124(6):2315–24. doi:10.1172/JCI72272
65. Fedeles SV, Tian X, Gallagher AR, Mitobe M, Nishio S, Lee SH, et al. A genetic interaction network of five genes for human polycystic kidney and liver diseases defines polycystin-1 as the central determinant of cyst formation. *Nat Genet* (2011) 43(7):639–47. doi:10.1038/ng.860
66. Piontek K, Menezes LF, Garcia-Gonzalez MA, Huso DL, Germino GG. A critical developmental switch defines the kinetics of kidney cyst formation after loss of Pkd1. *Nat Med* (2007) 13(12):1490–5. doi:10.1038/nm1675
67. Wei W, Hackmann K, Xu H, Germino G, Qian F. Characterization of cis-autoproteolysis of polycystin-1, the product of human polycystin kidney disease 1 gene. *J Biol Chem* (2007) 282(30):21729–37. doi:10.1074/jbc.M703218200

68. Yu S, Hackmann K, Gao J, He X, Piontek K, Garcia-Gonzalez MA, et al. Essential role of cleavage of Polycystin-1 at G protein-coupled receptor proteolytic site for kidney tubular structure. *Proc Natl Acad Sci U S A* (2007) 104(47):18688–93. doi:10.1073/pnas.0708217104
69. Gainullin VG, Hopp K, Ward CJ, Hommerding CJ, Harris PC. Polycystin-1 maturation requires polycystin-2 in a dose-dependent manner. *J Clin Invest* (2015) 125(2):607–20. doi:10.1172/JCI76972
70. Kim H, Xu H, Yao Q, Li W, Huang Q, Outeda P, et al. Ciliary membrane proteins traffic through the Golgi via a Rabep1/GGA1/Arl3-dependent mechanism. *Nat Commun* (2014) 5:5482. doi:10.1038/ncomms6482
71. Cai Y, Fedeles SV, Dong K, Anyatonwu G, Onoe T, Mitobe M, et al. Altered trafficking and stability of polycystins underlie polycystic kidney disease. *J Clin Invest* (2014) 124(12):5129–44. doi:10.1172/JCI67273
72. Fedeles SV, Gallagher AR, Somlo S. Polycystin-1: a master regulator of intersecting cystic pathways. *Trends Mol Med* (2014) 20(5):251–60. doi:10.1016/j.molmed.2014.01.004
73. Guay-Woodford L. Autosomal recessive polycystic kidney disease: the prototype of the hepato-renal fibrocystic diseases. *J Pediatr Genet* (2014) 3(2):89–101. doi:10.3233/PGE-14092
74. Li Y, Wright JM, Qian F, Germino GG, Guggino WB. Polycystin 2 interacts with type I inositol 1,4,5-trisphosphate receptor to modulate intracellular Ca2+ signaling. *J Biol Chem* (2005) 280(50):41298–306. doi:10.1074/jbc.M510082200
75. Anyatonwu GI, Estrada M, Tian X, Somlo S, Ehrlich BE. Regulation of ryanodine receptor-dependent calcium signaling by polycystin-2. *Proc Natl Acad Sci U S A* (2007) 104(15):6454–9. doi:10.1073/pnas.0610324104
76. Gallagher AR, Germino GG, Somlo S. Molecular advances in autosomal dominant polycystic kidney disease. *Adv Chronic Kidney Dis* (2010) 17(2):118–30. doi:10.1053/j.ackd.2010.01.002
77. Hooper KM, Boletta A, Germino GG, Hu Q, Ziegelstein RC, Sutters M. Expression of polycystin-1 enhances endoplasmic reticulum calcium uptake and decreases capacitative calcium entry in ATP-stimulated MDCK cells. *Am J Physiol Renal Physiol* (2005) 289(3):F521–30. doi:10.1152/ajprenal.00355.2004
78. Yamaguchi T, Pelling JC, Ramaswamy NT, Eppler JW, Wallace DP, Nagao S, et al. cAMP stimulates the in vitro proliferation of renal cyst epithelial cells by activating the extracellular signal-regulated kinase pathway. *Kidney Int* (2000) 57(4):1460–71. doi:10.1046/j.1523-1755.2000.00991.x
79. Belibi FA, Reif G, Wallace DP, Yamaguchi T, Olsen L, Li H, et al. Cyclic AMP promotes growth and secretion in human polycystic kidney epithelial cells. *Kidney Int* (2004) 66(3):964–73. doi:10.1111/j.1523-1755.2004.00843.x
80. Sussman CR, Ward CJ, Leightner AC, Smith JL, Agarwal R, Harris PC, et al. Phosphodiesterase 1A modulates cystogenesis in zebrafish. *J Am Soc Nephrol* (2014) 25(10):2222–30. doi:10.1681/ASN.2013040421
81. Gattone VH, Wang X, Harris PC, Torres VE. Inhibition of renal cystic disease development and progression by a vasopressin V2 receptor antagonist. *Nat Med* (2003) 9(10):1323–6. doi:10.1038/nm935
82. Torres VE, Wang X, Qian Q, Somlo S, Harris PC, Gattone VH. Effective treatment of an orthologous model of autosomal dominant polycystic kidney disease. *Nat Med* (2004) 10(4):363–4. doi:10.1038/nm1004
83. Torres VE, Chapman AB, Devuyst O, Gansevoort RT, Grantham JJ, Higashihara E, et al. Tolvaptan in patients with autosomal dominant polycystic kidney disease. *N Engl J Med* (2012) 367(25):2407–18. doi:10.1056/NEJMoa1205511
84. Torres VE, Harris PC. Strategies targeting cAMP signaling in the treatment of polycystic kidney disease. *J Am Soc Nephrol* (2014) 25(1):18–32. doi:10.1681/ASN.2013040398
85. Ibraghimov-Beskrovnaya O, Natoli TA. mTOR signaling in polycystic kidney disease. *Trends Mol Med* (2011) 17(11):625–33. doi:10.1016/j.molmed.2011.06.003
86. Tao Y, Kim J, Schrier RW, Edelstein CL. Rapamycin markedly slows disease progression in a rat model of polycystic kidney disease. *J Am Soc Nephrol* (2005) 16(1):46–51. doi:10.1681/ASN.2004080660
87. Shillingford JM, Murcia NS, Larson CH, Low SH, Hedgepeth R, Brown N, et al. The mTOR pathway is regulated by polycystin-1, and its inhibition reverses renal cystogenesis in polycystic kidney disease. *Proc Natl Acad Sci U S A* (2006) 103(14):5466–71. doi:10.1073/pnas.0509694103
88. Renken C, Fischer DC, Kundt G, Gretz N, Haffner D. Inhibition of mTOR with sirolimus does not attenuate progression of liver and kidney disease in PCK rats. *Nephrol Dial Transplant* (2011) 26(1):92–100. doi:10.1093/ndt/gfq384
89. Hogan MC, Masyuk TV, Page L, Holmes DR III, Li X, Bergstralh EJ, et al. Somatostatin analog therapy for severe polycystic liver disease: results after 2 years. *Nephrol Dial Transplant* (2012) 27(9):3532–9. doi:10.1093/ndt/gfs152
90. Chrispijn M, Nevens F, Gevers TJ, Vanslembrouck R, van Oijen MG, Coudyzer W, et al. The long-term outcome of patients with polycystic liver disease treated with lanreotide. *Aliment Pharmacol Ther* (2012) 35(2):266–74. doi:10.1111/j.1365-2036.2011.04923.x
91. Rowe I, Chiaravalli M, Mannella V, Ulisse V, Quilici G, Pema M, et al. Defective glucose metabolism in polycystic kidney disease identifies a new therapeutic strategy. *Nat Med* (2013) 19(4):488–93. doi:10.1038/nm.3092
92. Chiaravalli M, Rowe I, Mannella V, Quilici G, Canu T, Bianchi V, et al. 2-Deoxy-d-glucose ameliorates PKD progression. *J Am Soc Nephrol* (2016) 27(7):1958–69. doi:10.1681/ASN.2015030231
93. Zhou X, Fan LX, Sweeney WE Jr, Denu JM, Avner ED, Li X. Sirtuin 1 inhibition delays cyst formation in autosomal-dominant polycystic kidney disease. *J Clin Invest* (2013) 123(7):3084–98. doi:10.1172/JCI64401
94. Hajarnis S, Lakhia R, Yheskel M, Williams D, Sorourian M, Liu X, et al. microRNA-17 family promotes polycystic kidney disease progression through modulation of mitochondrial metabolism. *Nat Commun* (2017) 8:14395. doi:10.1038/ncomms14395
95. Chen L, Zhou X, Fan LX, Yao Y, Swenson-Fields KI, Gadjeva M, et al. Macrophage migration inhibitory factor promotes cyst growth in polycystic kidney disease. *J Clin Invest* (2015) 125(6):2399–412. doi:10.1172/JCI80467
96. Sweeney WE, Frost P, Avner ED. Tesevatinib ameliorates progression of polycystic kidney disease in rodent models of autosomal recessive polycystic kidney disease. *World J Nephrol* (2017) 6(4):188–200. doi:10.5527/wjn.v6.i4.188
97. Sweeney WE Jr, Avner ED. Emerging therapies for childhood polycystic kidney disease. *Front Pediatr* (2017) 5:77. doi:10.3389/fped.2017.00077

6

Many Genes—One Disease? Genetics of Nephronophthisis (NPHP) and NPHP-Associated Disorders

Shalabh Srivastava[1,2], Elisa Molinari[1], Shreya Raman[3] and John A. Sayer[1,4]*

[1] Institute of Genetic Medicine, Newcastle University, Newcastle upon Tyne, United Kingdom, [2] Renal Unit, City Hospitals Sunderland and South Tyneside NHS Foundation Trust, Sunderland, United Kingdom, [3] Department of Histopathology, Newcastle upon Tyne Hospitals NHS Foundation Trust, Newcastle upon Tyne, United Kingdom, [4] Renal Services, Newcastle upon Tyne Hospitals NHS Foundation Trust, Newcastle upon Tyne, United Kingdom

***Correspondence:**
John A. Sayer
john.sayer@ncl.ac.uk

Nephronophthisis (NPHP) is a renal ciliopathy and an autosomal recessive cause of cystic kidney disease, renal fibrosis, and end-stage renal failure, affecting children and young adults. Molecular genetic studies have identified more than 20 genes underlying this disorder, whose protein products are all related to cilia, centrosome, or mitotic spindle function. In around 15% of cases, there are additional features of a ciliopathy syndrome, including retinal defects, liver fibrosis, skeletal abnormalities, and brain developmental disorders. Alongside, gene identification has arisen molecular mechanistic insights into the disease pathogenesis. The genetic causes of NPHP are discussed in terms of how they help us to define treatable disease pathways including the cyclic adenosine monophosphate pathway, the mTOR pathway, Hedgehog signaling pathways, and DNA damage response pathways. While the underlying pathology of the many types of NPHP remains similar, the defined disease mechanisms are diverse, and a personalized medicine approach for therapy in NPHP patients is likely to be required.

Keywords: ciliopathy, molecular genetics, nephronophthisis, cilia, centrosome, DNA damage, cyclic adenosine monophosphate, Joubert syndrome

INTRODUCTION

Nephronophthisis (NPHP) is an autosomal recessive inherited kidney disease, which leads to end-stage renal disease (ESRD) typically within the first three decades of life (1). Traditionally, this disease was diagnosed using clinical and histological features. However, over recent years, many of the genetic causes underlying NPHP have been identified allowing both a precise molecular diagnosis to be made and some mechanistic insights into the underlying disease process. The known NPHP genes encode proteins that are almost all expressed in centrosomes and primary cilia. NPHP is therefore considered to be a ciliopathy disease (2), consistent with the fact that extrarenal manifestations, consistent will a ciliopathy syndrome, occur in around 20% of cases. Here we will review the clinical and histological features of the disease and its conventional classification before reviewing the underlying genetic causes and the ciliopathy syndromes associated with NPHP.

Based on the original histological descriptions, which included corticomedullary cysts, atrophy, and interstitial fibrosis, NPHP literally means disappearance or disintegration of nephrons (3). The clinical symptoms of NPHP, which reflect reduction in GFR and loss of distal tubular function (4), include polyuria, polydipsia, secondary enuresis, and growth retardation. Unfortunately, NPHP is associated with a progressive loss of kidney function and ESRD typically

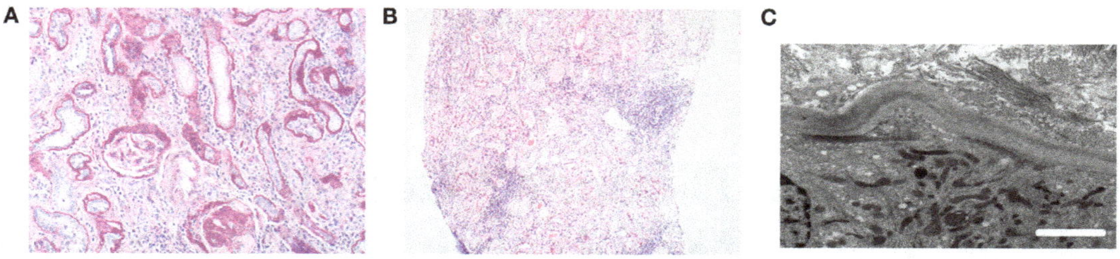

FIGURE 1 | Typical histological features of nephronophthisis. **(A)** Light microscopy image. PAS stain demonstrates a globally sclerosed glomerulus and some periglomerular fibrosis. There is moderate interstitial fibrosis with chronic inflammation and thickening of tubular basement membranes. **(B)** Light microscopy image. H&E stain shows tubular atrophy with hyaline casts, moderate interstitial fibrosis, and patchy mononuclear inflammation. **(C)** Electron microscopy image. Tubular basement membrane demonstrates thickening and multilayering. Scale bar 2 μm.

occurs before 30 years of age. Cases have historically been classified based on the age of onset of ESRD as infantile, juvenile, adolescent, and late onset. These are worth reviewing, although it is worth noting that a single genotype may present at a wide range of ages.

Juvenile NPHP is the classical form of NPHP and is characterized by polyuria and polydipsia symptoms and often anemia in patients within the first decade of life. Progressive loss of kidney function leads to ESRD at a median age of 13 years (5).

Kidneys affected by NPHP are grossly normal or have a shrunken appearance, typical of ESRD. There may be corticomedullary cysts that are up to 1.5 cm in size. Cysts often develop in later stages of the disease. The renal ultrasound scan appearances may often display a loss of corticomedullary differentiation.

Where renal biopsies have been performed in NPHP patients, distinct histological features have been reported. The histological changes can be divided into early or late stages of disease. In the early stages of the NPHP, there is interstitial fibrosis with sparse inflammation and lack of infiltration with neutrophils or monocytes. The tubules are tortuous and atrophic with segmented tubular basement membrane thickening (6). The distal tubules have focal diverticulum like protrusions. The glomeruli are usually normal but there may be periglomerular fibrosis that can extend into the glomerular tuft leading to focal or global collapse of the tuft and obsolescence of the glomeruli (7, 8). In later stages of the disease, the tubules may demonstrate basement membrane abnormalities with both atrophy and thickening. There often is cystic dilatation of the distal tubules, and the glomeruli may show collapse and severe periglomerular fibrosis (8, 9) (**Figure 1**). NPHP is not an immune mediated disease, and consequently there is no immune or complement deposition (6, 8). Electron microscopy may reveal tubular basement membrane duplication, thickening, and folding (6, 8). When examining clinical, pathological, and histological features of NPHP, it must be remembered that a separate disorder, known as medullary cystic kidney disease may share similar features. Medullary cystic kidney disease is an autosomal dominant condition, which is now classified under the term autosomal dominant tubulointerstitial kidney disease (ADTKD). Typical extrarenal manifestations include gout and anemia. A comparison of NPHP and ADTKD, alongside is given in **Table 1** and has been discussed elsewhere (10).

TABLE 1 | Comparison of nephronophthisis (NPHP) with autosomal dominant tubulointerstitial kidney disease (ADTKD).

Diagnosis	NPHP	ADTKD
Inheritance Gene(s)	Autosomal recessive *NPHP* genes	Autosomal dominant *MUC1* *UMOD* *REN* *SEC61A1*
Extrarenal associations	Retinal degeneration Cerebellar vermis aplasia, gaze palsy, liver fibrosis, situs inversus, and skeletal defects	Gout
Radiological features	Small or normal-sized hyperechogenic kidneys and corticomedullary cysts (except infantile variant)	Small or normal sized hyperechogenic kidneys and corticomedullary cysts
Median age of end-stage renal disease	Usually under 30 years	16–80 years (*MUC1*) 30–50 years (*UMOD*)

Infantile NPHP is rare, but is noteworthy, due to its severe phenotype with ESRD typically occurring during the first year of life (7). There may be antenatal presentations with oligohydramnios and bilateral enlarged cystic kidneys. Infantile NPHP is usually caused by mutations in *INVS* (11) and *NPHP3* (12) but has been reported for other genetic forms of NPHP such as *NEK8* (13) and *CEP83* (14). The macroscopic and histological kidney phenotype is markedly different from other varieties of NPHP, with enlarged cystic kidneys, as opposed to micro and small corticomedullary cysts. Histologically, infantile NPHP lacks the tubular basement membrane changes seen in other NPHP phenotypes and may resemble autosomal recessive polycystic kidney disease. There may also be severe cardiac anomalies including situs inversus and ventricular septal defects (15).

The adolescent form of NPHP was originally described in a large Venezuelan pedigree (16). Biallelic mutations in *NPHP3* were found in this family, resulting in ESRD at a median age of 19 years (16). It is now known that *NPHP3* mutations may lead to a broad range of phenotypes including perinatal lethal Meckel–Gruber syndrome and infantile presentations. The term "adolescent NPHP" is thus somewhat arbitrary and merely extends the phenotypic spectrum from juvenile NPHP.

A number of case reports have highlighted the fact that NPHP may first present later in life. Georges et al. reported three (genetically unsolved) families with retinal dystrophy, NPHP on renal biopsy and slowly progressive renal failure and ESRD between the ages of 42 and 56 years (17). In another family with a homozygous *NPHP1* deletion (18) ESRD was reported in three patients between 27 and 43 years of age. These cases of NPHP extend the age of ESRD from birth to up to the sixth decade of life.

AN APPROACH TO THE CLINICAL DIAGNOSIS OF NPHP

Clinical recognition of NPHP is important, and the renal and extrarenal features of a ciliopathy syndrome (discussed below) may allow a clinical diagnosis to be made. NPHP occurs in isolation in around 80% of cases and is associated with a variety of other ciliopathy phenotypes in 20% of cases. A detailed review with specific emphasis on the family history and extrarenal features known to be associated with NPHP is therefore an essential prerequisite to an exact diagnosis. NPHP is characterized by a urinary concentrating defect early on in life that leads to polyuria and polydipsia. The onset of the disease may be easily missed, as there is typically no severe hypertension, minimal or no proteinuria, and a bland urine sediment. Clinical spectrums of disease are wide and widening. Besides extensive investigations of renal function, clinical phenotyping should also encompass a full neurological screening to assess for cerebellar signs and fundoscopy to assess for retinal degeneration. A formal ophthalmological examination is advised. The role of renal biopsy in diagnosing NPHP is contentious and should be limited to cases where a tissue diagnosis will serve to distinguish it from other differential diagnoses. In most cases, a histopathological diagnosis should be superseded by a molecular genetic diagnostic approach, because genetic screening allows for early diagnosis and prevents complications of renal biopsy. *NPHP1* mutations and deletions are the most frequent genetic cause of NPHP and may be screened for using standard PCR assays (19). Given the large numbers of other NPHP genes involved multiplex PCR (20), targeted exon capture or whole-exome sequencing approaches are recommended (21).

EXTRARENAL MANIFESTATIONS OF NPHP

There are several important additional phenotypes that may be associated with NPHP (**Table 2**). These multisystem features are consistent with the fact that NPHP is a ciliopathy and may affect retina, brain, liver, and other tissues either by prenatal-onset dysplasia or by postnatal organ degeneration and fibrosis. Extrarenal manifestations are seen in ~20% of cases (22). In a recent study where 89 patients with NPHP mutations were analyzed, *NPHP1* mutations were the most common genetic cause and gave rise to typical renal presentations. These included increased echogenicity of the kidney and loss of corticomedullary differentiation, with cystic kidney disease presenting later in the disease course (median age 12.3 years) and ESRD at a median age of 12.8 years (23). Extrarenal manifestations of *NPHP1* mutations were seen more frequently than expected, with 8% presenting with liver symptoms, 19% having developmental delay and 7% epilepsy and seizures (23). The important syndromes associated with NPHP are briefly described below.

TABLE 2 | Extrarenal manifestations of nephronophthisis (NPHP) and their associated syndromes.

Extrarenal manifestation associated with NPHP	Syndrome
Retinitis pigmentosa/retinal dystrophy	Senior–Løken syndrome
	Alström syndrome
	Arima syndrome
Oculomotor apraxia	Cogan syndrome
Nystagmus	Joubert syndrome and related disorders
Ocular coloboma	Joubert syndrome and related disorders
Posterior encephalocele	Meckel–Gruber syndrome
Abnormal respiratory pattern	Joubert syndrome and related disorders
Cerebellar vermis aplasia/hypoplasia	Joubert syndrome and related disorders
Liver fibrosis	Joubert syndrome and related disorders
	Meckel–Gruber syndrome
	Arima syndrome
Postaxial polydactyly	Bardet–Biedl syndrome
	Joubert syndrome and related disorders
Skeletal dysplasia	Ellis–van Creveld syndrome
	Sensenbrenner syndrome
	Jeune syndrome
	Mainzer–Saldino syndrome
Situs inversus/cardiac malformation	Infantile NPHP

NPHP with Retinitis Pigmentosa (Senior–Løken Syndrome)

Retinal dysplasia and degeneration is seen in 10–15% of patients with NPHP and may lead to an early and severe visual loss resembling Leber congenital amaurosis (LCA) (24, 25). Later onset forms present initially with night blindness, which then progresses to visual loss.

Cerebellar Vermis Aplasia/Hypoplasia with NPHP (Joubert Syndrome)

Joubert syndrome is a developmental disorder characterized by cerebellar vermis hypoplasia (26). Brain imaging (MRI) reveals the typical sign known as the "molar tooth sign." Clinical features include hypotonia, cerebellar ataxia, neonatal tachypnea, and developmental delay. There may also be ocular coloboma, polydactyly, and hepatic fibrosis. NPHP is found in up to 30% of Joubert syndrome patients (27–29). Large cohorts of Joubert syndrome patients have been described, allowing some genotype/phenotype correlations to be made in the more frequent genetic causes. Mutations in *TMEM67* in Joubert syndrome are the most frequently associated with kidney disease, whereas mutations in *CEP290* were most likely to give retinal, renal, and brain phenotypes (28). In a recent cohort analysis of 97 patients with Joubert syndrome, renal phenotypes were detect in 30% of cases and was commonly associated with NPHP genes including *CEP290*, *TMEM67*, and *AHI1* (29). In this study, renal phenotypes in Joubert syndrome extended beyond classical NPHP and included an overlapping phenotype resembling autosomal recessive polycystic kidney disease and NPHP (mimicking infantile NPHP), unilateral multicystic dysplastic kidney and indeterminate cystic kidney disease phenotypes (29).

Oculomotor Apraxia (OMA) Type Cogan

Oculomotor apraxia type Cogan is an eye movement disorder. It is characterized by abnormal horizontal eye movements that include nystagmus and difficulty with saccades (smooth visual pursuits) and has been associated with NPHP (2, 30). OMA may be a mild form of Joubert syndrome, as cerebellar vermis aplasia has been described in this condition (31).

Perinatal Lethality (Meckel–Gruber Syndrome)

Meckel–Gruber syndrome is characterized by occipital encephalocele, polydactyly, bile ductal proliferation, and cystic kidney dysplasia. Typically, the condition is perinatally lethal. The syndrome is associated with severe biallelic mutations in NPHP genes that include *NPHP3*, *CEP290*, and *RPGRIP1L* (1, 32–35).

Skeletal Defects [Jeune Syndrome (JS), Sensenbrenner Syndrome, and Saldino-Mainzer Syndrome]

Various skeletal defects have been reported in association with NPHP. These include cone-shaped epiphyses (16, 36), shortening of limbs, and ribs, scoliosis, polydactyly, brachydactyly, and craniosynostosis. Mutations are in genes encoding intraflagellar transport (IFT) proteins including TTC21B and WDR19 (37–41).

Episodic Hyperpnea (Joubert Syndrome)

The original report of Joubert syndrome (42) described episodes of fast breathing followed by a period of apnea. This feature is demonstrable only when the patient is awake. Abnormal respiratory pattern is not a consistent feature of Joubert syndrome and the reported incidence varies (44–71%) (43).

Anosmia As an Extrarenal Manifestation of Renal Ciliopathies

Several renal ciliopathy syndromes have been associated with anosmia, secondary to olfactory cilia defects. This has been studied in most detail in Bardet–Biedl syndrome (BBS) (44, 45) but has been reported in patients with LCA secondary to mutations in *CEP290* and in a murine model of *Cep290* (46). Such data also suggest a link between ciliary defects in the olfactory neurons and kidney disease. Indeed, proteins that mediate olfactory-like chemosensory signaling pathways were found expressed in the renal tissue (47), including adenylate cyclase III, which is localized to the primary cilium (48). These pathways may be vital in tubuloglomerular feedback and blood pressure control. There is a real need now to assess patients with renal ciliopathies/NPHP (and indeed corresponding murine models) for defects in smell and to determine a role for olfactory-like signaling within the kidney.

KNOWN GENETIC CAUSES OF NPHP

There are now more than 20 genes that if mutated may lead to NPHP (**Table 3**). It is worth reviewing these genetic causes as they all point toward some mechanistic insights into the pathogenesis of NPHP. Finding commonality among the genetic causes relies on a connection to the centrosome/basal body/ primary cilium, although this may not be true for every genetic cause.

The most common genetic cause of NPHP is mutations in *NPHP1*, which account for around 20% of cases. The most common *NPHP1* gene defect is a large homozygous deletion affecting the whole gene (49, 79). Each of the remaining NPHP genes probably accounts for 1% or less of all cases of NPHP, meaning that around two-thirds of cases remain genetically unsolved (2). It is noteworthy that mutations in a single NPHP gene may give an extremely wide spectrum of clinical phenotypes that may include isolated NPHP, NPHP with additional features, such as Senior–Løken syndrome and Joubert syndrome and severe neonatal lethal forms, such as of Meckel–Gruber syndrome. Linkage studies and painstaking mapping approaches led to the identification of *NPHP1* in 1997 (49). Similar approaches for the next decade (sometimes combined with candidate gene screens) allowed the discovery of eight genes (at a rate of around one new gene per year). Since 2010, next-generation sequencing approaches have been utilized (80) allowing the detection of NPHP genes at a much faster rate.

NPHP1

NPHP1 encodes nephrocystin-1 (alias nephrocystin). It was shown to interact with p130cas, tensin, filamin, and focal adhesion kinase 2, all molecules involved in cell–cell adhesion and cell signaling (81–83). In the primary cilium, nephrocystin-1 interacts with nephrocystin-4 and RPGRIP1L at the transition zone and links it to inversin (77).

INVS

INVS causes ESRD in the first 2 years of life and presents typically as an infantile form of NPHP as described earlier. The frequency of *INVS* mutations has been reported to be as high as 78% in the group of patients reaching ESRD before 2 years of age (12). The kidney size in INVS is often enlarged unlike most other forms of NPHP in which the kidneys are normal in size or shrunken (12). The distribution of cysts is corticomedullary and is more reminiscent of autosomal recessive polycystic kidney disease, given the kidneys can be massively enlarged.

Inversin, the gene product of *INVS* interacts with nephrocystin-1 and nephrocystin-3 and plays a vital role in intercellular adhesion (84). It localizes to the cilium and serves as a switch between the canonical and non-canonical Wnt pathway (85). Otto et al. established a link between cystogenesis and the primary cilia in humans disease during the study of this disease in 2003 (11) establishing this as a landmark paper in the study of NPHP and ciliopathies. Inversin is also plays a role in planar cell polarity (PCP) processes, discussed below. Loss of inversin leads to abnormal mitotic spindle orientation (86), which may drive cystogenesis.

TABLE 3 | Genetic classification of NPHP, its related disorders and the key insights obtained.

HGNC gene symbol	NPHP type	Disorders associated with mutations	Key insights	Reference
NPHP1	NPHP1	NPHP/SLSN/JBTS	Localizes to microtubular organizing center, cell–cell junction, and ciliary transition zone protein	(49, 50)
INVS	NPHP2	NPHP/SLSN (including infantile NPHP) situs inversus	Localizes to primary cilium (inversin compartment). Protein possesses nuclear localization signals suggesting role in nucleus. Role in Wnt signaling and left–right determination	(11)
NPHP3	NPHP3	NPHP/SLSN/MKS (including infantile NPHP)	NPHP3 interacts with ANKS6, INVS, and NEK8 in a ciliary protein complex. Murine model *Pcy* has a hypomorphic *Nphp3* allele and has been utilized in pharmacological studies	(16, 51)
NPHP4	NPHP4	NPHP/SLSN	Localizes to primary cilia and cell–cell junctions. Role in transition zone of cilia	(52)
IQCB1	NPHP5	SLSN/LCA	Localizes to connecting cilium of photoreceptor cells and to primary cilia of renal tubular cells	(53)
CEP290	NPHP6	JBTS/BBS/MKS/LCA/SLSN	Centrosomal protein localizes to mother and daughter centrioles and to transition zone. Protein contains a nuclear localization signal and localizes to nucleus	(33, 54, 55)
GLIS2	NPHP7	NPHP	Localizes to nucleus and primary cilia. Increase in apoptosis and fibrosis in murine model Glis2	(56)
RPGRIP1L	NPHP8	JBTS/MKS	Ciliary transition zone protein and facilitates vesicular docking of ciliary proteins	(1, 57)
NEK8	NPHP9	NPHP (including infantile NPHP)	Localizes to primary cilium (inversin compartment). Links cilia and cell cycle defects in NPHP	(13)
SDCCAG8	NPHP10	SLSN/BBS	Localizes to centrosomes and cell–cell junctions. Localized in nucleus and implicated in DNA damage repair pathways	(58, 59)
TMEM67	NPHP11	NPHP/MKS/JBTS/COACH syndrome	Localizes to transition zone and to plasma membrane. Required for ciliogenesis and centriole migration	(60–62)
TTC21B	NPHP12	NPHP/JBTS	Intraflagellar transport (IFT) protein involved in retrograde transport. Localizes to cilia.	(37)
WDR19	NPHP13	NPHP/JBTS	IFT protein, involved in retrograde transport and ciliogenesis	(38, 39)
ZNF423	NPHP14	JBTS	Nuclear and centrosomal protein and role in DNA repair signaling. Znf423–/– mice exhibit cerebellar defects	(63, 64)
CEP164	NPHP15	NPHP/SLSN/JBTS	Centrosomal protein and role in DNA repair signaling. Plays a critical role in G2/M checkpoint and nuclear division. Localizes to nuclear foci	(63)
ANKS6	NPHP16	NPHP	Functional module with inversin and nephrocystin-3	(65, 66)
IFT172	NPHP17	NPHP/Jeune/Mainzer–Saldino syndrome	IFT protein (IFT-B module), defects affect both anterograde and retrograde IFT	(67)
CEP83	NPHP18	NPHP (including infantile NPHP)	Distal appendage protein of centriole, required for membrane contact during ciliogenesisis	(14, 68)
DCDC2	NPHP19	NPHP/liver fibrosis	Ciliary and mitotic spindle protein, mutations disrupt Wnt signaling	(69)
MAPKBP1	NPHP20	NPHP	Mitotic spindle pole protein	(70)
AHI1	JBTS3	NPHP/JBTS	Localized to basal bodies and cell–cell junctions. Important for cerebellar development	(71–74)
CC2D2A		JBTS/COACH syndrome/MKS	Transition zone protein, regulates cilia-directed cargo vesicle docking	(75)
XPNPEP3	NPHPL1	NPHP	Mitochondrial defect linking ciliopathies with mitochondria and potential novel pathways of disease	(76)
ATXN10		NPHP/spinocerebellar ataxia	Interacts with IQCB1. Nuclear and cytoplasmic localization	(77)
SLC41A1		NPHP-like/primary ciliary dyskinesia	Renal magnesium transporter defect. Ciliary localization not confirmed	(78)

BBS, Bardet–Biedl syndrome; COACH, cerebellar vermis hypo/aplasia, oligophrenia (mental retardation), ataxia, ocular coloboma, and hepatic fibrosis; JBTS, Joubert syndrome; LCA, Leber congenital amaurosis; MKS, Meckel syndrome; NPHP, nephronophthisis; SLNS, Senior–Løken syndrome.

NPHP3

Omran et al. first described mutations in *NPHP3* in a large Venezuelan family in 2000 (87). It is characterized by NPHP, situs inversus, and structural heart defects. Hoff et al. uncovered a link between nephrocystin-3, inversin, and NEK8 (65) in a report on the role of *ANKS6*, linking the above proteins at the proximal part of the primary cilium known as the inversin compartment. This may explain the overlap seen in the phenotype of patients with mutation in *INVS*, *NPHP3*, and *NEK8*.

NPHP4

NPHP4 was identified by homozygosity mapping and genome wide linkage analysis by Mollet et al. in patients with NPHP who did not have mutations in the *NPHP1*, *2*, and *3* genes. Nephrocystin-4 localizes to the primary cilia and cortical actin cytoskeleton in the polarized cells. In dividing cells, it localizes to the centrosomes. It has been shown to interact with p130 (Cas), tensin, and filamin (88).

IQCB1

Patients with *IQCB1* mutations are characterized by the presence of retinitis pigmentosa with NPHP (renal–retinal or Senior–Løken syndrome). In a study investigating the association of retinitis pigmentosa with NPHP, Otto et al. found a novel gene *IQCB1* that associates with retinitis pigmentosa GTPase regulator (RPGR) and calmodulin in the retinal connecting cilia, an analogous structure of the ciliary transition zone (53).

CEP290

Mutations in the *CEP290* gene underlie NPHP6 and are the leading cause of Joubert syndrome and related diseases, a cerebello–retinal–renal syndrome. The association of *CEP290* with NPHP was established in 2006 in a cohort of families with Joubert syndrome, Senior–Løken syndrome, and NPHP (54, 55). CEP290 was found to interact with the transcription factor ATF4, which is involved in cyclic adenosine monophosphate (cAMP) mediated cyst formation (54). *CEP290* mutations are the most common inherited cause of retinal degeneration (LCA). Mutations in *CEP290* may also cause BBS phenotypes (89).

TMEM67 (33, 90) and CC2D2A (91, 92) are both interacting partners of CEP290 and can cause severe ciliopathy phenotypes including Meckel–Gruber syndrome and Joubert syndrome. There is emerging evidence of the role of *CEP290* in ciliogenesis (93), cell signaling (94, 95), DNA damage response (DDR) (96), and consequently renal cystogenesis (97).

GLIS2

In 2007, Attanasio et al. reported a mutation in *GLIS2* as a novel cause for NPHP. The loss of this transcription factor leads to increased fibrosis and apoptosis (56). In a recent paper, *GLIS2* loss has been found to increase cell senescence. *Kif3a* null mice show increased cyst formation due to unrestrained proliferation, destabilization of p53 and increased DNA damage. This is partially rescued by ablation of *GLIS2* and pharmacological stabilization of p53 (98).

RPGRIP1L

Arts et al. identified mutations in *RPGRIP1L* as causative for Joubert syndrome in three families in 2007. This protein localizes to the basal body and interacts with NPHP4 (57).

NEK8

Otto et al. identified *NEK8* as the causative gene for Joubert syndrome after observing that the *jck* mouse harbors a mutation in the highly conserved RCC1 domain of Nek8. They performed a mutational analysis of a worldwide cohort of patients and established the pathogenic role of *NEK8* mutations in humans (13). More recently, *NEK8* loss was implicated in increased DNA damage in the pathogenesis of NPHP (99). This established one of the first associations between the role DDR and cystic kidney disease. Grampa et al. have recently described the association of *NEK8* with deregulation of the Hippo pathway and its role in severe syndromic renal cystic dysplasia (100). Al-Hamed et al. described a stillborn fetus with cystic kidneys, oligohydramnios, CVA and bilateral bowing of the femur secondary to *NEK8* mutation (101).

SDCCAG8

SDCCAG8 was the first NPHP gene to be identified using next-generation sequencing approaches (58). Patients with mutations in this gene were diagnosed with Senior–Løken syndrome, but may also have features suggestive of BBS (102). The encoded protein SDCCAG8 localizes to centrioles and directly interacts with the ciliopathy-associated protein OFD1. A recently described murine model of SDCCAG8 has implicated elevated levels of DDR signaling as a potential mechanism of kidney disease (59).

TMEM67

Otto et al. screened a cohort of 62 patients with NPHP and liver fibrosis and found hypomorphic mutations in *TMEM67* in 8% of the patients (61). *TMEM67* has been implicated in the pathogenesis of Meckel–Gruber syndrome, Joubert syndrome, and COACH syndrome (cerebellar vermis hypo/aplasia, oligophrenia, congenital ataxia, coloboma and congenital hepatic fibrosis) (33, 34). Liver fibrosis is a frequent feature of *TMEM67* mutations, and any patient with NPHP along with liver involvement should have tests for mutations in *TMEM67*. In a cohort of 100 patients with Joubert syndrome, mutations in *TMEM67* were most frequently associated with kidney disease (28).

TTC21B

Davis et al. reported the association of *TTC21B* mutations with both isolated NPHP and JS (37). *TTC21B* encodes the retrograde IFT protein IFT139, which has been shown to regulate Hedgehog signaling (103).

WDR19

WDR19 mutations have been reported in patients with ciliopathy syndromes including Sensenbrenner syndrome, Joubert syndrome, Senior–Løken syndrome, and isolated NPHP (38, 41, 104). *WDR19* encodes for IFT144, a protein that participates in retrograde IFT and is important for ciliogenesis.

ZNF423

ZNF423 mutations have shown to cause Joubert syndrome with NPHP (63). The encoded protein ZNF423 is a nuclear protein which functions as a DNA-binding transcription factor and interacts with DDR protein PARP1 [poly (ADP-ribose) polymerase 1] and also CEP290 (63).

CEP164

Mutations in *CEP164* may cause NPHP and related ciliopathy syndromes including Senior–Løken syndrome (63). The CEP164 protein is a regulator of ciliogenesis and is essential for the formation of the distal appendage of the centriole (105). Loss of *CEP164* induces DNA damage (63).

ANKS6

ANKS6 mutations lead to NPHP. ANKS6 localizes to the inversin compartment and links the NPHP proteins NPHP2, NPHP3, and NPHP9 to NEK8. This functional role of ANKS6 in an NPHP module may explain the phenotypic overlap that includes abnormalities in heart and liver, seen in the patients carrying individual mutations in these genes (65, 66).

IFT172

Intraflagellar transport is vital in maintaining the cilium and in executing its functions. IFT-A module has six components, and mutations in genes encoding these proteins have all been associated with ciliopathy diseases. IFT-B has 14 components. Halbritter et al. established the first link between IFT-B component IFT172 and skeletal ciliopathies. Some patients in this cohort had NPHP (67). Mutations in IFT172 may also cause BBS syndrome (106).

CEP83

CEP83 mutations have recently been described to cause infantile NPHP (14). *CEP83* encodes a centriolar distal appendage protein, CEP83. In the seven families so far described, the NPHP phenotype was early-onset (juvenile), and in some was also associated with hydrocephalus and learning difficulties (14).

DCDC2

Schueler et al. reported a novel mutation in the gene *DCDC2*, in patients presenting with an NPHP and hepatic fibrosis phenotype (69). DCDC2 localizes to the ciliary axoneme and the mitotic spindles. *DCDC2* knockdown inhibits ciliogenesis. It interacts with DVL, and *DCDC2* knockdown leads to defects in Wnt signaling and may contribute to the liver fibrosis (69).

MAPKBP1

Macia et al. have recently described a novel gene, *MAPKBP1*, in five families with eight individuals presenting with juvenile or late-onset NPHP with massive fibrosis. This gene encodes MAPKBP1, a scaffolding protein for JNK signaling. Interestingly, this protein does not localize to the primary cilium instead it localizes to the mitotic spindle pole. The authors also report increased DDR signaling in murine fibroblasts upon knockdown of *Mapkbp1* (70).

AHI1

Mutations in AHI1 were initially described in patients with Joubert syndrome and no kidney involvement (71, 72). However, AHI1 mutations may cause NPHP phenotypes (73) and may cause multicystic dysplastic kidneys also (29). AHI1 is localized to the basal body and cell–cell junctions (74).

CC2D2A

Mutations in *CC2D2A* have been reported to cause Joubert syndrome with and without cystic kidney disease (92). CC2D2A is localized to the basal body and colocalizes with CEP290 (92). Mutations in *CC2D2A* may also cause antenatal cystic kidney disease phenotypes and severe brain phenotypes (typical of Meckel–Gruber syndrome) leading to fetal death (101).

EVIDENCE OF OLIGOGENICITY AND TRIALLELISM IN NPHP

Alongside the novel findings relating to gene discovery in NPHP has been the continued theme of wide phenotypic variability, especially in extrarenal manifestations. The type of mutation may influence the phenotype in certain circumstances. Examples include *CC2D2A* (107, 108) and *TMEM67* (109) where two truncating mutations tend to lead to more severe phenotypes than missense mutations. With the now frequent sequencing of NPHP cohorts (110, 111) and the use of high-throughput genetic sequencing platforms (112), a few findings of oligogenicity and triallelism within NPHP have been reported; however, these are controversial as these findings are anecdotal. As an example, a heterozygous *AHI1* mutation when inherited with biallelic *NPHP1* mutations seems to lead to a more severe brain phenotype (111). Thus, a concept of mutation burden seems relevant to NPHP, and like BBS (113) it will be important that these variants are reported and that they are assessed in terms of their pathogenicity. Interestingly, *NPHP1* mutations and copy number variants, as well as causing NPHP and Joubert syndrome, may also contribute to the mutational burden of BBS (114, 115). More recent next-generation sequencing data studying Joubert syndrome suggest that rare disease variants are frequently found in addition to the causal biallelic variants. Typically, over one-third of affected individuals carry rare disease variants in addition to the causal mutations but importantly they did not correlate with disease severity (116). This study also found no evidence or support for triallelism. Discordant phenotypes between affected siblings were observed in 60% of subjects who shared causal mutations, suggesting that modifier alleles are important but elusive (116). Therefore, using third alleles and other NPHP gene variants of uncertain significance to determine additional phenotypes and disease severity and inform genetic counseling is not presently advised, or should only be done with the utmost care.

PATHOGENESIS OF NPHP

There are various theories behind the pathogenesis of the NPHP disease process. The very early hypotheses were based entirely on the histopathological description of the disease and led to the widespread belief that this disease was caused by some unknown nephrotoxic agent or an enzyme defect (8). The frequent finding of tubular basement membrane thickening led to a basement membrane hypothesis for the pathogenesis of NPHP. It was observed that nephrocystin-1, the protein product of *NPHP1* had a high degree of sequence conservation with CRK (a focal adhesion protein) (117), contained an SH3 domain and interacted with other proteins including p130Cas and ACK1 (49, 118). Nephrocystin-1 was shown to localize to adherens junctions and focal adhesions. This supported a hypothesis that nephrocystin-1 has an important role in the maintenance of the tubular epithelium and that abnormal cell–cell and cell–matrix interactions were the underlying defect in NPHP. Many years later, the debate of the initial pathogenic defect in NPHP continues, with the focus on NPHP as a ciliopathy (119). This hypothesis is strongly supported by multiple gene discoveries in NPHP with nearly all the affected genes coding for the components of the cilia, basal body or centrosome. Defects in primary cilia associated with cystic kidney disease were initially noted in *Ift88* mutant mice (120). This link between NPHP and cilia was confirmed in human disease established after the discovery that *INVS* mutations cause infantile NPHP and that the encoded protein inversin interacts with nephrocystin-1 and β-tubulin, colocalizing with them to the primary cilia of renal tubular cells (11). There is now almost universal agreement that the primary cilia are at the center of the disease process especially in terms of cystogenesis although it should not be forgotten that nephrocystins may have multiple subcellular localizations (54) and may play different roles in different tissues (1). There is an interesting overlap with the localization and function of NPHP genes and other "cystogenes" such as *PKD1*, *PKD2*, and the many other inherited causes of cystic kidney disease. The functional role of primary cilia in the human nephron is not fully understood. It was initially thought that the encoded proteins from *PKD1* and *PKD2*, namely, polycystin-1 and polycystin-2, were able to sense luminal flow of urine, and ciliary deflection stimulated calcium entry into the cell *via* the polycystin proteins leading to downstream signaling cascades (121). However, more recent studies have challenged this hypothesis (122, 123).

A COMPARISON OF NPHP AND ADPKD PATHOPHYSIOLOGY

A detailed discussion of the underlying pathophysiology of ADPKD has been recently published and is beyond the scope of this review (124). It is worth highlighting, however, that disease pathways in ADPKD involve cAMP, ciliary dysfunction, PCP and centrosome number as well as many others (124). Thus, these mechanisms of disease are shared with those of NPHP. Indeed, the development of tolvaptan, a vasopressin V2 receptor (V2R) antagonist for the use in patients with ADPKD was pioneered in murine models of NPHP (51). However, fluid secretion and proliferation seems less prominent in NPHP, while fibrosis and scarring are more prominent pathological features. The pairing of potential disease mechanisms in NPHP with targeted therapeutics will hopefully allow better treatments for NPHP in the near future (125).

OTHER KEY MOLECULAR PATHWAYS IMPLICATED IN NPHP

Planar Cell Polarity

Planar cell polarity is an evolutionary conserved mechanism by which cells maintain their orientation in a plane perpendicular to the apical-basal polarity of a cell layer. This is achieved by the correct alignment and orientation of cell division, orchestrated by the mitotic spindle and centrosomes. The maintenance of tubular diameter is dependent upon PCP signaling, and when this is defective, tubular dilatation rather than elongation is thought to contribute to cystogenesis (126, 127). Non-canonical Wnt signaling is vital for these signaling events and mutations in *INVS* are thought to lead to defective regulation of this pathway (84, 85). Mutations in *DCDC2*, leading to NPHP type 19 have also been implicated in this pathway, lending weight to this mechanism of cytogenesis and NPHP. Loss of Dcdc2 in IMCD3 cells led to an activation of Wnt signaling, leading to a loss of cilia, which was amenable to treatment with Wnt inhibitor treatment (69). Other connections to the Wnt pathway in NPHP includes CEP164 which interacts with disheveled protein 3 (DVL3) (63). The disheveled protein is a key component of the Wnt pathway, and part of the switch between canonical and non-canonical Wnt signaling. Defective Wnt signaling has also been demonstrated in murine models of Joubert syndrome. *Ahi1* mutant mice showed defect in cerebellar midline fusion in sites of reduced Wnt activity (128) while renal tissues from the same mice demonstrated abnormal Wnt signaling in late stages of NPHP (129). A murine gene trap model of *Cep290* similarly showed Wnt pathway changes (reduced Tcfl protein) only at later stages of the disease (murine kidney tissue aged 1 year) implicating this pathway in renal fibrosis (95). The relationship between Wnt signaling and cystic kidney disease has been recently reviewed (130).

cAMP Signaling

A huge amount of data have demonstrated the key role of elevated cAMP in mural epithelial cell proliferation and fluid secretion, which are the main drivers of cyst formation in polycystic kidney disease (131). However, some lines of evidence suggest that high cAMP levels are also implicated in junctional and polarity defects in NPHP. Levels of cAMP were found to be elevated in *Nphp3*-, *Nphp6*-, and *Nphp8*-stable knockdown mIMCD3 lines. When these cells were examined in a 3D spheroid culture system, they formed abnormal spheroids with no lumen and/or misaligned nuclei. Treatment with octreotide, an inhibitor of cAMP production, could rescue these structural abnormalities, linking high cAMP levels to cell polarity defects (132). Furthermore, it was shown that treatment with the cAMP analog 8-bromo-cAMP resulted in a dose-dependent loss of SDCCAG8 (NPHP10) protein in cell–cell junctions of the renal epithelial cell line MDCK-II, highlighting the potential role of high cAMP in perturbation of tissue architecture (58). Importantly, elevated cAMP levels and expression levels of the cAMP-dependent gene *Aquaporin-2* were found in the renal tissue of *Pcy* mice that carry a missense mutation in *Nphp3* (51).

mTOR Pathway

Increased mTOR (mechanistic target of rapamycin) activity was found in cystic kidney (133, 134) and in particular in cyst-lining epithelium (135) of several NPHP mouse models. mTOR is an atypical serine/threonine kinase that, by integrating a variety of signals from nutrients and growth factors, regulates cell growth and proliferation.

The detailed subcellular localization of mTOR pathway components is not clear but it has been showed that primary cilium is important for the regulation of mTOR pathway (136, 137). It has been proposed that the flow-dependent bending of primary cilium represents a mechanosensory signal that controls cell size through the regulation of mTOR activity (137). Consequently, cilia abnormalities may ultimately result in cell growth deregulation, which could be potentially critical for the tubular geometry of the kidney.

THE ROLE OF CILIA IN SONIC HEDGEHOG SIGNALING AND CELL CYCLE

The Hedgehog (Hh) signaling pathway is a key developmental pathway and was first discovered in *Drosophila* (138). There are three mammalian Hh homologs, Desert, Indian, and Sonic. The sonic Hh (Shh) pathway is essential for development (139), patterning, organogenesis, and cell signaling (140). It acts as a morphogen and a mitogen and dysregulation of the pathway can lead to severe developmental defects and can give rise to various cancers (141). Shh signaling is intimately related to the primary cilium (141). The receptor Patched (Ptch1) is 12-pass transmembrane protein localized to the primary cilium. It has an inhibitory effect on the translocation of Smoothened (Smo, a G-protein-coupled-like receptor). The secreted ligand Shh binds to Ptch1 and triggers internalization of Ptch1 into endocytic vesicles. This allows the translocation of Smo into the primary cilium and its stepwise activation (142). Downstream effector Glioma proteins (Gli2,3) remain in a neutral state under the effect of suppressor of fused and by sequential phosphorylation by protein kinase A, glycogen synthase kinase 3β, and casein kinase 1, they undergo proteolytic conversion to their repressor form. Smo, when enriched in the primary cilium and activated, promote the conversion of Gli repressor (Gli3r) forms into full-length activator forms. The Gli activators (Gli3a) induce the expression of Hh target genes *cyclin D1*, *Gli1*, *Gli2*, *N-myc*, and *Ptch1*. An intact Hh pathway is important for ciliogenesis. The evidence implicating the defects of the Hh signaling in NPHP, renal development and cystogenesis is evolving (77, 103). Loss of the transcription factor Glis2 (Gli-similar zinc finger protein) causes NPHP type 7 (56), Shh knockout mouse embryos showed either renal agenesis or cystic dysplasia (143) and upregulated Indian Hh has been implicated in cystogenesis (144). A subset of BBS proteins has been shown to modulate Shh signaling and interact with IFT proteins (145). More recently, Hh signaling has been shown to be dysregulated in models of cystic kidney disease including *Thm1*, *Pkd1*, *jck* (103) and *Cep290* (95).

THE CILIARY TRANSITION ZONE AND LINKS TO NPHP

Between the basal body and the ciliary axoneme lies the transition zone, a physical barrier between the ciliary membrane and the apical plasma membrane of the cell. Several genes causing NPHP encode transition zone components, including *NPHP1*, *RPGRIP1L*, *NPHP4*, and *CEP290*. The transition zone controls the protein entry into and exit from the primary cilium and the composition of the ciliary membrane, which directly impacts ciliary signaling pathways such as Hedgehog signaling. The hedgehog signaling molecule Smoothened has been shown to accumulate in discrete clusters in the transition zone, and RPGRIP1L mutations disrupted this localization, leading to disrupted signaling (146). These data support the hypothesis of the transition zone as a gatekeeper of the cilium and that defects can account for phenotypes such as NPHP.

DDR PATHWAYS AND NPHP

The DDR signaling pathway allows the cell to detect DNA damage, apply an arrest in cell cycle and promote repair of the DNA. Repair of double stranded DNA breaks is particularly important for the maintenance of chromosome integrity. The DNA damage pathway ensures that damaged cells do not progress through S phase and into mitosis before repair is complete. Recently, several of the proteins implicated in NPHP including NEK8 (99), CEP164 (147), ZNF423 (63), SDCCAG8 (58, 59), and CEP290 (96) have been implicated in this pathway, suggesting a nuclear (non-ciliary) role. Following DNA damage, ZNF423, CEP164, and SDCCAG8 proteins have been shown to colocalize to nuclear foci positive for TIP60, a marker of sites of DNA damage and knockdown of CEP164 or ZNF423 causes increased sensitivity to DNA damaging agents (63). These observations provided a hypothesis that may explain why some NPHP genes with null mutations (such as *NPHP3*, *CEP290*, and *RPGRIP1L*) present as severe congenital-onset dysplasia and malformation in multiple organs including the kidney, brain and eye while hypomorphic mutations in the same genes produce milder phenotypes, which include late-onset degeneration and fibrosis leading to NPHP in the kidney and retinal degeneration in the eye. During periods of high proliferation and replication stress such as morphogenesis, DDR signaling is essential, and defects may lead to tissue dysplasia. By contrast, during maintenance of tissues in postnatal life, low replication stress would be expected, and defects would produce a degenerative phenotype. This hypothesis may go some way to explain the organ specific phenotypes seen in Joubert syndrome and other syndromes associated with NPHP (63). DDR defects and replication stress may also be an explanation for the fibrosis seen in association with NPHP and represents drugable target for the disease, which may be independent from and more reversible than cystogenesis (96, 148).

AN INTEGRATION OF SIGNALING PATHWAYS IN THE DEVELOPMENT OF NPHP

It remains clear that given the genetic heterogeneity of NPHP and the numerous mechanistic pathways discussed that there is not one unifying pathology leading toward NPHP. The renal histology of NPHP points to a common endpoint of tubular damage and fibrosis, which may have multiple triggers. With each new gene discovery paper, there seems to be better clarity toward molecular diagnosis but more confusion regarding the signaling pathways underlying disease.

The clear themes concerning NPHP are that this disease is a manifestation of a renal ciliopathy with almost all NPHP-associated genes encoding gene products known to localize to primary cilia and regulate ciliary function and structure (149), with both the Hedgehog and Wnt signaling pathways implicated downstream from abnormal ciliary signaling. The function of the ciliary transition zone as a gatekeeper for ciliary protein entry and exit is clearly fundamental to ciliary signaling processes. Protein interaction studies of NPHP proteins now allow the proteins to be grouped into four distinct modules. These are the NPHP1-4-8 (NPHP1, NPHP4, and RPGRIP1L) module, the NPHP2-3-9-ANKS6 (INVS, NPHP3, NEK8, and ANKS6) module, the NPHP5-6 (IQCB1 and CEP290) module and the MKS module (MKS1, CC2D2A, and TCTN2). This points to the fact that each NPHP protein has a distinct localization and function within the centrosome/transition zone/cilium.

However, there is also growing evidence for a nuclear/DDR function of some NPHP-associated proteins, which may be important in disease initiation and progression. Whether this is independent of roles in the primary cilium is not known. It is possible that loss of ciliary function may be a downstream effect of nuclear events affecting cell cycle progression as a result of replication stress (148). The intimate relationship between ciliogenesis and DDR has recently been discussed (150). Centrosomal proteins including NEK8 and CEP290 that are mutated in ciliopathy disorders and are known to have functional roles in DDR are discussed in detail. Overall, it seems likely, given the body of evidence concerning cilia and cystic kidney disease that ciliary dysfunction is a relatively specific subcellular phenotype and final common pathway leading to NPHP, but other pathways may feed into this and be interrelated.

TREATMENT OF NPHP

Nephronophthisis is incurable at present, but a range of potential therapeutic interventions has arisen from several lines of investigation into the pathogenesis of NPHP. Elevated renal cAMP levels were found associated with the cystic phenotype of NPHP and the modulation of cAMP production has been extensively explored as a potential strategy in the treatment of cystic kidney disease (51, 151–154). V2R antagonists are able to slow the rate of cAMP production by inhibiting V2R that, by coupling with G proteins, regulates the activity of adenylate cyclase and mediates urine concentration. Indeed, V2R antagonists OPC31260 and tolvaptan were shown to be effective in reducing renal accumulation of cAMP and rescuing the cystic kidney phenotype in *Pcy* mice (a model of NPHP3) (16, 51, 153). The use of tolvaptan has now moved successfully from preclinical models, through clinical trials (155) and into clinical practice (156). Its use in childhood ADPKD is currently being investigated in clinical trials.

As discussed, several lines of evidence support a direct link between DNA damage and the loss of NPHP proteins. In particular, both the NPHP type nine associated protein NEK8 and Cep290 were shown to be important regulators of DNA damage as their loss leads to increased sensitivity to replication stress and increased levels of CDKs (96, 99). Interestingly, CDK inhibition is able to suppress the DNA damage caused by loss of NEK8 or Cep290, therefore providing a rationale for CDK inhibition as a potential strategy in the treatment of NPHP (96, 99). Indeed, the CDK inhibitor roscovitine and its analog S-CR8 significantly halted the progression of cystic phenotype and attenuated loss of kidney function in *jck* mice (carrying a mutation in *Nek8*) (99, 157). Furthermore, roscovitine was able to ameliorate the ciliary phenotype of renal epithelial cells derived from a patient with NPHP secondary to a mutation in *CEP290*. Interestingly, it was shown that the treatment with purmorphamine, an agonist of the Shh pathway, is not only as effective as roscovitine in rescuing the ciliary defect, but is also able to decrease CDK5 protein levels in patient cells, suggesting a possible convergence of these signaling pathways (158).

Given the pivotal role played by the primary cilium in the context of Hh pathway, a manipulation of Hh signaling appears as an appealing strategy in the treatment of ciliopathies such as NPHP. It has been shown that genetic deletion of *Gli2* can ameliorate the cystic kidney phenotype in an orthologous mouse model of TTC21B (56), while Hh agonism mediated by purmorphamine treatment is able to rescue the architectural defect displayed by 3D cultures of CEP290 renal epithelial cells (95).

Hyperactivation of mTOR (mechanistic target of rapamycin) pathway was found to be associated with cystic kidney disease and rapamycin has proven to be effective in several rodent [Han:SPRD rat (134, 159), LPK rat (135), *Pcy* mouse (133), and zebrafish models (*invs*, *iqcb1*, and *cep290* morphant) of NPHP (160)].

The zebrafish models of NPHP are proving also to be extremely useful for high-throughput drug screens to determine their effect on kidney development (161).

There is hope therefore that these and other animal models of NPHP will provide valuable insights for future personalized medicine treatments of NPHP in affected patients (162). However, despite the great number of promising interventions that has arisen from preclinical studies, no clinical trials have yet been conducted to test their therapeutic potential in NPHP patients, most of whom eligible for treatment would be less than 18 years of age (125).

To date, options for the treatment of NPHP remain supportive. Control of blood pressure is a priority in children and young adults affected. Management of complications arising from progressive renal failure such as anemia, symptoms of uremia and fluid overload are important alongside preparation for future renal replacement therapy. This disease does not recur in a transplant and renal transplantation remains the ideal mode of renal replacement therapy.

CONCLUSION

The clinical and pathological diagnosis of NPHP is important, given its progression to ESRD and its associated extrarenal manifestations. Molecular genetic investigations allows a diagnosis in around one-third of cases and can give insights into the associated disease features, the underlying mechanisms and hopefully pave the way for individualized treatments for the underlying kidney disease. As this review demonstrates, it is true that many genes cause NPHP and while most of the identified molecular causes implicate the primary cilium in the pathogenesis of NPHP, it has also become apparent that there are important differences in the underlying pathophysiology. The traditional descriptions of NPHP of infantile, juvenile, and adolescent may now seem dated; however, they highlight the fact that different genetic forms of the disease disrupt the kidney by different mechanisms, demanding a precision medicine approach to the diagnosis, understanding and treatment of NPHP and its associated syndromes.

AUTHOR CONTRIBUTIONS

JS conceived, drafted, and wrote the manuscript. SS and EM drafted and revised the manuscript. SR drafted the manuscript and provided figures.

ACKNOWLEDGMENTS

SS is a Kidney Research Clinical Training Fellow. EM is funded by Kids Kidney Research. JAS is funded by the MRC MR/M012212/1, the Newcastle upon Tyne Hospitals NHS Charity and Northern Counties Kidney Research Fund.

FUNDING

The authors gratefully acknowledge funding from Kidney Research UK, Kids Kidney Research, and Northern Counties Kidney Research Fund.

REFERENCES

1. Delous M, Baala L, Salomon R, Laclef C, Vierkotten J, Tory K, et al. The ciliary gene RPGRIP1L is mutated in cerebello-oculo-renal syndrome (Joubert syndrome type B) and Meckel syndrome. *Nat Genet* (2007) 39(7):875–81. doi:10.1038/ng2039
2. Hildebrandt F, Attanasio M, Otto E. Nephronophthisis: disease mechanisms of a ciliopathy. *J Am Soc Nephrol* (2009) 20(1):23–35. doi:10.1681/ASN.2008050456
3. Simms RJ, Eley L, Sayer JA. Nephronophthisis. *Eur J Hum Genet* (2008) 17(4):406–16. doi:10.1038/ejhg.2008.238
4. Krishnan R, Eley L, Sayer JA. Urinary concentration defects and mechanisms underlying nephronophthisis. *Kidney Blood Press Res* (2008) 31(3):152–62. doi:10.1159/000129648
5. Hildebrandt F, Strahm B, Nothwang HG, Gretz N, Schnieders B, Singh-Sawhney I, et al. Molecular genetic identification of families with juvenile nephronophthisis type 1: rate of progression to renal failure. APN Study Group. Arbeitsgemeinschaft fur Padiatrische Nephrologie. *Kidney Int* (1997) 51(1):261–9. doi:10.1038/ki.1997.31
6. Zollinger HU, Mihatsch MJ, Edefonti A, Gaboardi F, Imbasciati E, Lennert T. Nephronophthisis (medullary cystic disease of the kidney). A study using electron microscopy, immunofluorescence, and a review of the morphological findings. *Helv Paediatr Acta* (1980) 35(6):509–30.
7. Gagnadoux MF, Bacri JL, Broyer M, Habib R. Infantile chronic tubulo-interstitial nephritis with cortical microcysts: variant of nephronophthisis or new disease entity? *Pediatr Nephrol* (1989) 3(1):50–5. doi:10.1007/BF00859626
8. Waldherr R, Lennert T, Weber HP, Fodisch HJ, Scharer K. The nephronophthisis complex. A clinicopathologic study in children. *Virchows Arch A Pathol Anat Histol* (1982) 394(3):235–54. doi:10.1007/BF00430668
9. Gibson AA, Arneil GC. Nephronophthisis-report of 8 cases from Great Britain. *Arch Dis Child* (1972) 47:84–9. doi:10.1136/adc.47.251.84
10. Hildebrandt F, Otto E. Molecular genetics of nephronophthisis and medullary cystic kidney disease. *J Am Soc Nephrol* (2000) 11(9):1753–61.
11. Otto EA, Schermer B, Obara T, O'Toole JF, Hiller KS, Mueller AM, et al. Mutations in INVS encoding inversin cause nephronophthisis type 2, linking renal cystic disease to the function of primary cilia and left-right axis determination. *Nat Genet* (2003) 34(4):413–20. doi:10.1038/ng1217
12. Tory K, Rousset-Rouviere C, Gubler MC, Moriniere V, Pawtowski A, Becker C, et al. Mutations of NPHP2 and NPHP3 in infantile nephronophthisis. *Kidney Int* (2009) 75(8):839–47. doi:10.1038/ki.2008.662
13. Otto EA, Trapp ML, Schultheiss UT, Helou J, Quarmby LM, Hildebrandt F. NEK8 mutations affect ciliary and centrosomal localization and may cause nephronophthisis. *J Am Soc Nephrol* (2008) 19(3):587–92. doi:10.1681/ASN.2007040490
14. Failler M, Gee HY, Krug P, Joo K, Halbritter J, Belkacem L, et al. Mutations of CEP83 cause infantile nephronophthisis and intellectual disability. *Am J Hum Genet* (2014) 94(6):905–14. doi:10.1016/j.ajhg.2014.05.002
15. Wolf MT, Hildebrandt F. Nephronophthisis. *Pediatr Nephrol* (2011) 26(2):181–94. doi:10.1007/s00467-010-1585-z
16. Olbrich H, Fliegauf M, Hoefele J, Kispert A, Otto E, Volz A, et al. Mutations in a novel gene, NPHP3, cause adolescent nephronophthisis, tapeto-retinal degeneration and hepatic fibrosis. *Nat Genet* (2003) 34(4):455–9. doi:10.1038/ng1216
17. Georges B, Cosyns JP, Dahan K, Snyers B, Carlier B, Loute G, et al. Late-onset renal failure in Senior-Loken syndrome. *Am J Kidney Dis* (2000) 36(6):1271–5. doi:10.1053/ajkd.2000.19845
18. Hoefele J, Nayir A, Chaki M, Imm A, Allen SJ, Otto EA, et al. Pseudodominant inheritance of nephronophthisis caused by a homozygous NPHP1 deletion. *Pediatr Nephrol* (2011) 26(6):967–71. doi:10.1007/s00467-011-1761-9
19. Otto EA, Helou J, Allen SJ, O'Toole JF, Wise EL, Ashraf S, et al. Mutation analysis in nephronophthisis using a combined approach of homozygosity mapping, CEL I endonuclease cleavage, and direct sequencing. *Hum Mutat* (2008) 29(3):418–26. doi:10.1002/humu.20669
20. Halbritter J, Diaz K, Chaki M, Porath JD, Tarrier B, Fu C, et al. High-throughput mutation analysis in patients with a nephronophthisis-associated ciliopathy applying multiplexed barcoded array-based PCR amplification and next-generation sequencing. *J Med Genet* (2012) 49(12):756–67. doi:10.1136/jmedgenet-2012-100973
21. Gee HY, Otto EA, Hurd TW, Ashraf S, Chaki M, Cluckey A, et al. Whole-exome resequencing distinguishes cystic kidney diseases from phenocopies in renal ciliopathies. *Kidney Int* (2014) 85(4):880–7. doi:10.1038/ki.2013.450
22. Salomon R, Saunier S, Niaudet P. Nephronophthisis. *Pediatr Nephrol* (2009) 24(12):2333–44. doi:10.1007/s00467-008-0840-z
23. Konig J, Kranz B, Konig S, Schlingmann KP, Titieni A, Tonshoff B, et al. Phenotypic spectrum of children with nephronophthisis and related ciliopathies. *Clin J Am Soc Nephrol* (2017) 12(12):1974–83. doi:10.2215/CJN.01280217
24. Senior B, Friedmann AI, Braudo JL. Juvenile familial nephropathy with tapetoretinal degeneration: a new oculorenal dystrophy. *Am J Ophthalmol* (1961) 52:625–33. doi:10.1016/0002-9394(61)90147-7
25. Løken AC, Hanssen O, Halvorsen S, Jølster NJ. Hereditary renal dysplasia and blindness. *Acta Paediatr* (1961) 50:177–84. doi:10.1111/j.1651-2227.1961.tb08037.x
26. Parisi MA, Doherty D, Chance PF, Glass IA. Joubert syndrome (and related disorders) (OMIM 213300). *Eur J Hum Genet* (2007) 15(5):511–21. doi:10.1038/sj.ejhg.5201648

27. Bachmann-Gagescu R, Dempsey JC, Phelps IG, O'Roak BJ, Knutzen DM, Rue TC, et al. Joubert syndrome: a model for untangling recessive disorders with extreme genetic heterogeneity. *J Med Genet* (2015) 52(8):514–22. doi:10.1136/jmedgenet-2015-103087
28. Vilboux T, Doherty DA, Glass IA, Parisi MA, Phelps IG, Cullinane AR, et al. Molecular genetic findings and clinical correlations in 100 patients with Joubert syndrome and related disorders prospectively evaluated at a single center. *Genet Med* (2017) 19(8):875–82. doi:10.1038/gim.2016.204
29. Fleming LR, Doherty DA, Parisi MA, Glass IA, Bryant J, Fischer R, et al. Prospective evaluation of kidney disease in Joubert syndrome. *Clin J Am Soc Nephrol* (2017) 12(12):1962–73. doi:10.2215/CJN.05660517
30. Betz R, Rensing C, Otto E, Mincheva A, Zehnder D, Lichter P, et al. Children with ocular motor apraxia type Cogan carry deletions in the gene (NPHP1) for juvenile nephronophthisis. *J Pediatr* (2000) 136(6):828–31. doi:10.1067/mpd.2000.106225
31. Harris CM, Hodgkins PR, Kriss A, Chong WK, Thompson DA, Mezey LE, et al. Familial congenital saccade initiation failure and isolated cerebellar vermis hypoplasia. *Dev Med Child Neurol* (1998) 40(11):775–9. doi:10.1111/j.1469-8749.1998.tb12347.x
32. Bergmann C, Fliegauf M, Bruchle NO, Frank V, Olbrich H, Kirschner J, et al. Loss of nephrocystin-3 function can cause embryonic lethality, Meckel-Gruber-like syndrome, situs inversus, and renal-hepatic-pancreatic dysplasia. *Am J Hum Genet* (2008) 82(4):959–70. doi:10.1016/j.ajhg.2008.02.017
33. Baala L, Audollent S, Martinovic J, Ozilou C, Babron MC, Sivanandamoorthy S, et al. Pleiotropic effects of CEP290 (NPHP6) mutations extend to Meckel syndrome. *Am J Hum Genet* (2007) 81(1):170–9. doi:10.1086/519494
34. Baala L, Romano S, Khaddour R, Saunier S, Smith UM, Audollent S, et al. The Meckel-Gruber syndrome gene, MKS3, is mutated in Joubert syndrome. *Am J Hum Genet* (2007) 80(1):186–94. doi:10.1086/510499
35. Frank V, den Hollander AI, Bruchle NO, Zonneveld MN, Nurnberg G, Becker C, et al. Mutations of the CEP290 gene encoding a centrosomal protein cause Meckel-Gruber syndrome. *Hum Mutat* (2008) 29(1):45–52. doi:10.1002/humu.20614
36. Ellis DS, Heckenlively JR, Martin CL, Lachman RS, Sakati NA, Rimoin DL. Leber's congenital amaurosis associated with familial juvenile nephronophthisis and cone-shaped epiphyses of the hands (the Saldino-Mainzer syndrome). *Am J Ophthalmol* (1984) 97(2):233–9. doi:10.1016/S0002-9394(14)76095-7
37. Davis EE, Zhang Q, Liu Q, Diplas BH, Davey LM, Hartley J, et al. TTC21B contributes both causal and modifying alleles across the ciliopathy spectrum. *Nat Genet* (2011) 43(3):189–96. doi:10.1038/ng.756
38. Coussa RG, Otto EA, Gee HY, Arthurs P, Ren H, Lopez I, et al. WDR19: an ancient, retrograde, intraflagellar ciliary protein is mutated in autosomal recessive retinitis pigmentosa and in Senior-Loken syndrome. *Clin Genet* (2013) 84(2):150–9. doi:10.1111/cge.12196
39. Fehrenbach H, Decker C, Eisenberger T, Frank V, Hampel T, Walden U, et al. Mutations in WDR19 encoding the intraflagellar transport component IFT144 cause a broad spectrum of ciliopathies. *Pediatr Nephrol* (2014) 29(8):1451–6. doi:10.1007/s00467-014-2762-2
40. Perrault I, Saunier S, Hanein S, Filhol E, Bizet AA, Collins F, et al. Mainzer-Saldino syndrome is a ciliopathy caused by IFT140 mutations. *Am J Hum Genet* (2012) 90(5):864–70. doi:10.1016/j.ajhg.2012.03.006
41. Bredrup C, Saunier S, Oud MM, Fiskerstrand T, Hoischen A, Brackman D, et al. Ciliopathies with skeletal anomalies and renal insufficiency due to mutations in the IFT-A gene WDR19. *Am J Hum Genet* (2011) 89(5):634–43. doi:10.1016/j.ajhg.2011.10.001
42. Joubert M, Eisenring JJ, Robb JP, Andermann F. Familial agenesis of the cerebellar vermis. A syndrome of episodic hyperpnea, abnormal eye movements, ataxia, and retardation. *Neurology* (1969) 19(9):813–25. doi:10.1212/WNL.19.9.813
43. Pellegrino JE, Lensch MW, Muenke M, Chance PF. Clinical and molecular analysis in Joubert syndrome. *Am J Med Genet* (1997) 72(1):59–62. doi:10.1002/(SICI)1096-8628(19971003)72:1<59::AID-AJMG12>3.0.CO;2-T
44. Kulaga HM, Leitch CC, Eichers ER, Badano JL, Lesemann A, Hoskins BE, et al. Loss of BBS proteins causes anosmia in humans and defects in olfactory cilia structure and function in the mouse. *Nat Genet* (2004) 36(9):994–8. doi:10.1038/ng1418
45. Iannaccone A, Mykytyn K, Persico AM, Searby CC, Baldi A, Jablonski MM, et al. Clinical evidence of decreased olfaction in Bardet-Biedl syndrome caused by a deletion in the BBS4 gene. *Am J Med Genet A* (2005) 132A(4):343–6. doi:10.1002/ajmg.a.30512
46. McEwen DP, Koenekoop RK, Khanna H, Jenkins PM, Lopez I, Swaroop A, et al. Hypomorphic CEP290/NPHP6 mutations result in anosmia caused by the selective loss of G proteins in cilia of olfactory sensory neurons. *Proc Natl Acad Sci U S A* (2007) 104(40):15917–22. doi:10.1073/pnas.0704140104
47. Pluznick JL, Zou DJ, Zhang X, Yan Q, Rodriguez-Gil DJ, Eisner C, et al. Functional expression of the olfactory signaling system in the kidney. *Proc Natl Acad Sci U S A* (2009) 106(6):2059–64. doi:10.1073/pnas.0812859106
48. Ou Y, Ruan Y, Cheng M, Moser JJ, Rattner JB, van der Hoorn FA. Adenylate cyclase regulates elongation of mammalian primary cilia. *Exp Cell Res* (2009) 315(16):2802–17. doi:10.1016/j.yexcr.2009.06.028
49. Hildebrandt F, Otto E, Rensing C, Nothwang HG, Vollmer M, Adolphs J, et al. A novel gene encoding an SH3 domain protein is mutated in nephronophthisis type 1. *Nat Genet* (1997) 17(2):149–53. doi:10.1038/ng1097-149
50. Fliegauf M, Horvath J, von Schnakenburg C, Olbrich H, Muller D, Thumfart J, et al. Nephrocystin specifically localizes to the transition zone of renal and respiratory cilia and photoreceptor connecting cilia. *J Am Soc Nephrol* (2006) 17(9):2424–33. doi:10.1681/ASN.2005121351
51. Gattone VH II, Wang X, Harris PC, Torres VE. Inhibition of renal cystic disease development and progression by a vasopressin V2 receptor antagonist. *Nat Med* (2003) 9(10):1323–6. doi:10.1038/nm935
52. Otto E, Hoefele J, Ruf R, Mueller AM, Hiller KS, Wolf MT, et al. A gene mutated in nephronophthisis and retinitis pigmentosa encodes a novel protein, nephroretinin, conserved in evolution. *Am J Hum Genet* (2002) 71(5):1161–7. doi:10.1086/344395
53. Otto EA, Loeys B, Khanna H, Hellemans J, Sudbrak R, Fan S, et al. Nephrocystin-5, a ciliary IQ domain protein, is mutated in Senior-Loken syndrome and interacts with RPGR and calmodulin. *Nat Genet* (2005) 37(3):282–8. doi:10.1038/ng1520
54. Sayer JA, Otto EA, O'Toole JF, Nurnberg G, Kennedy MA, Becker C, et al. The centrosomal protein nephrocystin-6 is mutated in Joubert syndrome and activates transcription factor ATF4. *Nat Genet* (2006) 38(6):674–81. doi:10.1038/ng1786
55. Valente EM, Silhavy JL, Brancati F, Barrano G, Krishnaswami SR, Castori M, et al. Mutations in CEP290, which encodes a centrosomal protein, cause pleiotropic forms of Joubert syndrome. *Nat Genet* (2006) 38(6):623–5. doi:10.1038/ng1805
56. Attanasio M, Uhlenhaut NH, Sousa VH, O'Toole JF, Otto E, Anlag K, et al. Loss of GLIS2 causes nephronophthisis in humans and mice by increased apoptosis and fibrosis. *Nat Genet* (2007) 39(8):1018–24. doi:10.1038/ng2072
57. Arts HH, Doherty D, van Beersum SE, Parisi MA, Letteboer SJ, Gorden NT, et al. Mutations in the gene encoding the basal body protein RPGRIP1L, a nephrocystin-4 interactor, cause Joubert syndrome. *Nat Genet* (2007) 39(7):882–8. doi:10.1038/ng2069
58. Otto EA, Hurd TW, Airik R, Chaki M, Zhou W, Stoetzel C, et al. Candidate exome capture identifies mutation of SDCCAG8 as the cause of a retinal-renal ciliopathy. *Nat Genet* (2010) 42(10):840–50. doi:10.1038/ng.662
59. Airik R, Slaats GG, Guo Z, Weiss AC, Khan N, Ghosh A, et al. Renal-retinal ciliopathy gene Sdccag8 regulates DNA damage response signaling. *J Am Soc Nephrol* (2014) 25(11):2573–83. doi:10.1681/ASN.2013050565
60. Smith UM, Consugar M, Tee LJ, McKee BM, Maina EN, Whelan S, et al. The transmembrane protein meckelin (MKS3) is mutated in Meckel-Gruber syndrome and the wpk rat. *Nat Genet* (2006) 38(2):191–6. doi:10.1038/ng1713
61. Otto EA, Tory K, Attanasio M, Zhou W, Chaki M, Paruchuri Y, et al. Hypomorphic mutations in meckelin (MKS3/TMEM67) cause nephronophthisis with liver fibrosis (NPHP11). *J Med Genet* (2009) 46(10):663–70. doi:10.1136/jmg.2009.066613
62. Adams M, Simms RJ, Abdelhamed Z, Dawe HR, Szymanska K, Logan CV, et al. A meckelin–filamin A interaction mediates ciliogenesis. *Hum Mol Genet* (2012) 21(6):1272–86. doi:10.1093/hmg/ddr557
63. Chaki M, Airik R, Ghosh AK, Giles RH, Chen R, Slaats GG, et al. Exome capture reveals ZNF423 and CEP164 mutations, linking renal ciliopathies to

DNA damage response signaling. *Cell* (2012) 150(3):533–48. doi:10.1016/j.cell.2012.06.028

64. Cheng LE, Zhang J, Reed RR. The transcription factor Zfp423/OAZ is required for cerebellar development and CNS midline patterning. *Dev Biol* (2007) 307(1):43–52. doi:10.1016/j.ydbio.2007.04.005
65. Hoff S, Halbritter J, Epting D, Frank V, Nguyen TM, van Reeuwijk J, et al. ANKS6 is a central component of a nephronophthisis module linking NEK8 to INVS and NPHP3. *Nat Genet* (2013) 45(8):951–6. doi:10.1038/ng.2681
66. Taskiran EZ, Korkmaz E, Gucer S, Kosukcu C, Kaymaz F, Koyunlar C, et al. Mutations in ANKS6 cause a nephronophthisis-like phenotype with ESRD. *J Am Soc Nephrol* (2014) 25(8):1653–61. doi:10.1681/ASN.2013060646
67. Halbritter J, Bizet AA, Schmidts M, Porath JD, Braun DA, Gee HY, et al. Defects in the IFT-B component IFT172 cause Jeune and Mainzer-Saldino syndromes in humans. *Am J Hum Genet* (2013) 93(5):915–25. doi:10.1016/j.ajhg.2013.09.012
68. Stinchcombe JC, Randzavola LO, Angus KL, Mantell JM, Verkade P, Griffiths GM. Mother centriole distal appendages mediate centrosome docking at the immunological synapse and reveal mechanistic parallels with ciliogenesis. *Curr Biol* (2015) 25(24):3239–44. doi:10.1016/j.cub.2015.10.028
69. Schueler M, Braun DA, Chandrasekar G, Gee HY, Klasson TD, Halbritter J, et al. DCDC2 mutations cause a renal-hepatic ciliopathy by disrupting Wnt signaling. *Am J Hum Genet* (2015) 96(1):81–92. doi:10.1016/j.ajhg.2014.12.002
70. Macia MS, Halbritter J, Delous M, Bredrup C, Gutter A, Filhol E, et al. Mutations in MAPKBP1 cause juvenile or late-onset cilia-independent nephronophthisis. *Am J Hum Genet* (2017) 100(2):372. doi:10.1016/j.ajhg.2017.01.025
71. Ferland RJ, Eyaid W, Collura RV, Tully LD, Hill RS, Al-Nouri D, et al. Abnormal cerebellar development and axonal decussation due to mutations in AHI1 in Joubert syndrome. *Nat Genet* (2004) 36(9):1008–13. doi:10.1038/ng1419
72. Dixon-Salazar T, Silhavy JL, Marsh SE, Louie CM, Scott LC, Gururaj A, et al. Mutations in the *AHI1* gene, encoding jouberin, cause Joubert syndrome with cortical polymicrogyria. *Am J Hum Genet* (2004) 75(6):979–87. doi:10.1086/425985
73. Utsch B, Sayer JA, Attanasio M, Pereira RR, Eccles M, Hennies HC, et al. Identification of the first AHI1 gene mutations in nephronophthisis-associated Joubert syndrome. *Pediatr Nephrol* (2006) 21(1):32–5. doi:10.1007/s00467-005-2054-y
74. Tuz K, Hsiao YC, Juarez O, Shi B, Harmon EY, Phelps IG, et al. The Joubert syndrome-associated missense mutation (V443D) in the Abelson-helper integration site 1 (AHI1) protein alters its localization and protein-protein interactions. *J Biol Chem* (2013) 288(19):13676–94. doi:10.1074/jbc.M112.420786
75. Bachmann-Gagescu R, Dona M, Hetterschijt L, Tonnaer E, Peters T, de Vrieze E, et al. The ciliopathy protein CC2D2A associates with NINL and functions in RAB8-MICAL3-regulated vesicle trafficking. *PLoS Genet* (2015) 11(10):e1005575. doi:10.1371/journal.pgen.1005575
76. O'Toole JF, Liu Y, Davis EE, Westlake CJ, Attanasio M, Otto EA, et al. Individuals with mutations in XPNPEP3, which encodes a mitochondrial protein, develop a nephronophthisis-like nephropathy. *J Clin Invest* (2010) 120(3):791–802. doi:10.1172/JCI40076
77. Sang L, Miller JJ, Corbit KC, Giles RH, Brauer MJ, Otto EA, et al. Mapping the NPHP-JBTS-MKS protein network reveals ciliopathy disease genes and pathways. *Cell* (2011) 145(4):513–28. doi:10.1016/j.cell.2011.04.019
78. Hurd TW, Otto EA, Mishima E, Gee HY, Inoue H, Inazu M, et al. Mutation of the Mg2+ transporter SLC41A1 results in a nephronophthisis-like phenotype. *J Am Soc Nephrol* (2013) 24(6):967–77. doi:10.1681/ASN.2012101034
79. Saunier S, Calado J, Benessy F, Silbermann F, Heilig R, Weissenbach J, et al. Characterization of the *NPHP1* locus: mutational mechanism involved in deletions in familial juvenile nephronophthisis. *Am J Hum Genet* (2000) 66(3):778–89. doi:10.1086/302819
80. Sayer JA, Simms RJ. The challenges and surprises of a definitive molecular genetic diagnosis. *Kidney Int* (2014) 85(4):748–9. doi:10.1038/ki.2013.432
81. Donaldson JC, Dise RS, Ritchie MD, Hanks SK. Nephrocystin-conserved domains involved in targeting to epithelial cell-cell junctions, interaction with filamins, and establishing cell polarity. *J Biol Chem* (2002) 277(32):29028–35. doi:10.1074/jbc.M111697200
82. Donaldson JC, Dempsey PJ, Reddy S, Bouton AH, Coffey RJ, Hanks SK. Crk-associated substrate p130(Cas) interacts with nephrocystin and both proteins localize to cell-cell contacts of polarized epithelial cells. *Exp Cell Res* (2000) 256(1):168–78. doi:10.1006/excr.2000.4822
83. Benzing T, Gerke P, Hopker K, Hildebrandt F, Kim E, Walz G. Nephrocystin interacts with Pyk2, p130(Cas), and tensin and triggers phosphorylation of Pyk2. *Proc Natl Acad Sci U S A* (2001) 98(17):9784–9. doi:10.1073/pnas.171269898
84. Lienkamp S, Ganner A, Walz G. Inversin, Wnt signaling and primary cilia. *Differentiation* (2012) 83(2):S49–55. doi:10.1016/j.diff.2011.11.012
85. Simons M, Gloy J, Ganner A, Bullerkotte A, Bashkurov M, Kronig C, et al. Inversin, the gene product mutated in nephronophthisis type II, functions as a molecular switch between Wnt signaling pathways. *Nat Genet* (2005) 37(5):537–43. doi:10.1038/ng1552
86. Werner ME, Ward HH, Phillips CL, Miller C, Gattone VH, Bacallao RL. Inversin modulates the cortical actin network during mitosis. *Am J Physiol Cell Physiol* (2013) 305(1):C36–47. doi:10.1152/ajpcell.00279.2012
87. Omran H, Fernandez C, Jung M, Haffner K, Fargier B, Villaquiran A, et al. Identification of a new gene locus for adolescent nephronophthisis, on chromosome 3q22 in a large Venezuelan pedigree. *Am J Hum Genet* (2000) 66(1):118–27. doi:10.1086/302705
88. Mollet G, Silbermann F, Delous M, Salomon R, Antignac C, Saunier S. Characterization of the nephrocystin/nephrocystin-4 complex and subcellular localization of nephrocystin-4 to primary cilia and centrosomes. *Hum Mol Genet* (2005) 14(5):645–56. doi:10.1093/hmg/ddi061
89. Leitch CC, Zaghloul NA, Davis EE, Stoetzel C, Diaz-Font A, Rix S, et al. Hypomorphic mutations in syndromic encephalocele genes are associated with Bardet-Biedl syndrome. *Nat Genet* (2008) 40(4):443–8. doi:10.1038/ng.97
90. Brancati F, Iannicelli M, Travaglini L, Mazzotta A, Bertini E, Boltshauser E, et al. MKS3/TMEM67 mutations are a major cause of COACH syndrome, a Joubert syndrome related disorder with liver involvement. *Hum Mutat* (2009) 30(2):E432–42. doi:10.1002/humu.20924
91. Doherty D, Parisi MA, Finn LS, Gunay-Aygun M, Al-Mateen M, Bates D, et al. Mutations in 3 genes (MKS3, CC2D2A and RPGRIP1L) cause COACH syndrome (Joubert syndrome with congenital hepatic fibrosis). *J Med Genet* (2010) 47(1):8–21. doi:10.1136/jmg.2009.067249
92. Gorden NT, Arts HH, Parisi MA, Coene KL, Letteboer SJ, van Beersum SE, et al. CC2D2A is mutated in Joubert syndrome and interacts with the ciliopathy-associated basal body protein CEP290. *Am J Hum Genet* (2008) 83(5):559–71. doi:10.1016/j.ajhg.2008.10.002
93. Tsang WY, Bossard C, Khanna H, Peranen J, Swaroop A, Malhotra V, et al. CP110 suppresses primary cilia formation through its interaction with CEP290, a protein deficient in human ciliary disease. *Dev Cell* (2008) 15(2):187–97. doi:10.1016/j.devcel.2008.07.004
94. Singla V, Reiter JF. The primary cilium as the cell's antenna: signaling at a sensory organelle. *Science* (2006) 313(5787):629–33. doi:10.1126/science.1124534
95. Hynes AM, Giles RH, Srivastava S, Eley L, Whitehead J, Danilenko M, et al. Murine Joubert syndrome reveals Hedgehog signaling defects as a potential therapeutic target for nephronophthisis. *Proc Natl Acad Sci U S A* (2014) 111(27):9893–8. doi:10.1073/pnas.1322373111
96. Slaats GG, Saldivar JC, Bacal J, Zeman MK, Kile AC, Hynes AM, et al. DNA replication stress underlies renal phenotypes in CEP290-associated Joubert syndrome. *J Clin Invest* (2015) 125(9):3657–66. doi:10.1172/JCI80657
97. Waters AM, Beales PL. Ciliopathies: an expanding disease spectrum. *Pediatr Nephrol* (2011) 26(7):1039–56. doi:10.1007/s00467-010-1731-7
98. Lu D, Rauhauser A, Li B, Ren C, McEnery K, Zhu J, et al. Loss of Glis2/NPHP7 causes kidney epithelial cell senescence and suppresses cyst growth in the Kif3a mouse model of cystic kidney disease. *Kidney Int* (2016) 89(6):1307–23. doi:10.1016/j.kint.2016.03.006
99. Choi HJ, Lin JR, Vannier JB, Slaats GG, Kile AC, Paulsen RD, et al. NEK8 links the ATR-regulated replication stress response and S phase CDK activity to renal ciliopathies. *Mol Cell* (2013) 51(4):423–39. doi:10.1016/j.molcel.2013.08.006

100. Grampa V, Delous M, Zaidan M, Odye G, Thomas S, Elkhartoufi N, et al. Novel NEK8 mutations cause severe syndromic renal cystic dysplasia through YAP dysregulation. *PLoS Genet* (2016) 12(3):e1005894. doi:10.1371/journal.pgen.1005894
101. Al-Hamed MH, Kurdi W, Alsahan N, Alabdullah Z, Abudraz R, Tulbah M, et al. Genetic spectrum of Saudi Arabian patients with antenatal cystic kidney disease and ciliopathy phenotypes using a targeted renal gene panel. *J Med Genet* (2016) 53(5):338–47. doi:10.1136/jmedgenet-2015-103469
102. Schaefer E, Zaloszyc A, Lauer J, Durand M, Stutzmann F, Perdomo-Trujillo Y, et al. Mutations in SDCCAG8/NPHP10 cause Bardet-Biedl syndrome and are associated with penetrant renal disease and absent polydactyly. *Mol Syndromol* (2011) 1(6):273–81. doi:10.1159/000331268
103. Tran PV, Talbott GC, Turbe-Doan A, Jacobs DT, Schonfeld MP, Silva LM, et al. Downregulating Hedgehog signaling reduces renal cystogenic potential of mouse models. *J Am Soc Nephrol* (2014) 25(10):2201–12. doi:10.1681/ASN.2013070735
104. Halbritter J, Porath JD, Diaz KA, Braun DA, Kohl S, Chaki M, et al. Identification of 99 novel mutations in a worldwide cohort of 1,056 patients with a nephronophthisis-related ciliopathy. *Hum Genet* (2013) 132(8):865–84. doi:10.1007/s00439-013-1297-0
105. Graser S, Stierhof YD, Lavoie SB, Gassner OS, Lamla S, Le Clech M, et al. Cep164, a novel centriole appendage protein required for primary cilium formation. *J Cell Biol* (2007) 179(2):321–30. doi:10.1083/jcb.200707181
106. Schaefer E, Stoetzel C, Scheidecker S, Geoffroy V, Prasad MK, Redin C, et al. Identification of a novel mutation confirms the implication of IFT172 (BBS20) in Bardet-Biedl syndrome. *J Hum Genet* (2016) 61(5):447–50. doi:10.1038/jhg.2015.162
107. Mougou-Zerelli S, Thomas S, Szenker E, Audollent S, Elkhartoufi N, Babarit C, et al. CC2D2A mutations in Meckel and Joubert syndromes indicate a genotype-phenotype correlation. *Hum Mutat* (2009) 30(11):1574–82. doi:10.1002/humu.21116
108. Bachmann-Gagescu R, Ishak GE, Dempsey JC, Adkins J, O'Day D, Phelps IG, et al. Genotype-phenotype correlation in CC2D2A-related Joubert syndrome reveals an association with ventriculomegaly and seizures. *J Med Genet* (2012) 49(2):126–37. doi:10.1136/jmedgenet-2011-100552
109. Iannicelli M, Brancati F, Mougou-Zerelli S, Mazzotta A, Thomas S, Elkhartoufi N, et al. Novel TMEM67 mutations and genotype-phenotype correlates in meckelin-related ciliopathies. *Hum Mutat* (2010) 31(5):E1319–31. doi:10.1002/humu.21239
110. Hoefele J, Wolf MT, O'Toole JF, Otto EA, Schultheiss U, Deschenes G, et al. Evidence of oligogenic inheritance in nephronophthisis. *J Am Soc Nephrol* (2007) 18(10):2789–95. doi:10.1681/ASN.2007020243
111. Tory K, Lacoste T, Burglen L, Moriniere V, Boddaert N, Macher MA, et al. High NPHP1 and NPHP6 mutation rate in patients with Joubert syndrome and nephronophthisis: potential epistatic effect of NPHP6 and AHI1 mutations in patients with NPHP1 mutations. *J Am Soc Nephrol* (2007) 18(5):1566–75. doi:10.1681/ASN.2006101164
112. Hopp K, Heyer CM, Hommerding CJ, Henke SA, Sundsbak JL, Patel S, et al. B9D1 is revealed as a novel Meckel syndrome (MKS) gene by targeted exon-enriched next-generation sequencing and deletion analysis. *Hum Mol Genet* (2011) 20(13):2524–34. doi:10.1093/hmg/ddr151
113. Muller J, Stoetzel C, Vincent MC, Leitch CC, Laurier V, Danse JM, et al. Identification of 28 novel mutations in the Bardet-Biedl syndrome genes: the burden of private mutations in an extensively heterogeneous disease. *Hum Genet* (2010) 127(5):583–93. doi:10.1007/s00439-010-0804-9
114. Lindstrand A, Davis EE, Carvalho CM, Pehlivan D, Willer JR, Tsai IC, et al. Recurrent CNVs and SNVs at the NPHP1 locus contribute pathogenic alleles to Bardet-Biedl syndrome. *Am J Hum Genet* (2014) 94(5):745–54. doi:10.1016/j.ajhg.2014.03.017
115. Katsanis N. The continuum of causality in human genetic disorders. *Genome Biol* (2016) 17(1):233. doi:10.1186/s13059-016-1107-9
116. Phelps IG, Dempsey JC, Grout ME, Isabella CR, Tully HM, Doherty D, et al. Interpreting the clinical significance of combined variants in multiple recessive disease genes: systematic investigation of Joubert syndrome yields little support for oligogenicity. *Genet Med* (2017). doi:10.1038/gim.2017.94
117. Hildebrandt F. Identification of a gene for nephronophthisis. *Nephrol Dial Transplant* (1998) 13(6):1334–6. doi:10.1093/ndt/13.6.1334
118. Eley L, Moochhala SH, Simms R, Hildebrandt F, Sayer JA. Nephrocystin-1 interacts directly with Ack1 and is expressed in human collecting duct. *Biochem Biophys Res Commun* (2008) 371(4):877–82. doi:10.1016/j.bbrc.2008.05.016
119. Watnick T, Germino G. From cilia to cyst. *Nat Genet* (2003) 34(4):355–6. doi:10.1038/ng0803-355
120. Pazour GJ, Dickert BL, Vucica Y, Seeley ES, Rosenbaum JL, Witman GB, et al. *Chlamydomonas* IFT88 and its mouse homologue, polycystic kidney disease gene tg737, are required for assembly of cilia and flagella. *J Cell Biol* (2000) 151(3):709–18. doi:10.1083/jcb.151.3.709
121. Nauli SM, Alenghat FJ, Luo Y, Williams E, Vassilev P, Li X, et al. Polycystins 1 and 2 mediate mechanosensation in the primary cilium of kidney cells. *Nat Genet* (2003) 33(2):129–37. doi:10.1038/ng1076
122. Norris DP, Jackson PK. Cell biology: calcium contradictions in cilia. *Nature* (2016) 531(7596):582–3. doi:10.1038/nature17313
123. Delling M, Indzhykulian AA, Liu X, Li Y, Xie T, Corey DP, et al. Primary cilia are not calcium-responsive mechanosensors. *Nature* (2016) 531(7596):656–60. doi:10.1038/nature17426
124. Chang MY, Ong ACM. Targeting new cellular disease pathways in autosomal dominant polycystic kidney disease. *Nephrol Dial Transplant* (2017) 32(12):2144. doi:10.1093/ndt/gfx289
125. Molinari E, Sayer JA. Emerging treatments and personalised medicine for ciliopathies associated with cystic kidney disease. *Expert Opin Orphan Drugs* (2017) 5(10):785–98. doi:10.1080/21678707.2017.1372282
126. Fischer E, Legue E, Doyen A, Nato F, Nicolas JF, Torres V, et al. Defective planar cell polarity in polycystic kidney disease. *Nat Genet* (2006) 38(1):21–3. doi:10.1038/ng1701
127. Germino GG. Linking cilia to Wnts. *Nat Genet* (2005) 37(5):455–7. doi:10.1038/ng0505-455
128. Lancaster MA, Gopal DJ, Kim J, Saleem SN, Silhavy JL, Louie CM, et al. Defective Wnt-dependent cerebellar midline fusion in a mouse model of Joubert syndrome. *Nat Med* (2011) 17(6):726–31. doi:10.1038/nm.2380
129. Lancaster MA, Louie CM, Silhavy JL, Sintasath L, Decambre M, Nigam SK, et al. Impaired Wnt-beta-catenin signaling disrupts adult renal homeostasis and leads to cystic kidney ciliopathy. *Nat Med* (2009) 15(9):1046–54. doi:10.1038/nm.2010
130. Goggolidou P. Wnt and planar cell polarity signaling in cystic renal disease. *Organogenesis* (2014) 10(1):86–95. doi:10.4161/org.26766
131. Calvet JP. (2015). "The role of calcium and cyclic AMP in PKD," in *Polycystic Kidney Disease [Internet]*, ed. X. Li (Brisbane, AU: Codon Publications). doi:10.15586/codon.pkd.2015.ch8
132. Ghosh AK, Hurd T, Hildebrandt F. 3D spheroid defects in NPHP knockdown cells are rescued by the somatostatin receptor agonist octreotide. *Am J Physiol Renal Physiol* (2012) 303(8):F1225–9. doi:10.1152/ajprenal.00135.2012
133. Gattone VH II, Sinders RM, Hornberger TA, Robling AG. Late progression of renal pathology and cyst enlargement is reduced by rapamycin in a mouse model of nephronophthisis. *Kidney Int* (2009) 76(2):178–82. doi:10.1038/ki.2009.147
134. Wahl PR, Serra AL, Le Hir M, Molle KD, Hall MN, Wuthrich RP. Inhibition of mTOR with sirolimus slows disease progression in Han:SPRD rats with autosomal dominant polycystic kidney disease (ADPKD). *Nephrol Dial Transplant* (2006) 21(3):598–604. doi:10.1093/ndt/gfi181
135. Ta MH, Schwensen KG, Foster S, Korgaonkar M, Ozimek-Kulik JE, Phillips JK, et al. Effects of TORC1 inhibition during the early and established phases of polycystic kidney disease. *PLoS One* (2016) 11(10):e0164193. doi:10.1371/journal.pone.0164193
136. Bell PD, Fitzgibbon W, Sas K, Stenbit AE, Amria M, Houston A, et al. Loss of primary cilia upregulates renal hypertrophic signaling and promotes cystogenesis. *J Am Soc Nephrol* (2011) 22(5):839–48. doi:10.1681/ASN.2010050526
137. Boehlke C, Kotsis F, Patel V, Braeg S, Voelker H, Bredt S, et al. Primary cilia regulate mTORC1 activity and cell size through Lkb1. *Nat Cell Biol* (2010) 12(11):1115–22. doi:10.1038/ncb2117
138. Nusslein-Volhard C, Wieschaus E. Mutations affecting segment number and polarity in *Drosophila*. *Nature* (1980) 287(5785):795–801. doi:10.1038/287795a0

139. McMahon AP, Ingham PW, Tabin CJ. Developmental roles and clinical significance of Hedgehog signaling. *Curr Top Dev Biol* (2003) 53:1–114. doi:10.1016/S0070-2153(03)53002-2
140. Wong SY, Reiter JF. The primary cilium at the crossroads of mammalian Hedgehog signaling. *Curr Top Dev Biol* (2008) 85:225–60. doi:10.1016/S0070-2153(08)00809-0
141. Goetz SC, Anderson KV. The primary cilium: a signalling centre during vertebrate development. *Nat Rev Genet* (2010) 11(5):331–44. doi:10.1038/nrg2774
142. Milenkovic L, Scott MP, Rohatgi R. Lateral transport of Smoothened from the plasma membrane to the membrane of the cilium. *J Cell Biol* (2009) 187(3):365–74. doi:10.1083/jcb.200907126
143. Hu MC, Mo R, Bhella S, Wilson CW, Chuang PT, Hui CC, et al. GLI3-dependent transcriptional repression of Gli1, Gli2 and kidney patterning genes disrupts renal morphogenesis. *Development* (2006) 133(3):569–78. doi:10.1242/dev.02220
144. Chan SK, Riley PR, Price KL, McElduff F, Winyard PJ, Welham SJ, et al. Corticosteroid-induced kidney dysmorphogenesis is associated with deregulated expression of known cystogenic molecules, as well as Indian Hedgehog. *Am J Physiol Renal Physiol* (2010) 298(2):F346–56. doi:10.1152/ajprenal.00574.2009
145. Zhang Q, Seo S, Bugge K, Stone EM, Sheffield VC. BBS proteins interact genetically with the IFT pathway to influence SHH-related phenotypes. *Hum Mol Genet* (2012) 21(9):1945–53. doi:10.1093/hmg/dds004
146. Shi X, Garcia G III, Van De Weghe JC, McGorty R, Pazour GJ, Doherty D, et al. Super-resolution microscopy reveals that disruption of ciliary transition-zone architecture causes Joubert syndrome. *Nat Cell Biol* (2017) 19(10):1178–88. doi:10.1038/ncb3622
147. Slaats GG, Ghosh AK, Falke LL, Le Corre S, Shaltiel IA, van de Hoek G, et al. Nephronophthisis-associated CEP164 regulates cell cycle progression, apoptosis and epithelial-to-mesenchymal transition. *PLoS Genet* (2014) 10(10):e1004594. doi:10.1371/journal.pgen.1004594
148. Slaats GG, Giles RH. Are renal ciliopathies (replication) stressed out? *Trends Cell Biol* (2015) 25(6):317–9. doi:10.1016/j.tcb.2015.03.005
149. Braun DA, Hildebrandt F. Ciliopathies. *Cold Spring Harb Perspect Biol* (2017) 9(3):a028191. doi:10.1101/cshperspect.a028191
150. Johnson CA, Collis SJ. Ciliogenesis and the DNA damage response: a stressful relationship. *Cilia* (2016) 5:19. doi:10.1186/s13630-016-0040-6
151. Torres VE, Wang X, Qian Q, Somlo S, Harris PC, Gattone VH II. Effective treatment of an orthologous model of autosomal dominant polycystic kidney disease. *Nat Med* (2004) 10(4):363–4. doi:10.1038/nm1004
152. Wang X, Gattone V II, Harris PC, Torres VE. Effectiveness of vasopressin V2 receptor antagonists OPC-31260 and OPC-41061 on polycystic kidney disease development in the PCK rat. *J Am Soc Nephrol* (2005) 16(4):846–51. doi:10.1681/ASN.2004121090
153. Aihara M, Fujiki H, Mizuguchi H, Hattori K, Ohmoto K, Ishikawa M, et al. Tolvaptan delays the onset of end-stage renal disease in a polycystic kidney disease model by suppressing increases in kidney volume and renal injury. *J Pharmacol Exp Ther* (2014) 349(2):258–67. doi:10.1124/jpet.114.213256
154. Friedlander G, Amiel C. Somatostatin and alpha 2-adrenergic agonists selectively inhibit vasopressin-induced cyclic AMP accumulation in MDCK cells. *FEBS Lett* (1986) 198(1):38–42. doi:10.1016/0014-5793(86)81180-2
155. Torres VE, Chapman AB, Devuyst O, Gansevoort RT, Grantham JJ, Higashihara E, et al. Tolvaptan in patients with autosomal dominant polycystic kidney disease. *N Engl J Med* (2012) 367(25):2407–18. doi:10.1056/NEJMoa1205511
156. Müller R-U, Haas CS, Sayer JA. Practical approaches to the management of autosomal dominant polycystic kidney disease patients in the era of tolvaptan. *Clin Kidney J* (2017):sfx071. doi:10.1093/ckj/sfx071
157. Husson H, Moreno S, Smith LA, Smith MM, Russo RJ, Pitstick R, et al. Reduction of ciliary length through pharmacologic or genetic inhibition of CDK5 attenuates polycystic kidney disease in a model of nephronophthisis. *Hum Mol Genet* (2016) 25(11):2245–55. doi:10.1093/hmg/ddw093
158. Srivastava S, Ramsbottom SA, Molinari E, Alkanderi S, Filby A, White K, et al. A human patient-derived cellular model of Joubert syndrome reveals ciliary defects which can be rescued with targeted therapies. *Hum Mol Genet* (2017) 26(23):4657–67. doi:10.1093/hmg/ddx347
159. Tao Y, Kim J, Schrier RW, Edelstein CL. Rapamycin markedly slows disease progression in a rat model of polycystic kidney disease. *J Am Soc Nephrol* (2005) 16(1):46–51. doi:10.1681/ASN.2004080660
160. Tobin JL, Beales PL. Restoration of renal function in zebrafish models of ciliopathies. *Pediatr Nephrol* (2008) 23(11):2095–9. doi:10.1007/s00467-008-0898-7
161. Westhoff JH, Giselbrecht S, Schmidts M, Schindler S, Beales PL, Tonshoff B, et al. Development of an automated imaging pipeline for the analysis of the zebrafish larval kidney. *PLoS One* (2013) 8(12):e82137. doi:10.1371/journal.pone.0082137
162. Molinari E, Srivastava S, Sayer JA, Ramsbottom SA. From disease modelling to personalised therapy in patients with CEP290 mutations. *F1000Res* (2017) 6:669. doi:10.12688/f1000research.11553.1

7

Bartter Syndrome Type 3: Phenotype-Genotype Correlation and Favorable Response to Ibuprofen

*Xuejun Yang, Gaofu Zhang, Mo Wang, Haiping Yang and Qiu Li**

Department of Nephrology, Children's Hospital of Chongqing Medical University, Chongqing, China

***Correspondence:**
Qiu Li
liqiu809@126.com

Objective: To investigate the phenotype-genotype correlation in different genetic kinds of Bartter syndrome type 3 in children.

Methods: Clinical and genetic data of 2 patients with different mutations in Bartter syndrome type 3 was analyzed while the prognosis was compared after a 6-year follow-up or 2-year follow-up, respectively.

Results: Bartter syndrome is a kind of autosomal recessive inherited renal disorder. The manifestation and prognosis of Bartter syndrome change with mutation types, and severe mutation were often accompanied with unfavorable prognosis. Comprehensive therapy with ibuprofen, antisterone, captopril, and potassium have remarkable effect, while ibuprofen may improve growth retardation partly.

Conclusion: Bartter syndrome should be considered when children have unreasonable continuous electrolyte disturbance, metabolic alkalosis and growth retardation.As a genetic disease, its clinical features depend on the mutation type. It can be ameliorated by electrolyte supplementation, prostaglandin synthetase inhibitors, angiotensin-converting enzyme inhibitors and potassium-sparing diuretic. Considering the following electrolyte disturbances, infections, growth retardation, kidney failure and even death, Bartter syndrome need lifelong treatment, early diagnosis and treatment is the most important.

Keywords: Bartter syndrome, hypokalemia, alkalosis, children, *CLCNKB*

INTRODUCTION

In this study, we reported two cases of Chinese patients with Bartter syndrome type 3 caused by different mutations of *CLCNKB*, which lead to different symptoms and different response to therapeutic measures (the written informed consent was obtained from the parents to publish the case report).

BACKGROUND

Bartter syndrome is a rare diseases, which results from congenital defects in the renal tubular system regulating the reabsorption of sodium, potassium and chloride (1). Based on the different pathogenic genes, Bartter syndrome was classified into five types (Type 1–5) (2). Meanwhile, classical Bartter syndrome, neonatal Bartter syndrome and variant Bartter syndrome (Gitelman syndrome) are the three clinical types of Bartter syndrome (3). Hypokalemia, hypochloremia, metabolic alkalosis, and growth retardation are the most common manifestations of Bartter syndrome (4), while the manifestation and prognosis change with mutation types, and patients with severe mutation often have a unfavorable prognosis. Moreover, comprehensive therapy with electrolyte supplementation, adequate fluid intake, prostaglandin synthetase inhibitors, angiotensin-converting enzyme inhibitors, and potassium-sparing diuretic have remarkable effects (4, 5).

CASE PRESENTATION

Case 1

Clinical Features

A 4-month-old female baby was sent to a children's hospital because of repeated vomiting and growth retardation. Her vomiting, which was not bilious or projectile, had lasted for 2 months and became more and more forceful recently. The baby looked thin and week, with a weight of 3.5 kg (≤3SD), a height of 54 cm (≤3SD), and a head circumference of 37 cm (≤3SD) (6).

The infant was born to a healthy 25-year-old G1P1 mother via spontaneous vaginal delivery at 38 weeks gestational age without antenatal polyhydramnios, with a birth weight of 2.9 kg and height 49 cm, and the Apgar scores was 9, 8, 10, at 1, 5, and 10 min, respectively. The patient's parents and relatives did not have any apparent clinical symptoms such as vomiting. There's no family history of consanguineous marriage and hereditary disease.

After admission, physical examination on the baby was performed. This revealed dehydration and delayed development, which manifested as disability of rising her head. Her blood pressure was 80/60 mmHg, pulse was 139 beats/min, and respiratory rate was 46/min. No rash, edema or hepatosplenomegaly was found. Circulatory, respiratory and neurologic examination did not reveal other specific deficit. Ultrasound of the gastrointestinal tract was normal, while ultrasound of the kidneys showed echo enhancement in both kidney, compatoible with nephrocalcinosis. Electrocadiography showed a low and flat T wave, accompanied with U wave. Serum electrolytes revealed hyponatremia, hypokalemia, and hypochloremia as follows: Na^+ 122.5 mmol/l (normal range 135–145 mmol/l), K^+ 1.8 mmol/l (normal range 3.5–5.5 mmol/l), Cl^- 56.6 mmol/l (normal range 95–110 mmol/l), Mg^{2+} 1.22 mmol/l (normal range 0.8–1.6 mmol/l), Ca^{2+} 2.57 mmol/l (normal range 2.15–2.75 mmol/l). Blood gas analysis showed metabolic alkalosis (pH 7.8, HCO_3^- 35.7 mmol/L, pCO_2 5.6 Kpa). The serum aldosterone level was high (366 pg/ml, normal range 65–296 pg/ml), as well as the rennin activity (8.57 ng/ml/h, normal range 0.05–0.79 ng/ml/h), and the angiotensin II activity (1,084 pg/ml, normal range 28.2–52.5 pg/ml).

In consideration of vomiting, growth retardation, hypokalemia, hypochloremia, and metabolic alkalosis, the infant was treated as a suspect case of Bartter syndrome on the second day. Spironolactone (1 mg/kg/d), catopril (1 mg/kg/d) for oral and adequate intravenous fluid therapy were given. Since the parents refused, prostaglandin synthetase inhibitors such as ibuprofen or indomethacin were not given at that time. On day 6, on account of the discontinued vomiting, normal serum electrolytes and blood gas analysis, the intravenous therapy was replaced of oral KCl solution (10 mmol/kg/d). On day 11, the baby was dismissed from hospital in-patient care with the therapy of KCl and increased fluid intake with age, then started a regular follow-up from then on. During the first 2 years, the baby did not vomit again. Serum electrolytes and blood gas analysis checked every month were normal. In the third year of follow up, when the girl was 4 years old, obvious growth retardation [weight 8.5 kg (≤3SD), height 75 cm (≤3SD)] was still observed (6). After a conversation with her parents, they agreed to start treatment with ibuprofen (30 mg/kg/d, 3 times a day). This led to improved length and wait gain in the following period. However, at the age of 6 years, the girl's weight was 14.9 kg (−3SD∼−2SD) (**Figure 1A**), while the height was 105.4 cm (−2SD∼−SD) (6) (**Figure 1B**).

Mutation Analysis

Informed consent was obtained from the parents for mutational analysis of known Bartter syndrome genes. Genomic DNAs of the patients and their parents were extracted from peripheral blood, while DNA samples from 50 healthy unrelated Chinese people were severed as normal controls. Targeted sequencing using next-generation sequencing was conducted for genes responsible for Bartter syndrome (The detailed methods were in supplemental file 1).

As a result, two mutations of *CLCNKB* were identified. One is a homozygous transition (A–G) at the −2 position of the splicing acceptor site of intron 12 (NM_000085.4:C.1228-2A>G) from her mother (**Figure 2A**), which may resulted in the abnormal splice of exon 12. Another one is a heterozygous loss of exons 1–18(NM_000085.4: Ex1_18 del) from her father (**Figure 2B**). However, neither of these two mutations were detected in the control samples. Given the predicted devastating effect on protein structure of the 2 alleles, segregation within the family and no other mutations detected in known Bartter genes, we regarded the mutations as causative of Bartter syndrome type 3 (OMIM: 607364) in the baby.

Case 2

Clinical Features

A 42/12-year-old boy was brought to hospital because of persistent hypokalemia and growth retardation. His serum potassium was 2.1 mmol/L the day before in a local hospital. He was born to a healthy 20-year-old G1P1 mother via spontaneous vaginal delivery at 39^{+2} weeks gestational age without antenatal polyhydramnios, with a birth weight of 3.4 kg and height 50 cm, and the Apgar scorea were normal. However, the patient's parents were first cousins without family history of hereditary disease.

On admisssion, his weight was 9.9 kg (≤3SD) and height was 83.2 cm (≤3SD) (6). His blood pressure was 92/58 mmHg, pulse was 101 beats/min, and respiratory rate was 31/min. Besides dental enamel dysplasia, no rash, edema or hepatosplenomegaly was found. No disorder showed in circulatory, respiratory, or neurologic examination. Ultrasound of the gastrointestinal tract and electrocadiography were normal while renal ultrasound examination showed echo enhancement in both kidney similar

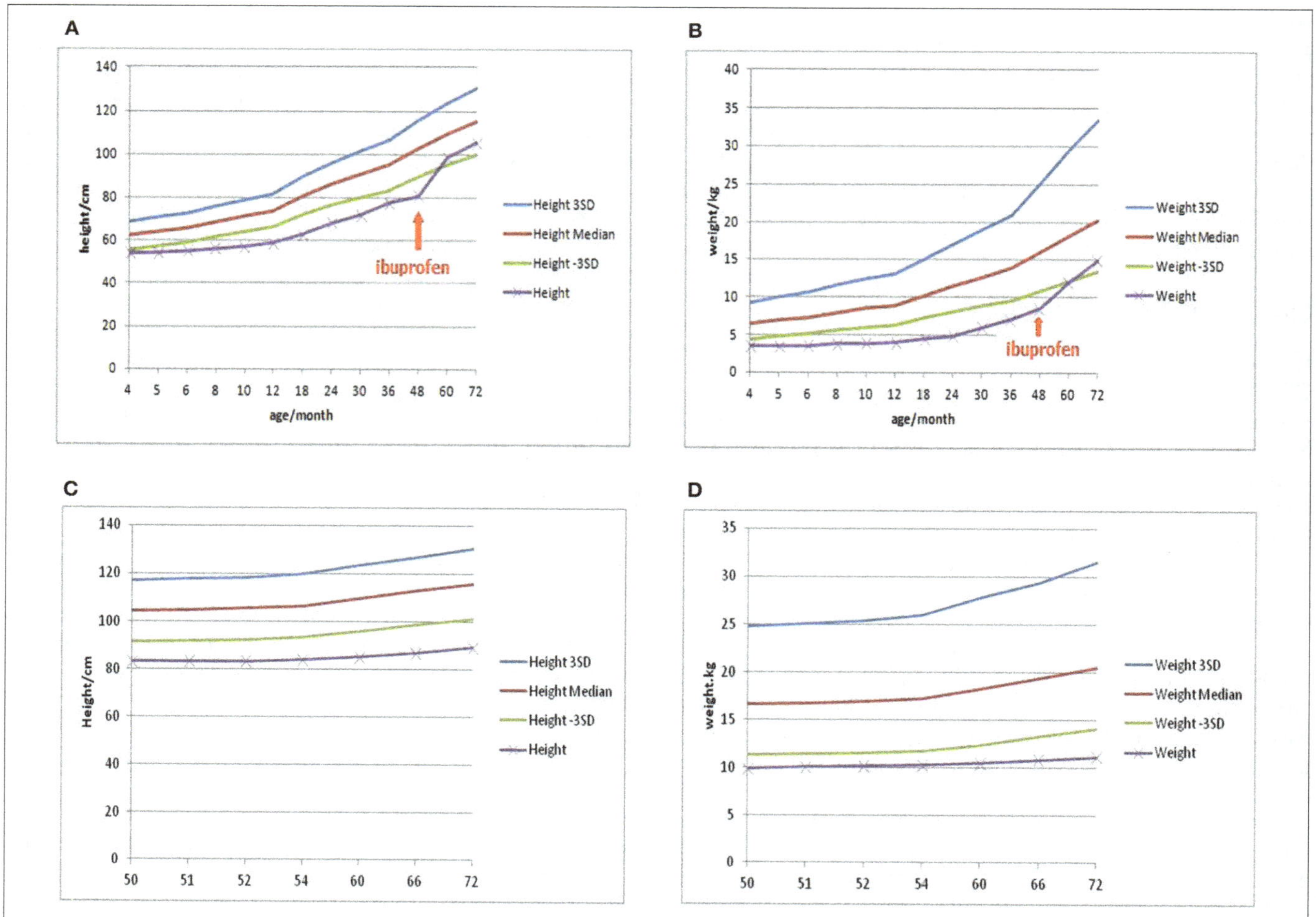

FIGURE 1 | Growth curve of patient 1 showed the effect of ibuprofen in improving weight and height **(A,B)**, while Growth curve of patient 2 showed persistent growth retardation **(C,D)**.

to what was observed in case 1 above. Serum electrolytes revealed hyponatremia, hypokalemia, and hypochloremia as follows: Na^+ 111.9, K^+ 2.3, Cl^- 70.3, Mg^{2+} 0.97, Ca^{2+} 2.52 mmol/L. Blood gas analysis showed metabolic alkalosis (pH 7.57, HCO_3^- 39.4 mmol/L, pCO_2 5.73 Kpa). The serum aldosterone level was high (422 pg/ml), as well as the rennin activity (11.15 ng/ml/h), and the angiotensin II activity (1,459 pg/ml).

With the presentations of growth retardation, hypokalemia and metabolic alkalosis, the boy was clinically diagnosed as Bartter syndrome type 3. Spironolactone (1 mg/kg/d), catopril (1 mg/kg/d), ibuprofen (30 mg/kg/d) for oral and intravenous fluid therapy were given. On day 3, on account of the corrective serum electrolytes and blood gas analysis, the intravenous therapy was replaced by oral KCl solution (10 mmol/kg/d). On day 7, the boy left the hospital with the therapy of KCl and increased fluid intake with age, then started a regular follow-up by telephone from then on (Since he lived in a small village far from our hospital, his parents arranged him to attend a local clinic and informed us about the results via telephone). During these 2 years, serum electrolytes and blood gas analysis checked every month showed that hypokalemia, hypochloremia (K^+ 2.8–4.0 mmol/L, Cl^- 84.1–100.5 mmol/L) and metabolic alkalosis (pH 7.37–7.58, HCO_3^- 28.6–35.7 mmol/L, pCO_2 4.0–6.0 Kpa) still existed. At the age of six, the boy came back to us, still suffering from a severe growth retardation [weight 11.2 kg (≤3SD), height 89.4 cm (≤3SD)] **(6)** (**Figures 1C,D**), hypokalemia, hypochloremia (K^+ 2.38 mmol/L, Cl^- 92.6 mmol/L) and metabolic alkalosis (pH 7.50, HCO_3^- 32.3 mmol/L, pCO_2 5.9 Kpa).

Mutation Analysis

In view of consanguineous marriage, NGS targeted sequencing of known Bartter syndrome genes and whole exome sequencing were both performed and revealed a mutation of CLCNKB. Unfortunately for the patient, since he descended from a consanguineous marriage, he inherited a large homozygous loss of exons 1–18 (NM_000085.4: Ex1_18 del) from his parents (**Figures 3A,B**), which was showed better by PCR electrophoresis of *CLCNKB* (**Figure 3C**). Meanwhile, another mutation of *FAM83H* was also identified, which was a homozygous transition

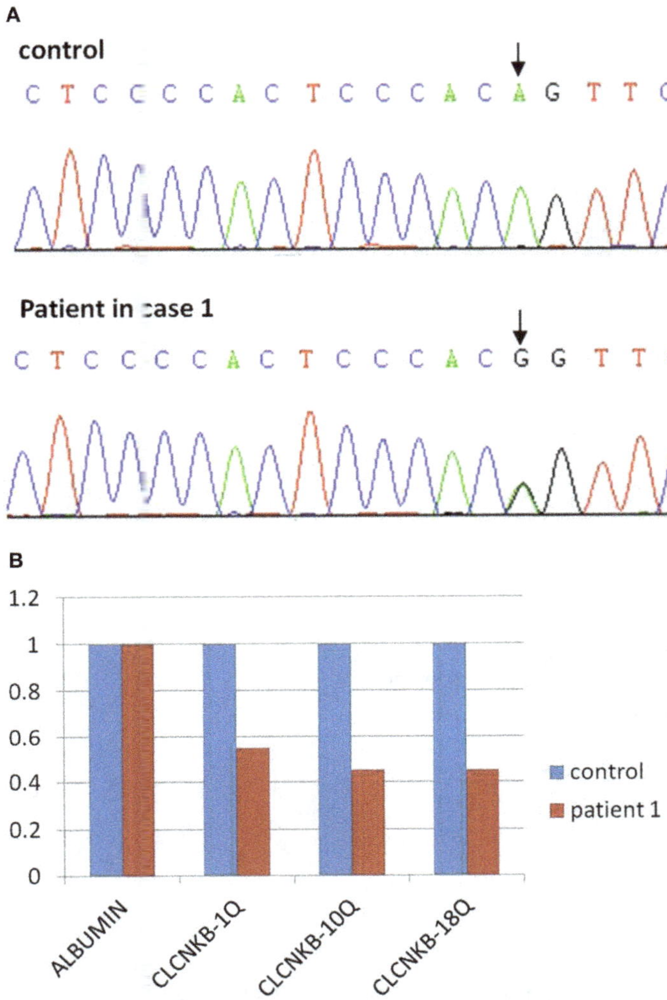

FIGURE 2 | Mutation analysis of patient 1 showed a point mutation of CLCNKB **(A)** and a loss of exons 1–18 **(B)**.

(G to A) in exon 2 (NM_198488.2:C.154G>A), leading to amelogenesis imperfecta type 3 (OMIM: 130900).

DISCUSSION

Bartter syndrome autosomal-recessively inherited and characterized by the association of hypokalemia, hypochloremia, metabolic alkalosis, growth retardation and the activation of the renin-aldosterone axis (4). Since first reported by Bartter et al. (4), more and more patients have been diagnosed. However, a report in 2008 showed its incidence was about 1/1,00,000 (7). Based on the different underlying disease causing genes, Bartter syndrome was classified into five types with mutations in *SLC12A1*, *KCNJ1*, *CLCNKB*, *BSND*, and *CASR* identified to date (8) (**Table 1**).

Bartter syndrome type 3, caused by the mutation in *CLCNKB*, which encodes a protein called ClC-Kb. ClC-Kb is a member of the voltage dependent chloride channel family (ClC), which is expressed in the thick ascending limb of Henle's loop, distal tubule and cortical collecting tubule and regulates the tubular reabsorption of chloride in the kidney (9). As a result, mutations inactivate ClC-Kb, reducing chloride as well as sodium reabsorption in the renal tubules. Moreover, the loss of sodium chloride and water activates the renin-angiotensin-aldosterone

TABLE 1 | Genetic classification of Bartter syndrome.

Type	Inheritance*	Gene	Affected Protein
1	AR	SLC12A1	Sodium-potassium-chloride cotransporter (NKCC2)
2	AR	KCNJ1	Rectified potassium channel (ROMK)
3	AR	CLCNKB	Chloride channel Kb (ClC-Kb)
4	AR	BSND	Barttin protein
5	AD	CASR	Calcium-sensing receptor (CaSR)

**AR, autosomal recessive inheritance; AD, autosomal dominant inheritance.*

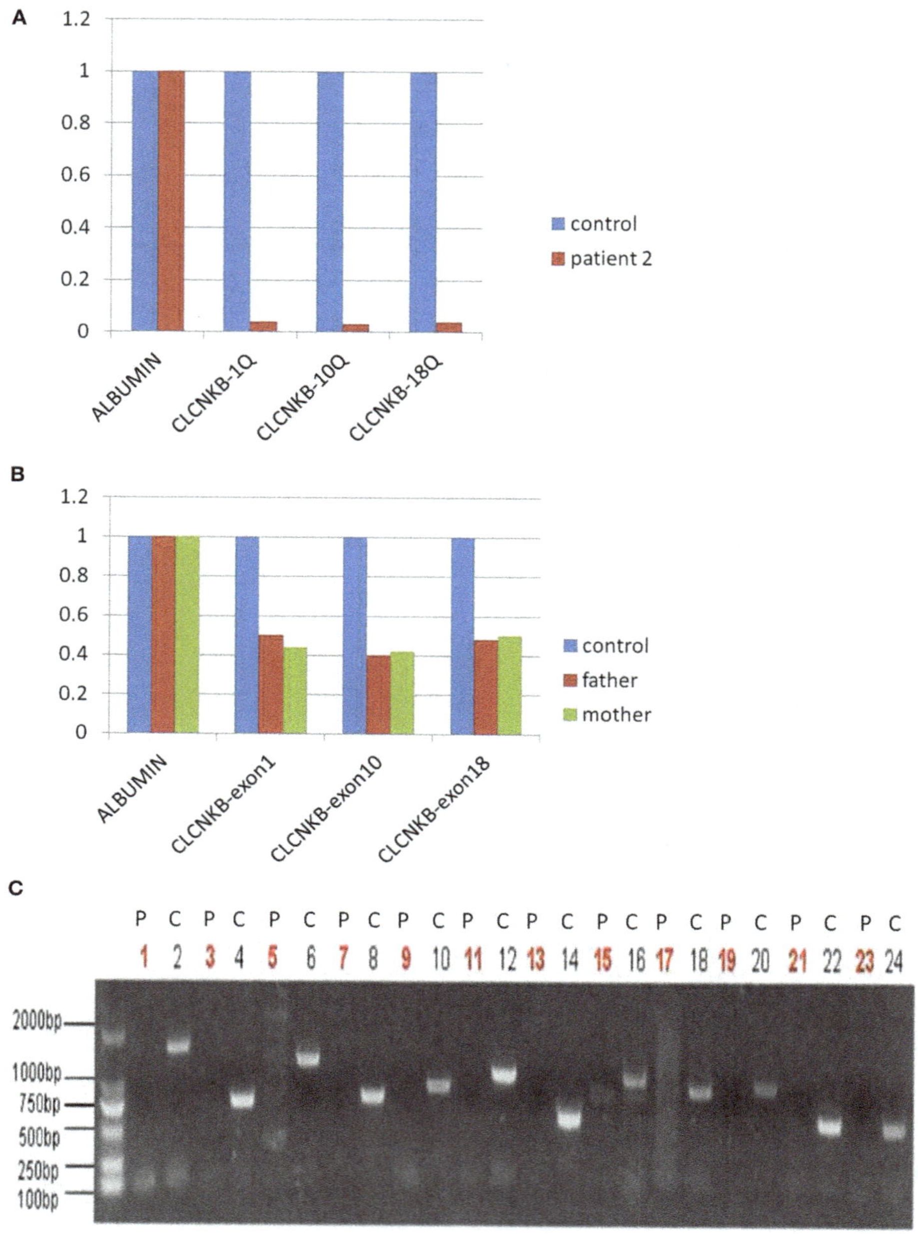

FIGURE 3 | *CLCNKB* q-PCR analysis of patient 2 showed a homozygous loss of exons 1–18 in *CLCNKB* **(A)** while both parents appeared heterozygous **(B)**. Homozygous loss of *CLCNKB* is also shown by absence of bands in gel-electrophoresis of *CLCNKB* specific PCR products specific compared to a control sample **(C)**. P, patient; C, control.

system (RAAS), which contributes to the loss of potassium and renal fibrosis (10, 11). Up to now, more than 50 mutations of *CLCNKB* have been identified, most of which have unclear functional effect (12). In the present study, we identified two different CLNCKB mutations with one individual being compound heterozygous for a splice site mutations and deletion of the entrie gene and the seocnd case being homozygous for the deletion. None of varaints has been found in control samples. Brochard et al. (13) reported a similar *CLCNKB* gene splice mutation at the +1 position of the splicing acceptor site of intron 11 (NM_000085.4:C.1107+1G>T), which may lead to the loss of splice donor site. For another, according to Simon et al. (10), many patients have homozygous *CLCNKB* deletions which result in loss of normal gene function. In view of the foregoing and the patients' clinical features, we believe these mutations are pathogenetic.

As classical Bartter syndrome, Bartter syndrome type 3 is always accompanied with the mildest presentation, begins in infancy or later and often manifests with dehydration, electrolyte imbalance, polyuria, polydipsia, vomiting, and growth retardation (14). However, in both cases, we found echo enhancement in kidney, which may suggest nephrocalcinosis. Nephrocalcinosis and nephrolithiasis are usually found in antenatal and neonatal Bartter syndrome. Nevertheless, recently some studies have mentioned nephrocalcinosis in classical Bartter syndrome (15, 16). It is considered that *CLCNKB* mutations most commonly cause the classic Bartter phenotype, but in a minority of patients, they can also cause phenotypes that overlap with either antenatal Bartter syndrome/neonatal Bartter syndrome or Gitelman sydrome, such as nephrocalcinosis and nephrolithiasis. Exactly what causes nephrocalcinosis is unknown, but several factors may contribute to the condition, such as hypercalciuria, marginal hyperuricosuria, and hyperoxaluria (15).

For all types of Bartter syndrome, phenotypes depend on genotypes (17). Serious mutations always bring severe damage to patients, as in our present cases. Comprehensive therapy with electrolyte supplementation, adequate fluid intake, prostaglandin synthetase inhibitors, angiotensin-converting enzyme inhibitors and potassium-sparing diuretic have remarkable effect (5). Futhermore, for the past few years, more and more studies have raised that, on the basis of salt substitution, prostaglandin synthetase inhibitors may play an important part in improving growth retardation (18–20), which was also suggested in case 1. According to long-term follow-up studies in Bartter Syndrome, with appropriate treatment, patients with Bartter syndrome can achieve normal electrolyte values and growth parameters (21, 22), as we also observed in case 1 regarding the electrolytes while growth retardation remained. Case 2 however still showed electrolyte imbalance, alkalosis and growth retardation even after treatment with salt substitution and prostaglandin synthetase inhibitors. The large homozygous deletion of 18 exons of CLCNKB in case 2 may cause more severe loss of function than the compound heterozygous mutations in case 1. Secondly, considering the parental consangouinous marriage, case 2 may carry additional modifiying alleles such as the mentioned mutation of FAM83H, which may exacerbate his condition. Flyybjerg et al. (23) suggested that hypokalemia is a causative factor of growth retardation, while Masanori et al. (24) stated that sometimes classical Bartter syndrome may be complicated with growth hormone deficiency which could also be the case in case 2. Thus, more laboratory examinations such as growth hormone, whole genome sequencing and longer follow up will be necessary to establish the exact cause for reduced treatment response in Bartter Syndrome patients such as case 2.

In summary, we reported different prognosis of two Chinese patients with different *CLCNKB* gene mutations leading to Bartter syndrome type 3, as well as the effect of prostaglandin synthetase inhibitors in improving growth retardation. Since only two cases are limited in estimating the correlation between phenotype and genotype, more cases should be collected and analyzed in the future. However, considering the patients like which in case 2 still suffer from unsatisfied prognosis, some new treatment such as renin inhibitor (25), as well as more functional study of the mutations, examinations and long follow-up should be taken into account.

ETHICS STATEMENT

This research was approved by the Ethics review committee of Chlidren's Hospital of Chongqing Medical University. Since this is a case report, no protocol or ethics committee was utilized for this report. Any identifiable information has been removed from the manuscript.

AUTHOR CONTRIBUTIONS

XY and GZ assumed clinical duties of this patient while he was hospitalized and drafted the initial manuscript. XY, HY, MW, and QL all reviewed and revised the manuscript. All authors approved the final case report as submitted and agree to be accountable for all aspects of the work.

REFERENCES

1. Chan JC, Gill JR, Bartter FC. Lack of evidence for a role of prostaglandin in the mediation of impaired urinary concentrating ability in Bartter's syndrome. *Nephron* (1983) **35**:116–9. doi: 10.1159/000183058
2. Naesensa M, Steelsb P, Verberckmoesa R, Vanrenterghem Y, Kuypers D. Barter's and Gitelman's syndrome from gene to clinic. *Nephron Physiol.* (2004) **96**:65–78. doi: 10.1159/000076752
3. Madigal G, Saborio P, Mora F, Rincon G, Guay-Woodford LM. Bartter syndrome in CostaRica: a description of 20 cases. *Pediatr Nephrol.* (1997) **11**:296–301. doi: 10.1007/s004670050280
4. Bartter FC, Pronove P, Gill JR Jr, MacCardle RC. Hyperplasia of the juxtaglomerular complex with hyperaldosteronism and hypokalemic alkalosis: a new syndrome. *Am J Med.* (1962) **33**:811–28.
5. Fremont OT, Chan JC. Understanding Bartter syndrome and Gitelman syndrome. *World J Pediatr.* (2012) **8**:25–30. doi: 10.1007/s12519-012-0333-9
6. WHO Multieemer Growth Referfence Study Group. *Who Child Growth Standards: Length/Height-for-Age, Weight-for-Age, Weight-for-Length, Weight-for-Height and Body Mass Inde-for-Age: Methods and Development.* Geneva: World Health Organization. Available online at: http://www.who.int/childgrowth/en/ (Accessed April 27, 2006).
7. Ji W, Foo JN, O'Roak BJ, Zhao H, Larson MG, Simon DB, et al. Rare independent mutations in renal salt handling genes contribute to blood pressure variation. *Nat Genet.* (2008) **40**:592–9. doi: 10.1038/ng.118

8. Kiran BV, Barman H, Iyengar A. Clinical profile and outcome of renal tubular disorders in children: a single center experience. *Indian J Nephrol.* (2014) **24**:362–6. doi: 10.4103/0971-4065.133002
9. Jentsch TJ, Stein V, Weinreich F, Zdebik AA. Molecular structure and physiological function of chloride channels. *Physiol Rev.* (2002) **82**:503–68. doi: 10.1152/physrev.00029.2001
10. Simon DB, Bindra RS, Mansfield TA, Nelson-Williams C, Mendonca E, Stone R, et al. Mutations in the chloride channel gene, CLCKNB, cause Bartter's syndrome type III. *Nat Genet.* (1997) **17**:171–8. doi: 10.1038/ng1097-171
11. Sun Y, Zhang J, Zhang JQ, Ramires FJ. Local angiotensin II and transforming growth factor-beta 1 in renal fibrosis of rats. *Hyperension* (2000) **35**:1078–4. doi: 10.1161/01.HYP.35.5.1078
12. Yu Y, Xu C, Pan X, Ren H, Wang W, Meng X, et al. Identification and functional analysis of novel mutations of the CLCNKB gene in Chinese patients with classic Bartter syndrome. *Clin Genet.* (2010) **77**:155–62. doi: 10.1111/j.1399-0004.2009.01288.x
13. Brochard K, Boyer O, Blanchard A, Loirat C, Niaudet P, Macher MA, et al. Phenotype-genotype correlation in antenatal and neonatal variants of Bartter syndrome. *Nephrol Dial Transplant.* (2009) **24**:1455–64. doi: 10.1093/ndt/gfn689
14. Rodriguez-Soriano J. Bartter and related syndromes: the puzzle is almost solved. *Pediatr Nephrol.* (1998) **12**:315–27. doi: 10.1007/s004670050461
15. Colussi G, De Ferrari ME, Tedeschi S, Prandoni S, Syrén ML, Civati G. Bartter syndrome type 3: an unusual cause of nephrolithiasis. *Nephrol Dial Transplant.* (2002) **17**:521–2. doi: 10.1093/ndt/17.3.521
16. García Castaño A, Pérez de Nanclares G, Madariaga L, Aguirre M, Madrid Á, Chocrón S, et al. Poor phenotype-genotype association in alarge series of patients with Type III Bartter syndrome. *PLoS ONE* (2017) **12**:e0173581. doi: 10.1371/journal.pone.0173581
17. Al Shibli A, Narchi H. Bartter and Gitelman syndromes: spectrum of clinical manifestations caused by different mutations. *World Methodol.* (2015) **5**:55–61. doi: 10.5662/wjm.v5.i2.55
18. Littlewood JM, Lee MR, Meadow SR. Treatment of Bartter's syndrome in early childhood with prostaglandin synthetase inhibitors. *Archiv Dis Child.* (1978) **53**:43–8.
19. Kleta R, Basoglu C, Kuwertz-Bröking E. New treatment options for Bartter's syndrome. *N Engl J Med.* (2000) **343**:661–2. doi: 10.1056/NEJM200008313430915
20. Ahmed HA, Khalifa M, Alnaimi L. An infant with poor weight gain and hypochloremic metabolic alkalosis: a case report. *Int J Gen Med.* (2014) **7**:389–91. doi: 10.2147/IJGM.S66550
21. Nakagawa Y, Toya K, Natsume H, Nasuda K, Takeuchi H, Kubota A, et al. Long-term follow-up of a girl with the neonatal form of Bartter's syndrome. *Endocr J.* (1997) **44**:275–81.
22. Puricelli E, Bettinell A, Borsa N, Sironi F, Mattiello C, Tammaro F, et al. Long-term follow-up of patients with Bartter syndrome type I and II. *Nephrol Dial Transplant.* (2010) **25**:2976–81. doi: 10.1093/ndt/gfq119
23. Flyybjerg A, Dorup I, Everts ME, Orskov H. Evidence that potassium deficiency induces growth retardation through reduced circulating levels of growth hormone and insulin-like growth factor I. *Metabolism* (1991) **40**:769–75. doi: 10.1016/0026-0495(91)90001-D
24. Masanori A, Toshiniro T, Koji Muroyal, Asakura Y. Classical Bartter syndrome complicated with profound growth hormone deficiency: a case report. *J Med Case Rep.* (2013) **7**:283–7. doi: 10.1186/1752-1947-7-283
25. Mendonça M1, Pinheiro A, Castro I. Bartter syndrome: a new therapeutic approach. *Acta Med Port.* (2011) **24**:671–4.

8

Zebrafish as a Model for Drug Screening in Genetic Kidney Diseases

Jochen Gehrig[1], Gunjan Pandey[1,2] and Jens H. Westhoff[2]*

[1] Acquifer is a Division of Ditabis, Digital Biomedical Imaging Systems AG, Pforzheim, Germany, [2] Department of Pediatrics I, University Children's Hospital Heidelberg, Heidelberg, Germany

***Correspondence:**
Jens H. Westhoff
jens.westhoff@med.uni-heidelberg.de

Genetic disorders account for a wide range of renal diseases emerging during childhood and adolescence. Due to the utilization of modern biochemical and biomedical techniques, the number of identified disease-associated genes is increasing rapidly. Modeling of congenital human disease in animals is key to our understanding of the biological mechanism underlying pathological processes and thus developing novel potential treatment options. The zebrafish (*Danio rerio*) has been established as a versatile small vertebrate organism that is widely used for studying human inherited diseases. Genetic accessibility in combination with elegant experimental methods in zebrafish permit modeling of human genetic diseases and dissecting the perturbation of underlying cellular networks and physiological processes. Beyond its utility for genetic analysis and pathophysiological and mechanistic studies, zebrafish embryos, and larvae are amenable for phenotypic screening approaches employing high-content and high-throughput experiments using automated microscopy. This includes large-scale chemical screening experiments using genetic models for searching for disease-modulating compounds. Phenotype-based approaches of drug discovery have been successfully performed in diverse zebrafish-based screening applications with various phenotypic readouts. As a result, these can lead to the identification of candidate substances that are further examined in preclinical and clinical trials. In this review, we discuss zebrafish models for inherited kidney disease as well as requirements and considerations for the technical realization of drug screening experiments in zebrafish.

Keywords: zebrafish, drug screening, compound screening, genetic kidney disease, high-throughput, high-content, automated microscopy

INTRODUCTION

Modern genetic diagnostics allow the rapid discovery of human disease-associated mutations. Moreover, human genetic disorders can often be mimicked in animal models that can be exploited in large-scale chemical investigations for the search of modifiers of disease-associated phenotypes and potentially therapeutic compounds. The zebrafish (*Danio rerio*) has become an increasingly accepted vertebrate model organism for biomedical research (1, 2).

Despite being a member of the teleost class of fish species, there is great homology in development as well as cell- and organ-specific structural and physiological properties between zebrafish and humans. Furthermore, even with the evolutionary distance, > 80% of human disease-associated genes have orthologs in the zebrafish genome (3). The embryonic and larval characteristics of zebrafish include small size, *ex utero* development, optical transparency, and rapidity of organogenesis. In combination with the high fecundity of adult zebrafish and a relatively simple and cost-effective animal husbandry, this enables large-scale *in vivo* investigations. The zebrafish genome has been completely sequenced, thus facilitating genetic and genomic analysis and manipulation (3, 4). For instance, reverse genetics allow for precise investigation of associated phenotypes, by e.g., transient gene knockdown using antisense morpholino oligos or by genome-editing technologies like the CRISPR/Cas9 system (5, 6).

Due to the simplicity of the pronephros that can be readily studied in embryonic and larval stages, the zebrafish is an applicable experimental model system for the analysis of renal development and disease (7). The pronephros, as the earliest nephric stage, contains two nephrons sharing numerous genetic, structural, and functional aspects with the mammalian nephron (8). Phenotypic changes upon genetic alterations can be easily analyzed within intact live animals (9). Large-scale mutagenesis screens have identified various mutants affecting kidney development allowing the exploration of genetic and molecular mechanisms underlying pronephros development and function (10, 11). Moreover, reverse genetics approaches enable researchers to specifically alter orthologous genetic elements potentially associated with human disease. To date, major fields of research where such zebrafish models are being employed include glomerular (i.e., podocytopathies) and cystic renal disorders (i.e., ciliopathies).

Phenotype-based screening for drug discovery applications is increasingly employed in biomedical and pharmaceutical research. In contrast to target-based screening, phenotype-based approaches do not require exact knowledge of the therapeutic target (7). In addition, whole-organism *in vivo* approaches have the advantage that they can unravel toxic and other side-effects of drugs at a very early stage of the study. Over the last years, due to the versatility and power of the model, the zebrafish has emerged as the main vertebrate model system for high-throughput and high-content chemical screening experiments and large-scale phenotypic scoring (12, 13). Clear and scalable readouts for *in vivo* large-scale experiments can be readily established and a plethora of mutant and transgenic models expressing fluorescent proteins driven by tissue-specific promoters is available. In combination with automation technologies and dedicated sample handling workflows, this has led to various biomedical screening assays in fields such as genetics (14, 15), toxicology (16, 17), immunology and infection biology (18, 19), cardiovascular research (20, 21), drug discovery and safety (12, 13, 22, 23), personalized medicine (24), non-coding-genome analysis (25) as well as behavioral analysis (26, 27). Notably, several compounds that were identified in the zebrafish model have made it to preclinical and clinical trials, including new substance classes and repurposed drugs (12). For instance, in a chemical genetic screen testing 2.480 compounds, prostaglandin E2 (PGE2) was identified as an evolutionarily conserved regulator of hematopoietic stem cell (HSC) number in zebrafish embryos (28). Based on these results, a chemical derivative of PGE2 (Prohema), has been developed with the aim of improving the efficiency of HSC transplants using umbilical cord blood. Prohema has meanwhile advanced to Phase II clinical trials.

GENETIC KIDNEY DISEASES IN ZEBRAFISH

Genetic kidney diseases can affect all parts of the kidney and its functions. To date, mutations in more than 150 genes have been identified that cause genetic human kidney diseases such as alterations of kidney development or specific glomerular and tubular diseases (29). Nephrogenesis in vertebrates is an intricate process that includes the successive formation of up to three kidneys depending on the species position in the phylogenetic tree: the pronephros, mesonephros, and metanephros (30). There is an increasing complexity with each successive kidney developing, however the structure and function of the basic renal units, the nephrons, remains largely unvaried across vertebrates (31).

In zebrafish, major vertebrate organ systems form within a few days after fertilization (32). The zebrafish pronephros is functional by 48 hpf (hours post fertilization) accomplishing the functions of blood filtration and osmoregulation (11, 33). It consists of two nephrons with a fused glomerulus at the midline (**Figure 1A**) (24). The tubular system consisting of the pronephric proximal and distal tubule and pronephric duct contains segment-specific conserved structural and physiological properties and spatio-temporal gene-expression patterns that are homologous to the human kidney (**Figure 1B**) (8, 35, 36). The zebrafish glomerulus is endowed with podocytes with extended and interdigitating foot processes and fenestrated endothelial cells forming a functional glomerular filtration barrier, analogous to the metanephric glomerulus of higher vertebrates (11).

At present, zebrafish is predominantly used as a genetic model for normal and abnormal kidney development, for hereditary glomerulopathies (i.e., podocytopathies) and for the study of ciliopathy-associated human cystic kidney diseases. These encompass polycystic kidney diseases and diseases of the nephronophthisis/medullary cystic kidney disease complex including more complex ciliopathies such as Joubert Syndrome, Meckel-Gruber Syndrome, and Bardet-Biedl-Syndrome (37). In this review, we focus on glomerulopathies and cystic kidney diseases.

ZEBRAFISH AS A MODEL FOR HUMAN HEREDITARY GLOMERULOPATHIES

Zebrafish models can recapitulate human genetic glomerulopathies, i.e., a variety of podocytopathies that clinically often manifest by steroid-resistant nephrotic syndrome (SRNS) due to podocyte foot process effacement. SRNS is mostly therapy-resistant and leads to end-stage renal disease (ESRD) within a few years of onset. A growing number of SRNS-causing mutations have been identified. For example, mutations in *NPHS1*, encoding Nephrin, cause congenital nephrotic syndrome of the Finnish type. Morpholino knockdown of *nphs1* in zebrafish results in edema and loss of slit-diaphragms with

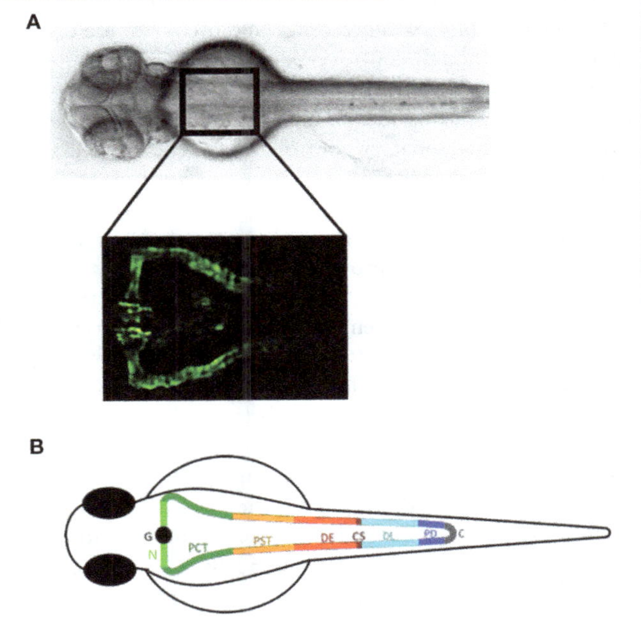

FIGURE 1 | The zebrafish pronephros: anatomical position and segmental organization. **(A)** Brightfield dorsal view of a 2 day post fertilization (dpf) zebrafish embryo (upper panel). The rectangle in the anterior trunk indicates the location of the proximal pronephric structures with a fused glomerulus at the midline that connects to the segmented pronephric tubules as labeled in the *Tg(wt1b:egfp)* zebrafish line by GFP expression (lower panel). **(B)** Schematic illustration of a zebrafish pronephros showing segmental organization of each nephron into glomerulus (G), neck (N), proximal convoluted tubule (PCT), proximal straight tubule (PST), distal early (DE), corpuscle of Stannius (CS), distal late (DL), and pronephric duct (PD) that fuse to the cloaca (C). Adapted from Wingert and Davidson (34).

abnormal podocyte foot processes (38, 39). Mutations in *WT1* (Wilms' tumor gene 1) have been associated with syndromic disorders such as Denys-Drash syndrome and Frasier syndrome, but also with diffuse mesangial sclerosis and early-onset isolated nephrotic syndrome (40). In zebrafish, knockdown of *wt1a* results in defects in podocyte development leading to glomerular injury and nephrosis (41). Mutations in *NPHS2*, Podocin, are the most relevant cause of autosomal-recessive SRNS of childhood. Zebrafish *nphs2* morphants display pronephric glomerular hypoplasia with pericardial edema and ultrastructural glomerular damage of the filtration barrier (38, 39). Mutations in *PLCE1* (Nephrocystin-3, NPHS3) have been identified in patients with SRNS and disease onset in the first year of life with a rapid progression to ESRD (42, 43). Zebrafish *plce1* morphants display an impairment of the kidney filtration barrier as measured by tubular uptake of filtered 500 kDa fluorescent dextran, accompanied by edema, and severe disorganization of slit diaphragms (43). Other rare human mutations that were mimicked in zebrafish include *ADCK4* (AarF domain containing kinase 4 gene) (44), *KANK1* (kidney ankyrin repeat-containing protein 1), *KANK2*, *KANK4* (45), *CRB2* (Crumbs homolog 2) (46), *NUP107* (Nuclear Pore Complex Subunit 107) (47), and *ARHGDIA* (48).

Whereas in many studies of genetic glomerulopathies the zebrafish has been used to model human disease-associated phenotypes, disruption of the glomerular filtration barrier can only be visualized by ultrastructural techniques like super-resolution or electron microscopy that are not compatible with large-scale chemical screens. Edema formation in zebrafish embryos can indirectly report glomerular barrier impairments; however, despite being easily observed in brightfield microscopy it is not exclusively linked to renal impairment (49). This restricts its value as a phenotypic readout parameter in chemical kidney screens. Functional assessment of glomerular filtration and barrier integrity can be achieved by monitoring the temporal reporter activity after microinjection of fluorescently labeled inulin (50) or dextrans of different molecular weight (51–53) into the vascular system; however, this method is laborious and incompatible with extensive screening experiments. Additionally, a transgenic zebrafish that expresses GFP (green fluorescent protein)-tagged vitamin D-binding protein (VDBP), which acts as a tracer for proteinuria, has been reported (54) and may serve as an attractive alternative for high-content and high-throughput screening (53).

ZEBRAFISH AS A MODEL FOR HUMAN CYSTIC KIDNEY DISEASES

Cystic diseases of the kidney are frequent monogenic disorders in humans (55, 56), with primary cilia dysfunction being the unifying cellular mechanism leading to most if not all cystic kidney diseases (56–58). Mutations in a variety of genes encoding the primary cilia/centrosome complex cause ciliopathies often associated with the development of renal cysts, in both human and zebrafish (59–64). However, it must be noted that cilia in the zebrafish pronephros are motile, whereas human renal cilia are thought to be non-motile (65, 66), suggesting a potential contribution of lack of fluid dynamics to cyst formation in the zebrafish model.

Mutations in polycystin-1 and polycystin-2 are responsible for autosomal dominant polycystic kidney disease (ADPKD), the most common human congenital renal disorder (67). In zebrafish, polycystin-2 morpholino knockdown or mutation of orthologous *pkd* genes induces kidney cysts, hydrocephalus, left/right asymmetry defects, and strong dorsal axis curvature (63, 68, 69). Autosomal recessive polycystic kidney disease (ARPKD) usually manifests perinatally or in childhood. In addition to *PKHD1* (polycystic kidney and hepatic disease 1), mutations in *DZIP1L* (DAZ interacting zinc finger protein 1 like) have recently been associated with ARPKD (70, 71). Other than *dzip1l* morphants and *dzip1l* CRISPR mutants, Lu et al. injected the *dzip1l* translation-blocking morpholino into *Tg(wt1b:egfp)* transgenic embryos expressing GFP under Wilms' tumor suppressor *(wt1b)* promoter in the pronephros (72), allowing for *in vivo* fluorescence imaging of the cystic pronephros.

Nephronophthisis (NPHP), an autosomal recessive cystic kidney disease, represents the most frequent genetic cause of ESRD in the first three decades of life (55). Nephronophthisis can be accompanied by anomalies in other organs, such as cerebellar vermis hypoplasia, laterality defects, intellectual disability, shortening of bones, retinal degeneration, and hepatobiliary disease (56). These features are represented in a variety of syndromes, including Senior–Løken syndrome, Joubert syndrome, Bardet–Biedl syndrome, and Jeune asphyxiating thoracic dystrophy (73, 74). To date, NPHP-causing mutations have been identified in more than 20 genes (56). Morpholino knockdown in zebrafish has been performed for *nphp2* to *6* (75–83) and *nphp11* (84). Zebrafish mutants for *arl13b/sco*^{hi459} (85), *ahi1*^{lri46} (86), and *cc2d2a* (87) develop pronephric cysts to varying degrees and serve as models for Joubert syndrome-related disease.

Intraflagellar transport (IFT) proteins are essential for the development and maintenance of motile and sensory cilia and localize to the cilium, basal body, and/or centrosome (88). Several zebrafish *ift* mutants demonstrating renal cysts were identified by forward genetic screens (63, 89). *IFT80* mutations underlie a subset of Jeune asphyxiating thoracic dystrophy cases, of which 20% are associated with kidney abnormalities including renal cysts (90). *Ift80* morphants show a dose-dependent phenotype with strong body curvature, large kidney cyst, and pericardial edema. *IFT172* mutations were initially reported in Jeune and Mainzer-Saldino syndromes, but have also been observed in patients with Bardet-Biedl syndrome (91, 92). Zebrafish mutants and morphants for *ift172* resemble these phenotypes, with renal cysts readily detectable in brightfield images (91). In our work, we have shown that morpholino knockdown of *ift80* and *ift172* in *Tg(wt1b:egfp)* with fluorescently labeled kidney structures allow for visualization of pronephric cysts, providing a model system for large-scale chemical screening studies to identify chemical modifiers of cyst formation (93).

CHEMICAL SCREENING IN ZEBRAFISH—TECHNICAL ASPECTS AND CONSIDERATIONS

The zebrafish can cost-effectively bridge the gap between high-throughput experimentation in cellular models lacking physiological context and low-throughput models such as rodents that are closer to human biology (12, 13, 23, 94). The optically transparent embryos and larvae fit into wells of microtiter plates rendering them amenable for automated microscopy applications using existing screening technologies (12, 13, 17, 23). Due to accessibility to genetic manipulation (37, 95), a plethora of zebrafish transgenic and mutant lines has been generated (www.zfin.org, www.ezrc.kit.edu, www.zebrafish.org) (96), complemented by transient labeling, knockdown and genome-editing techniques (97). This provides an extraordinary rich toolkit to model and visualize the biological processes underlying development and disease. Several transgenic lines labeling pronephric structures such as podocytes (98, 99), tubules, and ducts (98, 100–106) or both (72) have been established. In combination with genetic alteration, either by transient gene knockdown using antisense morpholino oligos or by genome-editing technologies, these lines can mimic e.g., ARPKD (71), ADPKD (107), and other cystic kidney diseases (93, 108) and enable *in vivo* fluorescence microscopy of the diseased pronephros. Although controversies exist regarding the use of morphants generated by morpholino knockdown (109–113), they remain a valuable tool in altering target gene expression, provided that all mandatory control experiments to validate the observed disease-associated phenotypes have been conducted (110, 111).

To our knowledge, large-scale screening experiments evaluating fluorescent pronephric phenotypes in models of genetic kidney diseases have not been demonstrated. In a chemical modifier screen using a custom library of 115 compounds in *pkd2*^{hi4166} and *ift172*^{hi2211} mutants displaying renal cysts (114), morphological parameters such as body axis curvature and/or laterality defects were scored. Histone deacetylase inhibitors Tricostatin A and valproic acid attenuated these phenotypes, and cyst size-reducing effects were confirmed in secondary assays. Additionally, a chemical screen of ~2,000 compounds identified histone deacetylase inhibitors to expand the pool of embryonic renal progenitor cells (115), a mechanism presumably involved in regeneration following acute kidney injury.

In combination with automated microscopy (116), zebrafish disease model systems allow performing large-scale phenotypic whole organism screening assays (117, 118). Phenotypic readouts encompass survival rates, overall morphology, physiological parameters, cell- and tissue-specific phenotypes, reporter gene expression patterns, and behavioral phenotypes (25, 27, 93, 119–123). Phenotypic screens within the context of a live vertebrate provide significant advantage over classical target-based *in vitro* assays as they do not require a priori knowledge about biochemical pathways affected, thus allowing unbiased identification of drug candidates or toxicological effects of substances. Furthermore, they intrinsically involve potential contributions of biodistribution, metabolism, and pharmacokinetics (1, 12, 13, 17, 95, 124).

Prior to large-scale zebrafish experiments careful planning and preparatory experiments are required to generate robust protocols and tailor conditions toward desired readouts in screening compatible disease models. In brief, handling of thousands of embryos causes logistical challenges, thus protocols for animal husbandry, micromanipulation, embryo culture, and treatment (e.g., anesthesia), and sample handling must be established. When image-based assays are carried out the usage of pigmentation mutant strains (e.g., casper line) or chemical treatment (e.g., 1-phenyl-2-thiourea, PTU) to block pigment formation is often necessary to adequately visualize internal structures. Moreover, to minimize false positive and negative results, non-specific developmental toxicity or off-target effects, control experiments must be carried out to titrate required compound concentration ranges as well as the treatment period during embryonic development. Importantly, controls should also be continuously carried out as a reference readout to benchmark observed phenotypic effects and normalize experimental variation. Finally, image acquisition routines must be balanced with analysis

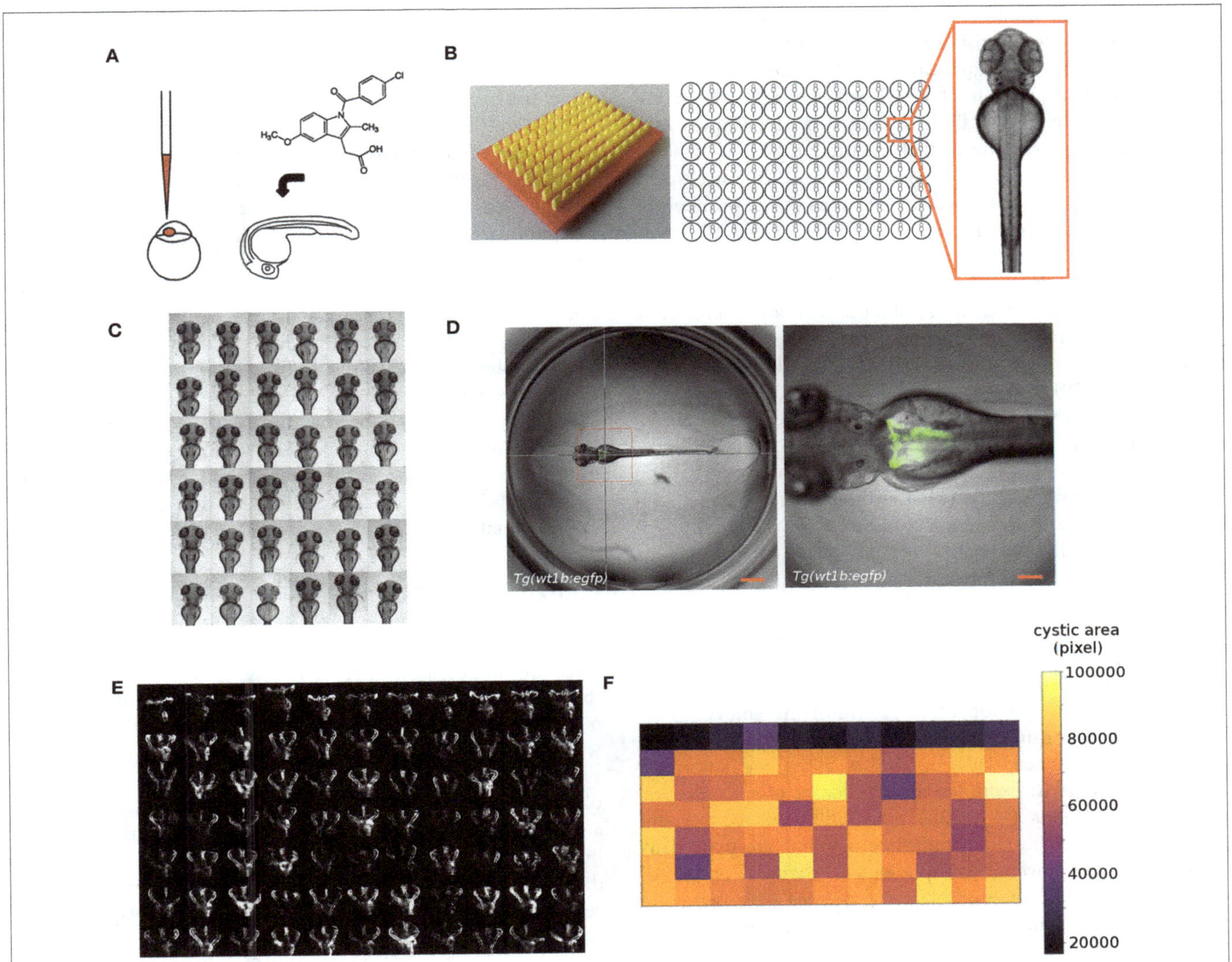

FIGURE 2 | Overview of screening workflows for organ specific phenotypic screening in zebrafish. Shown are examples from our screening work that illustrate the automatic acquisition of higher resolution datasets of embryonic kidneys in zebrafish embryos. **(A)** Experimental manipulation of embryos prior to mounting and automated imaging such as microinjection or compound treatment. **(B)** Mounting of zebrafish embryos in agarose coated microtiter plates generated using 3D printed orientation tools. Agarose layers contain cavities allowing for consistent alignment and orientation of specimen. **(C)** Automated acquisition of standardized views (e.g., dorsal) of zebrafish embryos arrayed in microtiter plates. **(D)** Automated acquisition of multidimensional image datasets using smart imaging techniques. Pronephric areas of the *Tg(wt1b:egfp)* zebrafish transgenic line are detected in low resolution datasets using image processing tools and are subsequently imaged at higher resolution. The hair cross indicates the detected position and the bounding box the field of view in subsequent higher resolution imaging. Scale bars indicate 600 μm (left panel) or 150 μm (right panel). **(E)** Detailed visualization of kidney regions enabling scoring of kidney phenotypes. Shown are wildtype (first row) or cystic (other rows) kidneys of 72 hpf *Tg(wt1b:egfp)* embryos. **(F)** Automated quantitative analysis and phenotypic scoring using image processing techniques. Heatmap shows quantitative measurements of cystic areas as shown in **(E)**. Figure panels are taken or modified from Westhoff et al. (93), Wittbrodt et al. (125), Pandey et al. (unpublished), and www.acquifer.de.

needs to ensure effective and robust scoring of phenotypic alterations.

Despite its amenability to large-scale experimentation, the full exploitation of the zebrafish model in screening assays is often hampered. While sample manipulation can be scaled efficiently, large-scale imaging, and phenotypic scoring remains challenging as available screening methodologies are usually optimized for *in vitro* assays (**Figure 2A**) (126). In comparison to cellular models, zebrafish embryos are large three-dimensional objects of complex morphology leading to random orientation of embryos within wells of microtiter plates (126, 127). This can obscure the view on target structures and leads to the generation of non-standardized image data. Therefore, novel sample preparations or automation strategies are needed, as it is unfeasible to upscale classical zebrafish mounting techniques. In our work, we developed orientation tools allowing the generation of agarose cavities within wells of microtiter plates for consistent positioning and orientation of zebrafish embryos (**Figure 2B**) (25, 93, 125). This enables the automated acquisition of consistent views of 48–96 hpf zebrafish larvae in large-scale screening scenarios (**Figure 2C**). For instance, we employed that methodology for imaging of embryonic kidneys in automated large-scale microscopy assays to score for morphological alterations of the pronephros upon compound exposure (93, 125, 128) (Westhoff et al. unpublished data) or capture phenotypic changes in cystic kidney disease models (129) (Pandey et al., unpublished data). Other more complex technical solutions employ microfluidic systems that combine automated detection and rotational orientation within glass capillaries followed by microscopic imaging (127, 130).

To date, the vast majority of zebrafish screens employ low magnification to capture the entire zebrafish embryo body, followed by subsequent analysis of phenotypic changes (13, 131). However, this significantly attenuates the power of using a fully developed live vertebrate embryo as *in vivo* visualization of morphological, physiological or genetic events on the cell- or tissue-specific level is hampered. The widespread usage of low resolution assays is largely due to the impracticality of positioning the regions of interest (ROI) within the small field of views of higher magnification objectives in combination with fixed scan-field coordinates of automated microscopes. Additionally, the spatiotemporal location of ROIs within the embryo body might be variable or unpredictable. To overcome that limitation, technologies have been developed that allow the automatic centering of ROIs in front of objective lenses of microscopes. Microfluidic systems (127, 130) can fulfill that requirement but usually require rather complex setups and are potentially challenged when overall morphological changes occur, or developmental and disease-associated processes are observed in time-lapse experiments. Several automated microscopy solutions for microplate-based screening have been reported that allow to teach or detect the position of ROIs followed by automatic centering and multidimensional image acquisition (126, 132–134). This can be an expert operator manually selecting target structures for subsequent automated imaging or more advanced methods employing automatic detection by image processing. These automated smart imaging approaches are based on interfacing the imaging device with external software tools that automatically detect coordinates of features of interest and send back machine commands containing instructions for re-centering, higher resolution imaging, or tracking of target structures. While several solutions have been reported, their application is usually restricted to cellular models and they are often characterized by a high level of complexity requiring expert knowledge in image processing, general programming and hard- and software interfacing. Therefore, to enable a widespread usage of such toolsets novel developments are needed that provide a simplified access to biomedical researchers. To this extent, we have developed a robotic microscopy platform (www.acquifer.de) with a smart imaging interface that allows to manually select ROIs, or to use any image processing software to send back human-readable script commands to the imaging device. We utilize this technique to e.g., acquire high-resolution datasets of cystic kidneys in a genetic zebrafish disease model to screen for modifiers of cystogenesis (**Figures 2D–F**) (129) (Pandey et al., unpublished data).

Due to the wide variety of potential zebrafish screening assays and thus phenotypic readouts there are myriad of potential quantitative descriptors that can be extracted from image-based datasets. This can include fluorescence intensity, morphological descriptors, or dynamic parameters and ranges from simple whole embryo signal intensity to spatiotemporal activity of fluorescent reporters or tissue dynamics and beyond. For instance, advanced segmentation techniques were used in the *Tg(cdh17:egfp)*^{pt305} zebrafish line to detect the fluorescently labeled tubular cells of the kidney (105). A full discussion of analysis strategies and development of automated image processing pipelines is beyond the scope of this manuscript (135). However, as post-acquisition analysis strategies are of vital importance for the success of any screening assay, the design of scoring pipelines needs careful consideration at early stages of experimental planning.

CONCLUSIONS

Phenotype-based, cost-effective whole-organism chemical screening in zebrafish offers a variety of advantages including the identification of disease-modifying drugs without knowledge of a validated target, the potential to identify compounds with polypharmacological efficacy, and the simultaneous assessment of compound efficacy, toxicity, biodistribution, and pharmacokinetics within a vertebrate model system. While a growing number of genes are being identified to cause human kidney diseases, therapeutic options to combat these diseases are often absent. Ideally, the use of genetically modified zebrafish mimicking human genetic disorders in conjunction with kidney-specific transgenic reporter lines or in conjunction with fluorescently-labeled functional reporter lines (or other secondary readouts), permit the implementation of chemical screening for disease-modifying substances in the field of genetic kidney diseases.

AUTHOR CONTRIBUTIONS

All authors listed have made a substantial, direct, and intellectual contribution to the work, and approved it for publication.

ACKNOWLEDGMENTS

We thank Franz Schaefer (University Children's Hospital Heidelberg), Felix Loosli (Karlsruhe Institute of Technology) and Jochen Wittbrodt (Centre for Organismal Studies (COS) Heidelberg) for general support. This work was partially funded by the RENALTRACT ITN project, that has received funding from the European Union's Horizon 2020 research and innovation programme under the Marie Sklodowska-Curie grant agreement N°642937. JHW has received funding from

Peter-Stiftung für die Nierenwissenschaft and Doktor Robert Pfleger-Stiftung. We acknowledge financial support by Deutsche Forschungsgemeinschaft within the funding programme Open Access Publishing, by the Baden-Württemberg Ministry of Science, Research and the Arts and by Ruprecht-Karls-Universität Heidelberg.

REFERENCES

1. Lieschke GJ, Currie PD. Animal models of human disease: zebrafish swim into view. *Nat Rev Genet.* (2007) 8:353–67. doi: 10.1038/nrg2091
2. Dooley K, Zon LI. Zebrafish: a model system for the study of human disease. *Curr Opin Genet Dev.* (2000) 10:252–6. doi: 10.1016/S0959-437X(00)00074-5
3. Howe K, Clark MD, Torroja CF, Torrance J, Berthelot C, Muffato M, et al. The zebrafish reference genome sequence and its relationship to the human genome. *Nature* (2013) 496:498–503. doi: 10.1038/nature12111
4. Ota S, Kawahara A. Zebrafish: a model vertebrate suitable for the analysis of human genetic disorders. *Congenit Anom.* (2014) 54:8–11. doi: 10.1111/cga.12040
5. Cong L, Ran FA, Cox D, Lin S, Barretto R, Habib N, et al. Multiplex genome engineering using CRISPR/Cas systems. *Science* (2013) 339:819–23. doi: 10.1126/science.1231143
6. Mali P, Yang L, Esvelt KM, Aach J, Guell M, DiCarlo JE, et al. RNA-guided human genome engineering via Cas9. *Science* (2013) 339:823–6. doi: 10.1126/science.1232033
7. Swanhart LM, Cosentino CC, Diep CQ, Davidson AJ, de Caestecker M, Hukriede NA. Zebrafish kidney development: basic science to translational research. *Birth Defects Res C Embryo Today* (2011) 93:141–56. doi: 10.1002/bdrc.20209
8. Wingert RA, Selleck R, Yu J, Song HD, Chen Z, Song A, et al. The cdx genes and retinoic acid control the positioning and segmentation of the zebrafish pronephros. *PLoS Genet.* (2007) 3:1922–38. doi: 10.1371/journal.pgen.0030189
9. Morales EE, Wingert RA. Zebrafish as a model of kidney disease. *Results Probl Cell Differ.* (2017) 60:55–75. doi: 10.1007/978-3-319-51436-9_3
10. Driever W, Solnica-Krezel L, Schier AF, Neuhauss SC, Malicki J, Stemple DL, et al. A genetic screen for mutations affecting embryogenesis in zebrafish. *Development* (1996) 123:37–46.
11. Drummond IA, Majumdar A, Hentschel H, Elger M, Solnica-Krezel L, Schier AF, et al. Early development of the zebrafish pronephros and analysis of mutations affecting pronephric function. *Development* (1998) 125:4655–67.
12. MacRae CA, Peterson RT. Zebrafish as tools for drug discovery. *Nat Rev Drug Discov.* (2015) 14:721–31. doi: 10.1038/nrd4627
13. Rennekamp AJ, Peterson RT. 15 years of zebrafish chemical screening. *Curr Opin Chem Biol.* (2015) 24:58–70. doi: 10.1016/j.cbpa.2014.10.025
14. Shah AN, Davey CF, Whitebirch AC, Miller AC, Moens CB. Rapid reverse genetic screening using CRISPR in zebrafish. *Nat Methods* (2015) 12:535–40. doi: 10.1038/nmeth.3360
15. Dang M, Fogley R, Zon LI. Identifying novel cancer therapies using chemical genetics and zebrafish. *Adv Exp Med Biol.* (2016) 916:103–24. doi: 10.1007/978-3-319-30654-4_5
16. Sipes NS, Padilla S, Knudsen TB. Zebrafish: as an integrative model for twenty-first century toxicity testing. *Birth Defects Res C Embryo Today* (2011) 93:256–67. doi: 10.1002/bdrc.20214
17. Yang L, Ho NY, Alshut R, Legradi J, Weiss C, Reischl M, et al. Zebrafish embryos as models for embryotoxic and teratological effects of chemicals. *Reprod Toxicol.* (2009) 28:245–53. doi: 10.1016/j.reprotox.2009.04.013
18. Sullivan C, Matty MA, Jurczyszak D, Gabor KA, Millard PJ, Tobin DM, et al. Infectious disease models in zebrafish. *Methods Cell Biol.* (2017) 138:101–36. doi: 10.1016/bs.mcb.2016.10.005
19. Astin JW, Keerthisinghe P, Du L, Sanderson LE, Crosier KE, Crosier PS, et al. Innate immune cells and bacterial infection in zebrafish. *Methods Cell Biol.* (2017) 138:31–60. doi: 10.1016/bs.mcb.2016.08.002
20. Kessler M, Rottbauer W, Just S. Recent progress in the use of zebrafish for novel cardiac drug discovery. *Expert Opin Drug Discov.* (2015) 10:1231–41. doi: 10.1517/17460441.2015.1078788
21. Vazao H, Rosa S, Barata T, Costa R, Pitrez PR, Honorio I, et al. High-throughput identification of small molecules that affect human embryonic vascular development. *Proc Natl Acad Sci USA.* (2017) 114:E3022–31. doi: 10.1073/pnas.1617451114
22. Eimon PM, Rubinstein AL. The use of *in vivo* zebrafish assays in drug toxicity screening. *Expert Opin Drug Metab Toxicol.* (2009) 5:393–401. doi: 10.1517/17425250902882128
23. Brady CA, Rennekamp AJ, Peterson RT. Chemical screening in Zebrafish. *Methods Mol Biol.* (2016) 1451:3–16. doi: 10.1007/978-1-4939-3771-4_1
24. Baxendale S, van Eeden F, Wilkinson R. The power of Zebrafish in personalised medicine. *Adv Exp Med Biol.* (2017) 1007:179–97. doi: 10.1007/978-3-319-60733-7_10
25. Gehrig J, Reischl M, Kalmar E, Ferg M, Hadzhiev Y, Zaucker A, et al. Automated high-throughput mapping of promoter-enhancer interactions in zebrafish embryos. *Nat Methods* (2009) 6:911–6. doi: 10.1038/nmeth.1396
26. Bruni G, Lakhani P, Kokel D. Discovering novel neuroactive drugs through high-throughput behavior-based chemical screening in the zebrafish. *Front Pharmacol.* (2014) 5:153. doi: 10.3389/fphar.2014.00153
27. Rihel J, Schier AF. Behavioral screening for neuroactive drugs in zebrafish. *Dev Neurobiol.* (2012) 72:373–85. doi: 10.1002/dneu.20910
28. North TE, Goessling W, Walkley CR, Lengerke C, Kopani KR, Lord AM, et al. Prostaglandin E2 regulates vertebrate haematopoietic stem cell homeostasis. *Nature* (2007) 447:1007–11. doi: 10.1038/nature05883
29. Eckardt KU, Coresh J, Devuyst O, Johnson RJ, Kottgen A, Levey AS, et al. Evolving importance of kidney disease: from subspecialty to global health burden. *Lancet* (2013) 382:158–69. doi: 10.1016/S0140-6736(13)60439-0
30. Drummond IA. Zebrafish kidney development. *Methods Cell Biol.* (2004) 76:501–30. doi: 10.1016/S0091-679X(04)76023-9
31. Desgrange A, Cereghini S. Nephron patterning: lessons from Xenopus, Zebrafish, and Mouse studies. *Cells* (2015) 4:483–99. doi: 10.3390/cells4030483
32. Ebarasi L, Oddsson A, Hultenby K, Betsholtz C, Tryggvason K. Zebrafish: a model system for the study of vertebrate renal development, function, and pathophysiology. *Curr Opin Nephrol Hypertens.* (2011) 20:416–24. doi: 10.1097/MNH.0b013e3283477797
33. Drummond IA. The zebrafish pronephros: a genetic system for studies of kidney development. *Pediatr Nephrol.* (2000) 14:428–35. doi: 10.1007/s004670050788
34. Wingert RA, Davidson AJ. The zebrafish pronephros: a model to study nephron segmentation. *Kidney Int.* (2008) 73:1120–7. doi: 10.1038/ki.2008.37
35. Anzenberger U, Bit-Avragim N, Rohr S, Rudolph F, Dehmel B, Willnow TE, et al. Elucidation of megalin/LRP2-dependent endocytic transport processes in the larval zebrafish pronephros. *J Cell Sci.* (2006) 119(Pt 10):2127–37. doi: 10.1242/jcs.02954
36. Nichane M, Van Campenhout C, Pendeville H, Voz ML, Bellefroid EJ. The Na+/PO4 cotransporter SLC20A1 gene labels distinct restricted subdomains of the developing pronephros in Xenopus and zebrafish embryos. *Gene Expr Patterns* (2006) 6:667–72. doi: 10.1016/j.modgep.2006.01.005
37. Santoriello C, Zon LI. Hooked! Modeling human disease in zebrafish. *J Clin Invest.* (2012) 122:2337–43. doi: 10.1172/JCI60434
38. Kramer-Zucker AG, Wiessner S, Jensen AM, Drummond IA. Organization of the pronephric filtration apparatus in zebrafish requires nephrin, podocin and the FERM domain protein mosaic eyes. *Dev Biol.* (2005) 285:316–29. doi: 10.1016/j.ydbio.2005.06.038
39. Fukuyo Y, Nakamura T, Bubenshchikova E, Powell R, Tsuji T, Janknecht R, et al. Nephrin and podocin functions are highly conserved between the zebrafish pronephros and mammalian metanephros. *Mol Med Rep.* (2014) 9:457–65. doi: 10.3892/mmr.2013.1844
40. Niaudet P, Gubler MC. WT1 and glomerular diseases. *Pediatr Nephrol.* (2006) 21:1653–60. doi: 10.1007/s00467-006-0208-1

41. Hall G, Gbadegesin RA, Lavin P, Wu G, Liu Y, Oh EC et al. A novel missense mutation of Wilms' Tumor 1 causes autosomal dominant FSGS. *J Am Soc Nephrol.* (2015) 26:831–43. doi: 10.1681/ASN.2013101053
42. Gbadegesin R, Hinkes BG, Hoskins BE, Vlangos CN, Heeringa SF, Liu J, et al. Mutations in PLCE1 are a major cause of isolated diffuse mesangial sclerosis (IDMS). *Nephrol Dial Transplant.* (2008) 23:1291–7. doi: 10.1093/ndt/gfm759
43. Hinkes B, Wiggins RC, Gbadegesin R, Vlangos CN, Seelow D, Nurnberg G, et al. Positional cloning uncovers mutations in PLCE1 responsible for a nephrotic syndrome variant that may be reversible. *Nat Genet.* (2006) 38:1397–405. doi: 10.1038/ng1918
44. Ashraf S, Gee HY, Woerner S, Xie LX, Vega-Warner V, Lovric S, et al. ADCK4 mutations promote steroid-resistant nephrotic syndrome through CoQ10 biosynthesis disruption. *J Clin Invest.* (2013) 123:5179–89. doi: 10.1172/JCI69000
45. Gee HY, Zhang F, Ashraf S, Kohl S, Sadowski CE, Vega-Warner V, et al. KANK deficiency leads to podocyte dysfunction and nephrotic syndrome. *J Clin Invest.* (2015) 125:2375–84. doi: 10.1172/JCI79504
46. Ebarasi L, Ashraf S, Bierzynska A, Gee HY, McCarthy HJ, Lovric S, et al. Defects of CRB2 cause steroid-resistant nephrotic syndrome. *Am J Hum Genet.* (2015) 96:153–61. doi: 10.1016/j.ajhg.2014.11.014
47. Miyake N, Tsukaguchi H, Koshimizu E, Shono A, Matsunaga S, Shiina M, et al. Biallelic mutations in nuclear pore complex subunit NUP107 cause early-childhood-onset steroid-resistant nephrotic syndrome. *Am J Hum Genet.* (2015) 97:555–66. doi: 10.1016/j.ajhg.2015.08.013
48. Gee HY, Saisawat P, Ashraf S, Hurd TW, Vega-Warner V, Fang H, et al. ARHGDIA mutations cause nephrotic syndrome via defective RHO GTPase signaling. *J Clin Invest.* (2013) 123:3243–53. doi: 10.1172/JCI69134
49. Hill AJ, Bello SM, Prasch AL, Peterson RE, Heideman W. Water permeability and TCDD-induced edema in zebrafish early-life stages. *Toxicol Sci.* (2004) 78:78–87. doi: 10.1093/toxsci/kfh056
50. Rider SA, Tucker CS, del-Pozo J, Rose KN, MacRae CA, Bailey MA, et al. Techniques for the *in vivo* assessment of cardio-renal function in zebrafish (*Danio rerio*) larvae. *J Physiol.* (2012) 590(Pt 8):1803–9. doi: 10.1113/jphysiol.2011.224352
51. Kotb AM, Muller T, Xie J, Anand-Apte B, Endlich K, Endlich N. Simultaneous assessment of glomerular filtration and barrier function in live zebrafish. *Am J Physiol Renal Physiol.* (2014) 307:F1427–34. doi: 10.1152/ajprenal.00029.2014
52. Hentschel DM, Park KM, Cilenti L, Zervos AS, Drummond I, Bonventre JV. Acute renal failure in zebrafish: a novel system to study a complex disease. *Am J Physiol Renal Physiol.* (2005) 288:F923–9. doi: 10.1152/ajprenal.00386.2004
53. Hanke N, King BL, Vaske B, Haller H, Schiffer M. A Fluorescence-based assay for proteinuria screening in larval zebrafish (*Danio rerio*). *Zebrafish* (2015) 12:372–6. doi: 10.1089/zeb.2015.1093
54. Zhou W, Hildebrandt F. Inducible podocyte injury and proteinuria in transgenic zebrafish. *J Am Soc Nephrol.* (2012). 23:1039–47. doi: 10.1681/ASN.2011080776
55. Hildebrandt F, Zhou W. Nephronophthisis-associated ciliopathies. *J Am Soc Nephrol.* (2007) 18:1855–71. doi: 10.1681/ASN.2006121344
56. Arts HH, Knoers NV. Current insights into renal ciliopathies: what can genetics teach us? *Pediatr Nephrol.* (2013) 28:863–74. doi: 10.1007/s00467-012-2259-9
57. Hildebrandt F, Otto E. Cilia and centrosomes: a unifying pathogenic concept for cystic kidney disease? *Nat Rev Genet.* (2005) 6:928–40. doi: 10.1038/nrg1727
58. Watnick T, Germino G. From cilia to cyst. *Nat Genet.* (2003) 34:355–6. doi: 10.1038/ng0803-355
59. Hostetter CL, Sullivan-Brown JL, Burdine RD. Zebrafish pronephros: a model for understanding cystic kidney disease. *Dev Dyn.* (2003) 228:514–22. doi: 10.1002/dvdy.10371
60. Liu S, Lu W, Obara T, Kuida S, Lehoczky J, Dewar K, et al. A defect in a novel Nek-family kinase causes cystic kidney disease in the mouse and in zebrafish. *Development* (2002) 129:5839–46. doi: 10.1242/dev.00173
61. Low SH, Vasanth S, Larson CH, Mukherjee S, Sharma N, Kinter MT, et al. Polycystin-1, STAT6, and P100 function in a pathway that transduces ciliary mechanosensation and is activated in polycystic kidney disease. *Dev Cell* (2006) 10:57–69. doi: 10.1016/j.devcel.2005.12.005
62. Otto EA, Schermer B, Obara T, O'Toole JF, Hiller KS, Mueller AM, et al. Mutations in INVS encoding inversin cause nephronophthisis type 2, linking renal cystic disease to the function of primary cilia and left-right axis determination. *Nat Genet.* (2003) 34:413–20. doi: 10.1038/ng1217
63. Sun Z, Amsterdam A, Pazour GJ, Cole DG, Miller MS, Hopkins N. A genetic screen in zebrafish identifies cilia genes as a principal cause of cystic kidney. *Development* (2004) 131:4085–93. doi: 10.1242/dev.01240
64. Tobin JL, Beales PL. Restoration of renal function in zebrafish models of ciliopathies. *Pediatr Nephrol.* (2008) 23:2095–9. doi: 10.1007/s00467-008-0898-7
65. Kramer-Zucker AG, Olale F, Haycraft CJ, Yoder BK, Schier AF, Drummond IA. Cilia-driven fluid flow in the zebrafish pronephros, brain and Kupffer's vesicle is required for normal organogenesis. *Development* (2005) 132:1907–21. doi: 10.1242/dev.01772
66. Satir P, Christensen ST. Structure and function of mammalian cilia. *Histochem Cell Biol.* (2008) 129:687–93. doi: 10.1007/s00418-008-0416-9
67. Le Corre S, Eyre D, Drummond IA. Modulation of the secretory pathway rescues zebrafish polycystic kidney disease pathology. *J Am Soc Nephrol.* (2014) 25:1749–59. doi: 10.1681/ASN.2013101060
68. Obara T, Mangos S, Liu Y, Zhao J, Wiessner S, Kramer-Zucker AG, et al. Polycystin-2 immunolocalization and function in zebrafish. *J Am Soc Nephrol.* (2006) 17:2706–18. doi: 10.1681/ASN.2006040412
69. Schottenfeld J, Sullivan-Brown J, Burdine RD. Zebrafish curly up encodes a Pkd2 ortholog that restricts left-side-specific expression of southpaw. *Development* (2007) 134:1605–15. doi: 10.1242/dev.02827
70. Bergmann C, Senderek J, Kupper F, Schneider F, Dornia C, Windelen E, et al. PKHD1 mutations in autosomal recessive polycystic kidney disease (ARPKD). *Hum Mutat.* (2004) 23:453–63. doi: 10.1002/humu.20029
71. Lu H, Galeano MCR, Ott E, Kaeslin G, Kausalya PJ, Kramer C, et al. Mutations in DZIP1L, which encodes a ciliary-transition-zone protein, cause autosomal recessive polycystic kidney disease. *Nat Genet.* (2017) 49:1025–34. doi: 10.1038/ng.3871
72. Perner B, Englert C, Bollig F. The Wilms tumor genes wt1a and wt1b control different steps during formation of the zebrafish pronephros. *Dev Biol.* (2007) 309:87–96. doi: 10.1016/j.ydbio.2007.06.022
73. Bergmann C. Educational paper: ciliopathies. *Eur J Pediatr.* (2012) 171:1285–300. doi: 10.1007/s00431-011-1553-z
74. Hildebrandt F, Benzing T, Katsanis N. Ciliopathies. *N Engl J Med.* (2011) 364:1533–43. doi: 10.1056/NEJMra1010172
75. Borgal L, Habbig S, Hatzold J, Liebau MC, Dafinger C, Sacarea I, et al. The ciliary protein nephrocystin-4 translocates the canonical Wnt regulator Jade-1 to the nucleus to negatively regulate beta-catenin signaling. *J Biol Chem.* (2012) 287:25370–80. doi: 10.1074/jbc.M112.385658
76. Burckle C, Gaude HM, Vesque C, Silbermann F, Salomon R, Jeanpierre C, et al. Control of the Wnt pathways by nephrocystin-4 is required for morphogenesis of the zebrafish pronephros. *Hum Mol Genet.* (2011) 20:2611–27. doi: 10.1093/hmg/ddr164
77. French VM, van de Laar IM, Wessels MW, Rohe C, Roos-Hesselink JW, Wang G, et al. NPHP4 variants are associated with pleiotropic heart malformations. *Circ Res.* (2012) 110:1564–74. doi: 10.1161/CIRCRESAHA.112.269795
78. Hoff S, Halbritter J, Epting D, Frank V, Nguyen TM, van Reeuwijk J, et al. ANKS6 is a central component of a nephronophthisis module linking NEK8 to INVS and NPHP3. *Nat Genet.* (2013) 45:951–6. doi: 10.1038/ng.2681
79. Schafer T, Putz M, Lienkamp S, Ganner A, Bergbreiter A, Ramachandran H, et al. Genetic and physical interaction between the NPHP5 and NPHP6 gene products. *Hum Mol Genet.* (2008) 17:3655–62. doi: 10.1093/hmg/ddn260
80. Simons M, Gloy J, Ganner A, Bullerkotte A, Bashkurov M, Kronig C, et al. Inversin, the gene product mutated in nephronophthisis type II, functions as a molecular switch between Wnt signaling pathways. *Nat Genet.* (2005) 37:537–43. doi: 10.1038/ng1552
81. Slanchev K, Putz M, Schmitt A, Kramer-Zucker A, Walz G. Nephrocystin-4 is required for pronephric duct-dependent cloaca formation in zebrafish. *Hum Mol Genet.* (2011) 20:3119–28. doi: 10.1093/hmg/ddr214

82. Zhao C, Malicki J. Nephrocystins and MKS proteins interact with IFT particle and facilitate transport of selected ciliary cargos. *EMBO J.* (2011) 30:2532–44. doi: 10.1038/emboj.2011.165
83. Zhou W, Dai J, Attanasio M, Hildebrandt F. Nephrocystin-3 is required for ciliary function in zebrafish embryos. *Am J Physiol Renal Physiol.* (2010) 299:F55–62. doi: 10.1152/ajprenal.00043.2010
84. Adams M, Simms RJ, Abdelhamed Z, Dawe HR, Szymanska K, Logan CV, et al. A meckelin-filamin A interaction mediates ciliogenesis. *Hum Mol Genet.* (2012) 21:1272–86. doi: 10.1093/hmg/ddr557
85. Duldulao NA, Lee S, Sun Z. Cilia localization is essential for *in vivo* functions of the Joubert syndrome protein Arl13b/Scorpion. *Development* (2009) 136:4033–42. doi: 10.1242/dev.036350
86. Lessieur EM, Fogerty J, Gaivin RJ, Song P, Perkins BD. The ciliopathy gene ahi1 is required for zebrafish cone photoreceptor outer segment morphogenesis and survival. *Invest Ophthalmol Vis Sci.* (2017) 58:448–60. doi: 10.1167/iovs.16-20326
87. Bachmann-Gagescu R, Phelps IG, Stearns G, Link BA, Brockerhoff SE, Moens CB, et al. The ciliopathy gene cc2d2a controls zebrafish photoreceptor outer segment development through a role in Rab8-dependent vesicle trafficking. *Hum Mol Genet.* (2011) 20:4041–55. doi: 10.1093/hmg/ddr332
88. Rosenbaum JL, Witman GB. Intraflagellar transport. *Nat Rev Mol Cell Biol.* (2002) 3:813–25. doi: 10.1038/nrm952
89. Amsterdam A, Nissen RM, Sun Z, Swindell EC, Farrington S, Hopkins N. Identification of 315 genes essential for early zebrafish development. *Proc Natl Acad Sci USA.* (2004) 101:12792–7. doi: 10.1073/pnas.0403929101
90. de Vries J, Yntema JL, van Die CE, Crama N, Cornelissen EA, Hamel BC. Jeune syndrome: description of 13 cases and a proposal for follow-up protocol. *Eur J Pediatr.* (2010) 169:77–88. doi: 10.1007/s00431-009-0991-3
91. Halbritter J, Bizet AA, Schmidts M, Porath JD, Braun DA, Gee HY, et al. Defects in the IFT-B component IFT172 cause Jeune and Mainzer-Saldino syndromes in humans. *Am J Hum Genet.* (2013) 93:915–25. doi: 10.1016/j.ajhg.2013.09.012
92. Schaefer E, Stoetzel C, Scheidecker S, Geoffroy V, Prasad MK, Redin C, et al. Identification of a novel mutation confirms the implication of IFT172 (BBS20) in Bardet-Biedl syndrome. *J Hum Genet.* (2016) 61:447–50. doi: 10.1038/jhg.2015.162
93. Westhoff JH, Giselbrecht S, Schmidts M, Schindler S, Beales PL, Tonshoff B, et al. Development of an automated imaging pipeline for the analysis of the zebrafish larval kidney. *PLoS ONE* (2013) 8:e82137. doi: 10.1371/journal.pone.0082137
94. Veldman MB, Lin S. Zebrafish as a developmental model organism for pediatric research. *Pediatr Res.* (2008) 64:470–6. doi: 10.1203/PDR.0b013e318186e609
95. Phillips JB, Westerfield M. Zebrafish models in translational research: tipping the scales toward advancements in human health. *Dis Model Mech.* (2014) 7:739–43. doi: 10.1242/dmm.015545
96. Geisler R, Borel N, Ferg M, Maier JV, Strahle U. Maintenance of Zebrafish Lines at the European Zebrafish Resource Center. *Zebrafish* (2016) 13(Suppl. 1):S19–23. doi: 10.1089/zeb.2015.1205
97. Sassen RW, Köster R. A molecular toolbox for genetic manipulation of zebrafish. *Adv Genom Genet.* (2015) 5:151–63. doi: 10.2147/AGG.S57585
98. Zhou W, Boucher RC, Bollig F, Englert C, Hildebrandt F. Characterization of mesonephric development and regeneration using transgenic zebrafish. *Am J Physiol Renal Physiol.* (2010) 299:F1040–7. doi: 10.1152/ajprenal.00394.2010
99. He B, Ebarasi L, Hultenby K, Tryggvason K, Betsholtz C. Podocin-green fluorescence protein allows visualization and functional analysis of podocytes. *J Am Soc Nephrol.* (2011) 22:1019–23. doi: 10.1681/ASN.2010121291
100. Seiler C, Pack M. Transgenic labeling of the zebrafish pronephric duct and tubules using a promoter from the enpep gene. *Gene Expr Patterns* (2011) 11:118–21. doi: 10.1016/j.gep.2010.10.002
101. Noonan HR, Metelo AM, Kamei CN, Peterson RT, Drummond IA, Iliopoulos O. Loss of vhl in the zebrafish pronephros recapitulates early stages of human clear cell renal cell carcinoma. *Dis Model Mech.* (2016) 9:873–84. doi: 10.1242/dmm.024380
102. Fisher S, Grice EA, Vinton RM, Bessling SL, McCallion AS. Conservation of RET regulatory function from human to zebrafish without sequence similarity. *Science* (2006) 312:276–9. doi: 10.1126/science.1124070
103. Vasilyev A, Liu Y, Mudumana S, Mangos S, Lam PY, Majumdar A, et al. Collective cell migration drives morphogenesis of the kidney nephron. *PLoS Biol.* (2009) 7:e9. doi: 10.1371/journal.pbio.1000009
104. Wang Y, Sun ZH, Zhou L, Li Z, Gui JF. Grouper tshbeta promoter-driven transgenic zebrafish marks proximal kidney tubule development. *PLoS ONE* (2014) 9:e97806. doi: 10.1371/journal.pone.0097806
105. Sanker S, Cirio MC, Vollmer LL, Goldberg ND, McDermott LA, Hukriede NA, et al. Development of high-content assays for kidney progenitor cell expansion in transgenic zebrafish. *J Biomol Screen* (2013) 18:1193–202. doi: 10.1177/1087057113495296
106. Cianciolo Cosentino C, Skrypnyk NI, Brilli LL, Chiba T, Novitskaya T, Woods C, et al. Histone deacetylase inhibitor enhances recovery after AKI. *J Am Soc Nephrol.* (2013) 24:943–53. doi: 10.1681/ASN.2012111055
107. Chang MY, Ma TL, Hung CC, Tian YC, Chen YC, Yang CW, et al. Metformin inhibits cyst formation in a zebrafish model of polycystin-2 deficiency. *Sci Rep.* (2017) 7:7161. doi: 10.1038/s41598-017-07300-x
108. Huang L, Xiao A, Wecker A, McBride DA, Choi SY, Zhou W, et al. A possible zebrafish model of polycystic kidney disease: knockdown of *wnt5a* causes cysts in zebrafish kidneys. *J Vis Exp.* (2014) e52156. doi: 10.3791/52156
109. Blum M, De Robertis EM, Wallingford JB, Niehrs C. Morpholinos: antisense and Sensibility. *Dev Cell* (2015) 35:145–9. doi: 10.1016/j.devcel.2015.09.017
110. Stainier DYR, Raz E, Lawson ND, Ekker SC, Burdine RD, Eisen JS, et al. Guidelines for morpholino use in zebrafish. *PLoS Genet.* (2017) 13:e1007000. doi: 10.1371/journal.pgen.1007000
111. Eisen JS, Smith JC. Controlling morpholino experiments: don't stop making antisense. *Development* (2008) 135:1735–43. doi: 10.1242/dev.001115
112. Kok FO, Shin M, Ni CW, Gupta A, Grosse AS, van Impel A, et al. Reverse genetic screening reveals poor correlation between morpholino-induced and mutant phenotypes in zebrafish. *Dev Cell* (2015) 32:97–108. doi: 10.1016/j.devcel.2014.11.018
113. Rossi A, Kontarakis Z, Gerri C, Nolte H, Holper S, Kruger M, et al. Genetic compensation induced by deleterious mutations but not gene knockdowns. *Nature* (2015) 524:230–3. doi: 10.1038/nature14580
114. Cao Y, Semanchik N, Lee SH, Somlo S, Barbano PE, Coifman R, et al. Chemical modifier screen identifies HDAC inhibitors as suppressors of PKD models. *Proc Natl Acad Sci USA.* (2009) 106:21819–24. doi: 10.1073/pnas.0911987106
115. de Groh ED, Swanhart LM, Cosentino CC, Jackson RL, Dai W, Kitchens CA, et al. Inhibition of histone deacetylase expands the renal progenitor cell population. *J Am Soc Nephrol.* (2010) 21:794–802. doi: 10.1681/ASN.2009080851
116. Pepperkok R, Ellenberg J. High-throughput fluorescence microscopy for systems biology. *Nat Rev Mol Cell Biol.* (2006) 7:690–6. doi: 10.1038/nrm1979
117. Mathias JR, Saxena MT, Mumm JS. Advances in zebrafish chemical screening technologies. *Future Med Chem.* (2012) 4:1811–22. doi: 10.4155/fmc.12.115
118. Yanik MF, Rohde CB, Pardo-Martin C. Technologies for micromanipulating, imaging, and phenotyping small invertebrates and vertebrates. *Annu Rev Biomed Eng.* (2011) 13:185–217. doi: 10.1146/annurev-bioeng-071910-124703
119. Burns CG, Milan DJ, Grande EJ, Rottbauer W, MacRae CA, Fishman MC. High-throughput assay for small molecules that modulate zebrafish embryonic heart rate. *Nat Chem Biol.* (2005) 1:263–4. doi: 10.1038/nchembio732
120. Kokel D, Bryan J, Laggner C, White R, Cheung CY, Mateus R, et al. Rapid behavior-based identification of neuroactive small molecules in the zebrafish. *Nat Chem Biol.* (2010) 6:231–7. doi: 10.1038/nchembio.307
121. Lin S, Zhao Y, Xia T, Meng H, Ji Z, Liu R, et al. High content screening in zebrafish speeds up hazard ranking of transition metal oxide nanoparticles. *ACS Nano* (2011) 5:7284–95. doi: 10.1021/nn202116p
122. Molina G, Vogt A, Bakan A, Dai W, Queiroz de Oliveira P, Znosko W, et al. Zebrafish chemical screening reveals an inhibitor of Dusp6 that expands cardiac cell lineages. *Nat Chem Biol.* (2009) 5:680–7. doi: 10.1038/nchembio.190
123. Pylatiuk C, Sanchez D, Mikut R, Alshut R, Reischl M, Hirth S, et al. Automatic zebrafish heartbeat detection and analysis for zebrafish embryos. *Zebrafish* (2014) 11:379–83. doi: 10.1089/zeb.2014.1002
124. Zon LI, Peterson RT. *In vivo* drug discovery in the zebrafish. *Nat Rev Drug Discov.* (2005) 4:35–44. doi: 10.1038/nrd1606

125. Wittbrodt JN, Liebel U, Gehrig J. Generation of orientation tools for automated zebrafish screening assays using desktop 3D printing. *BMC Biotechnol.* (2014) 14:36. doi: 10.1186/1472-6750-14-36
126. Peravali R, Gehrig J, Giselbrecht S, Lutjohann DS, Hadzhiev Y, Muller F, et al. Automated feature detection and imaging for high-resolution screening of zebrafish embryos. *Biotechniques* (2011) 50:319–24. doi: 10.2144/000113669
127. Pardo-Martin C, Chang TY, Koo BK, Gilleland CL, Wasserman SC, Yanik MF. High-throughput *in vivo* vertebrate screening. *Nat Methods* (2010) 7:634–6. doi: 10.1038/nmeth.1481
128. Westhoff JH, Steenbergen PJ, Wagner J, Tönshoff B, Liebel U, Gehrig J. *In vivo* high content screening in zebrafish to score developmental nephrotoxicity of approved drugs [abstract]. In: *10th European Zebrafish Meeting*. Budapest (2017) P-II-157.
129. Pandey G, Westhoff JH, Schaefer F, Gehrig J. An automated high content screening platform to identify cystic kidney disease-modifying substances in zebrafish [abstract]. In: *55th European Renal Association & European Dialysis and Transplant Association*. Copenhagen (2018) SuO018.
130. Pardo-Martin C, Allalou A, Medina J, Eimon PM, Wahlby C, Fatih Yanik M. High-throughput hyperdimensional vertebrate phenotyping. *Nat Commun.* (2013) 4:1467. doi: 10.1038/ncomms2475
131. Peterson RT, Fishman MC. Designing zebrafish chemical screens. *Methods Cell Biol.* (2011) 105:525–41. doi: 10.1016/B978-0-12-381320-6.00023-0
132. Conrad C, Wunsche A, Tan TH, Bulkescher J, Sieckmann F, Verissimo F, et al. Micropilot: automation of fluorescence microscopy-based imaging for systems biology. *Nat Methods* (2011) 8:246–9. doi: 10.1038/nmeth.1558
133. Gunkel M, Eberle JP, Erfle H. Fluorescence-based high-throughput and targeted image acquisition and analysis for phenotypic screening. *Methods Mol Biol.* (2017) 1563:269–80. doi: 10.1007/978-1-4939-6810-7_17
134. Tischer C, Hilsenstein V, Hanson K, Pepperkok R. Adaptive fluorescence microscopy by online feedback image analysis. *Methods Cell Biol.* (2014) 123:489–503. doi: 10.1016/B978-0-12-420138-5.00026-4
135. Mikut R, Dickmeis T, Driever W, Geurts P, Hamprecht FA, Kausler BX, et al. Automated processing of zebrafish imaging data: a survey. *Zebrafish* (2013) 10:401–21. doi: 10.1089/zeb.2013.0886

9

Nephropathic Cystinosis: Symptoms, Treatment and Perspectives of a Systemic Disease

Sören Bäumner* and Lutz T. Weber

Pediatric Nephrology, Children's and Adolescents' Hospital, University Hospital Cologne, Cologne, Germany

***Correspondence:**
Sören Bäumner
soeren.baeumner@uk-koeln.de

Cystinosis is a rare autosomal recessive lysosomal storage disorder caused by mutations in the *CTNS* gene. Main dysfunction is a defective clearance of cystine from lysosomes that leads to accumulation of cystine crystals in every tissue of the body. There are three different forms: infantile nephropathic cystinosis, which is the most common form, juvenile nephropatic, and non-nephropathic cystinosis. Mostly, first symptom in infantile nephropathic cystinosis is renal Fanconi syndrome that occurs within the first year of life. Another prominent symptom is photophobia due to corneal crystal deposition. Cystine depletion therapy with cysteamine delays end-stage renal failure but does not stop progression of the disease. A new cysteamine formulation with delayed-release simplifies the administration schedule but still does not cure cystinosis. Even long-term depletion treatment resulting in bypassing the defective lysosomal transporter cannot reverse Fanconi syndrome. A future perspective offering a curative therapy may be transplantation of *CTNS*-carrying stem cells that has successfully been performed in mice.

Keywords: nephropathic cystinosis, cysteamine, renal Fanconi syndrome, *CTNS* gene, hematopoietic stem cell therapy

INTRODUCTION

Nephropathic cystinosis is a rare autosomal recessive lysosomal storage disorder leading to end-stage renal disease and many extra-renal complications with crystal deposition in the conjunctiva and cornea being the most prominent. It is caused by mutations in the *CTNS* gene on chromosome 17p13, which encodes the lysosomal cystin transporter cystinosin (1). First descriptions date to the beginning of the twentieth century, when cystine crystals were found in liver and spleen of a toddler, who died from dehydration and failure to thrive (2). More insight gave studies in the 1980s, where a defective clearance of cystine from lysosomes could be demonstrated (3, 4). The encoding *CTNS* gene was found in 1998 (5). Since then more than 100 pathogenic mutations in the *CTNS* gene have been described (6).

Central column of treatment is a depletion therapy with cysteamine that has proven to slow down progression of renal failure and to prevent or slow down extra-renal manifestations, even though it is not a curative therapy.

There are three different forms of cystinosis, which differ in age at manifestation and severity of the symptoms: (i) infantile nephropathic cystinosis, which is the most common and severe form; (ii) juvenile nephropathic cystinosis, which is characterized by later onset of symptoms and slower progression; and (iii) non-nephropatic cystinosis, with a mainly ocular manifestation, also known as adult form. Each form shows different mutations in the *CTNS* gene (7). Cystinosis occurs approximately in 1–2 of 100,000 live births (6).

INFANTILE NEPHROPATHIC CYSTINOSIS

Neonates are clinically asymptomatic at birth with normal birthweight and normal length, even though cystine accumulation already starts *in utero*. First symptoms occur within the first year of life, usually presenting as renal Fanconi syndrome, a dysfunction of the proximal tubule that leads to polydipsia, polyuria, dehydration, proximal renal tubular acidosis, urinary loss of electrolytes, and growth retardation. In the urine, glucosuria and aminoaciduria can be found. In the case of glucosuria and normal serum glucose levels, one should always think of renal glucosuria or Fanconi syndrome. Glucosuria is the only parameter to be detected by urine dipstick in the Fanconi tubulopathy. The high protein turnover in the proximal tubule may explain why Fanconi syndrome is the first symptom of cystinosis.

Without treatment end-stage, renal failure occurs at a median age of 10 years. About 95% of cystinosis patients suffer from this type (6, 8). Historically cystinosis accounts for 5% of childhood renal failure (9).

JUVENILE NEPHROPATHIC CYSTINOSIS

Patients with the juvenile type of nephropathic cystinosis develop symptoms at an older age, often presenting with more unspecific symptoms than patients with infantile cystinosis like nephrotic syndrome or mild proximal tubulopathy, but not necessarily the complete picture of Fanconi syndrome. End-stage renal disease may occur. Most patients are diagnosed in the second decade of life, when onset of photophobia leads to ocular examination and cystine crystals in the cornea can be found. This form accounts for approximately 5% of all cases of cystinosis (7, 10).

NON-NEPHROPATHIC CYSTINOSIS

This type presents only with ocular symptoms, as deposits are limited to cornea and conjunctiva and is also known as the adult form of cystinosis. Of note, there might be a continuum between milder forms of cystinosis, since non-nephropathic and juvenile forms have been described within one family. Therefore, renal function of every patient with non-nephropathic cystinosis should be monitored closely (10, 11).

DIAGNOSIS

First clinical signs in patients with infantile nephropathic cystinosis are polyuria, polydipsia, and failure to thrive. These symptoms reflect renal Fanconi syndrome in combination with metabolic acidosis and loss of electrolytes, especially phosphate (1). Since cystinosis is the most common reason for renal Fanconi syndrome at this age, this differential diagnosis should always be considered. Less common reasons for secondary Fanconi syndrome may be Dent's disease, Lowe's syndrome, inherited fructose intolerance, galactosemia, or tyrosinemia (12). Corneal cystine deposits, which are pathognomonic in untreated cystinosis, can rarely be found in the first year of life but are visible in almost every untreated patient at the age of 16 months (13).

Confirmation of the diagnosis is made by measurement of elevated cystine levels in white blood cells followed by genetic testing for mutations in the *CTNS* gene (14). For cystine levels see **Table 1**.

GENETICS

Confirmation of the diagnosis can be made by genetic testing. The *CTNS* gene, which encodes for the lysosomal carrier cystinosin, is located on the short arm of chromosome 17 (p13) (5). The most frequent mutation in Northern Europe is a 57-kb deletion that accounts for approximately 75% of all cases of nephropathic cystinosis (7, 15). Up to now, more than 100 mutations are known in the *CTNS* gene (6, 14). Most mutations in the *CTNS* gene result in a total loss of transport activity of cystinosin. The phenotype is the infantile nephropathic cystinosis. Patients with the milder juvenile or non-nephropathic form show different mutations suggesting that there is a genotype–phenotype correlation (11, 16–18). Still the pathogenesis is not fully understood because no disease model explains the link between lysosomal cystine accumulation and renal Fanconi syndrome completely (19).

PATHOPHYSIOLOGY AND CLINICAL PRESENTATION

Cystine is a disulfide of the amino acid cysteine. It is generated by lysosomal protein hydrolysis. Because no enzymatic dysfunction was found in cystinotic cells, research focused on defect transporter proteins leading to the identification of the seven-domain transmembrane protein cystinosin, which provides the transport of cystine from lysosomes to cytoplasm (20). Defective transport leads to accumulation and crystallization of cystine in the lysosomal compartment. Affected cells suffer from mitochondrial dysfunction, oxidative stress, and inflammation and, in the end, undergo apoptosis. Since lysosomes are part of every cell type cystine accumulation occurs throughout the whole body, making cystinosis a systemic disease (2). Over time, further symptoms can be seen in virtually every organ. The following sections represent just a selection of cystinosis manifestations. See also **Figure 1**.

KIDNEY

Nonetheless, there is a different susceptibility of cell types to cystine accumulation with renal cells being especially susceptible. This is the reason why cystinosis presents primarily with renal symptoms (see above). Firstly impaired tissue is the proximal

TABLE 1 | Diagnosis of cystinosis by measuring cystine levels.

Normal	≤0.2 nmol hemicystine/mg protein
Nephropathic cystinosis	5.0–23.0 nmol hemicystine/mg protein
Non-nephropathic cystinosis	1.0–3.0 nmol hemicystine/mg protein
Heterozygous carrier	≤1.0 nmol hemicystine/mg protein
Target levels for treated nephropathic cystinosis	<0.5–1.0 nmol hemicystin/mg protein

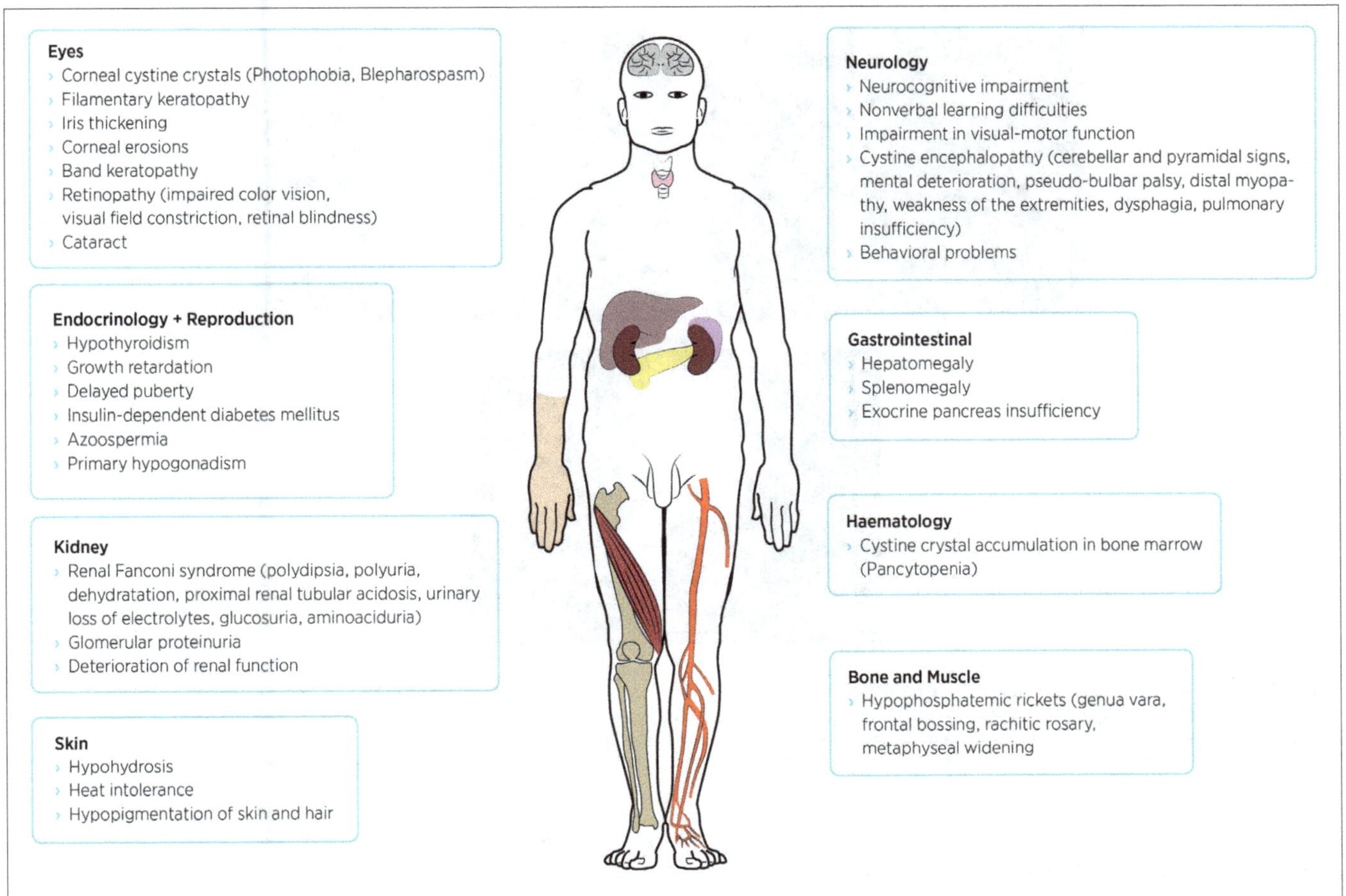

FIGURE 1 | Possible symptoms and disease manifestations of nephropathic cystinosis.

tubule leading to renal Fanconi syndrome, which is the major symptom of cystinosis. A characteristic histopathological sign is the so-called swan neck deformity, which describes the loss of proximal tubular cells. Electron microscopy shows cystine crystals in the tubular cells (10, 21, 22). Simultaneously, glomerular lesions occur due to involvement of podocytes that present histologically with the picture of focal and segmental sclerosis and lead clinically to glomerular proteinuria and progressive deterioration of renal function (2). Using electron microscopy, podocytes appear hypertrophic, multinucleate and have foot process effacement which is pathognomonic for cystinosis (23). Cystinosis does not recur in the kidney graft after transplantation has been performed.

EYE

Probably, the subjectively most impairing early problem is photophobia due to corneal deposition of cystine crystals (see **Figure 2**) which begins at a median age of 3–4 years, when no treatment is offered. The natural course of cystinosis in the eyes leads to blepharospams, corneal erosions, superficial punctuate keratopathy, and band keratopathy. Involvement of the retina, which can be seen constantly without treatment, causes loss of vision later in life (24, 25). Oral depletion treatment with cysteamine has no influence on the ocular manifestation since there is no vascularization in the cornea. So a topical treatment has been established, bearing new challenges for the patients because cysteamine eye drops have to be applied 6–12 times per day (26).

BONE AND MUSCLE

Increased urinary loss of phosphate, calcium, and disturbances in vitamin D metabolism cause hypophosphatemic rickets in cystinosis patients. Clinical signs are genua vara, frontal bossing, rachitic rosary, and metaphyseal widening on skeletal X-rays (12). However, there are patients who appear clinically similar without the laboratory findings of disturbed vitamin D metabolism mentioned above despite being treated with cysteamine. This finding might be explained by copper deficiency due to cysteamine toxicity, which may interfere with collagen cross-linking (28). Growth retardation is a frequent finding in cystinosis patients and is usually treated with growth hormone.

Even though X-ray absorptiometry shows bone densities within the normal range, bone fractures can be seen more often

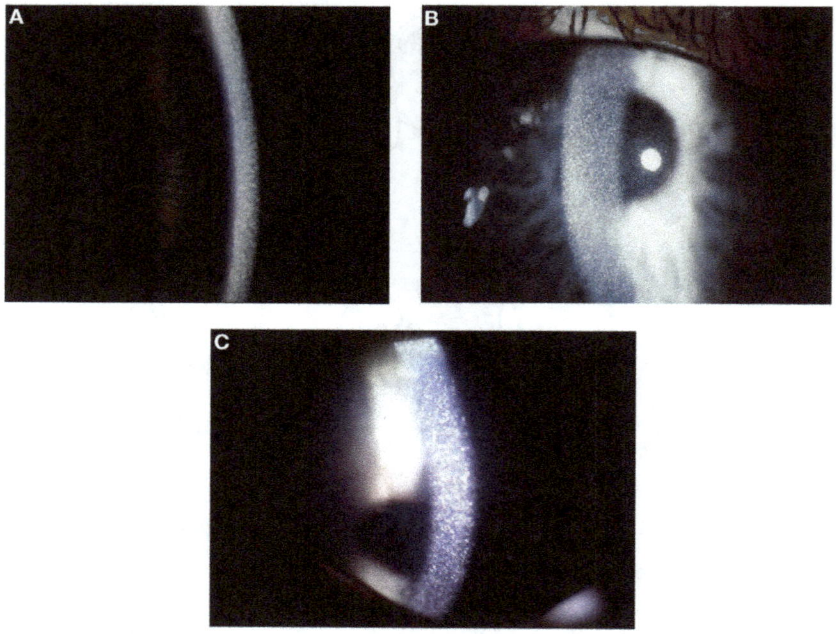

FIGURE 2 | Corneal slit-lamp examination of three patients with nephropathic cystinosis. **(A)** High magnificent slit beam view of cornea with cystine crystals. **(B)** Retroillumination showing marked diffuse crystals packed within the cornea. **(C)** Retroillumination with patient looking down showing the extent of crystal deposition up to the peripheral edge of the cornea. With friendly permission from Clinical Ophtalmology, Dove Press (27).

in cystinosis. Possibly, it might be that intra-osseous cystine crystals lead to falsely elevated X-ray absorptiometry levels making X-ray absorptiometry an ineffective tool to assess fracture risk in cystinosis patients (29). Three-dimensional peripheral computed tomography should be the preferred method to assess fracture risk in growth-retarded children with (chronic kidney) disease (30).

NEUROLOGY

Accumulation of cystine crystals in the brain leads to neurocognitive impairment. Early signs for brain involvement are nonverbal learning difficulties resulting in poor executive functions, whereas verbal and general intelligence are normal (6, 31). Cysteamine can cross the blood–brain barrier. Depletion treatment with cysteamine can improve neurological outcome even when patients are already symptomatic, but it has also been shown that impairment in visual-motor function occurs even if cysteamine treatment was started before neurologic impairment became noticeable. This suggests that it is not only accumulation, which causes learning difficulties in cystinosis patients (32, 33). Long-term neurological complications are cystine encephalopathy, presenting with cerebellar and pyramidal signs, mental deterioration and pseudo-bulbar palsy, as well as distal myopathy, which begins with weakness of the extremities and results in dysphagia and pulmonary insufficiency. Treatment with cysteamine has been shown to have a beneficial and potential reversible effect on both cystine encephalopathy and distal myopathy (34, 35).

ENDOCRINOLOGY

The most frequent endocrine finding is hypothyroidism, which appears approximately in half of all cystinosis patients and can easily be treated with substitution of thyroid hormones (6). Another frequent finding is hypogonadism. Male cystinosis patients are prone to be infertile due to azoospermia even if treated with cysteamine since early age. It has been shown that spermatogenesis at testicular level can be intact. The underlying mechanisms remain unclear (36). A successful conception after percutaneous epididymal sperm aspiration followed by intracytoplasmic sperm injection has recently been reported (37). Female cystinosis patients are fertile and several successful pregnancies have been described (38). Other affected endocrine organs are exocrine and endocrine pancreas resulting in diabetes mellitus in 5% of all patients (6, 12).

SYSTEMIC DEPLETION THERAPY

The first trials to deplete cystine from cells used 1,4-dithiothreitol (DTT) or ascorbic acid with moderate success (19). The cystine depleting therapy with cysteamine was first described in 1976 and is still the golden standard in cystinosis therapy (6, 39). Cysteamine induces a thiol-disulfide interchange reaction that generates equimolar amounts of cysteine and cysteine-cysteamine molecules from cystine (40). These molecules can exit the lysosomes using alternative cationic transporters and bypass the defective cystinosin transporter, as shown in **Figure 3** (41). Cysteamine treatment can be monitored by

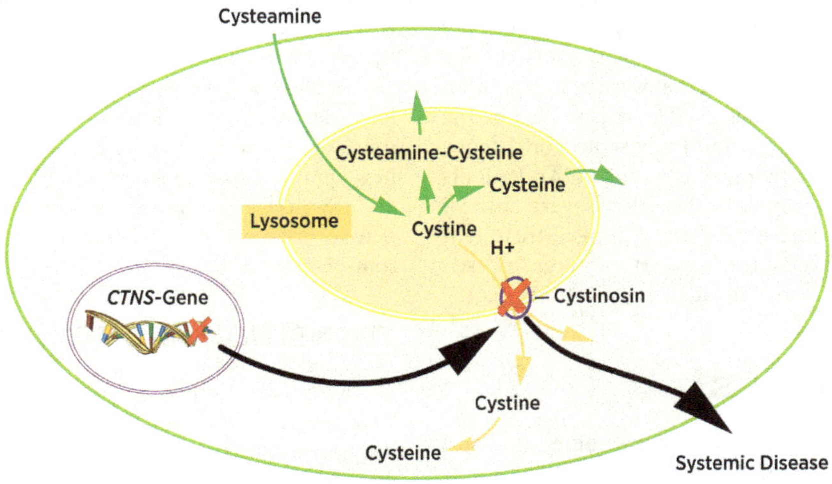

FIGURE 3 | Intracellular cystine metabolism. Cystine normally leaves the lysosome *via* cystinosin by cystine-proton symport (yellow arrows). Mutations in the *CTNS* gene cause cystine accumulation in the lysosome due to dysfunction of cystinosin (black arrows). Cystin accumulates and forms crystals inside the lysosome. Cysteamine induces a chemical reaction resulting in cysteamine–cysteine and cysteine. Both molecules exit the lysosome bypassing the cystinosin transporter protein (green arrows). Adapted from Ref. (6).

measuring intracellular cystine levels in white blood cells, which is considered to reflect the cystine concentration of the body's other tissues. Target levels are usually <1.0 nmol hemicystine/mg protein. Since cystine levels in healthy people are <0.2 nmol hemicystine/mg protein the optimal range for cystinosis patients is considered to be <0.5 nmol hemicystine/mg protein (12, 42, 43).

Cysteamine has been available as a commercial drug since 1997 in an immediate-release formulation that demands a strict 6-h administration schedule to maintain effective plasma levels. A new delayed-release formulation has been available since 2013 in the USA and since 2014 in Europe which must only be administered twice daily. Both formulas use cysteamine bitartrate since the bitartrate formulation needs lower doses to maintain plasma levels than cysteamine hydrochloride or phosphocysteamine (44). The new delayed-release formulation is composed of enteric-coated, microspheronised beads encapsulated in hard gelatin that allow to extend the intake up to 12 h (45). The maximum plasma levels of delayed-release cysteamine are reached about 3 h after administration, whereas maximum levels of the immediate formulation can be found after about 1 h already (46). Both extended- and immediate-release cysteamine have been proven to reach cystine target levels, which are thought necessary to slow down progress of cystinosis-related symptoms. The 12-h administration of the extended-release formulation supports therapy adherence by simplifying the administration schedule whereas experiences of side effects differ from center to center (43, 45, 47). Since new therapeutic strategies in many fields of pediatric diseases enabled patients to reach adolescence and adulthood, e.g., patients with cystic fibrosis or diabetes mellitus, new problems with therapy adherence at this age arose leading to the concept of a controlled transition from pediatric to adult health-care services. This can also be seen in cystinosis patients for whom special transition protocols are recommended (48, 49).

Most reported side effects of cysteamine therapy are halitosis, disagreeable sweat odor, and gastrointestinal side effects like nausea and abdominal pain. Proper dosing up to a maximum of 1.95 $g/m^2/day$ with a gradually increasing application schedule avoids side effects as lethargy, hyperthermia, and rash (50–52). Recent reports of new adverse events like bruise-like skin lesions, bone abnormalities, and muscle weakness in cystinosis patients with Fanconi syndrome showed that they have an increased urinary copper excretion under cysteamine therapy. This led to the hypothesis that cysteamine toxicity causes copper deficiency because of the structural similarity of cysteamine to D-penicillamine resulting in a reduced formation of aldehydes required for collagen cross-linking (28).

EYE DROPS

Systemic depletion therapy with cysteamine reduces posterior segment complications like pigmentary changes that can lead to retinopathy and loss of vision, but does not prevent deposition of cystine crystals in cornea and conjunctiva. It has been shown that photophobia is associated with crystal density, infiltration of inflammatory cells, and nerve damage within the cornea. Therefore, a topical treatment is necessary and has proven to be effective (24, 53, 54). Cysteamine eye drop formulations are aqueous solutions that have to be administered 6–12 times per day. Because cysteamine is unstable at room temperature and to light exposure, storage and transport of the eye drops are challenging making therapy adherence difficult. A new, gel-like viscous formulation with a fivefold higher concentration of cysteamine has been developed, which has to be administered only four times daily. The gel-like formulation increases the contact time to the cornea allowing the cysteamine to penetrate more deeply into the corneal layers. On the other hand, using the gel-like drops produce side effects like stinging, burning, and vision blurring that were more common compared to the aqueous formulation. The reason may be the higher cysteamine concentration and the viscous consistency but it did not lead to lower therapy adherence (24). Patients untreated with eye drops sometimes develop severe corneal lesions that require a corneal transplant. A topical treatment is necessary even after corneal transplantation because cystinosin-deficient host cells can reinvade into the transplanted cornea (14).

FUTURE PERSPECTIVES

Even though the depleting therapy with cysteamine—oral and topical—has improved the prognosis of cystinosis patients dramatically, it is still not a curative therapy because the defective lysosomal transport protein cystinosin is only bypassed. New formulations of oral and topic cysteamine can alleviate the medical schedule and through this support therapy adherence. But cysteamine has only a delaying effect on complications like end-stage renal failure. Evidence grows that dysfunction of the lysosomal transport protein cystinosin leads to several disturbed intracellular interactions that cannot be corrected by depleting cystine from the lysosomal compartment: for example, cystinotic cells show (i) impaired chaperone-mediated autophagy (55); (ii) reduced levels of transcription factor EB, a key factor in regulating lysosomal biogenesis and clearance (56); and (iii) downregulation of the mammalian target of rapamycin pathway in proximal tubular cells (57). All these mechanisms are not influenced by cysteamine treatment and are associated with the persistence of renal Fanconi syndrome (8). Also altered cellular energy homeostasis or increased oxidative stress found in cystinotic fibroblasts offer new potential targets for the treatment of cystinosis, but still do not offer a causal therapy (58, 59).

The most promising approach to cure cystinosis is the transplantation of hematopoietic *CTNS*-carrying stem cells. Stem cells from wild-type donors were transplanted into irradiated *CTNS*-knockout mice (60). Whereas transplantation of mesenchymal stem cells did not integrate efficiently, the transplantation of hematopoietic stem cells led to stable engraftment in mice. This resulted in a long-term improvement of renal function including Fanconi syndrome even though the stem cells did not reprogram proximal tubular cells. Confocal microscopy showed that most transplanted stem cells differentiated into interstitial lymphoid, dendritic, or fibroblastic cells and did not replace renal epithelium cells (61). The reduction of cystine content in different tissues reached up to 94% (60).

Transplantation of hematopoietic stem cells was still effective in older mice, suggesting that stem cell therapy might still be an option even if tissue injury is already manifested. The exact mechanism of stem cell therapy remains unclear. It is possible that stem cell therapy protects healthy tissue from being harmed by cystine crystals or that damaged tissue is being reversed (8). Further problems of allogeneic stem cell transplantation like graft-versus-host-disease, which cause high morbidity and mortality in transplanted patients, still need to be considered. A new approach uses genetically modified autologous hematopoietic stem cells. For transfer a self-inactivating-lentivirus vector is used in an attempt to lower the risks of allogeneic stem cell transplantation (62).

TRANSITION AND TRANSFER

The above-mentioned recommendations of structured transition programs (48, 49) must by no means attach little value but transition has paramount importance in rare diseases that require interdisciplinary lifelong care. Pediatric cystinosis patients in general experience comprehensive, interdisciplinary, and structured care led and coordinated by pediatric nephrologists with the Fanconi tubulopathy and chronic kidney disease being the leading symptoms. This coordinated guardian care may change when the patient is transferred to adult care. Lack of knowledge about rare diseases might be a problem just as appointments with separate professionals focusing on their own specialties resulting in "fragmented" care (48). Therefore, in Germany a current initiative aims to transfer pediatric cystinosis patients to adult Morbus Fabry centers. By this, young adult patients encounter a patient-centered care with high awareness of rare diseases that is led by an adult nephrologist and provides interdisciplinary resources and institutional support perfectly applicable to the needs of cystinosis patients.

CONCLUSION

Over the last decades, our knowledge and understanding of cystinosis has improved continuously. This led to new therapy options and simplified medicine formulations, which dramatically improved life expectancy and life quality of cystinosis patients. But still there is no curative therapy. The new approach of stem cell transplantation gives hope to become a curative treatment that would mean another big step for cystinosis patients to further improve life expectancy and quality.

AUTHOR CONTRIBUTIONS

SB and LW were responsible for concept and creation of this manuscript. Both authors revised the manuscript and approved the final version to be published.

ACKNOWLEDGMENTS

The authors thank Petra Kleinwächter for preparing the figures.

REFERENCES

1. Gahl WA, Thoene JG, Schneider JA. Cystinosis. *N Engl J Med* (2002) 347(2):111–21. doi:10.1056/NEJMra020552
2. Veys KR, Elmonem MA, Arcolino FO, van den Heuvel L, Levtchenko E. Nephropathic cystinosis: an update. *Curr Opin Pediatr* (2017) 29(2):168–78. doi:10.1097/MOP.0000000000000462
3. Gahl WA, Tietze F, Bashan N, Steinherz R, Schulman JD. Defective cystine exodus from isolated lysosome-rich fractions of cystinotic leucocytes. *J Biol Chem* (1982) 257(16):9570–5.
4. Steinherz R, Tietze F, Gahl WA, Triche TJ, Chiang H, Modesti A, et al. Cystine accumulation and clearance by normal and cystinotic leukocytes exposed to cystine dimethyl ester. *Proc Natl Acad Sci U S A* (1982) 79(14):4446–50. doi:10.1073/pnas.79.14.4446
5. Town M, Jean G, Cherqui S, Attard M, Forestier L, Whitmore SA, et al. A novel gene encoding an integral membrane protein is mutated in nephropathic cystinosis. *Nat Genet* (1998) 18(4):319–24. doi:10.1038/ng0498-319
6. Pape L, Pape A, Weber LT, Arbeiter K, Haffner D, Tönshoff B, et al. Cystinose. *Nephrologe* (2017) 12(3):223–9. doi:10.1007/s11560-017-0152-z
7. Al-Haggar M. Cystinosis as a lysosomal storage disease with multiple mutant alleles: phenotypic-genotypic correlations. *World J Nephrol* (2013) 2(4):94–102. doi:10.5527/wjn.v2.i4.94
8. Cherqui S, Courtoy PJ. The renal Fanconi syndrome in cystinosis: pathogenic insights and therapeutic perspectives. *Nat Rev Nephrol* (2017) 13:115. doi:10.1038/nrneph.2016.182
9. Middleton R, Bradbury M, Webb N, O'Donoghue D, Van't Hoff W. Cystinosis. A clinicopathological conference. "From toddlers to twenties and beyond" adult-paediatric nephrology interface meeting, Manchester 2001. *Nephrol Dial Transplant* (2003) 18(12):2492–5. doi:10.1093/ndt/gfg445
10. Servais A, Morinière V, Grünfeld J-P, Noel L-H, Goujon J-M, Chadefaux-Vekemans B, et al. Late-onset nephropathic cystinosis: clinical presentation, outcome, and genotyping. *Clin J Am Soc Nephrol* (2008) 3(1):27–35. doi:10.2215/CJN.01740407
11. Anikster Y, Lucero C, Guo J, Huizing M, Shotelersuk V, Bernardini I, et al. Ocular nonnephropathic cystinosis: clinical, biochemical, and molecular correlations. *Pediatr Res* (2000) 47(1):17–23. doi:10.1203/00006450-200001000-00007
12. Besouw MTP, Van Dyck M, Cassiman D, Claes KJ, Levtchenko EN. Management dilemmas in pediatric nephrology: cystinosis. *Pediatr Nephrol* (2015) 30(8):1349–60. doi:10.1007/s00467-015-3117-3
13. Gahl WA, Kuehl EM, Iwata F, Lindblad A, Kaiser-Kupfer MI. Corneal crystals in nephropathic cystinosis: natural history and treatment with cysteamine eyedrops. *Mol Genet Metab* (2000) 71(1–2):100–20. doi:10.1006/mgme.2000.3062
14. Emma F, Nesterova G, Langman C, Labbé A, Cherqui S, Goodyer P, et al. Nephropathic cystinosis: an international consensus document. *Nephrol Dial Transplant* (2014) 29(Suppl 4):iv87–94. doi:10.1093/ndt/gfu090
15. Touchman JW, Anikster Y, Dietrich NL, Maduro VVB, McDowell G, Shotelersuk V, et al. The genomic region encompassing the nephropathic cystinosis gene (CTNS): complete sequencing of a 200-kb segment and discovery of a novel gene within the common cystinosis-causing deletion. *Genome Res* (2000) 10(2):165–73. doi:10.1101/gr.10.2.165
16. Kalatzis V, Nevo N, Cherqui Sp, Gasnier B, Antignac C. Molecular pathogenesis of cystinosis: effect of CTNS mutations on the transport activity and subcellular localization of cystinosin. *Hum Mol Genet* (2004) 13(13):1361–71. doi:10.1093/hmg/ddh152
17. Attard M, Jean G, Forestier L, Cherqui S, van't Hoff W, Broyer M, et al. Severity of phenotype in cystinosis varies with mutations in the CTNS gene: predicted effect on the model of cystinosin. *Hum Mol Genet* (1999) 8(13):2507–14. doi:10.1093/hmg/8.13.2507
18. Thoene J, Lemons R, Anikster Y, Mullet J, Paelicke K, Lucero C, et al. Mutations of CTNS causing intermediate cystinosis. *Mol Genet Metab* (1999) 67(4):283–93. doi:10.1006/mgme.1999.2876
19. Wilmer MJ, Emma F, Levtchenko EN. The pathogenesis of cystinosis: mechanisms beyond cystine accumulation. *Am J Physiol* (2010) 299(5):F905–16. doi:10.1152/ajprenal.00318.2010
20. Kalatzis V, Cherqui S, Antignac C, Gasnier B. Cystinosin, the protein defective in cystinosis, is a H(+)-driven lysosomal cystine transporter. *EMBO J* (2001) 20(21):5940–9. doi:10.1093/emboj/20.21.5940
21. Joyce E, Ho J, El-Gharbawy A, Salgado CM, Ranganathan S, Reyes-Múgica M. Value of renal biopsy in diagnosing infantile nephropathic cystinosis associated with secondary nephrogenic diabetes insipidus. *Pediatr Dev Pathol* (2017) 20(1):72–5. doi:10.1177/1093526616683873
22. Larsen CP, Walker PD, Thoene JG. The incidence of atubular glomeruli in nephropathic cystinosis renal biopsies. *Mol Genet Metab* (2010) 101(4): 417–20. doi:10.1016/j.ymgme.2010.08.015
23. Wilmer MJ, Christensen EI, van den Heuvel LP, Monnens LA, Levtchenko EN. Urinary protein excretion pattern and renal expression of megalin and cubilin in nephropathic cystinosis. *Am J Kidney Dis* (2008) 51(6):893–903. doi:10.1053/j.ajkd.2008.03.010
24. Liang H, Labbé A, Le Mouhaer J, Plisson C, Baudouin C. A new viscous cysteamine eye drops treatment for ophthalmic cystinosis: an open-label randomized comparative phase III pivotal study. *Invest Ophthalmol Vis Sci* (2017) 58(4):2275–83. doi:10.1167/iovs.16-21080
25. Dufier JL, Dhermy P, Gubler MC, Gagnadoux MF, Broyer M. Ocular changes in long-term evolution of infantile cystinosis. *Ophthalmic Paediatr Genet* (1987) 8(2):131–7. doi:10.3109/13816818709028529
26. Kaiser-Kupfer MI, Fujikawa L, Kuwabara T, Jain S, Gahl WA. Removal of corneal crystals by topical cysteamine in nephropathic cystinosis. *N Engl J Med* (1987) 316(13):775–9. doi:10.1056/NEJM198703263161304
27. Shams F, Livingstone I, Oladiwura D, Ramaesh K. Treatment of corneal cystine crystal accumulation in patients with cystinosis. *Clin Ophthalmol* (2014) 8:2077–84. doi:10.2147/OPTH.S36626
28. Besouw MT, Schneider J, Janssen MC, Greco M, Emma F, Cornelissen EA, et al. Copper deficiency in patients with cystinosis with cysteamine toxicity. *J Pediatr* (2013) 163(3):754–60. doi:10.1016/j.jpeds.2013.03.078
29. Zimakas PJ, Sharma AK, Rodd CJ. Osteopenia and fractures in cystinotic children post renal transplantation. *Pediatr Nephrol* (2003) 18(4):384–90. doi:10.1007/s00467-003-1093-5
30. Weber LT, Mehls O. Limitations of dual x-ray absorptiometry in children with chronic kidney disease. *Pediatr Nephrol* (2010) 25(1):3–5. doi:10.1007/s00467-009-1248-0
31. Ballantyne AO, Spilkin AM, Trauner DA. Executive function in nephropathic cystinosis. *Cogn Behav Neurol* (2013) 26(1):14–22. doi:10.1097/WNN.0b013e31828b9f11
32. Viltz L, Trauner DA. Effect of age of treatment on cognitive performance in patients with cystinosis. *J Pediatr* (2013) 163(2):489–92. doi:10.1016/j.jpeds.2013.01.027
33. Besouw MTP, Hulstijn-Dirkmaat GM, van der Rijken REA, Cornelissen EAM, van Dael CM, Vande Walle J, et al. Neurocognitive functioning in school-aged cystinosis patients. *J Inherit Metab Dis* (2009) 33(6):787–93. doi:10.1007/s10545-010-9182-7
34. Broyer M, Tete MJ, Guest G, Bertheleme JP, Labrousse F, Poisson M. Clinical polymorphism of cystinosis encephalopathy. Results of treatment with cysteamine. *J Inherit Metab Dis* (1996) 19(1):65–75. doi:10.1007/BF01799350
35. Sonies BC, Almajid P, Kleta R, Bernardini I, Gahl WA. Swallowing dysfunction in 101 patients with nephropathic cystinosis: benefit of long-term cysteamine therapy. *Medicine* (2005) 84(3):137–46. doi:10.1097/01.md.0000164204.00159.d4
36. Besouw MT, Kremer JA, Janssen MC, Levtchenko EN. Fertility status in male cystinosis patients treated with cysteamine. *Fertil Steril* (2010) 93(6):1880–3. doi:10.1016/j.fertnstert.2008.12.113
37. Veys KR, D'Hauwers KW, van Dongen AJ, Janssen MC, Besouw MT, Goossens E, et al. First successful conception induced by a male cystinosis patient. *JIMD Rep* (2017). doi:10.1007/8904_2017_19
38. Haase M, Morgera S, Bamberg C, Halle H, Martini S, Hocher B, et al. A systematic approach to managing pregnant dialysis patients—the importance of an intensified haemodiafiltration protocol. *Nephrol Dial Transplant* (2005) 20(11):2537–42. doi:10.1093/ndt/gfi044
39. Thoene JG, Oshima RG, Crawhall JC, Olson DL, Schneider JA. Cystinosis. Intracellular cystine depletion by aminothiols in vitro and in vivo. *J Clin Invest* (1976) 58(1):180–9. doi:10.1172/JCI108448
40. Gahl WA, Tietze F, Butler JD, Schulman JD. Cysteamine depletes cystinotic leucocyte granular fractions of cystine by the mechanism of disulphide interchange. *Biochem J* (1985) 228(3):545–50. doi:10.1042/bj2280545

41. Pisoni RL, Thoene JG, Lemons RM, Christensen HN. Important differences in cationic amino acid transport by lysosomal system c and system y+ of the human fibroblast. *J Biol Chem* (1987) 262(31):15011–8.
42. Chabli A, Aupetit J, Raehm M, Ricquier D, Chadefaux-Vekemans B. Measurement of cystine in granulocytes using liquid chromatography-tandem mass spectrometry. *Clin Biochem* (2007) 40(9–10):692–8. doi:10.1016/j.clinbiochem.2007.02.005
43. Ahlenstiel-Grunow T, Kanzelmeyer NK, Froede K, Kreuzer M, Drube J, Lerch C, et al. Switching from immediate- to extended-release cysteamine in nephropathic cystinosis patients: a retrospective real-life single-center study. *Pediatr Nephrol* (2016) 32(1):91–7. doi:10.1007/s00467-016-3438-x
44. Belldina EB, Huang MY, Schneider JA, Brundage RC, Tracy TS. Steady-state pharmacokinetics and pharmacodynamics of cysteamine bitartrate in paediatric nephropathic cystinosis patients. *Br J Clin Pharmacol* (2003) 56(5):520–5. doi:10.1046/j.1365-2125.2003.01927.x
45. Langman CB, Greenbaum LA, Sarwal M, Grimm P, Niaudet P, Deschênes G, et al. Randomized controlled crossover trial with delayed-release cysteamine bitartrate in nephropathic cystinosis: effectiveness on white blood cell cystine levels and comparison of safety. *Clin J Am Soc Nephrol* (2012) 7(7):1112–20. doi:10.2215/CJN.12321211
46. Dohil R, Fidler M, Gangoiti JA, Kaskel F, Schneider JA, Barshop BA. Twice-daily cysteamine bitartrate therapy for children with cystinosis. *J Pediatr* (2010) 156(1):71–5.e1–3. doi:10.1016/j.jpeds.2009.07.016
47. Bäumner S, Weber LT. Conversion from immediate- to extended-release cysteamine may decrease disease control and increase additional side effects. *Pediatr Nephrol* (2017) 32(7):1281–2. doi:10.1007/s00467-017-3618-3
48. Ariceta G, Lara E, Camacho JA, Oppenheimer F, Vara J, Santos F, et al. Cysteamine (Cystagon®) adherence in patients with cystinosis in Spain: successful in children and a challenge in adolescents and adults. *Nephrol Dial Transplant* (2015) 30(3):475–80. doi:10.1093/ndt/gfu329
49. Raina R, Wang J, Krishnappa V. Structured transition protocol for children with cystinosis. *Front Pediatr* (2017) 5:191. doi:10.3389/fped.2017.00191
50. Brodin-Sartorius A, Tete MJ, Niaudet P, Antignac C, Guest G, Ottolenghi C, et al. Cysteamine therapy delays the progression of nephropathic cystinosis in late adolescents and adults. *Kidney Int* (2012) 81(2):179–89. doi:10.1038/ki.2011.277
51. Besouw MT, Bowker R, Dutertre JP, Emma F, Gahl WA, Greco M, et al. Cysteamine toxicity in patients with cystinosis. *J Pediatr* (2011) 159(6):1004–11. doi:10.1016/j.jpeds.2011.05.057
52. Corden BJ, Schulman JD, Schneider JA, Thoene JG. Adverse reactions to oral cysteamine use in nephropathic cystinosis. *Dev Pharmacol Ther* (1981) 3(1):25–30. doi:10.1159/000457418
53. Tsilou ET, Rubin BI, Reed G, Caruso RC, Iwata F, Balog J, et al. Nephropathic cystinosis: posterior segment manifestations and effects of cysteamine therapy. *Ophthalmology* (2006) 113(6):1002–9. doi:10.1016/j.ophtha.2005.12.026
54. Liang H, Baudouin C, Tahiri Joutei Hassani R, Brignole-Baudouin F, Labbe A. Photophobia and corneal crystal density in nephropathic cystinosis: an in vivo confocal microscopy and anterior-segment optical coherence tomography study. *Invest Ophthalmol Vis Sci* (2015) 56(5):3218–25. doi:10.1167/iovs.15-16499
55. Napolitano G, Johnson JL, He J, Rocca CJ, Monfregola J, Pestonjamasp K, et al. Impairment of chaperone-mediated autophagy leads to selective lysosomal degradation defects in the lysosomal storage disease cystinosis. *EMBO Mol Med* (2015) 7(2):158–74. doi:10.15252/emmm.201404223
56. Rega LR, Polishchuk E, Montefusco S, Napolitano G, Tozzi G, Zhang J, et al. Activation of the transcription factor EB rescues lysosomal abnormalities in cystinotic kidney cells. *Kidney Int* (2016) 89(4):862–73. doi:10.1016/j.kint.2015.12.045
57. Andrzejewska Z, Nevo N, Thomas L, Chhuon C, Bailleux A, Chauvet V, et al. Cystinosin is a component of the vacuolar H(+)-ATPase-Ragulator-Rag complex controlling mammalian target of rapamycin complex 1 signaling. *J Am Soc Nephrol* (2016) 27(6):1678–88. doi:10.1681/ASN.2014090937
58. Levtchenko EN, Wilmer MJG, Janssen AJM, Koenderink JB, Visch H-J, Willems PHGM, et al. Decreased intracellular ATP content and intact mitochondrial energy generating capacity in human cystinotic fibroblasts. *Pediatr Res* (2006) 59(2):287–92. doi:10.1203/01.pdr.0000196334.46940.54
59. Chol M, Nevo N, Cherqui S, Antignac C, Rustin P. Glutathione precursors replenish decreased glutathione pool in cystinotic cell lines. *Biochem Biophys Res Commun* (2004) 324(1):231–5. doi:10.1016/j.bbrc.2004.09.033
60. Syres K, Harrison F, Tadlock M, Jester JV, Simpson J, Roy S, et al. Successful treatment of the murine model of cystinosis using bone marrow cell transplantation. *Blood* (2009) 114(12):2542–52. doi:10.1182/blood-2009-03-213934
61. Yeagy BA, Harrison F, Gubler MC, Koziol JA, Salomon DR, Cherqui S. Kidney preservation by bone marrow cell transplantation in hereditary nephropathy. *Kidney Int* (2011) 79(11):1198–206. doi:10.1038/ki.2010.537
62. Harrison F, Yeagy BA, Rocca CJ, Kohn DB, Salomon DR, Cherqui S. Hematopoietic stem cell gene therapy for the multisystemic lysosomal storage disorder cystinosis. *Mol Ther* (2013) 21(2):433–44. doi:10.1038/mt.2012.214

10

Congenital Heart Defects and Ciliopathies Associated with Renal Phenotypes

George C. Gabriel[1], *Gregory J. Pazour*[2] *and Cecilia W. Lo*[1*]

[1] *Department of Developmental Biology, University of Pittsburgh School of Medicine, Pittsburgh, PA, United States,* [2] *Program in Molecular Medicine, University of Massachusetts Medical School, Worcester, MA, United States*

Correspondence:
Cecilia W. Lo
cel36@pitt.edu

Congenital heart disease (CHD) is one of the most common birth defects, and recent studies indicate cilia-related mutations play a central role in the genetic etiology of CHD. As cilia are also known to have important roles in kidney development and disease, it is not surprising that renal anomalies were found to be enriched among CHD mutant mice recovered in a large-scale mouse forward genetic screen. Indeed 42% of mutations identified to cause both CHD and renal anomalies were cilia-related. Many of these cilia mutations comprise cilia transition zone or inversin compartment components, consistent with the known role of these cilia proteins in a wide variety of ciliopathies. The high prevalence of CHD with congenital anomalies of the kidney and urinary tract (CAKUT) observed in mice was also corroborated with clinical studies that showed 20–30% of CHD patients have renal anomalies. Together these findings suggest CHD patients may benefit from early screening for renal anomalies to allow early diagnosis and intervention to improve outcome for this vulnerable patient population.

Keywords: cilia, CAKUT, congenital heart disease, congenital abnormalities, ciliopathies, genetic syndromes

Congenital heart disease (CHD) is the most common birth defect, occurring in up to 1% of live births (1). Interestingly, CHD often presents in combination with extra cardiac defects including congenital anomalies of the kidney and urinary tract (CAKUT) (2–4). In fact, renal or urinary system defects are associated with 23.1% of congenital heart defects (5). These findings suggest an overlapping genetic etiology for CHD and CAKUT. Consistent with this is the fact that several previously reported mouse models (not individually discussed in this review) have found genetic disruption of a single gene can affect both heart and kidney development, and that many genetic syndromes can present with both cardiac and renal anomalies (6–9). Hence, insights into the genetic etiology of CHD may help elucidate the etiology of CAKUT. Relevant to this is the recent unexpected finding from a large-scale forward genetic screen in mice indicating a significant role for cilia-related mutations in the pathogenesis of CHD (10). As cilia mutations are well-described in the context of CAKUT, this would suggest cilia defects may have a central role in mediating both CHD and CAKUT phenotypes. Below, we briefly discuss CAKUT and its association with CHD, and its shared genetic etiology involving cilia-related mutations.

ASSOCIATION OF HEART AND KIDNEY PHENOTYPES IN GENETIC SYNDROMES

CAKUT represent a broad range of kidney and urinary tract defects. This can include abnormalities in the shape, size, or structure of the kidney including kidney agenesis, kidney hypoplasia or dysplasia, horseshoe/fused kidney, cystic kidneys, or duplex/multiplex kidney, and multiple collecting ducts or ureters (11). These defects can occur in combination such as with the finding of cystic dysplastic kidneys. These structural abnormalities can result in vesicoureteral reflux, ureteropelvic junction obstruction, hydroureter, and hydronephrosis (10, 12). In humans, monogenic mutations in several genes have been implicated in CAKUT development; however, these mutations explain only 5–20% of patient disease (13). Additional causes of CAKUT phenotypes include genetic syndromes, which can present with a spectrum of phenotypes often involving defects in many organs including both the heart and the kidney.

In DiGeorge syndrome, heterozygous deletion of chromosome 22q11.2 is associated with multiple organ defects, including the heart, the kidney, the thymus, and the nervous system. It has an estimated prevalence of 1:3,000 to 1:4,000 live births, though prenatal chromosomal analysis suggests this may be an underestimate, and affected patients characteristically present with CHD, thymus hypoplasia or agenesis, and craniofacial defects (14–16). Approximately 20–30% of DiGeorge syndrome patients also exhibit CAKUT (17). Haploinsufficiency of *TBX1*, a transcription factor within the T-box family, has been shown to contribute to the cardiac phenotypes associated with this disorder (18, 19). More recently, another gene within the 22q11.2 locus, *CRKL*, an adaptor protein that regulates tyrosine kinase signaling, was found to contribute to developmental kidney defects in the context of DiGeorge syndrome (20, 21).

Another syndrome known as VACTERL association also presents with both congenital heart defects and renal abnormalities. Occurring in 1:10,000 to 1:40,000 live births, VACTERL association is a birth defect associated with at least 3 of the following phenotypes: vertebral defects, anal atresia, cardiac defects, trachea-esophageal fistula, renal defects, and limb defects (22). In a large study of patients diagnosed with VACTERL association, 80% exhibited kidney defects and 48% exhibited cardiac defects (23). In humans, several genes have been related to VACTERL association including *FGF8, FOXF1, HOXD13, LPP, TRAP1, and ZIC3,* all of which have been implicated in kidney developmental anomalies, with ZIC3 being an X-linked gene also shown to cause heterotaxy (24).

A rarer genetic disorder known as Fraser syndrome can also cause both CHD and genitourinary abnormalities. It is a recessive disorder with a prevalence of only 1 in 200,000 (25). Patients with Fraser syndrome can present with eye defects, syndactyly, kidney defects, most commonly kidney agenesis, and heart defects (25). Fraser syndrome is associated with mutations in *FRAS1*, *FREM2*, or *GRIP1*, all of which are known to interact to form a FRAS/FREM complex that is localized to the basement membrane (26, 27). Mutations in these genes cause loss of the FRAS/FREM complex that likely drives the disease phenotypes observed in Fraser syndrome, although the precise disease mechanism remains unclear (27, 28).

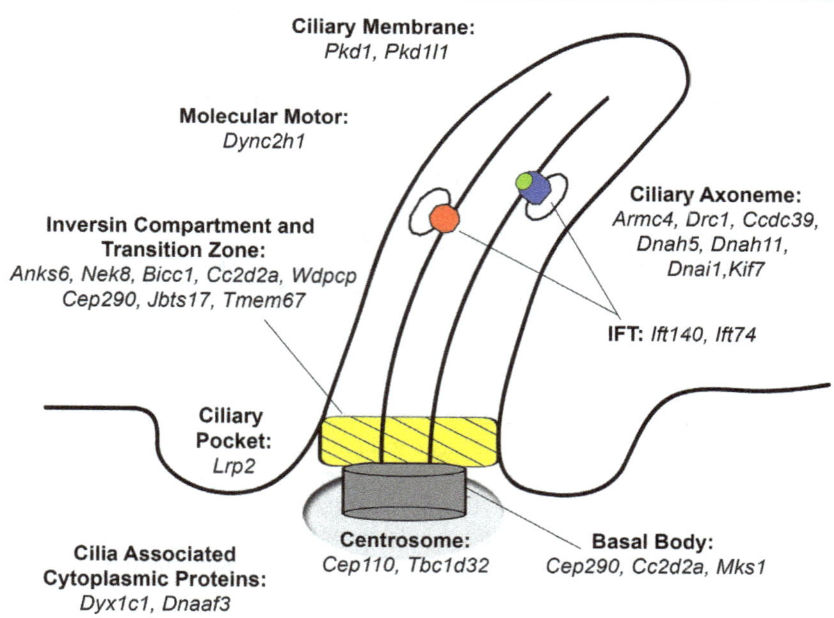

FIGURE 1 | Ciliary localization of proteins that when mutated cause congenital heart disease recovered from a large-scale screen. Mutations in several of these proteins can also cause CAKUT. Adapted from Damerla et al. (31).

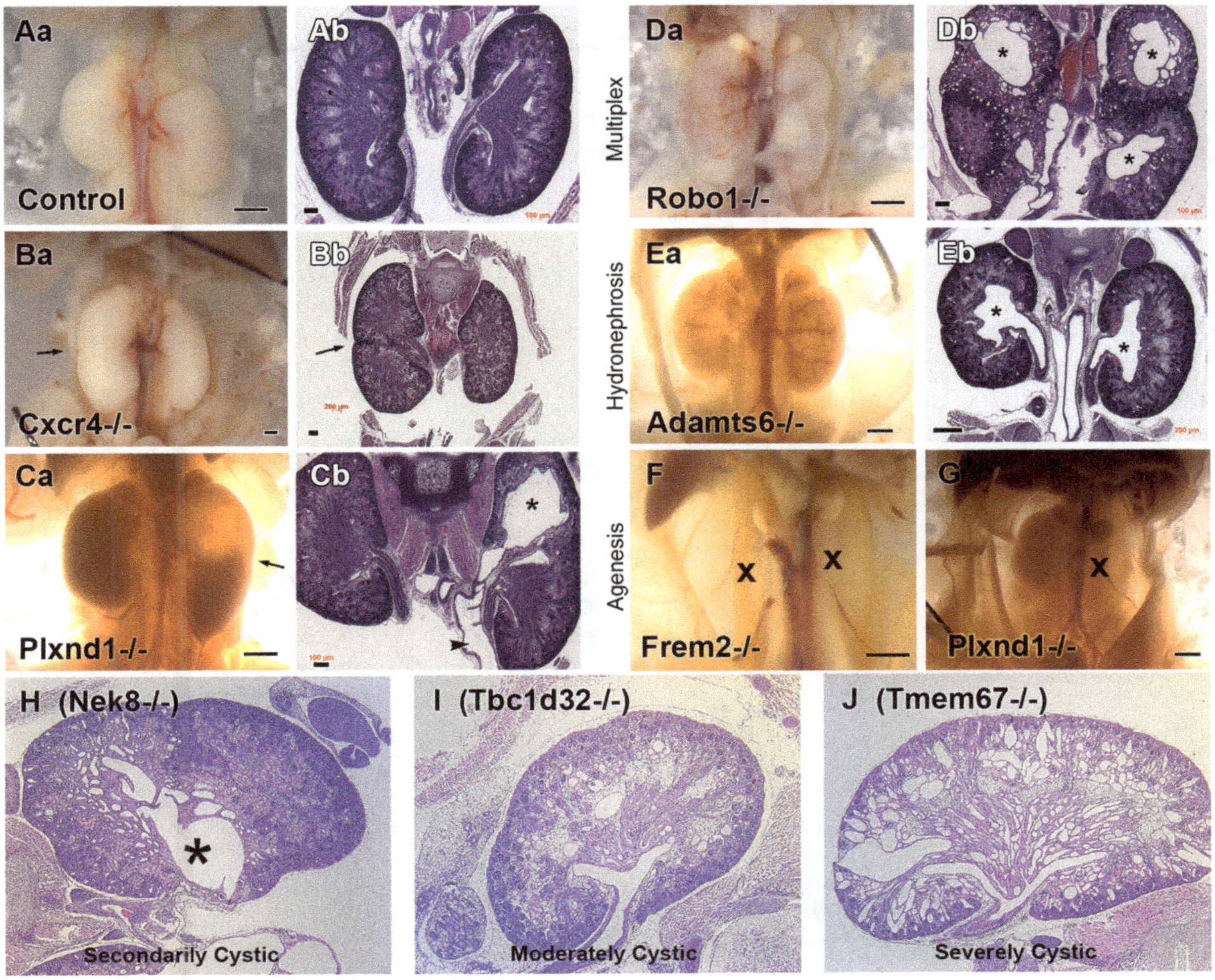

FIGURE 2 | Kidney Phenotypes Observed in Mice with Congenital Heart Disease. Representative examples of the kidney phenotypes observed in mice with congenital heart disease recovered from a large scale forward genetic screen. Phenotypes can be observed at necropsy and upon H&E staining. Adapted from San Agustin et al. (10). Control necropsy **(Aa)** and control H&E stained kidneys **(Ab)** can be compared with mutant necropsy **(Ba,Ca,Da,Ea,F,G)** and mutant H&E stained kidneys **(Bb,Cb,Db,Eb, H–J)**. *represents hydronephrosis.

CILIA AND THE GENETIC LANDSCAPE OF CHD

The close association of renal anomalies with CHD suggests insights into the genetics of CHD can yield significant insights into the mechanism of disease pathogenesis for CAKUT. Interestingly, the pursuit of a large-scale forward genetic screen in mice for mutations causing CHD yielded a large preponderance of mutations in cilia-related genes (29). From screening more than 100,000 ethylnitrosourea (ENU) mutagenized mice using *in utero* fetal ultrasound phenotyping, we recovered over 200 mouse lines with a wide spectrum of CHD. Using whole exome sequencing nearly 100 CHD-causing mutations were recovered in 61 genes, 34 (55.7%) of which were cilia-related (29). As this is a phenotype driven mutagenesis screen in which fetal echocardiography was used to identify mutants with CHD, these findings point to cilia as playing a central role in the pathogenesis of CHD. This is corroborated with the completion of the screen, showing over 50 genes are cilia-related among 100 genes recovered causing CHD. Moreover, analysis of de novo mutations identified in whole exome sequencing analysis from CHD patients also identified similar mutations contributing to CHD pathogenesis (30).

CILIA AND CILIOPATHIES IN CHD, RENAL ANOMALIES, AND OTHER HUMAN DISEASES

Cilia are microtubule-based organelles that have well-described compartments including an axoneme that projects from the apical cell surface, and a basal body base with an overlying transition zone and inversin compartment that regulate protein trafficking into and out of the cilium (**Figure 1**) (32). Cilia can

TABLE 1 | Renal anomalies associated with genes causing congenital heart defects.

Gene[a]	Duplex/multiplex	Hydro-nephrosis	Cystic	Agenesis/Hypoplasia	Cardiac phenotype
*Anks6** (10)	–	–	80%	–	DORV, TGA, AVSD, VSD
*Bicc1** (8)	–	–	100%	–	DORV, TGA, AVSD, IAA
*Cc2d2a** (5)	–	–	100%	–	TGA, PTA, DORV, AVSD, Pulmonary Atresia
Cep110 (5)	–	60%	–	–	DORV, AVSD, VSD
*Cep290** (13)	15%	–	100%	–	DORV, AVSD
*Dync2h1** (6)	50%	–	–	–	PTA/Pulmonary atresia, VSD, MAPCA
Lrp2 (3)	–	100%	100%	–	PTA, VSD, Ao arch defects
Pkd1 (4)	–	–	100%	–	Biventricular Hypertrophy
Ptk7 (3)	–	–	100%	–	DORV, VSD, Biventricular Hypertrophy
*Tbc1d32** (12)	25%	–	92%	–	PTA, DORV, TGA, AVSD
*Tmem67** (12)	42%	–	100%	–	DORV, AVSD, IAA
Adamts6 (16)	–	56%	–	–	DORV, OA
*Ap1b1** (10)	–	–	80%	–	AVSD, VSD, Atrial Isomerism
Ap2b1 (3)	–	–	75%	–	DORV/Taussig-Bing, AVSD, VSD, Ao arch defects
Bmp10 (2)	–	–	100%	–	DORV
Cxcr4 (5)	60%	–	–	–	VSD Ao atresia, Ao arch defects
Frem2 (10)	–	–	–	100%	Biventricular Hypertrophy
Lama5 (5)	–	–	–	60%	DORV
Plxnd1 (3)	–	–	–	63%	PTA, DORV, AVSD, RAA
Prdm1 (8)	38%	–	–	–	DORV, AVSD, VSD, Ao atresia, Ao arch defects
Qrich1 (3)	–	–	–	67%	DORV, AVSD, noncompaction
Robo1 (5)	100% (M)	–	–	–	VSD, Biventricular Hypertrophy
Slit2 (7)	100% (M)	–	–	–	DORV, VSD, Ao arch defects
Snx17 (3)	66%	–	–	–	DORV/OA, AVSD
Wnt5a (7)	43%	–	–	–	DORV, PTA, AVSD, VSD
Zbtb14 (4)	–	–	100%	–	DORV, AVSD, atrioventricular and semilunar valve defects

[a] Gene with dark highlighting are ciliary components based on proteomic and other studies.
*Gene names followed by * indicate mutations that cause situs defects.*
Parenthesis indicate the number of mutants analyzed.
Adapted from San Agustin et al. (10).

be motile with the expression of motor dyneins that drive ciliary motility, or nonmotile, termed primary cilia, which extend from almost all cell types in the body, including cells of the developing heart, and are known to serve important cell signaling functions by mediating various signal transduction processes (33–35). Motile cilia are required for left-right patterning as well as in mediating sperm motility, mucociliary clearance in the airway, and also cerebral spinal fluid flow in the brain. Importantly, it is now appreciated that cilia mutations can cause a wide spectrum of human diseases collectively known as ciliopathies (31). Many of these ciliopathies can present with renal anomalies, such as in nephronepthesis, Meckel-Gruber syndrome (MKS), Bardet-Biedl syndrome (BBS), Joubert syndrome, Alstrom syndrome and polycystic kidney disease among others (36). The renal defects observed may include CAKUT, polycystic kidney disease or progressive renal dysfunction. Other structural birth defects observed in the ciliopathies include CHD, cardiomyopathy, skeletal malformations, brain abnormalities, blindness, and obesity (31).

Many of the mutations known to cause renal anomalies within the ciliopathy spectrum are associated with proteins localized in the cilia transition zone or inversin compartment. Thus, among the 61 genes recovered causing CHD, half ($N = 34$) were cilia-related, including 11 affecting transition zone or inversin compartment components (29). While these are mainly thought to disrupt primary cilia function, recent studies showed ciliopathies generally considered to involve primary cilia defects may also impact motile cilia function. This is indicated by the observation of airway clearance defects in patients diagnosed with ciliopathies such as Leber congenital amaurosis or Sensenbrenner syndrome (37, 38). This is not unexpected given over 70% of proteins required for primary cilia function are also expressed in motile cilia (39). Indeed, airway clearance defects are the hallmark of a ciliopathy known as primary ciliary dyskinesia (PCD).

PCD patients have severe sinopulmonary disease and typically this is associated with mutations in genes required for motile cilia function, such as motor dyneins (40–42). It is interesting to note some isolated reports of bronchiectasis associated with polycystic kidney disease, although the connection with airway clearance defects is unknown (43). PCD patients also can exhibit laterality defects, a reflection of the requirement for

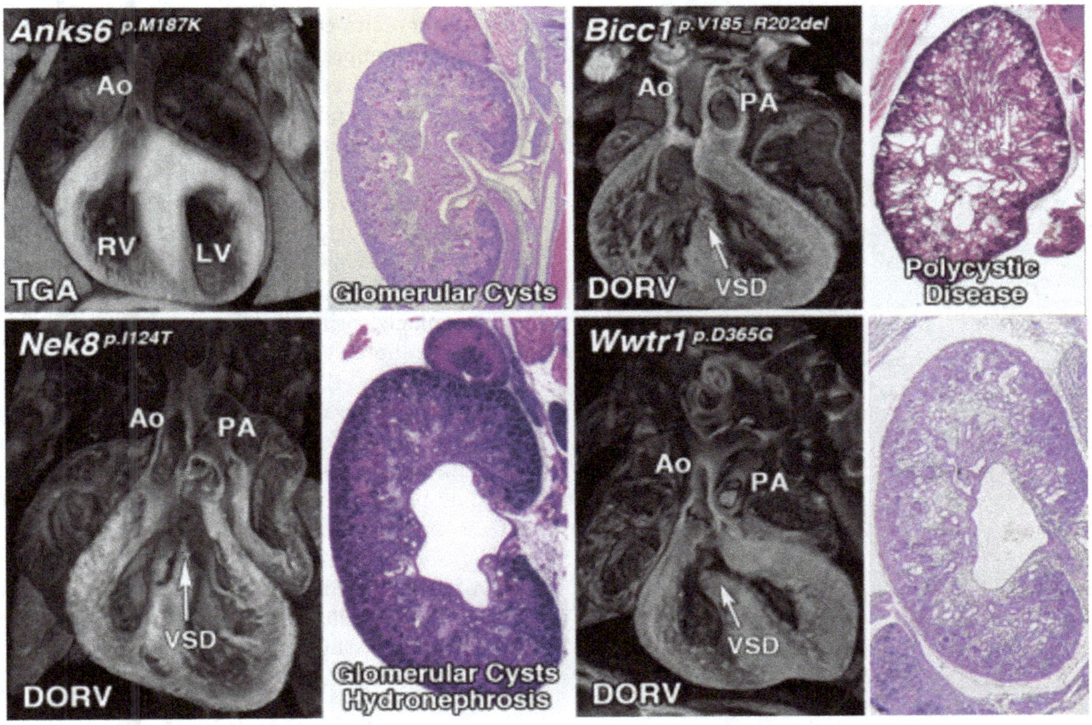

FIGURE 3 | Mutations in interacting proteins cause a similar spectrum of both heart and kidney phenotypes. Mutations in four interacting proteins, *Anks6, Bicc1, Nek8*, and *Wwtr1* cause similar phenotypes including both congenital heart disease and cystic kidney disease (Unpublished data).

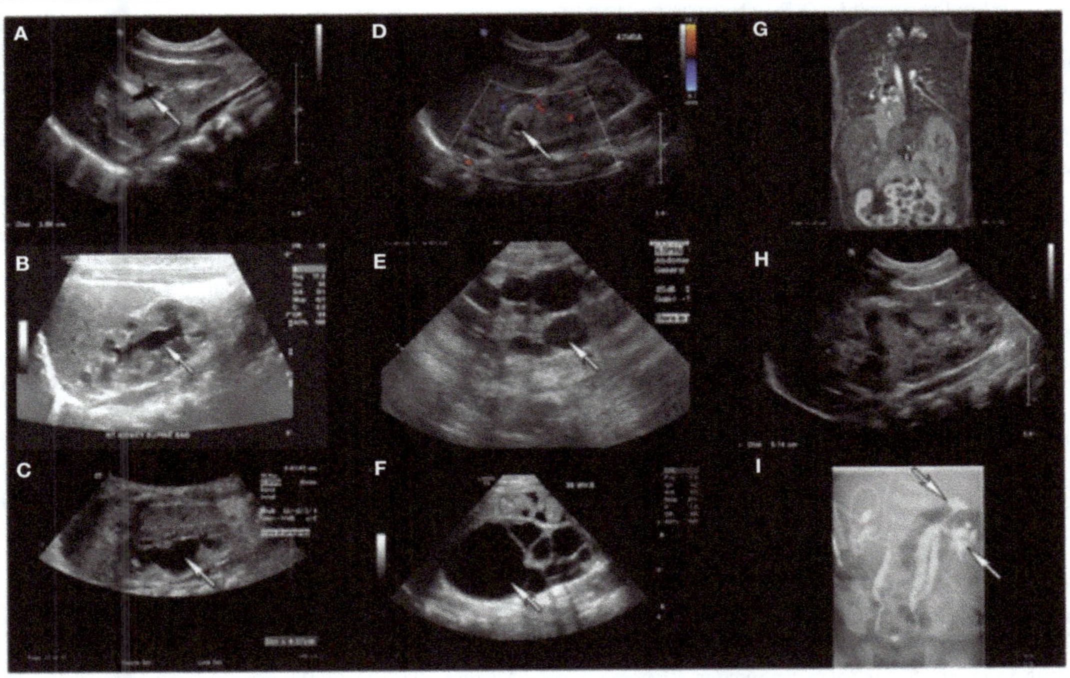

FIGURE 4 | Kidney Defects Observed in Patients with CHD. Renal ultrasound of patients with congenital heart disease unveils a spectrum of renal abnormalities including intrarenal collecting system dilation **(A–C)**, cystic-dysplastic abnormalities **(D–F)**, horseshoe kidney **(G)**, and duplicated collecting system depicted with renal ultrasound **(H)**, and voiding cystourethrogram **(I)**. Adapted from San Agustin et al. (10).

TABLE 2 | Clinical characteristics of congenital heart disease patients.

ID #	Kidney phenotypes	Cardiac phenotype*	Other phenotypes
7042	Abnormally rotated kidney, Pelvicaliectasis	HLHS	
7199	Caliectasis (dilation of the renal calices)	HLHS	Hypothyroidism
7351	Duplicated collecting duct system, Hydronephrosis	HLHS	
7208	Duplicated collecting system, Vesicoureteral reflux	D-TGA	
7319	Ectopic kidney	DORV, subaortic VSD	
7040	Ectopic kidney, vesicoureteral reflux	ASD, VSD	
7194	Horseshoe kidney	TOF, PA	
7035	Hydronephrosis	ASD, VSD	Tethered cord, hypothyroidism
7288	Mild Hydronephrosis	Truncus arteriosus	
7053	Pelvicaliectasis	D-TGA	
7302	Pelvicaliectasis	HLHS	
7306	Pelvicaliectasis	D-TGA	
7334	Pelvicaliectasis	ASD, VSD, PDA, Interrupted IVC	
7389	Pelvicaliectasis	HLHS	
7417	Pelvicaliectasis	VSD/PDA/ventricular hypertrophy	
7419	Pelvicaliectasis	DORV, PA, complete AVSD, supracardiac TAPVR	Heterotaxy, asplenia
7430	Pelvicaliectasis	Unbalanced AVSD, PA, supracardiac TAPVR	Heterotaxy, asplenia
7058	Pelvicaliectasis, Hydroureter	TOF	Tethered cord, exotropia, neurogenic bladder
7336	Pyelectasis (dilation of the renal pelvis)	D-TGA	
7289	Renal size asymmetry, Solitary cyst seen by ultrasound.	HLHS	
7474	Unilateral Agenesis	HLHS	Single testis
7027	Vesicoureteral reflux	D-TGA	Situs inversus totalis, seizures
7438	Vesicoureteral reflux	HLHS	Aspiration, hypospadias

**D-TGA, D-transposition of the great arteries; DORV, double outlet right ventricle; ASD, atrial septal defect; VSD, ventricular septal defect; HLHS, hypoplastic left heart syndrome; TOF, Tetralogy of Fallot; AVSD, atrioventricular septal defect; PA, pulmonary atresia; TAPVR, total anomalous pulmonary venous return. Adapted from San Agustin et al. (10).*

motile cilia in the specification of the left-right body axis (44, 45). Consistent with this, PCD patients can display a spectrum of phenotypes including situs solitus (normal visceral organ situs), situs inversus totalis also known as Kartagener's syndrome (reversed visceral organ situs), and heterotaxy, or the randomization of visceral organ situs. In this context, CHD is often associated with heterotaxy as a result of defects in motile cilia function.

Interestingly, some ciliopathies thought to affect only primary cilia function also can be associated with laterality defects, one prominent example being MKS, a ciliopathy that causes severe birth defects and is usually prenatal or neonatal lethal. Studies of *Mks1* mutant mice showed defects involving not only the primary cilia, but also laterality defects associated with the loss of motile cilia function in the embryonic node (46). Together, these findings suggest that the distinction of ciliopathies as either affecting motile or primary cilia can be problematic, given the promiscuity of cilia genes in having functional roles in both primary and motile cilia.

Intriguingly, primary cilia proteins can be found in other cellular locations, suggesting that they may have other non-ciliary functions (47). In fact, ciliary proteins are also involved in a wide range of cellular processes including cell cycle progression, cytoskeletal organization, and vesicular trafficking (48–50). Further, cilia themselves are involved in several cell signaling pathways including the sonic hedgehog, TGFβ, wnt, and notch pathways, and defects can arise in these pathways through defective cilia or pathway components outside of the cilium (51). Thus, future research will be important to determine the precise roles cilia and cilia associated proteins play in CHD and CAKUT development.

MUTATIONS CAUSING CHD AND CAKUT PHENOTYPES

Extra-cardiac phenotypes, including renal anomalies, were recovered in many CHD mutant mice even though the screen was entirely focused on CHD phenotyping. This included a spectrum of kidney phenotypes including duplex kidney, multiplex kidney, hydronephrosis, kidney agenesis, and cystic kidney (**Figure 2**), with the most commonly observed renal phenotype being duplex kidneys (10). Among the 39 mutant mouse lines recovered with congenital kidney abnormalities, the most common CHD phenotype is double outlet right ventricle (DORV), occurring in 19/39 lines (48.7%). This is followed by atrioventricular septal defect, which occurred in 15/39 lines (38.5%; **Table 1**). Other CHD phenotypes associated with kidney defects included transposition of the great arteries (TGA), persistent truncus arteriosus (PTA), ventricular septal defect (VSD), aortic arch anomalies, and biventricular hypertrophy (**Table 1**).

Previous attempts to recover CAKUT genes have been confounded by incomplete penetrance and the probable involvement of more complex genetics. The few CAKUT genes previously identified are largely those that mediate the early steps in kidney development and patterning. Other than *Pax2*, which causes renal coloboma syndrome, and *Hnf1b*, which causes renal cystic disease and diabetes, most genes identified to cause CAKUT are associated with disease in only a few patients and hence, the evidence supporting pathogenesis is limited (52). Among the 135 CHD mouse lines recovered, 39 (28.8%) had kidney defects caused by mutations in 26 genes, 11 (42%) being known cilia genes (**Table 1**, **Figure 1**) (10). Remarkably, this included four cilia genes that encoded known direct protein-protein interactors: *Anks6*, *Nek8*, *Bicc1*, and *Wwtr1* (53–56).

These mutations were found in four independent CHD mouse lines, with mutation in each gene causing a similar spectrum of kidney and heart defect phenotypes comprising double outlet right ventricle and cystic kidney disease (**Figure 3**).

CLINICAL STUDY SHOWING ASSOCIATION OF CHD WITH CAKUT PHENOTYPES

The relevance of CAKUT abnormalities in CHD was confirmed with a clinical study of 77 CHD patients recruited from the Children's Hospital of Pittsburgh. Retrospective review of the medical records of these 77 patients revealed 23 (30%) also had some form of renal defect such as renal cysts, kidney agenesis, cystic dysplastic kidneys, and horseshoe kidney (**Figure 4**, **Table 2**) (10). These findings are in agreement with a previous epidemiological study in the Atlanta metro area, which showed 23% of 8,000 subjects with CHD also had renal abnormalities (1). Thus, both the mouse and human studies point to a significant overlap in the genetic etiology of CHD and kidney abnormalities. This probably reflects the conservation of developmental pathways and cell signaling mechanisms that regulate cardiovascular and renal development, including a central role for cilia in the pathogenesis of CHD and renal birth defects. Together these findings suggest the routine evaluation of CHD patients for renal anomalies with simple non-invasive renal ultrasound may be warranted. This may allow early diagnosis and early therapeutic intervention to treat and manage any renal dysfunction that could negatively impact the long-term outcome of this high-risk patient population.

CONCLUSION

Studies in both CHD mutant mice and CHD patients showed CAKUT is highly associated with CHD. This is supported by the finding of CAKUT and CHD in various genetic syndromes, and the finding that many mutations identified to cause CHD can also cause CAKUT phenotypes. Among genes identified to cause both CHD and CAKUT there is a significant enrichment of cilia genes, indicating a central role for cilia in the pathogenesis of CHD and CAKUT phenotypes. However, as half of the mutations identified to cause CHD and renal anomalies are not known to be cilia-related, the association of CHD with renal anomalies likely extend beyond the role of cilia in heart and kidney development. The clinical relevance of these findings in mice were shown with the observation that 23–30% of CHD patients also exhibited renal anomalies. This would suggest CHD patients may benefit from routine evaluation for renal anomalies. This might improve the long-term outcome of this high-risk patient population by reducing potential renal complications with early diagnosis and therapeutic intervention.

AUTHOR CONTRIBUTIONS

All authors listed contributed intellectually to this work and approved it for publication.

ACKNOWLEDGMENTS

This work was supported by NIH grants HL098180, 1S10 OD010340, HL132024, and GM104412 to CL and GM060992 and DK103632 to GP.

REFERENCES

1. Reller MD, Strickland MJ, Riehle-Colarusso T, Mahle WT, Correa A. Prevalence of congenital heart defects in metropolitan Atlanta, 1998-2005. *J Pediatr.* (2008) 153:807–13. doi: 10.1016/j.jpeds.2008.05.059
2. Nedima Atić HB, Ibrahimović J, Zulić S, Osmanović E. Cardiac evaluation of children with congenital anomalies of the kidneys and urinary tract. *Paediatr Tdy* (2016) 12:169–75. doi: 10.5457/p2005-114.153
3. Egbe A, Lee S, Ho D, Uppu S, Srivastava S. Prevalence of congenital anomalies in newborns with congenital heart disease diagnosis. *Ann Pediatr Cardiol.* (2014) 7:86–91. doi: 10.4103/0974-2069.132474
4. Homsy J, Zaidi S, Shen Y, Ware JS, Samocha KE, Karczewski KJ, et al. *De novo* mutations in congenital heart disease with neurodevelopmental and other congenital anomalies. *Science* (2015) 350:1262–6. doi: 10.1126/science.aac9396
5. Miller A, Riehle-Colarusso T, Alverson CJ, Frias JL, Correa A. Congenital heart defects and major structural noncardiac anomalies, Atlanta, Georgia, 1968 to 2005. *J Pediatr.* (2011) 159:70–8.e2. doi: 10.1016/j.jpeds.2010.12.051
6. McCright B, Gao X, Shen L, Lozier J, Lan Y, Maguire M, et al. Defects in development of the kidney, heart and eye vasculature in mice homozygous for a hypomorphic Notch2 mutation. *Development* (2001) 128:491–502.
7. Riazi AM, Arsdell GV, Buchwald M. Transgenic expression of CECR1 adenosine deaminase in mice results in abnormal development of heart and kidney. *Transgen Res.* (2005) 14:333–6. doi: 10.1007/s11248-005-1174-2
8. Martinez-Estrada OM, Lettice LA, Essafi A, Guadix JA, Slight J, Velecela V, et al. Wt1 is required for cardiovascular progenitor cell formation through transcriptional control of Snail and E-cadherin. *Nat Genet.* (2010) 42:89–93. doi: 10.1038/ng.494
9. Boulter C, Mulroy S, Webb S, Fleming S, Brindle K, Sandford R. Cardiovascular, skeletal, and renal defects in mice with a targeted disruption of the Pkd1 gene. *Proc Natl Acad Sci USA.* (2001) 98:12174–9. doi: 10.1073/pnas.211191098
10. San Agustin JT, Klena N, Granath K, Panigrahy A, Stewart E, Devine W, et al. Genetic link between renal birth defects and congenital heart disease. *Nat Commun.* (2016) 7:11103. doi: 10.1038/ncomms 11103
11. Renkema KY, Winyard PJ, Skovorodkin IN, Levtchenko E, Hindryckx A, Jeanpierre C, et al. Novel perspectives for investigating congenital anomalies of the kidney and urinary tract (CAKUT). *Nephrol Dial Transplant.* (2011) 26:3843–51. doi: 10.1093/ndt/gfr655
12. Hwang DY, Dworschak GC, Kohl S, Saisawat P, Vivante A, Hilger AC, et al. Mutations in 12 known dominant disease-causing genes clarify many congenital anomalies of the kidney and urinary tract. *Kidney Int.* (2014) 85:1429–33. doi: 10.1038/ki.2013.508
13. van der Ven AT, Vivante A, Hildebrandt F. Novel insights into the pathogenesis of monogenic congenital anomalies of the kidney and urinary tract. *J Am Soc Nephrol.* (2018) 29:36–50. doi: 10.1681/ASN.20170 50561
14. Goodship J, Cross I, LiLing J, Wren C. A population study of chromosome 22q11 deletions in infancy. *Arch Dis Childhood* (1998) 79:348–51. doi: 10.1136/adc.79.4.348
15. Leana-Cox J, Pangkanon S, Eanet KR, Curtin MS, Wulfsberg EA. Familial DiGeorge/velocardiofacial syndrome with deletions of chromosome area22q11.2: report of five families with a review of the literature. *Am J Med Genet.* (1996) 65:309–16. doi: 10.1002/(sici)1096-8628(19961111)65:4<309::Aid-ajmg12>3.0.Co;2-y

16. Grati FR, Molina Gomes D, Ferreira JC, Dupont C, Alesi V, Gouas L, et al. Prevalence of recurrent pathogenic microdeletions and microduplications in over 9500 pregnancies. *Prenat Diagn.* (2015) 35:801–9. doi: 10.1002/pd.4613
17. Burnside RD. 22q11.21 deletion syndromes: a review of proximal, central, and distal deletions and their associated features. *Cytogenet Genome Res.* (2015) 146:89–99. doi: 10.1159/000438708
18. Lindsay EA, Vitelli F, Su H, Morishima M, Huynh T, Pramparo T, et al. Tbx1 haploinsufficieny in the DiGeorge syndrome region causes aortic arch defects in mice. *Nature* (2001) 410:97–101. doi: 10.1038/35065105
19. Yagi H, Furutani Y, Hamada H, Sasaki T, Asakawa S, Minoshima S, et al. Role of TBX1 in human del22q11.2 syndrome. *Lancet* (2003) 362:1366–73. doi: 10.1016/S0140-6736(03)14632-6
20. Haller M, Mo Q, Imamoto A, Lamb DJ. Murine model indicates 22q11.2 signaling adaptor CRKL is a dosage-sensitive regulator of genitourinary development. *Proc Natl Acad Sci USA.* (2017) 114:4981–6. doi: 10.1073/pnas.1619523114
21. Lopez-Rivera E, Liu YP, Verbitsky M, Anderson BR, Capone VP, Otto EA, et al. Genetic drivers of kidney defects in the DiGeorge syndrome. *N Engl J Med.* (2017) 376:742–54. doi: 10.1056/NEJMoa1609009
22. Hilger A, Schramm C, Pennimpede T, Wittler L, Dworschak GC, Bartels E, et al. *De novo* microduplications at 1q41, 2q37.3, and 8q24.3 in patients with VATER/VACTERL association. *Eur J Hum Genet.* (2013) 21:1377–82. doi: 10.1038/ejhg.2013.58
23. Botto LD, Khoury MJ, Mastroiacovo P, Castilla EE, Moore CA, Skjaerven R, et al. The spectrum of congenital anomalies of the VATER association: an international study. *Am J. Med. Genet.* (1997) 71:8–15. doi: 10.1002/(sici)1096-8628(19970711)71:1<8::aid-ajmg2>3.0.co;2-v
24. Reutter H, Hilger AC, Hildebrandt F, Ludwig M. Underlying genetic factors of the VATER/VACTERL association with special emphasis on the "Renal" phenotype. *Pediatr Nephrol.* (2016) 31:2025–33. doi: 10.1007/s00467-016-3335-3
25. Barisic I, Odak L, Loane M, Garne E, Wellesley D, Calzolari E, et al. Fraser syndrome: epidemiological study in a European population. *Am J Med Genet A* (2013) 161A:1012–8. doi: 10.1002/ajmg.a.35839
26. van Haelst MM, Maiburg M, Baujat G, Jadeja S, Monti E, Bland E, et al. Molecular study of 33 families with Fraser syndrome new data and mutation review. *Am J Med Genet A* (2008) 146A:2252–7. doi: 10.1002/ajmg.a.32440
27. Vogel MJ, van Zon P, Brueton L, Gijzen M, van Tuil MC, Cox P, et al. Mutations in GRIP1 cause Fraser syndrome. *J Med Genet.* (2012) 49:303–6. doi: 10.1136/jmedgenet-2011-100590
28. McGregor L, Makela V, Darling SM, Vrontou S, Chalepakis G, Roberts C, et al. Fraser syndrome and mouse blebbed phenotype caused by mutations in FRAS1/Fras1 encoding a putative extracellular matrix protein. *Nat Genet.* (2003) 34:203–8. doi: 10.1038/ng1142
29. Li Y, Klena NT, Gabriel GC, Liu X, Kim AJ, Lemke K, et al. Global genetic analysis in mice unveils central role for cilia in congenital heart disease. *Nature* (2015) 521:520–4. doi: 10.1038/nature14269
30. Zaidi S, Choi M, Wakimoto H, Ma L, Jiang J, Overton JD, et al. *De novo* mutations in histone-modifying genes in congenital heart disease. *Nature* (2013) 498:220–3. doi: 10.1038/nature12141
31. Rao Damerla R, Gabriel GC, Li Y, Klena NT, Liu X, Chen Y, et al. Role of cilia in structural birth defects: insights from ciliopathy mutant mouse models. *Birth Defects Res C Embryo Tdy* (2014) 102:115–25. doi: 10.1002/bdrc.21067
32. Satir P, Christensen ST. Overview of structure and function of mammalian cilia. *Annu Rev Physiol.* (2007) 69:377–400. doi: 10.1146/annurev.physiol.69.040705.141236
33. Pala R, Alomari N, Nauli SM. Primary cilium-dependent signaling mechanisms. *Int J Mol Sci.* (2017) 18:E2272. doi: 10.3390/ijms18112272
34. Reiter JF, Leroux MR. Genes and molecular pathways underpinning ciliopathies. *Nat Rev Mol Cell Biol.* (2017) 18:533–47. doi: 10.1038/nrm.2017.60
35. Slough J, Cooney L, Brueckner M. Monocilia in the embryonic mouse heart suggest a direct role for cilia in cardiac morphogenesis. *Dev Dyn.* (2008) 237:2304–14. doi: 10.1002/dvdy.21669
36. Mitchison HM, Valente EM. Motile and non-motile cilia in human pathology: from function to phenotypes. *J Pathol.* (2017) 241:294–309. doi: 10.1002/path.4843
37. Papon JF, Perrault I, Coste A, Louis B, Gerard X, Hanein S, et al. Abnormal respiratory cilia in non-syndromic Leber congenital amaurosis with CEP290 mutations. *J Med Genet.* (2010) 47:829–34. doi: 10.1136/jmg.2010.077883
38. Li Y, Garrod AS, Madan-Khetarpal S, Sreedher G, McGuire M, Yagi H, et al. Respiratory motile cilia dysfunction in a patient with cranioectodermal dysplasia. *Am J Med Genet A* (2015) 167A:2188–96. doi: 10.1002/ajmg.a.37133
39. Ishikawa H, Thompson J, Yates JR III, Marshall WF. Proteomic analysis of mammalian primary cilia. *Curr Biol.* (2012) 22:414–9. doi: 10.1016/j.cub.2012.01.031
40. Noone PG, Leigh MW, Sannuti A, Minnix SL, Carson JL, Hazucha M, et al. Primary ciliary dyskinesia: diagnostic and phenotypic features. *Am J Respir Crit Care Med.* (2004) 169:459–67. doi: 10.1164/rccm.200303-365OC
41. Horani A, Ferkol TW, Dutcher SK, Brody SL. Genetics and biology of primary ciliary dyskinesia. *Paediatr Respir Rev.* (2016) 18:18–24. doi: 10.1016/j.prrv.2015.09.001
42. Supp DM, Witte DP, Potter SS, Brueckner M. Mutation of an axonemal dynein affects left-right asymmetry in inversus viscerum mice. *Nature* (1997) 389:963–6. doi: 10.1038/40140
43. Driscoll JA, Bhalla S, Liapis H, Ibricevic A, Brody SL. Autosomal dominant polycystic kidney disease is associated with an increased prevalence of radiographic bronchiectasis. *Chest* (2008) 133:1181–8. doi: 10.1378/chest.07-2147
44. Leigh MW, Pittman JE, Carson JL, Ferkol TW, Dell SD, Davis SD, et al. Clinical and genetic aspects of primary ciliary dyskinesia/Kartagener syndrome. *Genet Med.* (2009) 11:473–87. doi: 10.1097/GIM.0b013e3181a53562
45. McGrath J, Somlo S, Makova S, Tian X, Brueckner M. Two populations of node monocilia initiate left-right asymmetry in the mouse. *Cell* (2003) 114:61–73. doi: 10.1016/s0092-8674(03)00511-7
46. Cui C, Chatterjee B, Francis D, Yu Q, SanAgustin JT, Francis R, et al. Disruption of Mks1 localization to the mother centriole causes cilia defects and developmental malformations in Meckel-Gruber syndrome. *Dis Model Mech.* (2011) 4:43–56. doi: 10.1242/dmm.006262
47. Hua K, Ferland RJ. Primary cilia proteins: ciliary and extraciliary sites and functions. *Cell Mol Life Sci.* (2018) 75:1521–40. doi: 10.1007/s00018-017-2740-5
48. Vertii A, Bright A, Delaval B, Hehnly H, Doxsey S. New frontiers: discovering cilia-independent functions of cilia proteins. *EMBO Rep.* (2015) 16:1275–87. doi: 10.15252/embr.201540632
49. McClure-Begley TD, Klymkowsky MW. Nuclear roles for cilia-associated proteins. *Cilia* (2017) 6:8. doi: 10.1186/s13630-017-0052-x
50. Yuan S, Sun Z. Expanding horizons: ciliary proteins reach beyond cilia. *Annu Rev Genet.* (2013) 47:353–76. doi: 10.1146/annurev-genet-111212-133243
51. Goetz SC, Anderson KV. The primary cilium: a signalling centre during vertebrate development. *Nat Rev Genet.* (2010) 11:331–44. doi: 10.1038/nrg2774
52. Nicolaou N, Renkema KY, Bongers EM, Giles RH, Knoers NV. Genetic, environmental, and epigenetic factors involved in CAKUT. *Nat Rev Nephrol.* (2015) 11:720–31. doi: 10.1038/nrneph.2015.140
53. Hoff S, Halbritter J, Epting D, Frank V, Nguyen TM, van Reeuwijk J, et al. ANKS6 is a central component of a nephronophthisis module linking NEK8 to INVS and NPHP3. *Nat Genet.* (2013) 45:951–6. doi: 10.1038/ng.2681
54. Stagner EE, Bouvrette DJ, Cheng J, Bryda EC. The polycystic kidney disease-related proteins Bicc1 and SamCystin interact. *Biochem Biophys Res Commun.* (2009) 383:16–21. doi: 10.1016/j.bbrc.2009.03.113

55. Czarnecki PG, Gabriel GC, Manning DK, Sergeev M, Lemke K, Klena NT, et al. ANKS6 is the critical activator of NEK8 kinase in embryonic situs determination and organ patterning. *Nat Commun.* (2015) 6:6023. doi: 10.1038/ncomms7023
56. Habbig S, Bartram MP, Sagmuller JG, Griessmann A, Franke M, Muller RU, et al. The ciliopathy disease protein NPHP9 promotes nuclear delivery and activation of the oncogenic transcriptional regulator TAZ. *Hum Mol Genet.* (2012) 21:5528–38. doi: 10.1093/hmg/dds408

11

Using the *Drosophila* Nephrocyte to Model Podocyte Function and Disease

Martin Helmstädter*[1,2], *Tobias B. Huber*[3] *and Tobias Hermle*[1,2]

[1] Renal Division, University Medical Center Freiburg, Freiburg, Germany, [2] Faculty of Medicine, University of Freiburg, Freiburg, Germany, [3] III. Department of Medicine, University Medical Center Hamburg-Eppendorf, Hamburg, Germany

***Correspondence:**
Tobias Hermle
tobias.hermle@uniklinik-freiburg.de

Glomerular disorders are a major cause of end-stage renal disease and effective therapies are often lacking. Nephrocytes are considered to be part of the *Drosophila* excretory system and form slit diaphragms across cellular membrane invaginations. Nehphrocytes have been shown to share functional, morphological, and molecular features with podocytes, which form the glomerular filter in vertebrates. Here, we report the progress and the evolving tool-set of this model system. Combining a functional, accessible slit diaphragm with the power of the genetic tool-kit in *Drosophila*, the nephrocyte has the potential to greatly advance our understanding of the glomerular filtration barrier in health and disease.

Keywords: nephrocyte, *Drosophila*, podocyte, glomerular disease, garland cell, endocytosis, renal disease

INTRODUCTION

Disorders that affect the glomerulus are the predominant cause of end-stage renal disease (ESRD) (1). Beyond renal replacement therapy, potent therapeutic options are not available for most of the disorders from this heterogeneous group. This underscores the unmet need for valid model systems that serve to understand the mechanisms of glomerular diseases.

The most established model system for the glomerulus is currently the mouse. Despite being the undeniable gold standard, this model has its inherent limitations in costs, speed, and considerations of animal welfare. Complementary systems are thus desirable. An excellent alternative can be found in the zebrafish model. But the aforementioned limitations of the mouse model are alleviated only in parts in zebrafish, while additional obstacles like the shortcomings of the morpholino technology need to be considered. Significant insights were also derived from *in vitro* studies, mainly by using cultured podocytes (2). However, here other significant limitations are arising. This is mainly a consequence of the complex glomerular architecture. The glomerular filter is three-layered, including the fenestrated endothelium, the glomerular basement membrane, and the podocytes that form the slit diaphragm. Podocytes are characterized by their most intricate cell shape that is paralleled only by neuronal cells. Cultured podocytes lack crucial features of their *in vivo* counterparts, most notably the formation of slit diaphragms. The *Drosophila* anatomy contains no structure whose analogy to the mammalian kidney appears obvious. Thus, it was unexpected that the *Drosophila* nephrocyte was identified as an invertebrate model that has the potential to meet the needs for a complementary model for glomerular disease (3, 4).

Discovered more than 150 years ago (5) and identified as storage kidneys, the nephrocyte received limited attention until after the discovery that their auto-cellular junctions need to be considered as slit diaphragms that are formed by the orthologs of the mammalian slit diaphragm proteins nephrin (*sns*) and *NEPH1 (kirre)* (3, 4). Loss-of-function of slit diaphragm proteins results in a smooth cell surface analogous to podocyte foot process effacement. Nephrocytes thus share molecular, ultrastructural, and functional features with podocytes (3, 4, 6, 7). This makes nephrocytes a unique model system with a functional slit diaphragm in a genetically highly tractable model organism. Now, nearly a decade after the introduction of the nephrocyte to a wider audience in the renal field, the purpose of this review is to examine the progress and the evolving tool-set of this model system for glomerular diseases that still has not reached its peak.

NEPHROCYTE BIOLOGY

Regarding the history and basic principles of nephrocyte biology, we refer to detailed previous reviews (8–10) in order to focus on the more recent findings.

Basic Concepts of Nephrocyte As an "Excretory" Organ

The two fundamental functional subunits of renal organs throughout vertebrate biology are the glomeruli that produce an ultrafiltrate and the tubules that process the ultrafiltrate further and finally feed the resulting urine into the disposal system. Together, they serve to eliminate toxins and waste products and maintain water, salt, and pH homeostasis. Following similar principles, *Drosophila* nephrocytes are considered to be part of the fly excretory system. The *Drosophila* renal system has two functional subunits as well: the nephrocytes, regarded as analogous to the glomeruli, and the Malpighian tubules, regarded as analogous to the renal tubular system. There are two distinct nephrocyte populations: the pericardial nephrocytes along the heart tube and the garland cell nephrocytes in a garland-like ring around

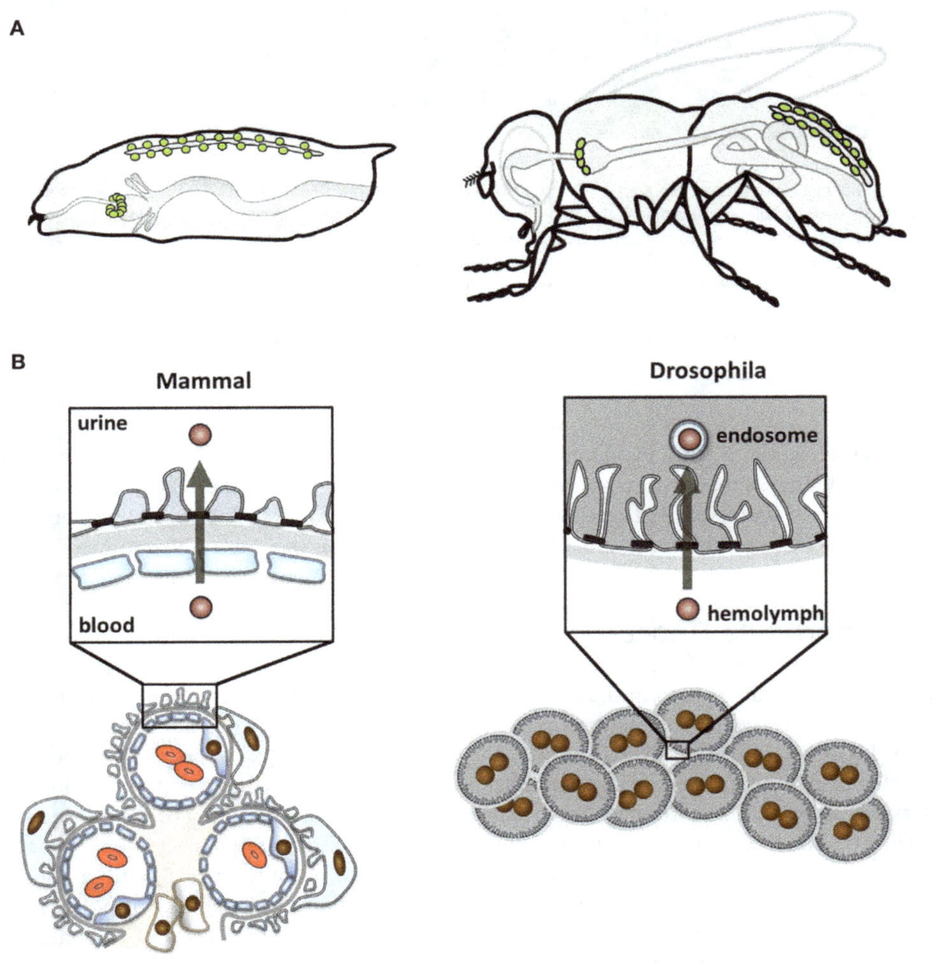

FIGURE 1 | Localization of nephrocytes and functional comparison with mammals. **(A)** The schematic shows the anatomical position of nephrocytes (green) within the larval body (left) and the adult fly (right). Garland cell nephrocytes localize within a ring around the esophagus and pericardial nephrocytes are found in pairs along the heart tube. **(B)** The schematic compares the glomerular function of mammals (left) and *Drosophila* (right). The mammalian glomerular filter is three-layered, consisting of the fenestrated endothelium, basement membrane, and the podocytes that form foot processes. Between these, the slit diaphragm is localized. Filtration occurs from the blood through the filter into the urinary space. In *Drosophila*, nephrocytes function as individual cells that are clustered. The glomerular filter is bi-layered, lacking the endothelium. Filtration occurs from the larval blood, the hemolymph, being destined for processing in endosomes.

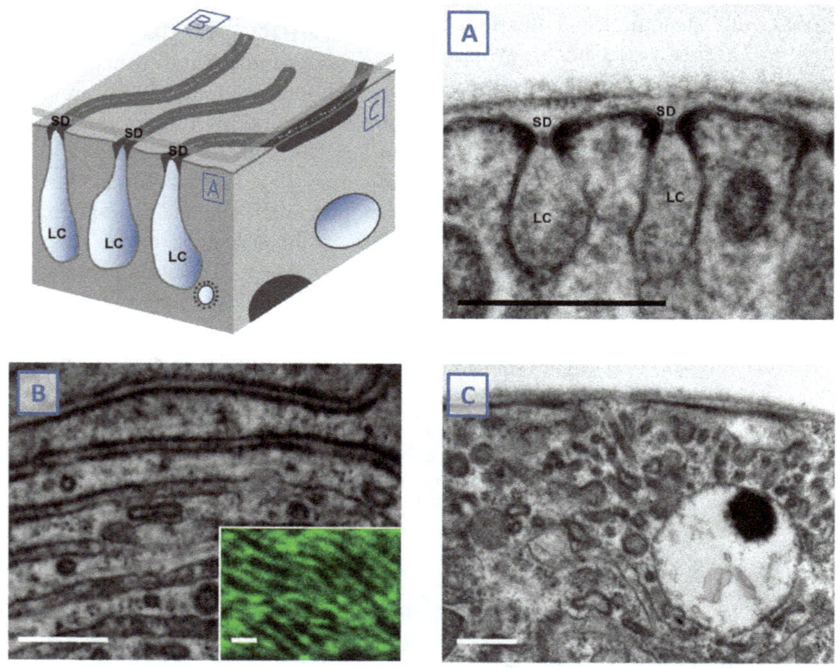

FIGURE 2 | Study of nephrocyte ultrastructural morphology using electron microscopy. The schematic illustrates a surface detail of a nephrocyte. Shown are labyrinthine channels as membrane invaginations that are sealed by the slit diaphragm. **(A)** The analogy to podocyte ultrastructure is most obvious in sections that are perpendicular to the nephrocyte surface. The slit diaphragm is recognizable as a fine line next to the electron-density around the entry to the membrane invagination. **(B)** Tangential sections through the surface show the slit diaphragm as continuous lines. This fine linear pattern correlates with the findings by confocal microscopy and staining of the ortholog of nephrin, sns (inset). **(C)** Perpendicular sections through the nephrocyte surface may be confusing when they cut through the nearly parallel lines of the slit diaphragms at an oblique angle. This results in an image that makes it difficult to identify the slit diaphragms and labyrinthine channels. Stretches of electron-density below the surface are mere indicators of their presence. SD indicates slit diaphragm, LC indicates labyrinthine channels, scale bars represent 500 nm.

the esophagus (**Figure 1A**). However, a substantial conceptual difference to the mammalian kidney is that nephrocytes have no connection to the tubular system of *Drosophila* that independently generates, modifies, and finally excretes urine into the intestinal lumen (8).

Brief History of Nephrocyte Research

Despite the divergence of anatomy and functional concepts, the role of nephrocytes was already discovered in the mid-19th century. The garland cell nephrocytes were first described in 1864 by August Weismann in Freiburg. Studying larvae from *Musca vomitoria*, he noted a string of cells reminiscent of a garland that was floating in the larval body cavity. Accordingly, he termed them "Guirlandenzellen" (German *Girlande* means garland) (11). The function of these cells was an utter mystery to their discoverer but not much later, in 1886, Kowalevsky intended to stain the intestinal mucosa of muscid larvae by feeding them carmine, methylene blue or silver. However, he noted that only nephrocytes took up and stored these tracers (12). He correctly concluded from the tracer experiments that these cells function like a storage kidney to clear the larval blood. This concept was later expanded by Hollande (13). The elaborate ultrastructure of *Drosophila* nephrocytes was described in the sixties of the last century (14, 15) and few years later Crossley (16) showed the size-selectivity of uptake and already noted the analogy of this ultrastructure to podocytes: membrane invaginations called labyrinthine channels are bridged by an auto-cellular slit diaphragm that controls their entry. Nephrocytes are covered by a basement membrane. Thus, two of the three layers of the glomerular filter in vertebrates are found in *Drosophila* nephrocytes (**Figures 1B** and **2A**).

After the discovery of nephrin (17), Skaer (3), Abmayr and colleagues (4), finally put the pieces together and proved a molecular analogy of podocytes and nephrocytes. They noted that the orthologs are both expressed in nephrocytes and that their absence results in nephrocyte loss of the complex invaginations and a smoothing of the cell surface (3, 4). Interestingly, this disruption of nephrocyte ultrastructure also follows treatment with puromycine (18) and protamine sulfate (7), both of which have the same effect in podocytes. Mammalian NEPH proteins have been shown to be functional within this invertebrate system (19). A most recent and surprising discovery is that nephrocytes potentially exhibit apico-basal polarity (20). Crumbs, a marker of apical polarity, was observed along the membrane of the labyrinthine channels. The presence of integrins on the nephrocyte surface may be suggestive of a basolateral compartment (7). This raises the possibility that despite being spherical cells, nephrocytes might be polarized within their complex ultrastructural morphology. Consequently, analogous to mammalian podocytes, apico-basal polarity may be a potential prerequisite for nephrocyte morphology and function (20). However, at this point it has not been ruled out that the functional role of these proteins in nephrocytes is independent from polarity.

Endocytosis As an Essential Nephrocyte Function

It is astounding that nephrocytes can exert their function as an "excretory" organ without a connection to the outside world. This feat is performed by endocytosis. The first step is endocytic uptake of material from the blood of the fly that is called hemolymph. Nephrocytes then sort the endocytic cargo for either degradation in the lysosome or recycling back to the hemolymph. Unwanted cargo that cannot be destroyed, will be stored intracellularly. In that way, nephrocytes detoxify the hemolymph and nephrocyte dysfunction reduces survival upon toxin exposure (3). Nephrocytes thus do not contribute to urine formation in any way but nevertheless the high endocytic activtity can be regarded as "excretory" activity (**Figure 1B**). To be optimized for that purpose, they increase their surface area by forming invaginations from the cell surface called labyrinthine channels. Endocytic uptake may occur from the cell surface but the major site of endocytosis is from within the labyrinthine channels (21, 22). These regularly spaced furrows cover the entire nephrocyte surface (4, 7). The high endocytic activity attracted researchers to use nephrocytes as a model to study mechanisms of endocytosis (22–26). Endocytic uptake is at least in part dependent on the ortholog of Cubilin (7, 27, 28). In face of this conceptual similarity to the proximal tubular function, it has been proposed that nephrocytes are also a model for the proximal tubule (28). Nephrocytes have been shown to regulate the hemolymph composition through their endocytic activity (29).

Developmental Aspects

Like podocytes, both subsets of nephrocytes are derived from the mesoderm. Differentiation and maintenance of nephrocytes requires *dKLF15* as a nephrocyte-restricted growth factor (30). *dKLF15* is the ortholog of Krüppel-Like Factor 15 which plays a role in podocyte development (31). The expression of *sns* and *kirre* and the formation of slit diaphragms begin during mid-embryogenesis and are maintained through larval development into adulthood (3, 4, 7, 32). Garland cell nephrocytes undergo a fusion process between embryonic stage E13 and E18, resulting in binucleate cells (4). For unknown reasons, the cell number decreases for both, garland cell and pericardial nephrocytes throughout development. About a quarter of the 25 garland cell nephrocytes and 120 pericardial nephrocytes that are present at the end of embryogenesis are maintained during development into adulthood (4, 7, 8, 33). Adult garland cell nephrocytes exhibit tracer uptake and show regular ultrastructural morphology, supporting these to be functional cells (7).

Frontiers of Nephrocyte Research

Despite the considerable interest nephrocytes have gained in the recent past, we do not fully understand the significance of nephrocytes within the adult fly organism. Ivy et al. (30) recorded the life-span of adult flies that lack nephrocytes due to the absence of *Klf15* in comparison with wild-type. In contrast to the observations in larval stages, the absence of nephrocytes did not affect survival of adult flies, not even under toxin stress. Further work will be required to determine the functional role of nephrocytes in the organism of adult flies.

A secretory function of nephrocytes that is suggested by the abundance of rough endoplasmic reticulum has been shown for lysozyme (16) but this functional aspect has not been further explored.

Regarding the two subsets of nephrocytes, i.e., pericardial and garland cell nephrocytes, it has become overwhelmingly clear that both cells share critical features. This includes gene expression patterns of the slit diaphragm proteins and other genes like *dKlf15, hand, rudhira*, or *Amnionless*. On the other hand, obvious differences define them as distinct cell lineages, beginning with the number of nuclei. These differences are still not explored in detail. Currently, garland cell and pericardial nephrocytes are best considered to be complementary.

READOUTS AND STRATEGIES OF NEPHROCYTE RESEARCH

The functional tool-set for nephrocytes is still evolving. As a consequence, there is no defined optimal strategy or established gold standard. However, a general rule emerges that a functional and a morphological assay need to be combined. We will discuss the merits and pitfalls of different strategies to give an overview.

Tracer Endocytosis As a Readout of Nephrocyte Function

Tracer endocytosis stood at the very beginning of nephrocyte research when they enabled Kowalevski to identify clearance of the larval circulation as their functional role. Until present time, virtually any manuscript regarding nephrocytes employs tracer uptake as a functional readout. This is based on the fact that the "excretory" function of nephrocytes occurs *via* endocytosis. An analogous effect has also been shown for endogenous proteins like *imaginal disk growth factor 2* (34).

A broad array of tracers has been used since Kowalevsky, who introduced AgNO3 that is still in use today. The most commonly used tracers are proteins like GFP-derivates (6), albumin (7), avidin (26), wheat germ agglutinin (22), or Horseradish peroxidase (HRP) (16). Another common approach uses polysaccharids like dextrans (3). Less commonly employed are colloidal substances like Coomassie Brilliant Blue (35). The choice of tracer may follow personal preference but it is important to consider the basic principles for these experiments that became clear through recent findings.

The broad range of possible tracer substances is astonishing. This reflects that the uptake of at least some tracers occurs *via* the scavenger receptor Cubilin (7), whose mammalian ortholog shows affinity for a broad range of ligands as well (36). Aside from the drastic reduction of tracer endocytosis upon silencing of Cubilin/Amnionless, this concept is supported by experiments that suggest that tracer uptake occurs receptor-mediated (7). The observation by Crossley (16) that Lanthanum-dioxide and HRP both enter the labyrinthine channels, while only the latter is taken up, indicates a certain extent of selectivity for the entry mechanism which most likely reflects the receptor affinity.

Being dependent on the scavenger receptor, measurements of nephrocyte tracer endocytosis for most tracers thus do not simply reflect the surface area of nephrocytes. The interpretation of experiments applying tracer endocytosis in nephrocytes should always take possible effects on receptor abundance, function, or specificity into account.

Filtration of tracers across the nephrocyte slit diaphragm is an important concept that directly relates to the functional analogy to podocytes and thus also underlines the significance of such experiments. Crossley (16) was able to show that in nephrocytes, tracers may be excluded size-dependently by the basement membrane and the slit membrane, thus defining a cut-off of about 12 nm. More recently, receptor competition experiments revealed that this size cut-off is comparable with the mammalian glomerulus around 70 kDa (7). Basement membrane thickening occurring upon loss of slit diaphragm proteins (3) mainly affects tracers with a high molecular weight while this effect is not directly related to the nephrocyte ultrastructure or filtration. This became obvious when it was shown using a rapid intervention like protamine treatment that perturbs the ultrastructure without thickening the basement membrane. This treatment has no effect on tracers with a high molecular weight while a tracer that is below the filtration cut-off is strongly reduced (7). In light of these findings, a tracer that is smaller than 70 kDa appears to be preferable. Another potential confounding effect comes with the saturability of tracer endocytosis (7). Choosing an excessive tracer concentration or incubation period thus may even blur the effect of silencing *sns* despite using tracers that are small enough to pass the slit diaphragm (3).

The two major alternative strategies are a pulsed uptake by exposing nephrocytes to tracers *ex vivo* or using an endogenous tracer *in vivo*. The latter strategy was first described by Han and colleagues (6). It employs a transgenic fusion protein of red fluorescent protein with the atrial natriuretic factor from rat. This transgenic tracer is expressed endogenously by muscle cells, secreted into the larval circulation followed by endocytosis and degradation by nephrocytes. The fluorescence intensity of larval pericardial nephrocytes can be observed by transcutaneous imaging. This elegant approach is fast and enabled large-scale genetic screens (6). Studying nephrocytes *in vivo*, this approach appears superior to *ex vivo* interventions. On the other hand, one has to be conscious of certain limitations that nevertheless may favor a decision for an *ex vivo* setting. Imaging fluorescence through the larval cuticle may entail weak and variable signal intensity. True *in vivo* imaging is complicated by larval movements that usually require measures to reduce larval motility. The continuous tracer expression furthermore inherently renders the net result from uptake and degradation as readout. A block in degradation and an increase in uptake thus may have the same outcome. Possible variations in tracer production, distribution, and alternative degradation are difficult to control. The *ex vivo* incubation on the other hand, is able to exclusively reflect rapid uptake under controlled conditions with direct imaging of the nephrocytes. These experiments do not require the presence of a transgene that controls the expression of the endogenous tracer and thus can be immediately applied in any genetic background that allows larval survival. This approach further allows the combination with additional interventions like drug exposure. The dissection of garland cell nephrocytes can be accomplished within few seconds which minimizes the impact of an *ex vivo* setting. An intermediate strategy by dissecting nephrocytes from transgenic animals that express a tracer endogenously may allow to combine some of the advantages of both approaches like speed and precision of direct imaging. Then again, this also retains disadvantages from both sides like the confounders entailed by continuous tracer production and the invasiveness of dissection. In summary, application of either strategy needs to be tailored to the experimental question and the available resources.

Finally, an important consideration for any uptake experiment is that it is hard to interpret without additional morphological studies. As we can learn from loss-of-function of endosomal proteins, reduced tracer uptake may occur while the slit diaphragms are maintained (25, 26) (or potentially also *vice versa* in different settings).

Electron Microscopy As a Readout of Nephrocyte Morphology

The major advantage of nephrocytes lies in the formation of functional slit diaphragms that are easily accessible. These slit diaphragms can be observed directly by transmission electron microscopy (TEM) providing the most unequivocal evidence. That way the ultrastructural analysis is an important complement for the tracer studies whose interpretation can be more difficult but that still are indispensable as a rapid functional assay. Although the technique is well established after many decades of research, study of nephrocytes still holds challenges that entail the complex ultrastructural architecture of these cells. The labyrinthine channels are nearly parallel furrows that are observed across the whole nephrocyte surface (**Figure 2**). The slit diaphragms seal these invaginations like a ceiling. Tangential sections through slit diaphragms therefore impress as parallel lines (4, 7) (**Figure 2B**). The interpretation of equatorial cross sections is more difficult, as they are dependent on their orientation in regard to the lines formed by the slit diaphragm. A cross-section that cuts through the slit diaphragms at an approximately perpendicular angle renders the classical image (**Figure 2A**). However, if the section cuts through the parallel lines of the slit diaphragms at an angle that is too oblique (**Figure 2C**), the slit diaphragms and labyrinthine channels will be distorted and difficult to identify. For that reason, such a section may even be mistaken for a smoothing of the nephrocyte surface. However, these oblique sections are marked by elongated stretches of electron-density (**Figure 2C**) that clearly distinguish them from a true phenotype. Unfortunately, examples for this error can even be found in the literature.

Analogous to the observations regarding the mammalian slit diaphragm (37), one can assume that fixation and sample preparation may influence the resulting image.

Scanning electron microscopy (SEM) can be most useful to gather information regarding cell shape and number (4, 19), while this may be achieved by using approaches involving light microscopy as well. The assessment of the nephrocyte ultrastructure through this approach is complicated as the labyrinthine channels are concealed by the basement membrane. Specific protocols like protease treatments can overcome this limitation but need to be considered carefully to avoid artefact.

Immunofluorescence (IF) As Complementary Strategy

Immunofluorescence of slit diaphragm proteins facilitated the discovery of nephrocytes as a model for glomerular diseases (3, 4). Still, this assay is regarded a complementary strategy that was omitted in a number of manuscripts. A significant recent observation concerns highly resolved tangential confocal sections of nephrocytes stained for Sns or Kirre. These stainings reveal a fingerprint-like pattern that correlates with the picture obtained in tangential sections in TEM (**Figure 2A** inset) (7). This not only implies that findings obtained with TEM can be backed up by stainings of the slit diaphragm proteins but also that significant information about ultrastructural aberrations can be obtained before applying TEM. Combined with the opportunity of co-IF, this allows a more comprehensive analysis for a number of questions. IF with 3D reconstruction also revealed that the entire cell body is covered by slit diaphragms (7). In a similar fashion, IF can be regarded as an alternative to SEM.

It remains to be seen, if super resolution imaging using stimulated emission depletion microscopy or stochastic optical reconstruction microscopy will be able to render additional information.

Readouts of Mortality

Observing survival under the exposure to toxins like silver nitrate in larvae has been described as a possible assay that directly relates to nephrocyte function. That way it may be a suitable complement for tracer strategies that documents the effect on the larval physiology. Another assay that has been introduced more recently is to record adult life-span (38). This appears a logical addition to the spectrum of investigations. However, at this point in time, it is difficult to connect reduced adult survival with nephrocyte functions due to the findings by Hartley and colleagues (30). They did not observe an altered life-span when nephrocytes were even entirely absent entirely due to lack of *dKlf15*. Potential confounders for fly survival can result from expression in other tissues. The commonly used *GAL4*-drivers to control expression of RNAi do not follow anatomic structures but are dependent on gene expression patterns. It is very difficult to rule out that temporary or very limited expression in other tissues contributes to a broad compound readout like survival. At least until the role of nephrocytes in the physiology of the adult animal is better understood, in our opinion it appears prudent to rather make use of assays that are more specifically tailored to nephrocytes.

Loss-of-Function Strategies

The virtually genome-wide availability of cost-effective, off-the-shelf RNAi libraries is a major advantage of *Drosophila* as a model system. Loss-of-function strategies that employ RNAi are inherently limited by potential off-targets or inefficient knock-down. This may result in contradicting results between different RNAi-transgenes. A common strategy in the *Drosophila* field consists in analyzing at least two independent RNAi stocks to confirm the findings. Further confirmation often remains desirable. This can be achieved by utilizing genetic null alleles. However, lethality frequently impedes this strategy like in the case of *sns*. Nephrocytes are not amenable to the classic mosaic analysis in *Drosophila* as they are non-dividing cells. The CRISPR/Cas9 technology allows to introduce a conditional loss-of-function that is not RNAi dependent (7). This can be accomplished by transgenic *Drosophila* that combine nephrocyte-restricted expression of Cas9 in conjunction with ubiquitous expression of a directed guide RNA. In this approach, individual cells may have divergent phenotypes dependent on individual CRISPR/Cas-induced mutations. Possible draw backs of this strategy are off-targets, inefficient gene disruption, and persistence of mRNA. Therefore, it is reasonable to either use two independent guide RNAs or combine this with an RNAi approach. For both methods, RNAi and CRISPR/Cas, loss-of-function best is further verified, e.g., by IF using a specific antibody or rescue experiments with an RNAi/CRISPR-resistant transgene.

A number of different *GAL4*-driver lines have been utilized to control the expression of transgenes to induce loss-of-function in nephrocytes. These include *Dorothy-GAL4* (6, 39), *sns*-GCN-*GAL4* (4, 40), and *Hand-GAL4* (41). While these lines express *GAL4* in both subsets of nephrocytes, the equally common *prospero-GAL4* (3, 42) has predominantly been used for garland cell nephrocytes. A garland cell nephrocyte-restricted expression has been described for *Aug21-GAL4* (43). All commonly used driver lines appear to exhibit robust expression during the larval stage. *G447.2-GAL4* (3) was used to direct expression in embryonic garland cell nephrocytes. *Dorothy-GAL4* (7, 44, 45), *Hand-GAL4* (46), and *sns*-GCN-*GAL4* (47) have been employed in nephrocytes dissected from adult animals. A systematic comparison of the available *GAL4* lines regarding onset, continuation, and intensity of transgene expression is currently lacking. The same is true for a characterization of the extra-nephrocytic expression that almost certainly occurs in all the *GAL4*-drivers.

NEPHROCYTE AS DISEASE MODEL

Monogenic Forms of Nephrotic Syndrome

Drosophila shows a surprising extent of conservation of disease genes and this model organism has proven to be appropriate for the investigation of monogenic diseases. These disorders are characterized by mutation of a single gene as the molecular cause of a disease. The role of nephrocytes as a model for genetic kidney disease has recently been reviewed in more detail (48). Nephrocytes are suitable to study the functional role of candidate genes that were identified in genetic studies and also elucidate the involved functional pathways which is facilitated by the low redundancy of the fly genome. The speed, cost-effectiveness, and reliability of this model make it well equipped to handle the considerable number of candidate variants that may result from contemporary sequencing efforts like whole exome sequencing. Beyond that, nephrocytes can also be applied to assess the significance of individual candidate mutations using transgenic rescue constructs. In the near future, *Drosophila* nephrocytes may further facilitate the development of targeted therapies and personalized medicine.

The most extensive work in *Drosophila* nephrocytes concerns steroid resistant nephrotic syndrome (SRNS). This disorder is characterized by childhood onset of edema, massive proteinuria, and progression to ESRD. SRNS is the second most frequent cause of ESRD within the first two decades of life and monogenic mutations explain a significant fraction of cases that manifest before 25 years of age (49). By now, more than 50 different genes have been implicated as a single gene cause for this disorder (50, 51) and more genes are likely to be discovered. The large number of known SRNS genes prompted systematic analyses that showed that about 60–80% of the studied orthologs of human disease genes resulted in a reduction of tracer uptake (7, 38) including genes that are involved in the slit diaphragm complex, actin regulation, CoQ_{10}-biosynthesis, or interaction with the extracellular matrix. This bears testimony to the surprising extent of evolutionary conservation and underlines that central pathomechanisms of podocytopathies can be studied in nephrocytes. This is most obvious for *COQ2*-nephropathy (52) where findings in *Drosophila* indicate formation of reactive oxygen species as a critical event in the pathogenesis. Successful drug treatment of flies further provides evidence for Vanillic acid as a potential treatment (7). Importantly, these data further support that *COQ2*-nephropathy may be treatable (53) and that treatment strategies can be tested in nephrocytes. Some of these findings were confirmed in a recent manuscript that furthermore implicated autophagy and mitophagy as pathomechanistically relevant (54).

For the identification of several of the SRNS genes, studies in nephrocytes were instrumental by providing functional evidence supporting the genetic findings. This includes the KANK proteins (55), *ARHGDIA* (56), *ADCK4* (57), and most extensively *SGPL1* (58). For the ortholog of *SGPL1*, rescue constructs that reflect the mutations from SRNS patients were shown to be inefficient in contrast to a rescue with wild-type constructs. *Drosophila* nephrocytes also exhibited an altered lipid metabolism reflecting the observations in the SRNS patients.

Diabetic Nephropathy

Diabetic nephropathy represents the single most significant cause of ESRD (1). Targeted therapies are unavailable and the current regimes are only sufficient to slow down the progress of disease. It is thus noteworthy that nephrocytes were found to be a model for diabetic nephropathy (59). High-glucose diet was shown to induce nephrocyte dysfunction and decrease the amount of Sns, which represents the ortholog of nephrin. The authors identified a transcriptional downregulation by a pathway that includes *Knot*, the ortholog of *EBF2*, to be responsible for the reduction of Sns in nephrocytes. Interestingly, the authors were able to validate their findings in *Drosophila* nephrocytes in mouse models of diabetic nephropathy.

APOL1-Associated Nephropathies

Incidence of ESRD is nearly fourfold in African Americans compared with those of European descent. Much of the excess risk is attributable to two risk alleles of the *APOL1* gene. The study of *APOL1* is hampered by its poor evolutionary conservation as orthologs are lacking in most model organisms. Transgenic expression of the human *APOL1* in nephrocytes has been shown to result in a cellular toxicity that was more pronounced upon expression of the human *APOL1* risk alleles (44, 45). Nephrocyte dysfunction and loss was observed with increasing age of the flies, involving a mechanism connected to endosomal trafficking. More recently, the findings in *Drosophila* were confirmed by transgenic expression of the human gene in mouse (60). Essential features of the human disease were recapitulated in this model. It is intriguing, that the role of a common risk allele was studied successfully in *Drosophila* nephrocytes.

Endocytosis and Proximal Tubular Diseases

Imerslund–Gräsbeck syndrome is characterized by Cobalamin-deficiency and tubular proteinuria while renal function is usually preserved. Mutations of Cubilin (61) and Amnionless (62) have been shown to be causative for this disorder. The orthologs of both genes are expressed in *Drosophila* nephrocytes, exercising an analogous role for nephrocyte function (28). Megalin, that may cause Donnai–Barrow syndrome (63) that also involves tubular proteinuria in humans, does not seem to be required for nephrocyte function (7, 27). A megalin-indepdendent role of Cubilin/Amnionless has also been described in humans for the absorption of vitamin B_{12} in the terminal ileum (64).

Organ Crosstalk

Drosphila is an appropriate model to study communication between organs. In an effort to identify renal cardiomodulatory factors, Hartley and colleagues induced nephrocyte disruption and observed signs of a cardiomyopathy in the fly. Analyzing the hemolymph composition, they were able to identify *secreted protein acidic and cysteine rich* (SPARC), whose circulating levels are downregulated by nephrocytes. Reducing the gene dosage of this factor independently, through a heterozygous null allele, ameliorated the cardiomyopathy. Interestingly, *SPARC* has been linked to cardiac aging and metabolic syndrome in humans.

Translational Applications

The genetic tool-kit of Drosophila combined with the cost-effectiveness and speed inherent to this model offer great opportunities for a translational approach. Only a glimmer of these opportunities can be recognized in the effect of Vanillic acid on defective CoQ_{10}-biosynthesis (7). Screening platforms have been introduced that already enable large-scale genetic screens. These protocols need to be optimized to facilitate the discovery of treatment options for glomerular diseases.

OUTLOOK

We have seen significant progress in the last decade, and the nephrocyte currently emerges from the phase of experimental establishment to a driving force of glomerular discovery research. Combining a functional, accessible slit diaphragm with the power of the genetic tool-kit in *Drosophila*, the nephrocyte as a complementary model system is well equipped to reveal mechanisms of podocyte function and glomerular diseases. Once the enormous potential for translational applications is unlocked, the nephrocyte will play its role in the identification of targeted therapies that are urgently needed in nephrology.

AUTHOR CONTRIBUTIONS

The manuscript was written by TH with help from MH, MH designed the figures with help from TH, TBH critically reviewed and edited the manuscript and gave relevant additional insight. The title was suggested by TBH.

ACKNOWLEDGMENTS

TH is supported by the Deutsche Forschungsgemeinschaft (DFG, HE 7456/1-1, CRC 1140/associated member) and the Faculty of Medicine of the University of Freiburg. TBH is supported by the DFG (CRC 1140, CRC 992, HU 1016/8-1), by the BMBF (01GM1518C), by the European Research Council—ERC grant 616891, and by the H2020-IMI2 consortium BEAt-DKD. We thank Maria Ericsson (Harvard Medical School Electron Microscopy Facility) for technical assistance.

REFERENCES

1. United States Renal Data System. *2016 USRDS Annual Data Report: Epidemiology of Kidney Disease in the United States*. Bethesda, MD: National Institutes of Health, National Institute of Diabetes and Digestive and Kidney Diseases (2016).
2. Saleem MA, O'Hare MJ, Reiser J, Coward RJ, Inward CD, Farren T, et al. A conditionally immortalized human podocyte cell line demonstrating nephrin and podocin expression. *J Am Soc Nephrol* (2002) 13:630–8.
3. Weavers H, Prieto-Sanchez S, Grawe F, Garcia-Lopez A, Artero R, Wilsch-Brauninger M, et al. The insect nephrocyte is a podocyte-like cell with a filtration slit diaphragm. *Nature* (2009) 457:322–6. doi:10.1038/nature07526
4. Zhuang S, Shao H, Guo F, Trimble R, Pearce E, Abmayr SM. Sns and Kirre, the *Drosophila* orthologs of Nephrin and Neph1, direct adhesion, fusion and formation of a slit diaphragm-like structure in insect nephrocytes. *Development* (2009) 136:2335–44. doi:10.1242/dev.031609
5. Kowalevsky A. Ein Beitrag zur Kenntnis der Excretionsorgane. *Biol Centralbl* (1889) 9:74–9.
6. Zhang F, Zhao Y, Han Z. An in vivo functional analysis system for renal gene discovery in *Drosophila* pericardial nephrocytes. *J Am Soc Nephrol* (2013) 24:191–7. doi:10.1681/ASN.2012080769
7. Hermle T, Braun DA, Helmstadter M, Huber TB, Hildebrandt F. Modeling monogenic human nephrotic syndrome in the *Drosophila* garland cell nephrocyte. *J Am Soc Nephrol* (2017) 28:1521–33. doi:10.1681/ASN.2016050517
8. Denholm B, Skaer H. Bringing together components of the fly renal system. *Curr Opin Genet Dev* (2009) 19:526–32. doi:10.1016/j.gde.2009.08.006
9. Simons M, Huber TB. Flying podocytes. *Kidney Int* (2009) 75:455–7. doi:10.1038/ki.2008.653
10. Cagan RL. The *Drosophila* nephrocyte. *Curr Opin Nephrol Hypertens* (2011) 20:409–15. doi:10.1097/MNH.0b013e328347ae02
11. Weismann A. Die nachembryonale Entwicklung der Musciden nach Beobachtungen an Musca vomitoria und Sarcophaga carnaria. *Zeitschrift für wissenschaftliche Zoologie* (1864) 14:187–336.
12. Kowalevsky A. Zum Verhalten des Rückengefäßes und des guirlandenförmigen Zellstranges der Musciden während der Metamorphose. *Biol Centralbl* (1886) 6:74–9.
13. Hollande A. La cellule péricardiale des insectes. Cytologie, histochemie, role physiologique. *Archiv Anat Mic* (1921) 18:85–307.
14. Mills RP, King RC. The pericardial cells of *Drosophila melanogaster*. *Q J Microsc Sci* (1965) 106:261–8.
15. Aggarwal SK, King RC. The ultrastructure of the wreath cells of *Drosophila melanogaster* larvae. *Protoplasma* (1967) 63:343–52. doi:10.1007/BF01252944
16. Crossley AC. The ultrastructure and function of pericardial cells and other nephrocytes in an insect: calliphora erythrocephala. *Tissue Cell* (1972) 4:529–60. doi:10.1016/S0040-8166(72)80029-6
17. Kestila M, Lenkkeri U, Mannikko M, Lamerdin J, McCready P, Putaala H, et al. Positionally cloned gene for a novel glomerular protein – nephrin – is mutated in congenital nephrotic syndrome. *Mol Cell* (1998) 1:575–82. doi:10.1016/S1097-2765(00)80057-X
18. Tutor AS, Prieto-Sanchez S, Ruiz-Gomez M. Src64B phosphorylates Dumbfounded and regulates slit diaphragm dynamics: *Drosophila* as a model to study nephropathies. *Development* (2014) 141:367–76. doi:10.1242/dev.099408
19. Helmstadter M, Luthy K, Godel M, Simons M, Ashish, Nihalani D, et al. Functional study of mammalian Neph proteins in *Drosophila melanogaster*. *PLoS One* (2012) 7:e40300. doi:10.1371/journal.pone.0040300
20. Hochapfel F, Denk L, Mendl G, Schulze U, Maassen C, Zaytseva Y, et al. Distinct functions of Crumbs regulating slit diaphragms and endocytosis in *Drosophila* nephrocytes. *Cell Mol Life Sci* (2017) 74(24):4573–86. doi:10.1007/s00018-017-2593-y
21. Kosaka T, Ikeda K. Reversible blockage of membrane retrieval and endocytosis in the garland cell of the temperature-sensitive mutant of *Drosophila melanogaster*, shibirets1. *J Cell Biol* (1983) 97:499–507. doi:10.1083/jcb.97.2.499
22. Narita K, Tsuruhara T, Koenig JH, Ikeda K. Membrane pinch-off and reinsertion observed in living cells of *Drosophila*. *J Cell Physiol* (1989) 141:383–91. doi:10.1002/jcp.1041410220
23. Lloyd TE, Atkinson R, Wu MN, Zhou Y, Pennetta G, Bellen HJ. Hrs regulates endosome membrane invagination and tyrosine kinase receptor signaling in *Drosophila*. *Cell* (2002) 108:261–9. doi:10.1016/S0092-8674(02)00611-6
24. Kim S, Wairkar YP, Daniels RW, DiAntonio A. The novel endosomal membrane protein Ema interacts with the class C Vps-HOPS complex to promote endosomal maturation. *J Cell Biol* (2010) 188:717–34. doi:10.1083/jcb.200911126
25. Lorincz P, Lakatos Z, Varga A, Maruzs T, Simon-Vecsei Z, Darula Z, et al. MiniCORVET is a Vps8-containing early endosomal tether in *Drosophila*. *Elife* (2016) 5:e14226. doi:10.7554/eLife.14226
26. Vijayakrishnan N, Woodruff EA III, Broadie K. Rolling blackout is required for bulk endocytosis in non-neuronal cells and neuronal synapses. *J Cell Sci* (2009) 122:114–25. doi:10.1242/jcs.036673
27. Gleixner EM, Canaud G, Hermle T, Guida MC, Kretz O, Helmstadter M, et al. V-ATPase/mTOR signaling regulates megalin-mediated apical endocytosis. *Cell Rep* (2014) 8:10–9. doi:10.1016/j.celrep.2014.05.035
28. Zhang F, Zhao Y, Chao Y, Muir K, Han Z. Cubilin and amnionless mediate protein reabsorption in *Drosophila* nephrocytes. *J Am Soc Nephrol* (2013) 24:209–16. doi:10.1681/ASN.2012080795
29. Hartley PS, Motamedchaboki K, Bodmer R, Ocorr K. SPARC-dependent cardiomyopathy in *Drosophila*. *Circ Cardiovasc Genet* (2016) 9:119–29. doi:10.1161/CIRCGENETICS.115.001254
30. Ivy JR, Drechsler M, Catterson JH, Bodmer R, Ocorr K, Paululat A, et al. Klf15 is critical for the development and differentiation of *Drosophila* nephrocytes. *PLoS One* (2015) 10:e0134620. doi:10.1371/journal.pone.0134620
31. Mallipattu SK, Liu R, Zheng F, Narla G, Ma'ayan A, Dikman S, et al. Kruppel-like factor 15 (KLF15) is a key regulator of podocyte differentiation. *J Biol Chem* (2012) 287:19122–35. doi:10.1074/jbc.M112.345983

32. Tepass U, Hartenstein V. The development of cellular junctions in the *Drosophila* embryo. *Dev Biol* (1994) 161:563–96. doi:10.1006/dbio.1994.1054
33. Sellin J, Albrecht S, Kolsch V, Paululat A. Dynamics of heart differentiation, visualized utilizing heart enhancer elements of the *Drosophila melanogaster* bHLH transcription factor Hand. *Gene Expr Patterns* (2006) 6:360–75. doi:10.1016/j.modgep.2005.09.012
34. Broz V, Kucerova L, Rouhova L, Fleischmannova J, Strnad H, Bryant PJ, et al. *Drosophila* imaginal disc growth factor 2 is a trophic factor involved in energy balance, detoxification, and innate immunity. *Sci Rep* (2017) 7:43273. doi:10.1038/srep43273
35. Das D, Aradhya R, Ashoka D, Inamdar M. Macromolecular uptake in *Drosophila* pericardial cells requires rudhira function. *Exp Cell Res* (2008) 314:1804–10. doi:10.1016/j.yexcr.2008.02.009
36. Nielsen R, Christensen EI, Birn H. Megalin and cubilin in proximal tubule protein reabsorption: from experimental models to human disease. *Kidney Int* (2016) 89:58–67. doi:10.1016/j.kint.2015.11.007
37. Grahammer F, Wigge C, Schell C, Kretz O, Patrakka J, Schneider S, et al. A flexible, multilayered protein scaffold maintains the slit in between glomerular podocytes. *JCI Insight* (2016) 1(9):e86177. doi:10.1172/jci.insight.86177
38. Fu Y, Zhu JY, Richman A, Zhao Z, Zhang F, Ray PE, et al. A *Drosophila* model system to assess the function of human monogenic podocyte mutations that cause nephrotic syndrome. *Hum Mol Genet* (2017) 26:768–80. doi:10.1093/hmg/ddw428
39. Kimbrell DA, Hice C, Bolduc C, Kleinhesselink K, Beckingham K. The Dorothy enhancer has Tinman binding sites and drives hopscotch-induced tumor formation. *Genesis* (2002) 34:23–8. doi:10.1002/gene.10134
40. Kocherlakota KS, Wu JM, McDermott J, Abmayr SM. Analysis of the cell adhesion molecule sticks-and-stones reveals multiple redundant functional domains, protein-interaction motifs and phosphorylated tyrosines that direct myoblast fusion in *Drosophila melanogaster*. *Genetics* (2008) 178:1371–83. doi:10.1534/genetics.107.083808
41. Albrecht S, Wang S, Holz A, Bergter A, Paululat A. The ADAM metalloprotease Kuzbanian is crucial for proper heart formation in *Drosophila melanogaster*. *Mech Dev* (2006) 123:372–87. doi:10.1016/j.mod.2006.03.005
42. Ohshiro T, Yagami T, Zhang C, Matsuzaki F. Role of cortical tumour-suppressor proteins in asymmetric division of *Drosophila* neuroblast. *Nature* (2000) 408:593–6. doi:10.1038/35046087
43. Andreenkova OV, Karpova EK, Menshanov PN, Rauschenbach IY. Knockdown of InR gene in ventral nephrocytes promotes resistance to toxic stress in *Drosophila melanogaster* females. *Genetika* (2015) 51:263–5. doi:10.1134/S1022795415020027
44. Kruzel-Davila E, Shemer R, Ofir A, Bavli-Kertselli I, Darlyuk-Saadon I, Oren-Giladi P, et al. APOL1-mediated cell injury involves disruption of conserved trafficking processes. *J Am Soc Nephrol* (2017) 28:1117–30. doi:10.1681/ASN.2016050546
45. Fu Y, Zhu JY, Richman A, Zhang Y, Xie X, Das JR, et al. APOL1-G1 in nephrocytes induces hypertrophy and accelerates cell death. *J Am Soc Nephrol* (2017) 28:1106–16. doi:10.1681/ASN.2016050550
46. Davis EE, Zhang Q, Liu Q, Diplas BH, Davey LM, Hartley J, et al. TTC21B contributes both causal and modifying alleles across the ciliopathy spectrum. *Nat Genet* (2011) 43:189–96. doi:10.1038/ng.756
47. Na J, Musselman LP, Pendse J, Baranski TJ, Bodmer R, Ocorr K, et al. A *Drosophila* model of high sugar diet-induced cardiomyopathy. *PLoS Genet* (2013) 9:e1003175. doi:10.1371/journal.pgen.1003175
48. Helmstadter M, Simons M. Using *Drosophila* nephrocytes in genetic kidney disease. *Cell Tissue Res* (2017) 369:119–26. doi:10.1007/s00441-017-2606-z
49. Sadowski CE, Lovric S, Ashraf S, Pabst WL, Gee HY, Kohl S, et al. A single-gene cause in 29.5% of cases of steroid-resistant nephrotic syndrome. *J Am Soc Nephrol* (2015) 26:1279–89. doi:10.1681/ASN.2014050489
50. Lovric S, Ashraf S, Tan W, Hildebrandt F. Genetic testing in steroid-resistant nephrotic syndrome: when and how? *Nephrol Dial Transplant* (2016) 31:1802–13. doi:10.1093/ndt/gfv355
51. Bierzynska A, Soderquest K, Dean P, Colby E, Rollason R, Jones C, et al. MAGI2 mutations cause congenital nephrotic syndrome. *J Am Soc Nephrol* (2017) 28:1614–21. doi:10.1681/ASN.2016040387
52. Diomedi-Camassei F, Di Giandomenico S, Santorelli FM, Caridi G, Piemonte F, Montini G, et al. COQ2 nephropathy: a newly described inherited mitochondriopathy with primary renal involvement. *J Am Soc Nephrol* (2007) 18:2773–80. doi:10.1681/ASN.2006080833
53. Desbats MA, Lunardi G, Doimo M, Trevisson E, Salviati L. Genetic bases and clinical manifestations of coenzyme Q10 (CoQ 10) deficiency. *J Inherit Metab Dis* (2015) 38:145–56. doi:10.1007/s10545-014-9749-9
54. Zhu JY, Fu Y, Richman A, Zhao Z, Ray PE, Han Z. A personalized model of COQ2 nephropathy rescued by the wild-type COQ2 allele or dietary coenzyme Q10 supplementation. *J Am Soc Nephrol* (2017) 28:2607–17. doi:10.1681/ASN.2016060626
55. Gee HY, Zhang F, Ashraf S, Kohl S, Sadowski CE, Vega-Warner V, et al. KANK deficiency leads to podocyte dysfunction and nephrotic syndrome. *J Clin Invest* (2015) 125:2375–84. doi:10.1172/JCI79504
56. Gee HY, Saisawat P, Ashraf S, Hurd TW, Vega-Warner V, Fang H, et al. ARHGDIA mutations cause nephrotic syndrome via defective RHO GTPase signaling. *J Clin Invest* (2013) 123:3243–53. doi:10.1172/JCI69134
57. Ashraf S, Gee HY, Woerner S, Xie LX, Vega-Warner V, Lovric S, et al. ADCK4 mutations promote steroid-resistant nephrotic syndrome through CoQ10 biosynthesis disruption. *J Clin Invest* (2013) 123:5179–89. doi:10.1172/JCI69000
58. Lovric S, Goncalves S, Gee HY, Oskouian B, Srinivas H, Choi WI, et al. Mutations in sphingosine-1-phosphate lyase cause nephrosis with ichthyosis and adrenal insufficiency. *J Clin Invest* (2017) 127:912–28. doi:10.1172/JCI89626
59. Na J, Sweetwyne MT, Park AS, Susztak K, Cagan RL. Diet-induced podocyte dysfunction in *Drosophila* and mammals. *Cell Rep* (2015) 12:636–47. doi:10.1016/j.celrep.2015.06.056
60. Beckerman P, Bi-Karchin J, Park AS, Qiu C, Dummer PD, Soomro I, et al. Transgenic expression of human APOL1 risk variants in podocytes induces kidney disease in mice. *Nat Med* (2017) 23:429–38. doi:10.1038/nm.4287
61. Aminoff M, Carter JE, Chadwick RB, Johnson C, Grasbeck R, Abdelaal MA, et al. Mutations in CUBN, encoding the intrinsic factor-vitamin B12 receptor, cubilin, cause hereditary megaloblastic anaemia 1. *Nat Genet* (1999) 21:309–13. doi:10.1038/6831
62. Tanner SM, Aminoff M, Wright FA, Liyanarachchi S, Kuronen M, Saarinen A, et al. Amnionless, essential for mouse gastrulation, is mutated in recessive hereditary megaloblastic anemia. *Nat Genet* (2003) 33:426–9. doi:10.1038/ng1098
63. Kantarci S, Al-Gazali L, Hill RS, Donnai D, Black GC, Bieth E, et al. Mutations in LRP2, which encodes the multiligand receptor megalin, cause Donnai-Barrow and facio-oculo-acoustico-renal syndromes. *Nat Genet* (2007) 39:957–9. doi:10.1038/ng2063
64. Jensen LL, Andersen RK, Hager H, Madsen M. Lack of megalin expression in adult human terminal ileum suggests megalin-independent cubilin/amnionless activity during vitamin B12 absorption. *Physiol Rep* (2014) 2(7):e12086. doi:10.14814/phy2.12086

12

Novel Aspects of Renal Magnesium Homeostasis

Paula Giménez-Mascarell[1], Carlotta Else Schirrmacher[2], Luis Alfonso Martínez-Cruz[1] and Dominik Müller[2]**

[1] CIC bioGUNE, Bizkaia Science and Technology Park, Derio, Spain, [2] Department of Pediatric Gastroenterology, Nephrology and Metabolism, Charité – Universitätsmedizin Berlin, Berlin, Germany

***Correspondence:**
Luis Alfonso Martínez-Cruz
amartinez@cicbiogune.es;
Dominik Müller
dominik.mueller@charite.de

Magnesium (Mg^{2+}) is indispensable for several vital functions, such as neurotransmission, cardiac conductance, blood glucose, blood pressure regulation, and proper function of more than 300 enzymes. Thus, Mg^{2+} homeostasis is subject to tight regulation. Besides the fast and immediate regulation of plasma Mg^{2+}, a major part of Mg^{2+} homeostasis is realized by a concerted action of epithelial molecular structures that tightly control intestinal uptake and renal absorption. This mechanism is provided by a combination of para- and transcellular pathways. Whereas the first pathway provides the organism with a maximal amount of vital substances by a minimal energy expenditure, the latter enables controlling and fine-tuning by means of local and regional regulatory systems and also, hormonal control. The paracellular pathway is driven by an electrochemical gradient and realized in principal by the tight junction (TJ), a supramolecular organization of membrane-bound proteins and their adaptor and scaffolding proteins. TJ determinants are claudins (CLDN), a family of membrane spanning proteins that generate a barrier or a pore between two adjacent epithelial cells. Many insights into molecular mechanisms of Mg^{2+} handling have been achieved by the identification of alterations and mutations in human genes which cause disorders of paracellular Mg^{2+} pathways (CLDN10, CLDN14, CLDN16, CLDN19). Also, in the distal convoluted tubule, a basolateral protein, CNNM2, causes if mutated, familial dominant and also recessive renal Mg^{2+} wasting, albeit its true function has not been clarified yet, but is assumed to play a key role in the transcellular pathway. Moreover, mutations in human genes that are involved in regulating these proteins directly or indirectly cause, if mutated human diseases, mostly in combination with comorbidities as diabetes, cystic renal disease, or metabolic abnormalities. Generation and characterization of animal models harboring the corresponding mutations have further contributed to the elucidation of physiology and pathophysiology of Mg^{2+} disorders. Finally, high-end crystallization techniques allow understanding of Mg^{2+} handling in more detail. As this field is rapidly growing, we describe here the principles of physiology and pathophysiology of epithelial transport of renal Mg^{2+} homeostasis with emphasis on recently identified mechanisms involved.

Keywords: magnesium, crystallography, CNNM2, kidney, genetics

INTRODUCTION

Magnesium (in its ionized and biologically active form: Mg^{2+}) belongs to the group of alkaline earth metals and is the second most abundant intracellular divalent cation. It is the eleventh most abundant element by mass in the human body. Mg^{2+} is indispensable for several vital functions, such as neurotransmission, cardiac conductance, blood glucose control, and blood pressure regulation.

In muscle, Mg^{2+} regulates contraction by antagonizing calcium (1–4). Mg^{2+} has also been identified as a second messenger, e.g., in T-Cells, where mutations in the gene MAGT1 have been linked to human immunodeficiency. There, mutations disable transient Mg^{2+} influx induced by the activation of the T-cell receptor (5).

Adenosine triphosphosphate (ATP) is the major source of cell energy, and must bind Mg^{2+} in order to be biologically active. The resulting complex, Mg^{2+}-ATP is vital for the stability of all polyphosphate compounds in cells, including those associated with synthesis of DNA and RNA. More than 300 enzymes are dependent on Mg^{2+} for their biocatalytic function, including those that utilize or synthesize ATP, or those that use other nucleotides to synthesize DNA and RNA (6). In plants, Mg^{2+} is the central ion of chlorophyll and, therefore, vital for photosynthesis. In higher organisms, hemoglobin, the essential O_2 carrier, has high structural similarities with chlorophyll but here, Fe^{2+} replaced Mg^{2+} as the central ion. Magnesium is an essential mineral nutrient (i.e., element) and is present in every cell type and in every organism. In the blood and serum, Mg^{2+} is mostly bound to serum albumin (like the most abundant divalent cation, Ca^{2+}) and stored in muscle fibers and in bone. The biologically active form is the ionized form and dietary sources rich of magnesium are plants [Almonds, Cashews, Cocoa, Pumpkin Seeds, Spinach, and Fish (Halibut, Mackeral)]. Clinically, deficiency of Mg^{2+} causes nausea, appetite loss, fatigue, and general weakness. At a later stage, patients present with numbness, tingling, muscle cramps, cerebral seizures, and cardiac arrhythmias. Moreover, Mg^{2+} deficiency can lead to hypocalcemia and hypokalemia (7). On the other hand, little is known about the consequences of hypermagnesemia as can be encountered, e.g., in patients with end stage renal disease (8). However, Mg^{2+} complexes are involved in the development of vascular calcifications, a major cause of morbidity and mortality of patients with chronic kidney disease (9).

Compared to Ca^{2+} storage (around 1000 g in adults), the whole body content of Mg^{2+} only sums up to 20 g. In addition, Mg^{2+} stores are not as readily accessible as Ca^{2+} stores by, e.g., PTH action. Therefore, the organisms' intra- and extracellular Mg^{2+} levels are kept tightly within narrow limits. Likewise, the available, ionized, biologically active and relevant form (Mg^{2+}) is dependent on a more or less a continuous nutritional supply. Mg^{2+} serum concentrations in adults range from 0.7 to 1.1 mmol/l, while newborns and toddlers can have lower limit serum concentrations (e.g., from 0.45 mmol/l on). The daily need of Mg^{2+} in adults is around 300–350 mg/day and fractional intestinal uptake varies depending on the amount of intake. Fine et al. found that intestinal Mg^{2+} absorption increases with intake but also that fractional Mg^{2+} absorption fells progressively (from 65% at low to 11% at high intake) (10). The authors described the intestinal absorption by an equation containing a hyperbolic function plus a linear function. They concluded that Mg^{2+} absorption must, therefore, be realized by a twin-mechanism that simultaneously reaches an absorptive maximum, and in addition a mechanism that endlessly absorbs a defined fraction (7%, as the authors concluded) (10). Although the molecular mechanisms have not been identified at that time, their and the findings of other groups later, predicted the coexistence of two distinct mechanisms of Mg^{2+} absorption, the trans- and paracellular transport in the intestine. Moreover, as we know nowadays, the same holds true for the kidney.

In both organs, the intestine and the kidney, Mg^{2+} is absorbed *via* paracellular as well as by transcellular routes. Whereas the first pathway is in principal driven by an existing electrochemical gradient, the latter requires energy-consuming mechanisms in order to conduct apical uptake, buffering, transport, and basolateral extrusion (**Figure 1**). The paracellular route guarantees the organism to retrieve a considerable amount of vital substances with a minimal energetic expenditure. On the other side, the

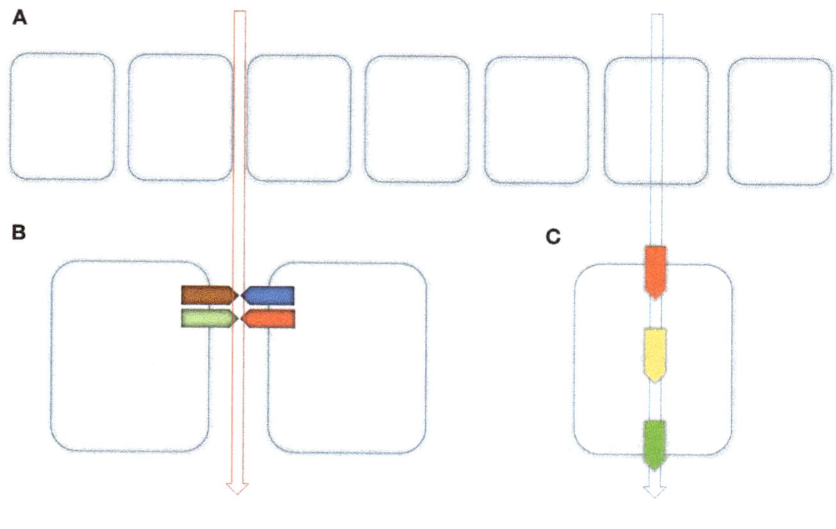

FIGURE 1 | Routes of epithelial transport. **(A)** Epithelial transport is performed by two different routes. Paracellular (left) and transcellular (right) as indicated by the vertical arrows. **(B)** The paracellular transport is realized through the tight Junction (TJ) which is composed of several Proteins mainly by Claudins. Together with their adaptor and scaffolding proteins, they make up as hetero- or homodimers dimers the main part of the TJ. **(C)** Paracellular transport is realized by apical uptake (red), intracellular buffering and transport (yellow), and basolateral extrusion (green).

energy-consuming transcellular route provides a fine-tuning at the several steps of transport and is, therefore, subject to precise local, regional, or global regulation. This can be realized by hormones such as $1,25(OH)D_2$ or parathyroid hormone according to the basic but also the actual needs of the organism (e.g., growth).

In the kidney, the driving force of transepithelial Mg^{2+} absorption is provided by a continuously maintained electrochemical gradient between the apical (tubular fluid) and the basolateral (blood) compartment. This process is realized by a battery of transcellular (and apical to basolateral) and paracellular transport mechanisms. As a principle, paracellular transport mainly takes place where the transepithelial concentration gradient is high, i.e., the proximal jejunum in the gut and in the proximal tubule (PT) as well the thick ascending loop of Henle in the kidney. By contrast, transcellular transport takes place in the late ileum, colon, and the distal part of the renal tubule (11, 12).

MAGNESIUM HANDLING ALONG THE NEPHRON

After glomerular filtration, the non-protein-bound fraction, Mg^{2+} is absorbed along the nephron before it is finally lost irretrievable for the organism within the urine. Under normal conditions (Glomerular filtration rate >90 ml/min/1.73 m^2), more than 95% of filtered Mg^{2+} in the pro-urine is reabsorbed along the tubular system by several coordinated transport processes (13). Besides their anatomical localization, regulatory mechanisms of renal Mg^{2+} homeostasis can also be classified by their involvement in the hierarchy of transport. Therefore, we classify here the mechanisms of Mg^{2+} transport and homeostasis according to their involvement in the network of Mg^{2+} handling (**Table 1**). The first category comprises proteins or elements that transport Mg^{2+} by itself, e.g., a direct Mg^{2+} transport mechanism. The second category includes proteins and mechanisms that regulate elements of category 1. The third category comprises members that influence Mg^{2+} handling in a more remote way, e.g., by regulating ions, other than Mg^{2+} but thereby influence Mg^{2+} handling. To the latter category belong also proteins that influence Mg^{2+} homeostasis, e.g., by causing polyuria and thereby a "wash out" of Mg^{2+} by reducing the time of contact of absorbing mechanisms with the corresponding substance (as can be seen by the treatment with furosemide). With this newly proposed classification, we aim to focus on the current knowledge on Mg^{2+} handling toward a more interactive model, the magnesiome, and the Mg^{2+} interactome.

TABLE 1 | Protein classification based on the role played by each molecule in renal magnesium handling.

Category	Role in Mg^{2+} handling	Proteins
1	Direct transport of Mg^{2+}	Claudin-16[a]; Claudin-19[a]; TRPM6[b]; CNNM2[c,b]; SLC41A3[c,b]
2	Regulation of a direct transporter/channel of Mg^{2+}	Claudin-14[a]; EGF[b]; CNNM2[c,b]
3	Contribution to Mg^{2+} homeostasis by indirect means	NKCC2[a], Claudin-10[a]; ROMK[a,b]; PCBD[a,b], HNF1B[a,b], Barttin[a,b]; Na^+-K^+-ATPase[a,b]/FXYD2a,b[a,b]; CaSR[a,b]; ClC-Kb[a,b]; Kir4.1[b]; Kv1.1[b]; NCC[b]

[a]*Proteins expressed in the TAL.*
[b]*Proteins expressed in the DCT.*
[c]*Proteins which role is under debate.*

Anatomically, the major sites of renal Mg^{2+} reabsorption are, besides the PT (10–20%), the thick ascending loop of Henle (TAL, 65–70%) and the distal convoluted tubule (DCT, 10%) (**Figure 2**). Beyond the DCT, no significant mechanisms of Mg^{2+} absorption have been described so far (11, 12).

PT and Thick Ascending Part of Henle's Loop

Mg^{2+} absorption in the PT and TAL occurs mainly *via* paracellular route and in the DCT the transcellular route (13). The paracellular route is mainly determined by the Tight Junction (TJ), a supramolecular organization of membrane-bound proteins and their intracellular adaptor- and scaffolding proteins. The major proteins of the TJ comprise Claudins (from lat. *claudere*: to seal), a protein family consisting of at least 24 members in Eukaryotes enabling the TJ to function as either (a) barrier, (b) fence, or (c) channel (**Figure 3**). The *Barrier* function of the TJ enables the organism to increase transepithelial resistance (TER; $\Omega \times cm^2$) where needed. As such, the PT has a low resistance (6–10 $\Omega \times cm^2$) whereas downstream, toward TAL (11–34 $\Omega \times cm^2$) and the Collecting Duct (60 $\Omega \times cm^2$; MDCK cells) TER is constantly increasing (14, 15). The bladder, in order to fulfill its function of a tight reservoir, has the highest epithelial resistance [>300 k$\Omega \times cm^2$ (16); **Figure 3A**]. The *Fence* function of the TJ is a key element that contributes to the apical-to-basolateral orientation of epithelial cells. In order to guarantee a coordinated, regulated transcellular transport, membrane-bound proteins must be oriented stable at either apical or the basolateral side. This principal requirement of all epithelial tissues is mainly realized by the TJ (17). Likewise, the loss of the apical-to-basolateral orientation, i.e., the loss of polarity and even cell-to-cell contact is an early event in tumor development. Several claudins have been shown to be potential markers of gastrointestinal tumors and their progression (18). Moreover, other Claudins (e.g., Claudin-3) have been demonstrated to be involved, in men and animals in tumor invasiveness and in autoimmune disorders (18, 19). Also, several Claudins are vital for teeth development in mice and humans (20). A great step toward the determination of the role of Claudins has been achieved by the resolution of the crystal structure of the Claudin protein Claudin-15 (21, 22) (**Figure 3B**). Although their contribution to human disease has been demonstrated, proteins that directly interfere with Claudins have only been preliminarily characterized (23, 24). The *Channel* function of the TJ is crucial for ions (like Mg^{2+} and Ca^{2+}) and H_20 absorption and is dependent on an existing electro-chemical gradient (17). The *Channel* function is realized by a surplus of one charge on one side of the epithelial layer than on the other side (e.g., apical vs. basolateral or vice versa) or on the surplus of a molecule or substance over the epithelial layer. Although the TJ does not possess pumps or antiporters, transport can nevertheless be selective by the variation and regulation of TJ composition and protein expression (25). Thus, the expression of different Claudins along epithelial

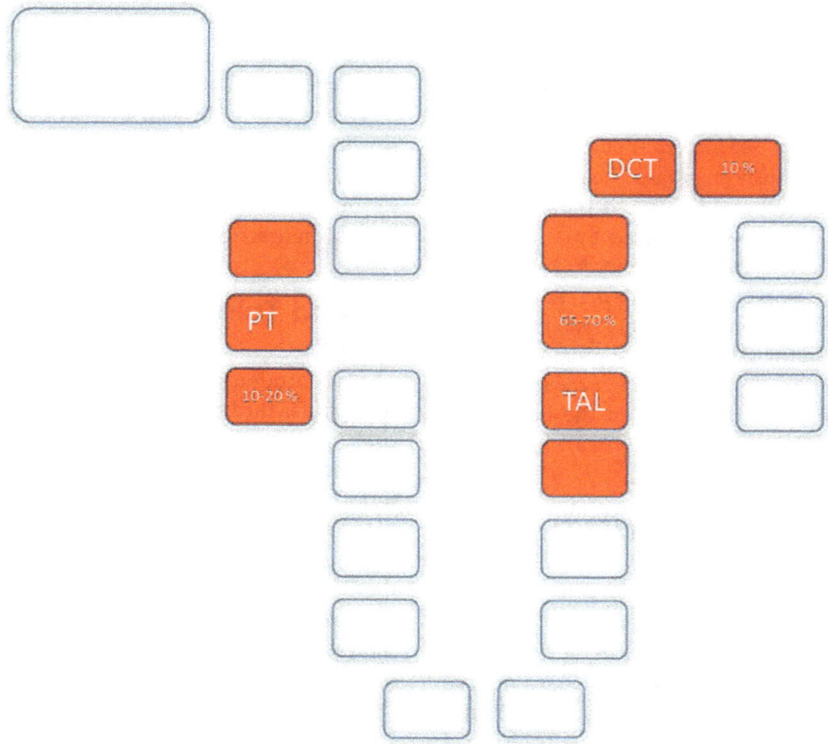

FIGURE 2 | Mg^{2+} absorption along the nephron: Uptake along the nephron is realized by the proximal tubule (PT) (10–20%), the TAL (65–70%) and the distal convoluted tubule (DCT, 10%).

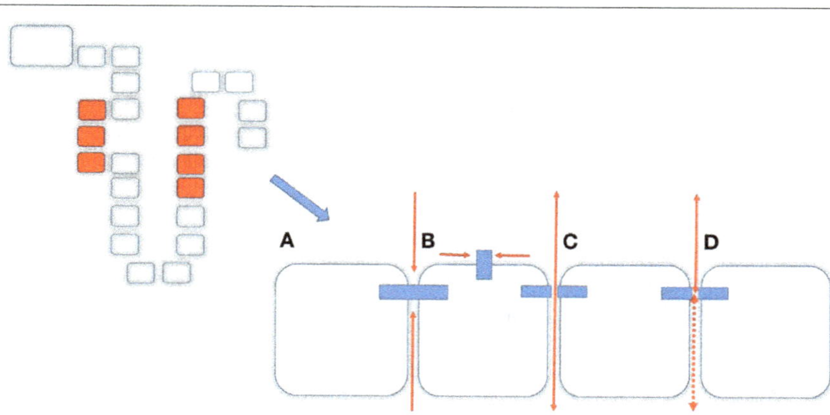

FIGURE 3 | Transcellular transport. Tight junctions (TJs) and Caudins are responsible for different functions **(A)** Barrier, i.e., no transit in any direction, **(B)** Fence, enabling a cell apical-to-basolateral orientation, **(C)** Channel function, allowing molecules to pass from apical to basolateral and *vice versa*, and **(D)** depending on the composition of the TJ.

tissues and their regulation and expression can determine Mg^{2+} spatial and temporal reabsorption (26) (**Figure 4**).

Although our knowledge on Mg^{2+} handling in the more distal nephron has increased significantly, little is known about Mg^{2+} transport in the PT, where it is believed to be transported by the paracellular way. There, terminus "bulk reabsorption" is used widely although this phenomenon has not been elucidated in detailed molecular or physiological context.

Bartter's Syndrome, first described by the endocrinologist Frederick Bartter, is characterized by renal wasting of Na^+, K^+, and polyuria. Clinically, hyperaldosteronism in preterm borns, polyhydramnion and prematurity became a hallmark. The seminal work of the Lifton and Hildebrandt groups showed that mutations in the genes that code for the apical transport in the TAL of Na^+, K^+ and Cl^- (NKCC2, ROMK2) as well as the basolateral extrusion mechanisms (ClC-Ka, Barttin) are essential for Na^+ K^+ and Cl^- handling in the TAL (Bartter's Syndrome types 1–4)

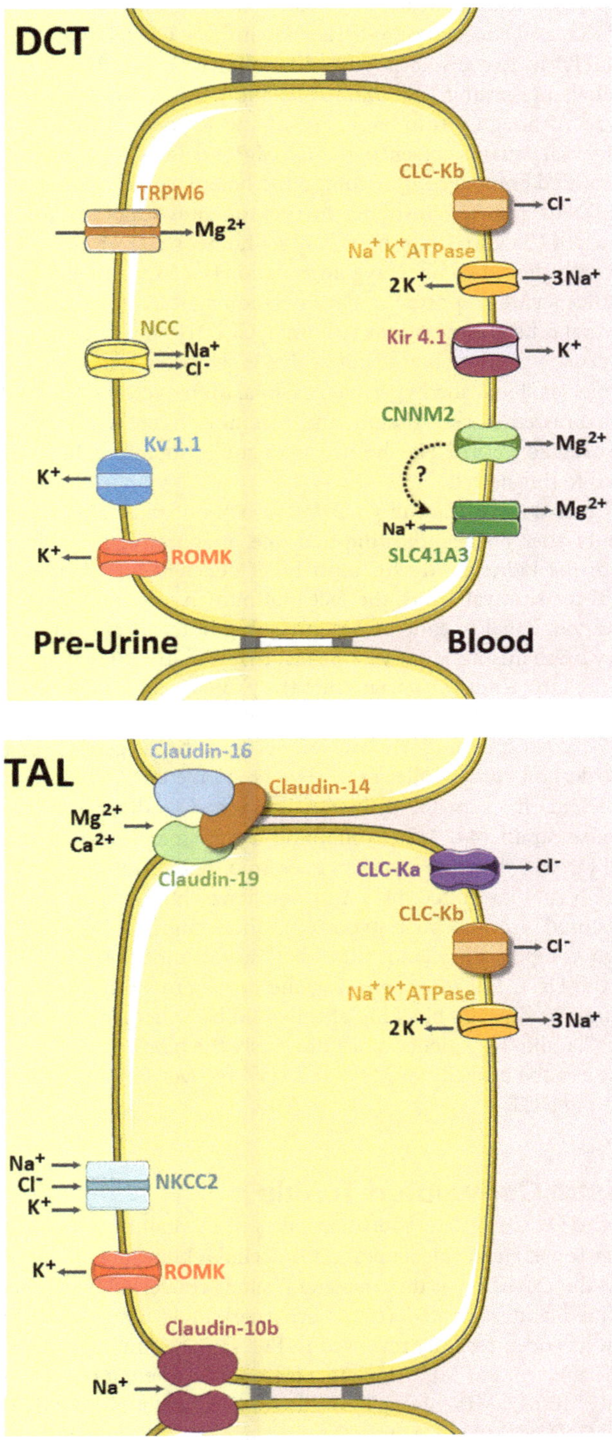

FIGURE 4 | Continued

FIGURE 4 | Mg^{2+} handling network along the TAL and distal convoluted tubule (DCT). In the TAL (bottom), Mg^{2+} and Ca^{2+} are absorbed *via* the permeable channel formed by Claudin-16 and Claudin-19, which is inhibited by Claudin-14 (light brown). Claudin-10b is a cation-selective channel with high preference for Na^+. The apical force needed for Mg^{2+} reabsorption is created by the cooperative activities of the basolateral Na^+ K^+ ATPase pump, the Chloride channels ClC-Ka and ClC-Kb, and the apical Na^+ K^+ $2Cl^-$ cotransporter (NKCC2) and the K^+ extruder, ROMK. (up) In the DCT, Mg^{2+} is mainly absorbed by transcellular routes. The Mg^{2+} ions enter into the cell through the apical TRPM6 channel and are then extruded by either CNNM2 and/or SLC41A3 (still under debate). The apical force needed for Mg^{2+} transport is created by the cooperative action of the basolateral Na^+ K^+ ATPase, the Cl^- channel ClC-Kb, the K^+ transporter Kir 4.1 and the apical Na^+ Cl^- cotransporter (NCC) and the K^+ extruders, ROMK and Kv 1.1 (5, 27).

(28–33) Here, Mg^{2+} wasting is not caused by a direct mechanisms, and likewise Mg^{2+} wasting is a clinical hint, but not a mandatory feature of Bartter's syndrome. Mg^{2+} wasting in Bartter's Syndrome is also believed to be secondary to polyurias (and polydipsia) present in these patients. Thus, all the proteins are classified into Category 3 (**Table 1**) supported by the fact that also mice with a targeted deletion of NKCC2 show a Bartter-like phenotype but no hypomagnesemia (34). Interestingly, a transient form of Bartter's syndrome has been described in several patients recently. Patients displayed the prenatal (Polyhydramnion, Prematurity) and post-natal (Hyponatrimia, Hypokalemia) clinical hallmarks of Bartter's syndrome. The authors have shown that these disorders are caused by mutations in the gene encoding melanoma-associated antigen D2, explaining that fact that only males were affected (35, 36). Although the authors have not reported on Mg^{2+} levels, it is intriguing that this disorder is a more common cause of neonatal hypomagnesemia than anticipated that far.

The TAL is separated anatomically but also by its functional elements in the medullary and the cortical part (mTAL and cTAL). An important driving force in epithelial tissues and, therefore, also in the TAL, in order to maintain a transepithelial gradient is generated by the basolateral Na^+ K^+ ATPase. Mutations in the gene (FYXD2) coding for the γ-subunit of this protein have been shown to cause dominant familial Hypomagnesemia. Thus, it has been shown that this protein is a "conditio-sine-qua-non" for generating the necessary transepithelial gradient for transport systems and, thus, also for renal Mg^{2+} handling (11, 12, 37), this protein can be classified into the Category 2.

During the last years, several proteins have been shown to be involved in renal paracellular ion transport. However, a clear phenotype–genotype correlation has established in some but not in all of the genes and proteins involved. An example is provided by CLDN14. Mutations in CLDN14 cause non-syndromic deafness in men and mice (38, 39). Affected human individuals do not display overt renal abnormalities and the same holds true for mice with targeted deletions in CLDN14 (38). On the other hand, genome-wide association studies identified CLDN14 variants as a major risk gene associated with hypercalciuric stone disease (4, 40, 41). Furthermore, in the TAL, mutations in human genes (CLDN10, CLDN14, CLDN16, and CLDN19), that define the paracellular pathway (**Figure 4**) of Mg^{2+} absorption have been shown to cause rare human disorders. In the TAL, where significant Mg^{2+} and Ca^{2+} transcellular transport is absent, paracellular transport is of vital importance and is driven by a lumen-positive potential. Mutations in CLDN16 cause an autosomal-recessive disorder called "Familial Hypomagnesemia with Hypercalciuria and Nephrocalcinosis" (FHHNC) (42). Patients affected display renal Mg^{2+} and Ca^{2+} wasting accompanied by nephrocalcinosis. This disorder causes in most of the cases end stage renal disease, leading in many, but not all cases to the need for renal transplantation (43). A clinical significant problem is given by the fact that there currently is no general screening procedure at the neonatal stage or later for toddles and schoolchildren on hypercalciuria or hypermagnesemia. Thus, if such patients are referred to a secondary or tertiary center, respectively, chronic renal insufficiency and calcifications have often already progressed to a severe and often, irreversible state. In contrast to the human situation, mice with targeted deletion of CLDN16 recapitulate human renal Mg^{2+} and Ca^{2+} wasting, but do not show any signs of overt renal calcifications and, moreover, no signs of apparent or progressing renal insufficiency (44). There is currently no explanation for this significant difference; however, it is intriguing that solving this striking difference, a possible route for treatment of patients may be opened. A novel recent finding was that the absence of CLDN16 in ameloblasts explains the clinical finding of amelogenesis imperfecta in FHHNC patients and mice with CLDN16 deficiency (45). A similar finding was reported for patients with mutations in the genes coding for CLDN19 and similar for mice (CLDN3) (20, 46).

In 2006, Konrad et al. reported that mutations in human CLDN19 also lead to renal Mg^{2+} and Ca^{2+} wasting, clinically an almost phenocopy of patients with CLDN16 mutations (47). Although still a matter of debate, it is believed that CLDN16 and CLDN19 interact and form a heteromeric paracellular channel, with a cation selectivity including Ca^{2+} and Mg^{2+} (48) (**Figure 4**). However, they could also show that patients harboring CLDN19 mutations suffer from severe ocular involvement, as Claudin-19, but not Claudin-16 is expressed in the retinal pigment epithelium TJs, leading besides the renal Mg^{2+} and Ca^{2+} wasting to major vision problems (47, 49).

Another Claudin (Claudin-10) that contributes to Mg^{2+} handling exists at least in two principal forms. Claudin-10a and -10b, both confer different electrophysiological properties (anion-selective channel vs. cation-selective channel with a high preference for Na^+) and their tissue distribution (Kidney and Uterus for Claudin-10a and ubiquitously for Claudin-10b) (50–52) (**Figure 4**). The expression of the Claudin-10b in almost every epithelial tissue might explain that mice with a targeted deletion die soon after birth. In sharp contrast, the generation of a kidney specific CLDN10-KO mouse (by the use of a ksp-Cre deleter strain) led to a vital mouse model. However, these mice displayed hypermagnesemia, hypocalciuria, nephrocalcinosis, and polyuria (53). Isolated mouse tubules of the TAL demonstrated a decreased paracellular Na^+ permeability as well as higher expression of Claudin-16. Interestingly, recently four independent groups have reported mutations in human CLDN10 (54–57). Bongers et al. reported on two non-related patients presenting with alkalosis, hypokalemia, hypocalciuria, and hypercalcemia and a serum Mg^{2+} in the upper range of normal. They identified heterozygous mutations (P149R, Glu157_Tyr192del, and D73N) in two unrelated families. Hadj-Rabia et al. reported mutations in six patients from two unrelated families (S131L, M1T), resulting in an absence of CLDN10 at the plasma membrane. Affected members had high serum Mg^{2+} levels and renal loss of K^+, Na^+ and Cl^-. Of interest is that patients also suffered from a variety of skin and teeth disorders (hypolacrymia, ichthyosis, xerostomia, and severe enamel wear). A similar renal phenotype was reported by Klar and colleagues (55). They identified a CLDN10 Mutation (N48K) in two distantly related families with 13 affected individuals presenting with anhidrosis and the inability to produce tears. Although serum levels of Na^+ and K^+ were in the normal range, all patients present with high Mg^{2+} serum levels. All groups identified homozygous or compound heterozygous mutations in CLDN10 and demonstrated thereby unequivocally the importance of Claudin-10 for human Mg^{2+} homeostasis. However, the recently described homozygote mutation (G163A) in a patient by Terliesner was reported to have normomagnesemia (57). So far, several different mutations in human CLDN10 have been shown to cause a renal tubular disorder that is characterized by hypokalemia, alkalosis, and hypermagnesemia. Moreover, as Claudin-10 is expressed in skin tissues, and several different symptoms of disordered dermal Na^+ homeostasis could, therefore, be attributed to this defect.

Interestingly, the full CLDN10 knock-out mouse dies a few hours after birth, indicating that one or more organs different than the kidney and skin must be, if deficient for Claudin-10, vital for survival. Thus, the fact that human mutation does not lead to a lethal phenotype are intriguing in terms of compensatory mechanisms. However, the fact that Claudin-10 is expressed in the lung leads to spectate that the primary cause of postnatal death is caused by the absence of Claudin-10 in the lung (58, 59).

A corresponding mouse model has been generated by Breiderhoff and colleagues, by crossbreeding Claudin-16-deficient mice with a kidney-specific Claudin-10-deficient mouse strain (44, 53). Combining a hypomagnesemic model ($CLDN16^{-}/^{-}$) with a hypermagnesemic model (kidney specific $CLDN10^{-/-}$) resulted in a normomagnesemic mouse, thus a "restored" normal phenotype (60). These findings point at the high compensatory, and more than so far anticipated capacity of the DCT. Put in perspective, the development of a selective renal Claudin-10b blocking agent could be a therapeutic option for Claudin-16 patients, since obviously the block of a Na^+ pore restores the capacity of Mg^{2+} and Ca^{2+} recovery more distantly, i.e., the DCT.

Distal Convoluted Tubule

In the DCT, Mg^{2+} reabsorption takes place mainly by transcellular route. Here, apical uptake, intracellular buffering, transport, and the extrusion at the basolateral site is concerted by a highly defined and regulated (e.g., hormonal) molecular machinery that has been recently reviewed in Ref. (5, 27). Among the eight different types of Mg^{2+} transport factors identified in eukaryotes (TRPM6/M7, Mrs2, MMgT, MagT1, SLC41 family, NIPA, HIP14, and CNNMs) (61–67), only three are expressed at the DCT. The selected list includes (1) the transient receptor potential channel melastatin member 6 (TRPM6) (68), (2) the third member of the solute carrier SLC41A family (SLC41A3) (69), and (3) the "Cyclin and CBS Domain Divalent Metal Cation Transport Mediator-2" (CNNM2), also referred to as ACDP2 (ancient conserved domain protein-2) (63, 65) (**Figure 4**).

These three proteins are classified in the first category of **Table 1** as they are directly involved in Mg^{2+} transport or have been related to direct Mg^{2+} handling in the DCT.

TRPM6 was the first molecularly identified protein involved in active Mg^{2+} reabsorption (68). This channel, which associates in homotetramers, and may also interact with its closest homolog TRPM7 to form heterotetrameric species (70), is five times more permeable to Mg^{2+} than to Ca^{2+}, and permits the reabsorption of these cations through the apical membrane of the epithelial cells (68). The three-dimensional structure of TRPM6 still remains unsolved, but its domain distribution is known and includes a cytosolic N-terminus followed by a transmembrane region of six α-helices and a long intracellular C-terminus that contains a serine-threonine active kinase domain similar to that present in α-kinases. The ion pore is putatively located between the fifth and sixth α-helices of the transmembrane section (71). Interestingly, mutations that impair the phosphorylation of threonine at position 1851 (72) decrease the protein transport activity. These findings have led to propose that autophosphorylation is a key step in the regulatory mechanism of Mg^{2+} transport through this channel (73). Clinical or genetical disturbances in TRPM6 are linked to different diseases. For example, mutations in its amino acid sequence cause the rare autosomal-recessive familial hypomagnesemia with secondary hypocalcemia (74–76). Other variants have been linked to hypoparathyroidism (77) and breast cancer (78). Of note, genetic ablation of the TRPM6 gene in mice results in early embryonic lethality (79). Interestingly, $TRPM6^{\pm}$ mice showed reduced expression of the channel in kidney and colon, resulting in mild hypomagnesemia with no hypocalcemia (80).

A set of other mutations in genes that are not primarily associated with Mg^{2+}, but relevant for the establishment of the apical membrane potential to drive Mg^{2+} entry through TRPM6 (and, therefore, classified in categories 2 and 3 in **Table 1**), have been identified causing secondary Mg^{2+} wasting. The corresponding genes code for transcriptional factors (HNF1B and PCBD1), growth factors (EGF), (co)-transporters (NCC, encoded by gene SLC12A3), or even ion-channels (Kir4.1 encoded by KCNJ10) (66, 81–84) (**Figure 4**). According to the gene mutated, the resulting phenotype comprises cystic kidney disease, diabetes, electrolyte disturbances other than Mg^{2+}, or seizures. Clinically, hypomagnesemia is, compared to coexisting diabetes (MODY5), the chronic kidney disease and the hyperphenylinaemia a subordinated problem to the patient. However, identifying hypomagnesemia might be of value to identify the comorbidities at an early stage (85). Furthermore, elucidating the mechanisms that contribute to the disordered handling of Mg^{2+} in these patients may also enable a better understanding and treatment of diabetes, cyctic kidney disease, and hyperphenylinemia.

Inactivating mutations in SLC12A3 cause Gitelman syndrome, the most frequent cause of hereditary hypomagnesemia and characterized by hypokalemic metabolic alkalosis with hypomagnesemia and hypocalciuria. It has been proposed that a decrease activity of the NCC protein affects the membrane potential necessary for Mg^{2+} reabsorption in the apical membrane of DCT by TRPM6 (86–89).

SLC41A3 was originally described by Quamme as part of the solute carrier family 41 (65), which encompasses three integral cytoplasmic membrane putative Mg^{2+} transporters (SLC41A1, -A2, and -A3) (90). Mutations in this family are linked to Parkinson's disease (91), diabetes (92), and nephrolithiasis (93). As in the case of TRPM6, the three-dimensional structure of these transporters remains unsolved, but is known to be built up of 10 or 11 transmembrane α-helices (94). SLC41A3, whose molecular function and interaction partners remain also elusive, is the highest enriched member in the DCT. Recently, de Baaij et al. found that, a $Slc41a3^{-/-}$ knockout mice suffer from hypomagnesemia and normomagnesiuria, accompanied by upregulation of TRPM6 and SLC41A (69). These results underlined the relevant role played by SLC41A3 in Mg^{2+} reabsorption.

The third identified Mg^{2+} transport mediator expressed in the DCT is CNNM2, which belongs to the Cyclin M family. This family encompasses four different members (CNNM1-4). Mutations in CNNM2 cause dominant familial hypomagnesemia (67), and have been linked to brain development anomalies (95), hypertension, diabetes, and obesity (96, 97). Moreover, the CNNM2 locus has been linked by GWAS to neuro-psychiatric disorders (e.g., Schizophrenia) (98, 99). In 2014, Arjona et al. found that knockdown of CNNM2 orthologs in zebrafish results in brain abnormalities, increase of spontaneous contractions, and Mg^{2+} waste (95). These authors also identified five new families with mutations in CNNM2 that suffered hypomagnesemia with mental retardation and seizures. These findings suggested an essential role of CNNM2 in Mg^{2+} homeostasis and brain development. The relevant role of CNNM2 is underlined by the fact that mice lacking CNNM2 are embryonic lethal (100). Heterozygous ($Cnnm2^{+/-}$) mice show lower Mg^{2+} levels in serum, thus suggesting defects in Mg^{2+} reabsorption in kidney. In addition, these animals showed lower blood pressure than compared to control mice. These results highlighted the importance of Mg^{2+} and its reabsorption in the kidney to maintain blood pressure (100).

The CNNMs represent the least-studied members across the mammalian transporters and share with MgtE and with the CLC family of chloride channels the presence of a cystathionine β-synthase (CBS) domain pair in their amino acid sequence (101–103). The four CNNM family members were first identified in 2003 by Wang et al. (61, 104) and show very strong homology to the bacterial CorC protein [which is involved in Mg^{2+} and cobalt (Co^{2+}) efflux (63)], and with the Mam3p proteins (67, 105). It was initially suggested that CNNMs might be involved in cell-cycle regulation (61), as they contain a cyclin box-like motif and are located in the plasma membrane. However, the cyclin M function has that far not been proved *in vivo*.

The second member of the Cnnm family, CNNM2, is abundant in brain and kidney (64, 65), and shows a complex modular architecture composed by four structural domains (**Figure 5**) (106). The N-terminal section (likely to be an extracellular compoment) consists of a β-stranded enriched region (residues 1–250) and precedes a DUF21 domain (residues 251–400, Pfam code PF01595) with three or four transmembrane α-helices (107).

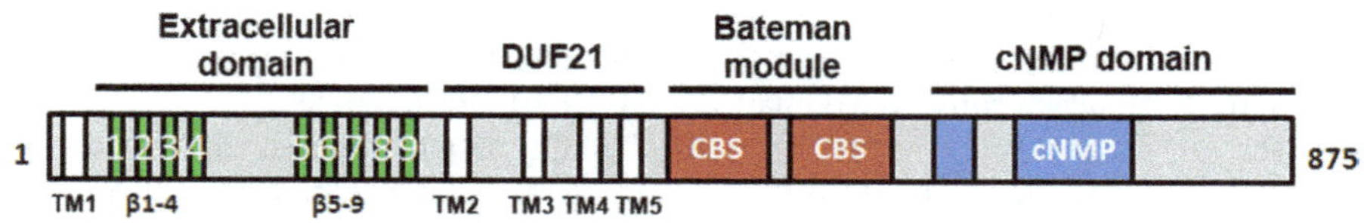

FIGURE 5 | Domain distribution of CNNM2. CNNM2 is a 97 kDa protein of 875 amino acid residues, formed by four different domains: (i) the N-terminal extracellular region is enriched in β-strands and presents a large cleavage signal peptide of approximately 65 residues. This zone is preceded by a transmembrane α-helix (TM1); (ii) the following DUF21 domain includes 3 or 4 transmembrane helices (TM1-4) that are putatively responsible for Mg^{2+} transport across the membrane; the intracellular part includes two domains: (iii) a Bateman module consisting of two consecutive CBS domains and (iv) a cyclic nucleotide monophosphate (cNMP)-like domain. CNNM2 shows two isoforms (Iso1 and Iso2). Iso2_CNNM2 lacks residues 721–742.

The following intracellular region includes a CBS domain pair (so called "Bateman" module; Pfam code PF00571) (106) and a C-terminal cyclic nucleotide monophosphate (cNMP) like binding domain (Pfam code PF00027) (106) (**Figure 5**). Although the concrete function of each domain remains unknown, recent biophysical and structural data supports a regulatory role for the Bateman module.

Mechanisms of Mg^{2+} Transport in the DCT and CNNM2

Despite the universally recognized relevance of magnesium in maintaining key life processes as mentioned above, current knowledge about the CNNMs and their role in the DCT, as well as the molecular mechanisms involved in its transport across the cellular membranes remain still to be explored. This is largely due to the scarce structural information available on Mg^{2+} transporters and channels, that so far was limited to the crystal structures of two prokaryotic proteins: (i) CorA from *Thermotoga maritima* (108–111) and (ii) MgtE from *Thermus thermophilus* (112–115). These proteins are homologs of two eukaryotic Mg^{2+} transport mediators: the mitochondrial Mg^{2+} channel Mrs2 and the solute carrier (SLC) family 41 members (homologs of CorA and MgtE, respectively). CorA represents the major transport machinery responsible for Mg^{2+} uptake in bacteria and it translocates Mg^{2+} by using an inwardly biased electrochemical gradient that serves as the driving force for Mg^{2+} permeation (108, 109, 111, 116).

MgtE is a dimeric Mg^{2+} selective channel (117) that permeates Mg^{2+} ions and maintains the intracellular Mg^{2+} homeostasis in bacteria. MgtE shares with CNNM2 (but not with SLC41) the presence of an intracellular CBS domain pair (101, 102). An ATP/Mg-dependent open-to-close gating process that involves binding of the nucleotide at this region defines the threshold of intracellular Mg^{2+} for the channel inactivation and provides sensory capacity to this protein (113, 114, 118).

The recent elucidation of the crystal structure of the Bateman module of CNNM2 (119, 120) has shed new light on the molecular mechanisms underlying Mg^{2+} transport through the basolateral membrane of the DCT (**Figure 6**). We and others recently confirmed that this region may host ATP in a Mg^{2+}-dependent manner, as well as independent Mg^{2+} atoms that interact with some acidic clusters located in the CBS1 motifs (106, 119). The fact that the Mg^{2+} independent sites are far away from the nucleotide suggest that, as observed in MgtE (114), binding of

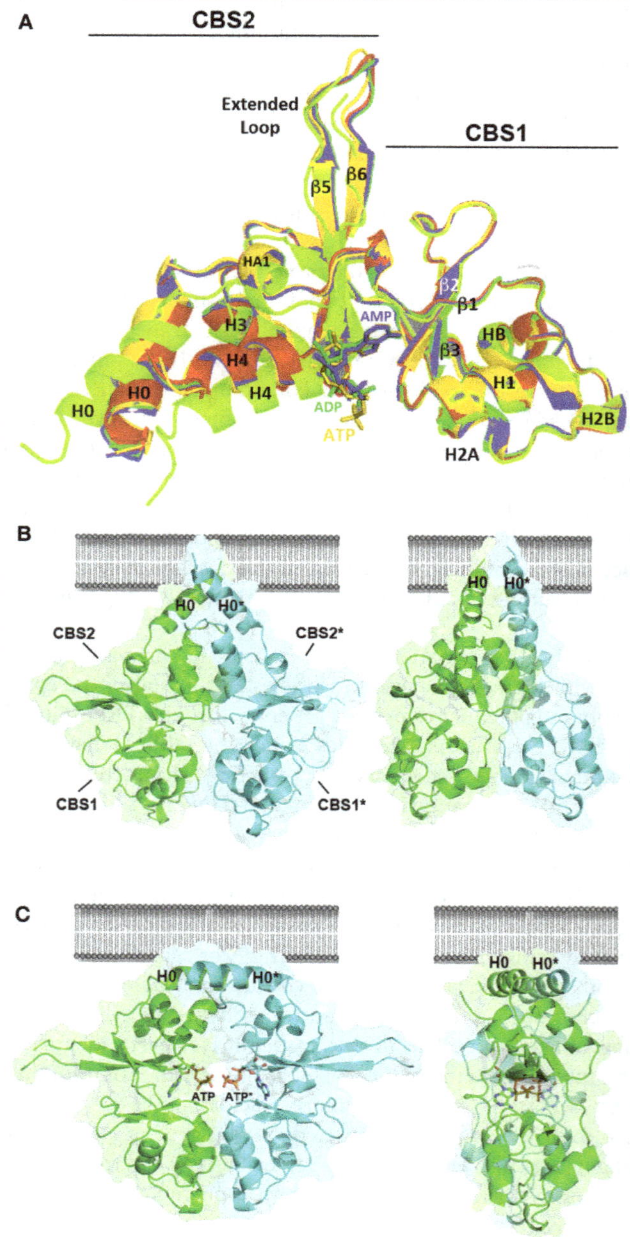

FIGURE 6 | Continued

FIGURE 6 | Crystal structure of the Bateman module of CNNM2. **(A)** The Bateman module of CNNM2 consists of two consecutive cystathionine β-synthase (CBS) motifs (CBS1, residues 445–508; CBS2, residues 509–578). A long extended loop links strands β5 and β6 in the CBS2 motif. The H0 helix connects CBS1 with the DUF21 transmembrane domain in the full-length protein. The H4 helix connects CBS2 with the cyclic nucleotide monophosphate domain. Nucleotides, ca. AMP (blue), ADP (green), or adenosine triphosphosphate (ATP) (orange) bind independently at the S2 site, thus disrupting the interactions formerly existing in the cavity between residues of the CBS1 and CBS2 motifs. This induces a displacement of helices H0, H1, and H4 in each Bateman subunit. The apo- and the nucleotide-bound Bateman module are represented in green and marine, respectively. The crystal structure of the T568I protein variant is in red. As shown, the T568I mutation mimics the structural effect of ATP binding; although in the first case, the structural change is irreversible, thus locking the protein in the nucleotide-bound like conformation. **(B,C)** *Conformational changes induced by ATP*. The Bateman module of CNNM2 associates in disk-like dimers known as "CBS modules," which adopt a *twisted* **(B)** or a *flat* **(C)** state depending on whether the site S2 of each subunit is empty or hosts an ATP (or MgATP) molecule, respectively. Note that the H0 helices connecting the CBS2 motif with the DUF21 domain are differently oriented in each case, thus likely transmitting the transformation suffered by the Bateman module to the transmembrane region.

Mg^{2+} at concrete positions may not be directly coupled with ATP binding, although it may complement its effect in conformational transformations suffered by the whole module (106, 121).

The Bateman module of CNNM2 features two major cavities (named as S1 and S2) that are located at opposite ends of the central β-sheets of the CBS motifs. In contrast with S1, which is partially occluded and full of bulky residues, the site S2 is fully accessible and can accommodate phospho-nucleotides, such as AMP, ADP, or ATP (106, 121) (**Figure 6**). Site S2 is built by three different structural blocks: (i) the central residues from the linker preceding the first β-strand (β1) of the CBS1 domain, (ii) the C-terminal residues from the last β-strand (β6) of the CBS2 motif, and (iii) the first two turns of helix H4 of CBS2 (**Figure 6**). The upper and right walls of the cavity are mainly hydrophobic and help accommodating the bulky adenine ring of ATP (106, 121). By contrast, the left wall of the cleft is hydrophilic and is built from the last β-strand and the following α-helix (H4) of the CBS2 motif. A conserved threonine (T568) and an aspartate residue (D571) from this helix are key in help orienting the ribose ring of the nucleosides inside the cavity, and if mutated, impede the allocation of ATP inside (106). Interestingly, the repulsive effect otherwise exerted by the acidic cluster formed by residues E570, D571, and E574 (at the first turn of α-helix H4 of CBS2) over the polyphosphate chain of ATP (106) is neutralized by the Mg atom that accompanies the ATP molecule. The positive dipole end of helix H4 and the nearby arginine residue, R480, complement the neutralizing effect (106). The Bateman module of CNNMs associates in head-to-head oriented disk-like dimers known as *CBS modules* (**Figures 6B,C**) (106, 121).

At low concentrations of Mg^{2+} and in the absence of MgATP, the CBS module adopts a "twisted" shape (**Figure 6B**), in which the CBS2 domains from complementary subunits remain in contact while the CBS1 motifs are separated and retain only scarce hydrophobic interactions. Binding of MgATP at site S2 disrupts a network of H-bonds centered on the conserved threonine at

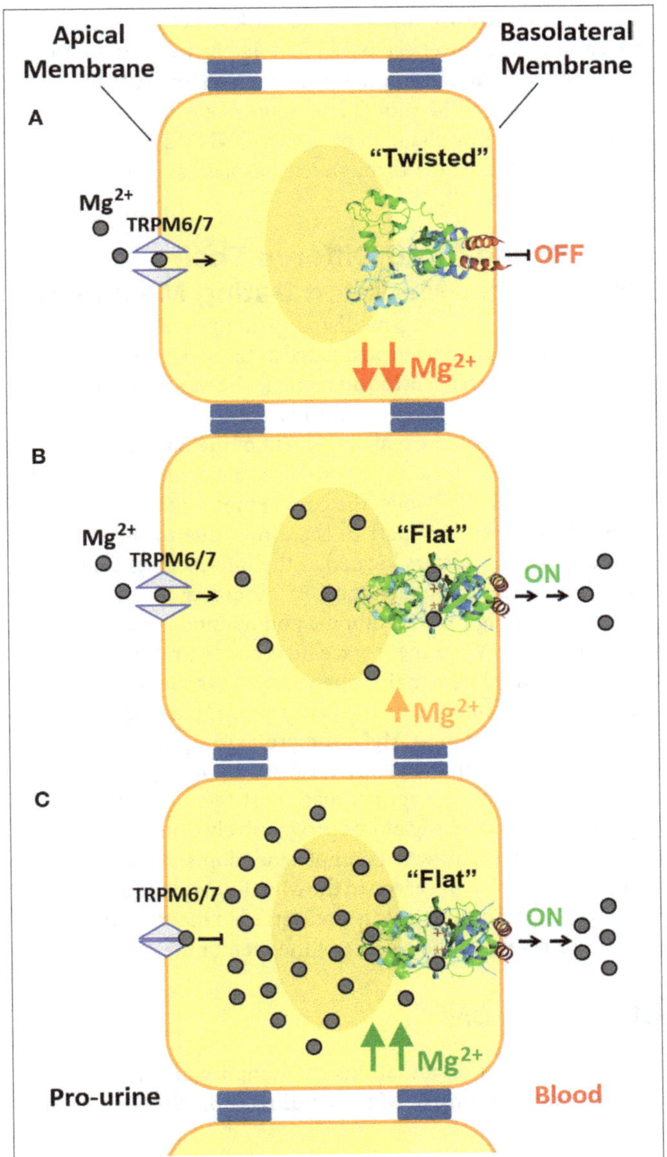

FIGURE 7 | Mechanism of Mg^{2+} transport at the distal convoluted tubule (DCT). **(A)** Mg^{2+} enters into the DCT epithelial cells through the apical membrane with the help of TRPM6/7 channels. At low Mg^{2+} concentrations, the cystathionine β-synthase (CBS) module of CNNM2, located at the basolateral membrane, remains in its twisted conformation. **(B,C)** Upon increasing the intracellular concentration of Mg^{2+}, binding of these cations and of MgATP to CNNM2, triggers the progression of the CBS module toward its flat state, and the transport of Mg^{2+} through the basolateral membrane toward the blood torrent. In addition, an increased intracellular Mg^{2+} concentration inhibits apical transport by TRPM6.

position 568 (T568) as well as a salt bridge between R480 and E570 and causes the displacement the C-terminal helix of the CBS2 domain (helix H4) as well as of the long α-helix (helix H0) that connects the Bateman module with the DUF21 domain (**Figure 5**). These structural changes, which occur concomitantly in the two complementary subunits of the dimer, trigger an overall rearrangement of the CBS module that makes it to evolve from a "twisted" (**Figure 6B**) toward a "flat" disk structure (**Figure 6C**). The conformational effect of ATP is likely transferred to the DUF21 transmembrane domain through helix (H0) that connects it with the CBS2 motif. This sequence of events has been postulated as the mechanism by which CNNM2 might regulate the gating of Mg^{2+} ions through the basolateral cell membrane (106, 121) (**Figure 7**).

CNNM2 and MgtE Differ in Their CBS-Domain-Mediated Gating Mechanism

Interestingly, an ATP/Mg-mediated gating process ruled out by CBS domains has also been postulated as the mechanism by which the MgtE transporter senses and regulate the Mg^{2+} homeostasis in bacteria (114). In contrast with the twisted-to-flat transformation observed in CNNM, the rearrangement of the Bateman modules of MgtE responds to an open-to-close mechanism (113–115). In the absence of Mg^{2+} ions, the complementary CBS2 motifs of MgtE subunits remain apart in the dimer due to the repulsion exerted by acidic clusters located at the interfacial helices of the CBS2 domains. In this state, the CBS module impairs the transport of Mg through the membrane and maintains the protein in an "open" state. While the intracellular concentration of Mg^{2+} is low, the CBS module remains open and allows the influx of Mg^{2+} ions toward the interior of the cell. Upon increasing the intracellular concentration of Mg^{2+}, the pre-existing repulsive acidic clusters become sequentially neutralized by newly bound Mg^{2+} ions, thus allowing the approximation of the CBS2 motifs. The sequential binding of Mg atoms progressively causes a closure of the CBS module that, when completed, adopts a "flat" disk-like arrangement as that observed in the MgATP/Mg^{2+} bound form of CNNM2 (106). The new state is transferred to the transmembrane region and results in the closure of the membrane pore (114).

CONCLUSION

The identification of mutations in human genes has led to a deeper understanding of Mg^{2+} handling in health and disease. On that basis, technologies, such as mouse genetic engineering as well as crystallography, have contributed in this field of physiology and pathophysiology. However, our current knowledge of the molecular mechanisms underlying magnesium transport through the cell membranes is very scarce, and represents an incipient field of research that will mature, as we are able to identify new molecular partners involved in this process. Proteins involved in trans- and paracellular pathways have the potential of being key players in Magnesium Homeostasis and also other disorders, such as diabetes, hypertension, and schizophrenia, thus being a potential target for pharmaceutical interventions.

AUTHOR CONTRIBUTIONS

All authors listed have made a substantial, direct, and intellectual contribution to the work and approved it for publication.

FUNDING

This work was supported in part by Departamento de Educación, Universidades e Investigación del Gobierno Vasco Grant PI2010-17, Departamento de Industria, Innovación, Comercio y Turismo del Gobierno Vasco Grants ETORTEK IE05-14 and IE07-202, Diputación Foral de Bizkaia Grants 7/13/08/2006/11 and 7/13/08/2005/14, Spanish Ministerio de Ciencia e Innovación (MICINN), Grant BFU2010-17857, Spanish Ministry of Economy and Competitiveness Grant BFU2013-47531-R, BFU2016-77408-R from Spanish Ministry of Economy and Competitiveness (MINECO) and Ministerio de Ciencia e Innovación CONSOLIDER-INGENIO 2010 Program Grant CSD2008-00005 (to LM-C). We also thank MINECO for the Severo Ochoa Excellence Accreditation (SEV-2016-0644) and by a PhD fellowship from MINECO (REF BES-2014-068464) awarded to PG-M. DM was supported by the German Research Foundation (DFG, Graduate School 2318) and by The Berlin Institute of Health (BIH) G(CRG 12.01.134).

REFERENCES

1. Rude RK. Magnesium. 11th ed. In: Ross AC, Caballero B, Cousins RJ, Tucker KL, Ziegler TR, editors. *Modern Nutrition in Health and Disease*. Baltimore, MA: Lippincott Williams & Wilkins (2012). p. 159–75.
2. Romani AM. Chapter 3. Magnesium in health and disease. In: Sigel A, Sigel H, Sigel RKO, editors. *Interrelations between Essential Metal Ions and Human Diseases. Metal Ions in Life Sciences*. (Vol. 13), Dordrecht: Springer (2013). p. 49–79.
3. Kass L, Weekes J, Carpenter L. Effect of magnesium supplementation on blood pressure: a meta-analysis. *Eur J Clin Nutr* (2012) 66(4):411–8. doi:10.1038/ejcn.2012.4
4. Corre T, Arjona FJ, Hayward C, Youhanna S, de Baaij JHF, Belge H, et al. Genome-wide meta-analysis unravels interactions between magnesium homeostasis and metabolic phenotypes. *J Am Soc Nephrol* (2018) 29(1): 335–48. doi:10.1681/ASN.2017030267
5. Li H, Sun S, Chen J, Xu G, Wang H, Qian Q. Genetics of Magnesium Disorders. *Kidney Dis (Basel)* (2017) 3(3):85–97. doi:10.1159/000477730
6. Cowan JA. *Introduction to the Biological Chemistry of Magnesium. The Biological Chemistry of Magnesium*. New York, NY: VCH (1995).
7. Rude RK. Magnesium. 2nd ed. In: Coates PM, Betz JM, Blackman MR, Cragg GM, Levine M, Moss J, et al., editors. *Encyclopedia of Dietary Supplements*. New York, NY: Informa Healthcare (2010). p. 527–37.
8. Kanbay M, Goldsmith D, Uyar ME, Turgut F, Covic A. Magnesium in chronic kidney disease: challenges and opportunities. *Blood Purif* (2010) 29(3):280–92. doi:10.1159/000276665
9. Verberckmoes SC, Persy V, Behets GJ, Neven E, Hufkens A, Zebger-Gong H, et al. Uremia-related vascular calcification: more than apatite deposition. *Kidney Int* (2007) 71(4):298–303. doi:10.1038/sj.ki.5002028
10. Fine KD, Santa Ana CA, Porter JL, Fordtran JS. Intestinal absorption of magnesium from food and supplements. *J Clin Invest* (1991) 88(2):396–402. doi:10.1172/JCI115317
11. de Baaij JH, Hoenderop JG, Bindels RJ. Magnesium in man: implications for health and disease. *Physiol Rev* (2015) 95(1):1–46. doi:10.1152/physrev.00012.2014
12. de Baaij JH, Dorresteijn EM, Hennekam EA, Kamsteeg EJ, Meijer R, Dahan K, et al. Recurrent FXYD2 p.Gly41Arg mutation in patients with isolated dominant hypomagnesaemia. *Nephrol Dial Transplant* (2015) 30(6):952–7. doi:10.1093/ndt/gfv014
13. Blaine J, Chonchol M, Levi M. Renal control of calcium, phosphate, and magnesium homeostasis. *Clin J Am Soc Nephrol* (2015) 10(7):1257–72. doi:10.2215/CJN.09750913
14. Seely JF. Variation in electrical resistance along length of rat proximal convoluted tubule. *Am J Physiol* (1973) 225(1):48–57.
15. Burg M, Good D. Sodium chloride coupled transport in mammalian nephrons. *Annu Rev Physiol* (1983) 45:533–47. doi:10.1146/annurev.ph.45.030183.002533

16. Reuss L, Finn AL. Passive electrical properties of toad urinary bladder epithelium. Intercellular electrical coupling and transepithelial cellular and shunt conductances. *J Gen Physiol* (1974) 64(1):1–25. doi:10.1085/jgp.64.1.1
17. Zihni C, Mills C, Matter K, Balda MS. Tight junctions: from simple barriers to multifunctional molecular gates. *Nat Rev Mol Cell Biol* (2016) 17(9):564–80. doi:10.1038/nrm.2016.80
18. Ahmad R, Kumar B, Chen Z, Chen X, Müller D, Lele SM, et al. Loss of claudin-3 expression induces IL6/gp130/Stat3 signaling to promote colon cancer malignancy by hyperactivating Wnt/β-catenin signaling. *Oncogene* (2017) 36(47):6592–604. doi:10.1038/onc.2017.259
19. Kooij G, Kopplin K, Blasig R, Stuiver M, Koning N, Goverse G, et al. Disturbed function of the blood-cerebrospinal fluid barrier aggravates neuro-inflammation. *Acta Neuropathol* (2014) 128(2):267–77. doi:10.1007/s00401-013-1227-1
20. Bardet C, Ribes S, Wu Y, Diallo MT, Salmon B, Breiderhoff T, et al. Loss-of-function disrupts tight junctions and impairs amelogenesis. *Front Physiol* (2017) 8:326. doi:10.3389/fphys.2017.00326
21. Suzuki H, Nishizawa T, Tani K, Yamazaki Y, Tamura A, Ishitani R, et al. Crystal structure of a claudin provides insight into the architecture of tight junctions. *Science* (2014) 344(6181):304–7. doi:10.1126/science.1248571
22. Suzuki H, Tani K, Fujiyoshi Y. Crystal structures of claudins: insights into their intermolecular interactions. *Ann N Y Acad Sci* (2017) 1397(1):25–34. doi:10.1111/nyas.13371
23. Müller D, Kausalya PJ, Claverie-Martin F, Meij IC, Eggert P, Garcia-Nieto V, et al. A novel claudin 16 mutation associated with childhood hypercalciuria abolishes binding to ZO-1 and results in lysosomal mistargeting. *Am J Hum Genet* (2003) 73(6):1293–301. doi:10.1086/380418
24. Liu F, Koval M, Ranganathan S, Fanayan S, Hancock WS, Lundberg EK, et al. Systems proteomics view of the endogenous human claudin protein family. *J Proteome Res* (2016) 15(2):339–59. doi:10.1021/acs.jproteome.5b00769
25. Milatz S, Himmerkus N, Wulfmeyer VC, Drewell H, Mutig K, Hou J, et al. Mosaic expression of claudins in thick ascending limbs of Henle results in spatial separation of paracellular Na^+ and Mg^{2+} transport. *Proc Natl Acad Sci U S A* (2017) 114(2):E219–27. doi:10.1073/pnas.1611684114
26. Gong Y, Hou J. Claudins in barrier and transport function-the kidney. *Pflugers Arch* (2017) 469(1):105–13. doi:10.1007/s00424-016-1906-6
27. Viering DHHM, de Baaij JHF, Walsh SB, Kleta R, Bockenhauer D. Genetic causes of hypomagnesemia, a clinical overview. *Pediatr Nephrol* (2017) 32(7):1123–35. doi:10.1007/s00467-016-3416-3
28. Bartter FC, Pronove P, Gill JR Jr, MacCardle RC. Hyperplasia of the juxtaglomerular complex with hyperaldosteronism and hypokalemic alkalosis. A new syndrome. *Am J Med* (1962) 33:811–28. doi:10.1016/0002-9343(62)90214-0
29. Simon DB, Karet FE, Hamdan JM, DiPietro A, Sanjad SA, Lifton RP. Bartter's syndrome, hypokalaemic alkalosis with hypercalciuria, is caused by mutations in the Na-K-2Cl cotransporter NKCC2. *Nat Genet* (1996) 13(2):183–8. doi:10.1038/ng0696-183
30. Simon DB, Karet FE, Rodriguez-Soriano J, Hamdan JH, DiPietro A, Trachtman H, et al. Genetic heterogeneity of Bartter's syndrome revealed by mutations in the K^+ channel, ROMK. *Nat Genet* (1996) 14(2):152–6. doi:10.1038/ng1096-152
31. Simon DB, Bindra RS, Mansfield TA, Nelson-Williams C, Mendonca E, Stone R, et al. Mutations in the chloride channel gene, CLCNKB, cause Bartter's syndrome type III. *Nat Genet* (1997) 17(2):171–8. doi:10.1038/ng1097-171
32. Birkenhäger R, Otto E, Schürmann MJ, Vollmer M, Ruf EM, Maier-Lutz I, et al. Mutation of BSND causes Bartter syndrome with sensorineural deafness and kidney failure. *Nat Genet* (2001) 29(3):310–4. doi:10.1038/ng752
33. Estévez R, Boettger T, Stein V, Birkenhäger R, Otto E, Hildebrandt F, et al. Barttin is a Cl- channel beta-subunit crucial for renal Cl- reabsorption and inner ear K^+ secretion. *Nature* (2001) 414(6863):558–61. doi:10.1038/35107099
34. Kemter E, Rathkolb B, Bankir L, Schrewe A, Hans W, Landbrecht C, et al. Mutation of the $Na^{(+)}$-$K^{(+)}$-2Cl(-) cotransporter NKCC2 in mice is associated with severe polyuria and a urea-selective concentrating defect without hyperreninemia. *Am J Physiol Renal Physiol* (2010) 298(6):F1405–15. doi:10.1152/ajprenal.00522.2009
35. Laghmani K, Beck BB, Yang SS, Seaayfan E, Wenzel A, Reusch B, et al. Polyhydramnios, transient antenatal Bartter's syndrome, and MAGED2 mutations. *N Engl J Med* (2016) 374(19):1853–63. doi:10.1056/NEJMoa1507629
36. Kömhoff M, Laghmani K. Pathophysiology of antenatal Bartter's syndrome. *Curr Opin Nephrol Hypertens* (2017) 26(5):419–25. doi:10.1097/MNH.0000000000000346
37. Meij IC, Koenderink JB, van Bokhoven H, Assink KF, Groenestege WT, de Pont JJ, et al. Dominant isolated renal magnesium loss is caused by misrouting of the $Na^{(+)}$, $K^{(+)}$-ATPase gamma-subunit. *Nat Genet* (2000) 26(3):265–6. doi:10.1038/81543
38. Ben-Yosef T, Belyantseva IA, Saunders TL, Hughes ED, Kawamoto K, Van Itallie CM, et al. Claudin 14 knockout mice, a model for autosomal recessive deafness DFNB29, are deaf due to cochlear hair cell degeneration. *Hum Mol Genet* (2003) 12:2049–61. doi:10.1093/hmg/ddg210
39. Wilcox ER, Burton QL, Naz B, Riazuddin S, Smith TN, Ploplis B, et al. Mutations in the gene encoding tight junction claudin-14 cause autosomal recessive deafness DFNB29. *Cell* (2001) 104:165–72. doi:10.1016/S0092-8674(01)00200-8
40. Corre T, Olinger E, Harris SE, Traglia M, Ulivi S, Lenarduzzi S, et al. Common variants in CLDN14 are associated with differential excretion of magnesium over calcium in urine. *Pflugers Arch* (2017) 469(1):91–103. doi:10.1007/s00424-016-1913-7
41. Thorleifsson G, Holm H, Edvardsson V, Walters GB, Styrkarsdottir U, Gudbjartsson DF, et al. Sequence variants in the CLDN14 gene associate with kidney stones and bone mineral density. *Nat Genet* (2009) 41(8):926–30. doi:10.1038/ng.404
42. Simon DB, Lu Y, Choate KA, Velazquez H, Al-Sabban E, Praga M, et al. Paracellin-1, a renal tight junction protein required for paracellular Mg^{2+} resorption. *Science* (1999) 285(5424):103–6. doi:10.1126/science.285.5424.103
43. Konrad M, Hou J, Weber S, Dötsch J, Kari JA, Seeman T, et al. CLDN16 genotype predicts renal decline in familial hypomagnesemia with hypercalciuria and nephrocalcinosis. *J Am Soc Nephrol* (2008) 19(1):171–81. doi:10.1681/ASN.2007060709
44. Will C, Breiderhoff T, Thumfart J, Stuiver M, Kopplin K, Sommer K, et al. Targeted deletion of murine Cldn16 identifies extra- and intrarenal compensatory mechanisms of Ca^{2+} and Mg^{2+} wasting. *Am J Physiol Renal Physiol* (2010) 298(5):F1152–61. doi:10.1152/ajprenal.00499.2009
45. Bardet C, Courson F, Wu Y, Khaddam M, Salmon B, Ribes S, et al. Claudin-16 deficiency impairs tight junction function in ameloblasts, leading to abnormal enamel formation. *J Bone Miner Res* (2016) 31(3):498–513. doi:10.1002/jbmr.2726
46. Yamaguti PM, Neves FA, Hotton D, Bardet C, de La Dure-Molla M, Castro LC, et al. Amelogenesis imperfecta in familial hypomagnesaemia and hypercalciuria with nephrocalcinosis caused by CLDN19 gene mutations. *J Med Genet* (2017) 54(1):26–37. Erratum in: *J Med Genet* (2017) 54(11):786. doi:10.1136/jmedgenet-2016-103956
47. Konrad M, Schaller A, Seelow D, Pandey AV, Waldegger S, Lesslauer A, et al. Mutations in the tight-junction gene claudin 19 (CLDN19) are associated with renal magnesium wasting, renal failure, and severe ocular involvement. *Am J Hum Genet* (2006) 79:949–57. doi:10.1086/508617
48. Hou J, Renigunta A, Gomes AS, Hou M, Paul DL, Waldegger S, et al. Claudin-16 and claudin-19 interaction is required for their assembly into tight junctions and for renal reabsorption of magnesium. *Proc Natl Acad Sci U S A* (2009) 106:15350–5. doi:10.1073/pnas.0907724106
49. Claverie-Martín F, García-Nieto V, Loris C, Ariceta G, Nadal I, Espinosa L, et al. Claudin-19 mutations and clinical phenotype in Spanish patients with familial hypomagnesemia with hypercalciuria and nephrocalcinosis. *PLoS One* (2013) 8(1):e53151. doi:10.1371/journal.pone.0053151
50. Van Itallie CM, Rogan S, Yu A, Vidal LS, Holmes J, Anderson JM. Two splice variants of claudin-10 in the kidney create paracellular pores with different ion selectivities. *Am J Physiol Renal Physiol* (2006) 291(6):F1288–99. doi:10.1152/ajprenal.00138.2006
51. Günzel D, Stuiver M, Kausalya PJ, Haisch L, Krug SM, Rosenthal R, et al. Claudin-10 exists in six alternatively spliced isoforms that exhibit distinct localization and function. *J Cell Sci* (2009) 122(Pt 10):1507–17. doi:10.1242/jcs.040113
52. Milatz S, Breiderhoff T. One gene, two paracellular ion channels-claudin-10 in the kidney. *Pflugers Arch* (2017) 469(1):115–21. doi:10.1007/s00424-016-1921-7
53. Breiderhoff T, Himmerkus N, Stuiver M, Mutig K, Will C, Meij IC, et al. Deletion of claudin-10 (Cldn10) in the thick ascending limb impairs

paracellular sodium permeability and leads to hypermagnesemia and nephrocalcinosis. *Proc Natl Acad Sci U S A* (2012) 109(35):14241–6. doi:10.1073/pnas.1203834109

54. Bongers EMHF, Shelton LM, Milatz S, Verkaart S, Bech AP, Schoots J, et al. A novel hypokalemic-alkalotic salt-losing tubulopathy in patients with *CLDN10* mutations. *J Am Soc Nephrol* (2017) 28(10):3118–28. doi:10.1681/ASN.2016080881
55. Klar J, Piontek J, Milatz S, Tariq M, Jameel M, Breiderhoff T, et al. Altered paracellular cation permeability due to a rare CLDN10B variant causes anhidrosis and kidney damage. *PLoS Genet* (2017) 13(7):e1006897. doi:10.1371/journal.pgen.1006897
56. Hadj-Rabia S, Brideau G, Al-Sarraj Y, Maroun RC, Figueres ML, Leclerc-Mercier S, et al. Multiplex epithelium dysfunction due to CLDN10 mutation: the HELIX syndrome. *Genet Med* (2018) 20(2):190–201. doi:10.1038/gim.2017.71
57. Terliesner N, Halbritter J, Bergmann C, Schitke J, Dittrich K. Phänotyp einer neuartigen CLDN10-*Mutation*. Nieren- und Hochdruckkrankheiten, Jahrgang 47, Nr. 2/2018, S. 1–61. (2018).
58. Merikallio H, Pääkkö P, Harju T, Soini Y. Claudins 10 and 18 are predominantly expressed in lung adenocarcinomas and in tumors of nonsmokers. *Int J Clin Exp Pathol* (2011) 4(7):667–73.
59. Ohta H, Chiba S, Ebina M, Furuse M, Nukiwa T. Altered expression of tight junction molecules in alveolar septa in lung injury and fibrosis. *Am J Physiol Lung Cell Mol Physiol* (2012) 302(2):L193–205. doi:10.1152/ajplung.00349.2010
60. Breiderhoff T, Himmerkus N, Drewell H, Plain A, Günzel D, Mutig K, et al. Deletion of claudin-10 rescues claudin-16-deficient mice from hypomagnesemia and hypercalciuria. *Kidney Int* (2018) 93(3):580–588. doi:10.1016/j.kint.2017.08.029
61. Wang C-Y, Shi J-D, Yang P, Kumar PG, Li Q-Z, Run Q-G, et al. Molecular cloning and characterization of a novel gene family of four ancient conserved domain proteins (ACDP). *Gene* (2003) 306:37–44. doi:10.1016/S0378-1119(02)01210-6
62. Rainier S, Chai JH, Tokarz D, Nicholls RD, Fink JK. NIPA1 gene mutations cause autosomal dominant hereditary spastic paraplegia (SPG6). *Am J Hum Genet* (2003) 73(4):967–71. doi:10.1086/378817
63. Wang C-Y, Yang P, Shi J-D, Purohit S, Guo D, An H, et al. Molecular cloning and characterization of the mouse Acdp gene family. *BMC Genomics* (2004) 5:7. doi:10.1186/1471-2164-5-7
64. Goytain A, Quamme GA. Functional characterization of ACDP2 (ancient conserved domain protein), a divalent metal transporter. *Physiol Genomics* (2005) 22:82–9. doi:10.1152/physiolgenomics.00058.2005
65. Quamme GA. Molecular identification of ancient and modern mammalian magnesium transporters. *Am J Physiol Cell Physiol* (2010) 298:C407–29. doi:10.1152/ajpcell.00124.2009
66. Ferre S, Hoenderop JG, Bindels RJ. Insight into renal Mg^{2+} transporters. *Curr Opin Nephrol Hypertens* (2011) 20:169–76. doi:10.1097/MNH.0b013e3283435ee4
67. Stuiver M, Lainez S, Will C, Terryn S, Günzel D, Debaix H, et al. CNNM2, encoding a basolateral protein required for renal Mg^{2+} handling, is mutated in dominant hypomagnesemia. *Am J Hum Genet* (2011) 88(3):333–43. doi:10.1016/j.ajhg.2011.02.005
68. Voets T, Nilius B, Hoefs S, van der Kemp AW, Droogmans G, Bindels RJ, et al. TRPM6 forms the Mg^{2+} influx channel involved in intestinal and renal Mg^{2+} absorption. *J Biol Chem* (2004) 279(1):19–25. doi:10.1074/jbc.M311201200
69. de Baaij JH, Arjona FJ, van den Brand M, Lavrijsen M, Lameris AL, Bindels RJ, et al. Identification of SLC41A3 as a novel player in magnesium homeostasis. *Sci Rep* (2016) 6:28565. doi:10.1038/srep28565
70. Schmitz C, Dorovkov MV, Zhao X, Davenport BJ, Ryazanov AG, Perraud AL. The channel kinases TRPM6 and TRPM7 are functionally nonredundant. *J Biol Chem* (2005) 280:37763–71. doi:10.1074/jbc.M509175200
71. Schlingmann KP, Waldegger S, Konrad M, Chubanov V, Gudermann T. TRPM6 and TRPM7 – Gatekeepers of human magnesium metabolism. *Biochim Biophys Acta* (2007) 1772(8):813–21. doi:10.1016/j.bbadis.2007.03.009
72. Cao G, Thébault S, van der Wijst J, van der Kemp A, Lasonder E, Bindels RJ, et al. RACK1 inhibits TRPM6 activity via phosphorylation of the fused alpha-kinase domain. *Curr Biol* (2008) 18:168–76. doi:10.1016/j.cub.2007.12.058
73. Zhang Z, Yu H, Huang J, Faouzi M, Schmitz C, Penner R, et al. The TRPM6 kinase domain determines the Mg·ATP sensitivity of TRPM7/M6 heteromeric ion channels. *J Biol Chem* (2014) 289(8):5217–27. doi:10.1074/jbc.M113.512285
74. Schlingmann KP, Weber S, Peters M, Niemann Nejsum L, Vitzthum H, Klingel K, et al. Hypomagnesemia with secondary hypocalcemia is caused by mutations in TRPM6, a new member of the TRPM gene family. *Nat Genet* (2002) 31(2):166–70. doi:10.1038/ng889
75. Walder RY, Landau D, Meyer P, Shalev H, Tsolia M, Borochowitz Z, et al. Mutation of TRPM6 causes familial hypomagnesemia with secondary hypocalcemia. *Nat Genet* (2002) 31(2):171–4. doi:10.1038/ng901
76. Coulter M, Colvin C, Korf B, Messiaen L, Tuanama B, Crowley M, et al. Hypomagnesemia due to two novel TRPM6 mutations. *J Pediatr Endocrinol Metab* (2015) 28(11–12):1373–8. doi:10.1515/jpem-2014-0394
77. Astor MC, Løvås K, Wolff AS, Nedrebø B, Bratland E, Steen-Johnsen J, et al. Hypomagnesemia and functional hypoparathyroidism due to novel mutations in the Mg-channel TRPM6. *Endocr Connect* (2015) 4(4):215–22. doi:10.1530/EC-15-0066
78. Zhang Y, Cai Q, Shu XO, Gao YT, Li C, Zheng W, et al. Whole-exome sequencing identifies novel somatic mutations in chinese breast cancer patients. *J Mol Genet Med* (2015) 9(4):183. doi:10.4172/1747-0862.1000183
79. Komiya Y, Runnels LW. TRPM channels and magnesium in early embryonic development. *Int J Dev Biol* (2015) 59(7–9):281–8. doi:10.1387/ijdb.150196lr
80. Woudenberg-Vrenken TE, Sukinta A, van der Kemp AW, Bindels RJ, Hoenderop JG. Transient receptor potential melastatin 6 knockout mice are lethal whereas heterozygous deletion results in mild hypomagnesemia. *Nephron Physiol* (2011) 117(2):11–9. doi:10.1159/000320580
81. Samite D, Kofent J, Gong M, Rüschendorf F, Jia S, Arn P, et al. Recessive mutations in PCBD1 cause a new type of early-onset diabetes. *Diabetes* (2014) 63(10):3557–64. doi:10.2337/db13-1784
82. Kompatscher A, de Baaij JHF, Aboudehen K, Hoefnagels APWM, Igarashi P, Bindels RJM, et al. Loss of transcriptional activation of the potassium channel Kir5.1 by HNF1β drives autosomal dominant tubulointerstitial kidney disease. *Kidney Int* (2017) 92(5):1145–56. doi:10.1016/j.kint.2017.03.034
83. Glaudemans B, van der Wijst J, Scola RH, Lorenzoni PJ, Heister A, van der Kemp AW, et al. A missense mutation in the Kv1.1 voltage-gated potassium channel-encoding gene KCNA1 is linked to human autosomal dominant hypomagnesemia. *J Clin Invest* (2009) 119(4):936–42. doi:10.1172/JCI36948
84. Groenestege WM, Thébault S, van der Wijst J, van den Berg D, Janssen R, Tejpar S, et al. Impaired basolateral sorting of pro-EGF causes isolated recessive renal hypomagnesemia. *J Clin Invest* (2007) 117(8):2260–7. doi:10.1172/JCI31680
85. van der Made CI, Hoorn EJ, de la Faille R, Karaaslan H, Knoers NV, Hoenderop JG, et al. Hypomagnesemia as first clinical manifestation of ADTKD-HNF1B: a case series and literature review. *Am J Nephrol* (2015) 42(1):85–90. doi:10.1159/000439286
86. Knoers NV, Levtchenko EN. Gitelman syndrome. *Orphanet J Rare Dis* (2008) 3:22. doi:10.1186/1750-1172-3-22
87. Nijenhuis T, Vallon V, van der Kemp AW, Loffing J, Hoenderop JG, Bindels RJ. Enhanced passive Ca^{2+} reabsorption and reduced Mg^{2+} channel abundance explains thiazide-induced hypocalciuria and hypomagnesemia. *J Clin Invest* (2005) 115(6):1651–8. doi:10.1172/JCI24134
88. Yogi A, Callera GE, O'Connor SE, He Y, Correa JW, Tostes RC, et al. Dysregulation of renal transient receptor potential melastatin 6/7 but not paracellin-1 in aldosterone-induced hypertension and kidney damage in a model of hereditary hypomagnesemia. *J Hypertens* (2011) 29(7):1400–10. doi:10.1097/HJH.0b013e32834786d6
89. Pham PC, Pham PA, Pham SV, Pham PT, Pham PM, Pham PT. Hypomagnesemia: a clinical perspective. *Int J Nephrol Renovasc Dis* (2014) 7:219–30. doi:10.2147/IJNRD.S42054
90. Schweigel-Röntgen M, Kolisek M. SLC41 transporters – molecular identification and functional role. *Curr Top Membr* (2014) 73:383–410. doi:10.1016/B978-0-12-800223-0.00011-6
91. Kolisek M, Sponder G, Mastrototaro L, Smorodchenko A, Launay P, Vormann J, et al. Substitution p.A350V in Na^{+}/Mg^{2+} exchanger SLC41A1, potentially associated with Parkinson's disease, is a gain-of-function mutation. *PLoS One* (2013) 8(8):e71096. doi:10.1371/journal.pone.0071096
92. Chan KH, Chacko SA, Song Y, Cho M, Eaton CB, Wu WC, et al. Genetic variations in magnesium-related ion channels may affect diabetes risk

among African American and Hispanic American women. *J Nutr* (2015) 145:418–24. doi:10.3945/jn.114.203489
93. Hurd TW, Otto EA, Mishima E, Gee HY, Inoue H, Inazu M, et al. Mutation of the Mg transporter SLC41A1 results in a nephronophthisis-like phenotype. *J Am Soc Nephrol* (2013) 24:967–77. doi:10.1681/ASN.2012101034
94. Fleig A, Schweigel-Röntgen M, Kolisek M. Solute carrier family SLC41, what do we really know about it? *Wiley Interdiscip Rev Membr Transp Signal* (2013) 2(6). doi:10.1002/wmts.95
95. Arjona FJ, de Baaij JHF, Schlingmann KP, Lameris ALL, van Wijk E, Flik G, et al. CNNM2 mutations cause impaired brain development and seizures in patients with hypomagnesemia. *PLoS Genet* (2014) 10(4):e1004267. doi:10.1371/journal.pgen.1004267
96. Kieboom BC, Ligthart S, Dehghan A, Kurstjens S, de Baaij JH, Franco OH, et al. Serum magnesium and the risk of prediabetes: a population-based cohort study. *Diabetologia* (2017) 60(5):843–53. doi:10.1007/s00125-017-4224-4
97. Lv WQ, Zhang X, Zhang Q, He JY, Liu HM, Xia X, et al. Novel common variants associated with body mass index and coronary artery disease detected using a pleiotropic cFDR method. *J Mol Cell Cardiol* (2017) 112:1–7. doi:10.1016/j.yjmcc.2017.08.011
98. Ohi K. Influences of schizophrenia risk variant rs7914558 at CNNM2 on brain structure. *Br J Psychiatry* (2015) 206(4):343–4. doi:10.1192/bjp.206.4.343b
99. Duarte RRR, Troakes C, Nolan M, Srivastava DP, Murray RM, Bray NJ. Genome-wide significant schizophrenia risk variation on chromosome 10q24 is associated with altered cis-regulation of BORCS7, AS3MT, and NT5C2 in the human brain. *Am J Med Genet B Neuropsychiatr Genet.* (2016) 171(6):806–14. doi:10.1002/ajmg.b.32445
100. Funato Y, Yamazaki D, Miki H. Renal function of cyclin M2 Mg^{2+} transporter maintains blood pressure. *J Hypertens* (2017) 35(3):585–92. doi:10.1097/HJH.0000000000001211
101. Ignoul S, Eggermont J. CBS domains: structure, function, and pathology in human proteins. *Am J Physiol Cell Physiol* (2005) 289(6):C1369–78.
102. Biemans-Oldehinkel E, Mahmood NA, Poolman B. A sensor for intracellular ionic strength. *Proc Natl Acad Sci U S A* (2006) 103(28):10624–9.
103. Ereño-Orbea J, Oyenarte I, Martínez-Cruz LA. CBS domains: ligand binding sites and conformational variability. *Arch Biochem Biophys* (2013) 540(1–2):70–81. doi:10.1016/j.abb.2013.10.008
104. Ochoa B. Can a congenital dysfunctional bladder be diagnosed from a smile? The Ochoa syndrome updated. *Pediatr Nephrol* (2004) 19:6–12. doi:10.1007/s00467-003-1291-1
105. Yang M, Jensen LT, Gardner A, Culotta VC. Manganese toxicity and *Saccharomyces cerevisiae* Mam3p, a member of the ACDP (ancient conserved domain protein) family of proteins. *Biochem J* (2005) 383:479–87. doi:10.1042/BJ20041582
106. Corral-Rodríguez MA, Stuiver M, Abascal-Palacios G, Diercks T, Oyenarte I, Ereño-Orbea J, et al. Nucleotide binding triggers a conformational change of the CBS module of the magnesium transporter CNNM2 from a twisted towards a flat structure. *Biochem J* (2014) 464(1):23–34. doi:10.1042/BJ20140409
107. de Baaij JH, Stuiver M, Meij IC, Lainez S, Kopplin K, Venselaar H, et al. Membrane topology and intracellular processing of cyclin M2 (CNNM2). *J Biol Chem* (2012) 287(17):13644–55. doi:10.1074/jbc.M112.342204
108. Eshaghi S, Niegowski D, Kohl A, Martinez Molina D, Lesley SA, Nordlund P. Crystal structure of a divalent metal ion transporter CorA at 2.9 angstrom resolution. *Science* (2006) 313:354–7. doi:10.1126/science.1127121
109. Lunin VV, Dobrovetsky E, Khutoreskaya G, Zhang R, Joachimiak A, Doyle DA, et al. Crystal structure of the CorA Mg^{2+} transporter. *Nature* (2006) 440:833–7. doi:10.1038/nature04642
110. Payandeh J, Pai EF. A structural basis for Mg^{2+} homeostasis and the CorA translocation cycle. *EMBO J* (2006) 25:3762–73. doi:10.1038/sj.emboj.7601269
111. Matthies D, Dalmas O, Borgnia MJ, Dominik PK, Merk A, Rao P, et al. Cryo-EM structures of the magnesium channel CorA reveal symmetry break upon gating. *Cell* (2016) 164(4):747–56. doi:10.1016/j.cell.2015.12.055
112. Smith RL, Thompson LJ, Maguire ME. Cloning and characterization of MgtE, a putative new class of Mg^{2+} transporter from *Bacillus firmus* OF4. *J Bacteriol* (1995) 177(5):1233–8. doi:10.1128/jb.177.5.1233-1238.1995
113. Hattori M, Tanaka Y, Fukai S, Ishitani R, Nureki O. Crystal structure of magnesium transporter MgtE. *Nature* (2007) 448:1072–5. doi:10.1038/nature06093
114. Tomita A, Zhang M, Jin F, Zhuang W, Takeda H, Maruyama T, et al. Crystal structure of the Mg^{2+} channel MgtE in complex with ATP. *Nat Commun* (2017) 8:148–148. doi:10.1038/s41467-017-00082-w
115. Takeda H, Hattori M, Nishizawa T, Yamashita K, Shah ST, Caffrey M, et al. Structural basis for ion selectivity revealed by high-resolution crystal structure of Mg^{2+} channel MgtE. *Nat Commun* (2014) 5:5374. doi:10.1038/ncomms6374
116. Dalmas O, Sompornpisut P, Bezanilla F, Perozo E. Molecular mechanism of Mg^{2+}-dependent gating in CorA. *Nat Commun* (2014) 5:3590. doi:10.1038/ncomms4590
117. Moomaw AS, Maguire ME. The unique nature of Mg^{2+} channels. *Physiology (Bethesda)* (2008) 23:275–85. doi:10.1152/physiol.00019.2008
118. Ishitani R, Sugita Y, Dohmae N, Furuya N, Hattori M, Nureki O. Mg^{2+}-sensing mechanism of Mg^{2+} transporter MgtE probed by molecular dynamics study. *Proc Natl Acad Sci U S A* (2008) 105(40):15393–8. doi:10.1073/pnas.0802991105
119. Hirata Y, Funato Y, Takano Y, Miki H. Mg^{2+}-dependent interactions of ATP with the cystathionine-β-synthase (CBS) domains of a magnesium transporter. *J Biol Chem* (2014) 289(21):14731–9. doi:10.1074/jbc.M114.551176
120. Gómez-García I, Stuiver M, Ereño J, Oyenarte I, Corral-Rodríguez MA, Müller D, et al. Purification, crystallization and preliminary crystallographic analysis of the CBS-domain pair of cyclin M2 (CNNM2). *Acta Crystallogr Sect F Struct Biol Cryst Commun* (2012) 68(Pt 10):1198–203. doi:10.1107/S1744309112035348
121. Giménez-Mascarell P, Oyenarte I, Hardy S, Breiderhoff T, Stuiver M, Kostantin E, et al. Structural basis of the oncogenic interaction of phosphatase PRL-1 with the magnesium transporter CNNM2. *J Biol Chem* (2017) 292(3):786–801. doi:10.1074/jbc.M116.759944

13

Managing Bardet–Biedl Syndrome—Now and in the Future

Elizabeth Forsythe, Joanna Kenny, Chiara Bacchelli and Philip L. Beales*

Genetics and Genomic Medicine Programme, UCL Great Ormond Street Institute of Child Health, University College London, London, United Kingdom

***Correspondence:**
Elizabeth Forsythe
elizabeth.forsythe@ucl.ac.uk

Bardet–Biedl syndrome is a rare autosomal recessive multisystem disorder caused by defects in genes encoding for proteins that localize to the primary cilium/basal body complex. Twenty-one disease-causing genes have been identified to date. It is one of the most well-studied conditions in the family of diseases caused by defective cilia collectively known as ciliopathies. In this review, we provide an update on diagnostic developments, clinical features, and progress in the management of Bardet–Biedl syndrome. Advances in diagnostic technologies including exome and whole genome sequencing are expanding the spectrum of patients who are diagnosed with Bardet–Biedl syndrome and increasing the number of cases with diagnostic uncertainty. As a result of the diagnostic developments, a small number of patients with only one or two clinical features of Bardet–Biedl syndrome are being diagnosed. Our understanding of the syndrome-associated renal disease has evolved and is reviewed here. Novel interventions are developing at a rapid pace and are explored in this review including genetic therapeutics such as gene therapy, exon skipping therapy, nonsense suppression therapy, and gene editing. Other non-genetic therapies such as gene repurposing, targeted therapies, and non-pharmacological interventions are also discussed.

Keywords: Bardet–Biedl syndrome, genetic therapies, pharmacogenomics, genome editing, targeted therapies, drug repurposing

INTRODUCTION

Bardet–Biedl syndrome (BBS), sometimes known as Laurence–Moon–Bardet-Biedl syndrome, is a rare autosomal recessive ciliopathy characterized by rod-cone dystrophy, learning difficulties, polydactyly, obesity, genital malformations, and renal abnormalities.

In the 1880s, a family with retinitis pigmentosa, obesity, and intellectual impairment was described by doctors Laurence and Moon. The affected family members later went on to develop a spastic paraparesis. In 1920 and 1922, respectively, doctors Bardet and Biedl independently described two families with obesity, retinitis pigmentosa, and polydactyly. From 1925, the syndrome was known as Laurence–Moon–Bardet–Biedl syndrome, but there was disagreement as to whether they were the same entity. Later, it was considered as two entities, Laurence–Moon and Bardet–Biedl syndromes, but mutations in known BBS genes have been seen in families with both syndromes (1, 2). Today, it is most usually known as BBS.

It is a pleiotropic disorder and has a prevalence of around 1:100,000 in North America and Europe, but it is significantly more common in certain isolated communities including Newfoundland (1:18,000) (2) and Kuwaiti Bedouins (1: 13,500) (3, 4). In the last 2 decades, 21 BBS genes (BBS1–BBS21) (5–7) have been identified, mutations in which account for 80% of cases with a clinical diagnosis of BBS (1). **Table 1** outlines the 21 BBS genes.

Mutations in *BBS1* and *BBS10* account for the majority of genotypes (~51 and ~20%, respectively) in Northern Europe and North America (4).

Bardet–Biedl syndrome proteins localize to the primary cilium/basal body complex, a ubiquitously expressed highly evolutionarily conserved organelle functioning primarily for cell-to-cell signaling. The genes that cause BBS can also cause other ciliopathies, with the classic example being *CEP290*, which can cause Joubert syndrome, Leber congenital amaurosis, Meckel syndrome, and Senior-Loken syndrome in addition to BBS (8).

DIAGNOSING BBS

Bardet–Biedl syndrome is a pleiotropic disorder and diagnosis is based on the presence of at least four major features or three major features and at least two minor features in accordance with the diagnostic criteria published by Beales et al. (9). **Figure 1** demonstrates the clinical features associated with BBS and highlights the relative frequencies at which these features are observed.

TABLE 1 | Known genes causing BBS.

BBS type	Gene name
BBS1	*BBS1*
BBS2	*BBS2*
BBS3	*ARL6*
BBS4	*BBS4*
BBS5	*BBS5*
BBS6	*MKKS*
BBS7	*BBS7*
BBS8	*TTC8*
BBS9	*BBS9*
BBS10	*BBS10*
BBS11	*TRIM32*
BBS12	*BBS12*
BBS13	*MKS1*
BBS14	*CEP290*
BBS15	*WDPCP*
BBS16	*SDCCA8*
BBS17	*LZTFL1*
BBS18	*BBIP1*
BBS19	*IFT27*
BBS20	*IFT172*
BBS21	*C8orf37*

Molecular confirmation of BBS has evolved over the last decade from targeted sequencing of common genetic variants, including the common *BBS1* p.M390R, *BBS2* p.Y24X, *BBS2* p.R275X, and *BBS10* c.91fsX5 mutations to next-generation sequencing gene panels containing all known BBS genes. The frequency at which molecular confirmation is achieved has increased accordingly from approximately 40–80% (1).

The age at which patients are diagnosed is extremely variable and is driven by the age of onset of symptomatic rod-cone dystrophy. While this may manifest in infancy, it is more usually seen between the ages of 5 and 10 years of age and typically presents with night blindness (9). Isolated polydactyly at birth or obesity, generally seen from infancy, do not usually prompt referral. Siblings of affected children are generally diagnosed earlier. Antenatal diagnosis is extremely rare in the absence of a family history, but BBS may be suspected from the identification of echogenic kidneys and polydactyly on ultrasound scanning. Children presenting with renal anomalies or renal failure may be diagnosed earlier than those without, but there are insufficient data to confirm this. A subset of individuals present with isolated rod-cone dystrophy with notable absence of other BBS-related features and are often diagnosed in adulthood. These individuals are now being picked up because of the introduction of panel-based genetic testing and major diagnostic studies such as the UK 100,000 genomes project (10) and the Deciphering Developmental Disorders (exome) study (11). They were previously overlooked as there are many causes of rod-cone dystrophy, and it was not understood that BBS genes could cause this feature in isolation.

Currently, diagnostic gene panels are the diagnostic tool of choice. The use of whole exome sequencing (WES) and whole genome sequencing (WGS) may increase coverage, aid in the discovery of novel genes, and allow for the identification of

i. Clinical features of Bardet-Biedl syndrome

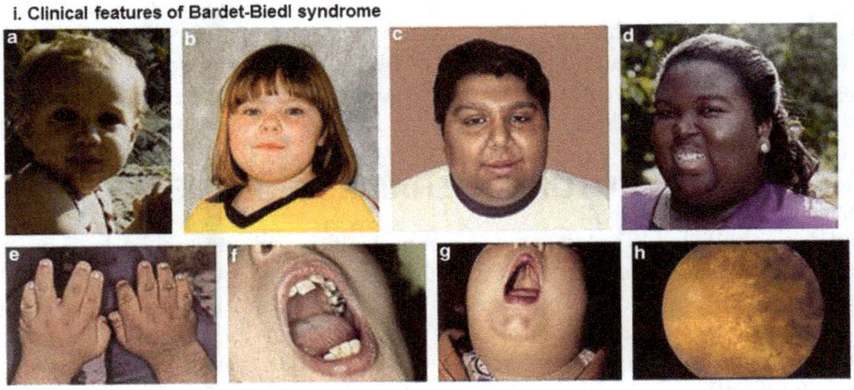

ii. Diagnostic features

Primary features	*Frequency*
Rod-cone dystrophy	93%
Polydactyly	63–81%
All four limbs:	21%
Upper limbs only:	9%
Lower limbs only:	21%
Obesity	72–92%
Genital anomalies	59–98%
Renal anomalies	53%
Learning difficulties	61%
Secondary features	
Speech delay	54–81%
Developmental delay	50–91%
Diabetes mellitus	6–48%
Dental anomalies	51%
Congenital heart disease	7%
Brachydactyly/ syndactyly	46–100%/8–95%
Ataxia/ poor coordination	40–86%
Anosmia/hyposmia	60%

FIGURE 1 | Clinical and diagnostic features of Bardet–Biedl syndrome. (i) Clinical features associated with Bardet–Biedl syndrome. **(A–D)** Typical facial features are often subtle and not always present. Typical facial features include malar hypoplasia, a depressed nasal bridge, deep set eyes, and retrognathia. **(E)** Brachydactyly. **(F)** Dental crowding. **(G)** High palate. **(H)** Rod-cone dystrophy. (ii) Diagnostic features of Bardet–Biedl syndrome. At least four major features or three major and two minor features are required to make a clinical diagnosis. Informed consent was obtained and republished with permission (4).

non-coding variants. However, along with increased expense, disadvantage of the more advanced diagnostic sequencing techniques is the identification of pathogenic variants in non-BBS genes and of variants of unknown significance (VUS) in BBS genes (12). This can result in a diagnostic conundrum in particular where patients manifest only one or two non-specific major diagnostic criteria such as obesity and/or learning difficulties. The use of WES and WGS requires careful consenting of patients and having a plan in place to deal with VUS and unlooked for results.

Variable expressivity is the hallmark of BBS (8); patients with the same genotype and even siblings frequently manifest symptoms differently. As a result, although genotype–phenotype correlations exist on a population basis, it is not possible to make individual predictions about symptomatic manifestations (13). As a group, patients with mutations in *BBS1* are usually less severely affected than patients with mutations in other BBS genes. On average, they develop visual deterioration later in life (14), are less likely to develop renal disease (13), and more likely to have a better endocrine biochemical profile (15) with a lower prevalence of metabolic syndrome (16, 17). It is not possible to delineate if this is a consequence of the common missense mutation *BBS1* p.M390R identified in 80% of Northern European patients (4) or if the milder phenotype is representative of an overall less severe phenotype associated with *BBS1* mutations (17).

Suggestion that BBS would be a candidate for triallelic inheritance, whereby a third mutation is required to either manifest the condition or adding mutational load, has gathered limited evidence (18–20). In practice, the phenotypic variability observed in patients with the same genotype and within families is likely to reflect a complex interplay between multiple genetic factors and environmental influences.

In the future, it may be possible to identify phenotypic modifiers and further elucidate the cause for variability through analysis of the "Omics" (genomics, epigenomics, transcriptomics, proteomics, and metabolomics) whereby the complex interplay of genes, transcription, protein expression, and metabolism is considered as part of the phenotypic analysis (21, 22).

RENAL DISEASE IN BBS

Bardet–Biedl syndrome has classically been associated with polycystic kidney disease, a typical feature of ciliopathies with renal manifestations (13, 16, 23–29). The prevalence of renal disease in BBS has been estimated at 53–82% (13, 16, 25). A recent study of 350 patients from the United Kingdom estimated that 50% of patients will develop functional renal disease and demonstrated that cystic or dysplastic disease only accounts for 30% of patients with renal disease, where the remainder have hydronephrosis, scarred or atrophic kidneys, loss of corticomedullary function, or developmental abnormalities (13). Around 8% of patients go on to develop end-stage renal disease requiring dialysis or transplantation (13). The majority of patients who develop end-stage renal disease do so in early childhood (before the age of 5), and in most cases, deterioration is rapid with frequent requirement for dialysis within the first year of life (13). Some patients develop sudden renal failure in adulthood for unknown reasons, and a further group of patients develop end-stage kidney disease as a result of comorbidities including type 2 diabetes and hypertension (13). The prevalence of these comorbidities is thought to be higher in BBS patients than the normal population and in 1 study of 69 patients were found in 22 and 35%, respectively (17). The risk of type 2 diabetes relates to obesity and is treated using standard protocols. Many patients with structural renal abnormalities do not go on to develop functional renal disease (17).

The molecular mechanistic pathways leading to renal disease in BBS remain unelucidated (29). It has been suggested that aberrant mTOR signaling may contribute to the development of cystic kidney disease (28). Another theory proposes that ciliary dysfunction leads to aberrant non-canonical Wnt signaling and planar cell polarity, which may contribute to the development of cysts (30). Molecular evidence supporting these theories remains limited. Furthermore, they do not explain why only some patients develop renal dysplasia or indeed the heterogeneous types of renal disease developed by patients.

CURRENT MANAGEMENT OF BBS

Bardet–Biedl syndrome is currently treated symptomatically focusing in particular on aggressive management of diabetes, hypertension, and metabolic syndrome to minimize the secondary impact that these conditions have on vulnerable organ systems already affected by BBS, in particular the eyes and kidneys (17). Weight management is a continual struggle for the majority of patients (31). Some elect to have bariatric surgery (32) while others take antiobesity medication, but for the majority of patients, dietetic input provides the safest and most effective weight loss strategy (33).

In the UK, patients who attend the national BBS clinics are invited to attend a multidisciplinary clinic for annual review by a geneticist, ophthalmologist, nephrologist, endocrinologist, psychologist, dietitian, speech and language therapist, nurse, and a patient support group representative. This provides a platform for regular review and individualized risk assessment in particular with reference to renal and endocrine deterioration. All patients are genotyped using a service-developed diagnostic gene panel. The clinic also provides an opportunity for research into the natural progression of BBS, and it is expected that patients will eventually be stratified according to genotype and their need for clinical follow-up.

FUTURE THERAPIES FOR BBS

The last decade has seen significant advances in the development of therapeutic modalities, which could potentially be applicable to patients with BBS and related ciliopathies. However, the large number of disease-causing genes and private mutations, which are those seen in only a single family, present a unique challenge in developing genetic therapies for BBS (34). **Figure 2** outlines potential future therapies, which are likely to benefit patients with BBS in the future.

Genetic Therapies

A particular focus for therapeutic intervention in the ciliopathies has been the development of therapy for rod-cone dystrophy

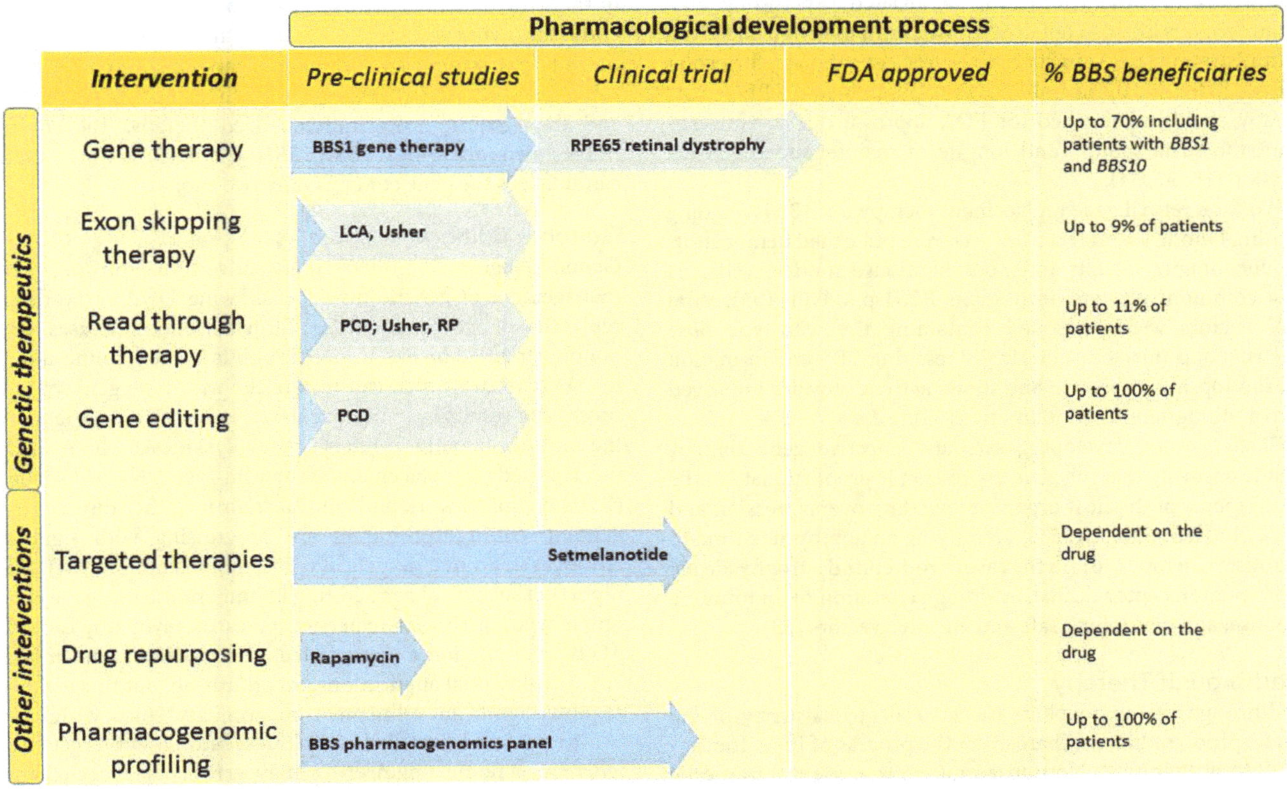

FIGURE 2 | Future interventions and stage in the pharmacological development process. Genetic therapies and other pharmacological interventions are under development for BBS. Dark blue arrows demonstrate the stage to which BBS-specific interventions have been developed. Other ciliopathy relevant developments are indicated in light blue. The last column indicates the percentage of BBS patients who could benefit from this type of intervention. BBS, Bardet–Biedl syndrome; LCA, leber congenital amaurosis; PCD, primary ciliary dyskinesia; RP, retinitis pigmentosa; US, Usher syndrome.

(34–36). The eye offers an attractive organ for therapeutic intervention in BBS due to the ease of access, the presence of a control (other) eye, the small amount of tissue that needs to be infiltrated, and a window of opportunity to develop treatment as patients typically do not develop symptoms before mid to late childhood (37).

Novel disease models are being generated with the potential to develop *in vitro* organ systems for the assessment of new therapies. A promising development is the generation of induced pluripotent stem cells (38–43). These cells are generated when adult cells are reprogrammed and subsequently differentiated into another cell type through the addition of growth factors (41). A number of cell types have been used for reprogramming including dermal fibroblasts (44), renal epithelial cells (45), keratinocytes (46), and peripheral blood cells (47).

Urine-derived renal epithelial cells have been used to model ciliopathies, such as Joubert syndrome to assess the effect of potential therapeutics (48, 49) and BBS to derive mechanistic insights into disease pathogenesis (unpublished data). This is a particularly attractive model for many ciliopathies including BBS as it is non-invasive and offers an organ-specific relevant disease model.

To our knowledge, currently, there are no efforts in progress to develop genetic therapies targeted to the renal manifestations of BBS. This is likely to be a function of a number of issues including that the onset of renal manifestations is often antenatal precluding a therapeutic window of opportunity. Furthermore, the natural history of renal disease in BBS is not well understood, and the cause of renal disease can be both primary (e.g., cystic renal disease) and secondary to metabolic syndrome, hypertension, or diabetes all of which occur more frequently in BBS than the general population (13). In addition, the kidney is more difficult to target with genetic therapies but may prove to be a more amenable target for pharmacological therapies.

Gene Therapy

Traditional gene replacement therapy has achieved significant success in the treatment of ciliopathy-related eye diseases including Usher syndrome and Leber congenital amaurosis in recent years (50–52). The premise involves the generation of viral or non-viral vectors carrying a wild-type gene of choice with the aim of integrating the gene into the host genome. The highest chance of success is achieved in diseases where only a small amount of healthy gene expression is required to generate a phenotypic effect (53).

A major challenge in developing genetic therapies for BBS is the generation of a long lasting therapy. A successful example of this is the retinal gene therapy (Luxturna), which has been successfully developed for RPE65-associated Leber congenital amaurosis. It is likely to obtain approval from the Food and Drug Administration (FDA) in 2018 as the first gene therapy for ocular disease. Extensive optimization was required before RPE65 gene therapy could be launched for FDA approval due to concerns about the sustainability and long-term maintenance of visual function (36, 37, 54).

Work on retinal gene replacement therapy for BBS is ongoing in animal models, and recent efforts were published demonstrating encouraging results in knock-in mouse models with the most common genotype in humans *BBS1* p.M390R (55). Viral AAV vectors were generated containing the wild-type *Bbs1* construct and injected subretinally rescuing BBSome formation and rhodopsin localization and showing trends toward improved electroretinogram function in mice (55).

Challenges of developing safe and effective gene therapy include ensuring that the gene expression is proportionate to the requirements of the host organism avoiding overexpression and thus cell toxicity (36, 51, 55), identifying an appropriate time to administer therapy (36) (in the case of rod-cone dystrophy ideally before photoreceptor death), avoiding generation of an immune response, and developing safe and effective vectors (53).

Readthrough Therapy

Readthrough therapy exploits the natural inconsistency of the genetic proofreading mechanism in the process of RNA translation into protein (56). Nonsense mutations account for an estimated 11% of the total mutational load in BBS (own unpublished data) and lead to premature termination of protein synthesis and subsequent degradation via nonsense mediated decay (57). Readthrough therapy acts by destabilizing the translational ribosome's response to a nonsense mutation, hence allowing the insertion of a near cognate amino-acyl-tRNA. This allows translation to continue and a full-length protein to be produced (58). The effect mimics that of a missense mutation in the same locus, which may result in a less severe clinical phenotype. Readthrough therapy has been applied to a number of different conditions and been tested in clinical trials for both cystic fibrosis (59–61) and Duchenne muscular dystrophy (62, 63). The effect of readthrough therapy has been assessed on some ciliopathies at the preclinical stage including primary ciliary dyskinesia (64), Usher syndrome (65), and retinitis pigmentosa (RP2) (66).

Exon Skipping Therapy

Exon skipping therapy operates at the level of RNA transcription allowing the transcriptional machinery to "skip" exons containing undesirable genetic sequences (67, 68). Antisense oligonucleotides are designed to target an exon/intron of interest. This allows for a novel splicing product that may retain much of its wild-type function depending on the quantity and importance of functional motifs coded for by the exon. This form of genetic therapy is often used to target mutations, which disrupt the genetic reading frame and may otherwise result in a complete lack of functional protein. Successful application of exon skipping therapy has been developed to the level of clinical trials for Duchenne muscular dystrophy and spinal muscular atrophy (69, 70). Exon skipping therapy for ciliopathies has been developed to the stage of preclinical trials for Leber Congenital Amaurosis and Usher syndrome (67, 71). In BBS, this form of therapy could benefit up to 9% of patients. The primary challenge is that many mutations suitable for exon skipping therapy in BBS are private and thus require truly individualized therapy. The common frameshift mutation in BBS (*BBS10* c.91fsX5) is not a suitable candidate as the gene contains only two exons.

Genome Editing

Genome engineering offers an attractive future prospect in the management of genetic diseases, allowing DNA to be deleted, replaced, or corrected (72). Targeted endonucleases create double-stranded breaks at specific points in the genome allowing for DNA repair, which can restore the wild-type genotype (43). Promising results have been achieved in cells from patients with the motile ciliopathy primary ciliary dyskinesia where ciliation was restored on replacement of the wild-type *DNAH11* sequence (73). Preclinical work and clinical trials for other diseases using genome editing techniques are progressing with significant advances in animal models of epidermolysis bullosa (74). Initial reports of successful gene editing in humans include gene editing on embryos at risk for hypertrophic cardiomyopathy caused by *MYBPC3* mutation (75) and treatment-resistant leukemia (75, 76). The potential applications are promising, but this technique requires significant refinement in specificity, efficacy, and safety before this can be applied in a clinical setting. Off target effects, whereby genome engineering may erroneously occur on an unintended gene causing DNA damage are a major challenge in bringing this technique forward (72).

While genome editing can be used to target specific organ systems, it can also be applied *ex vivo* to correct or insert mutations to directly comparable cell types which apart from the mutation of interest are genetically identical, thus eliminating genetic background noise and providing an ideal model system (77).

Non-Genetic Personalized Therapies

Targeted Therapies

A novel development in the therapeutic landscape for BBS is the application of targeted drug therapies. An example of this is the ongoing work on the melanocortin receptor agonists as potential therapeutic intervention against obesity in BBS (78). Our understanding of how aberrant BBS proteins cause signal disruption is still evolving; however, there is emerging evidence suggesting that BBS results in defects in the hypothalamic leptin–melanocortin axis (79). This in turn causes leptin resistance culminating in obesity (78).

Seo et al. demonstrated that intravenous administration of a melanocortin receptor agonist decreased both body weight and food intake in wild-type and *Bbs* knockout mice (78). A phase 2/3 clinical trial is in process assessing the effect of novel melanocortin receptor agonist setmelanotide on obesity in BBS and other forms of syndromic obesity (80).

Drug Repurposing

Future therapies may include repurposing of drugs, which are already FDA approved. Early work on *Bbs* zebrafish indicated that rapamycin may be a candidate for rectifying the renal cystic phenotype (81). Further work on higher animals has not been published, but drug repurposing offers an attractive and economical option for management in a clinical setting since the cost and failure rate of developing novel therapeutics remain high.

NON-PHARMACOLOGICAL FUTURE INTERVENTIONS

A major challenge in any clinical service is harnessing the advances in technology and managing increasing clinical pressures. To this end, the UK National BBS clinic is implementing several new strategies to meet the increasing need for transparency and access to clinical services.

There is an increasing move to offer patients easy access to their medical notes and to data sharing within the UK National Health Service to optimize patient management (82). These issues are being addressed in the UK National BBS clinic through the development of a cloud-based medical notes system, which is accessible to all clinicians in the service. In the future, patients will be able to access their personal medical records through smart phones or other devices, so that medical information can be accessed wherever they are.

Telemedicine and virtual clinics, whereby patient consultations can take place *via* a screen in the patient's own home, are an attractive alternative for BBS patients who are stable and in particular for those with visual impairment where travel can present a considerable obstacle to attending hospital appointments. It also offers an advantage to clinicians where hospital resources and clinic space are at a premium.

PHARMACOGENOMICS

Pharmacogenomic profiling, whereby the effect of the genome on drug response is determined, could offer significant advantages to those patients with complex medical needs who are subject to polypharmacy (83) including BBS patients. Although several private companies offer pharmacogenomics gene panels, this is not currently available in the UK National Health Service, and the evidence base is unclear for many of these private initiatives. However, there is a growing evidence base supporting pharmacogenomic profiling, and this is likely to become available in the National Health Service in the coming years.

CONCLUSION

Bardet–Biedl syndrome provides a robust model disease for future opportunities in genetic and non-genetic therapeutic management of rare diseases. A significant advantage in the United Kingdom is the presence of the national BBS clinics, which offer a centralized hub for clinical and scientific expertise. The multiorgan effects and wide range of genes and mutation types mean that a number of different genetic therapeutic modalities must be considered, as well as non-genetic pharmacological interventions and non-pharmacological approaches to optimize management of this rare disease in the future.

AUTHOR CONTRIBUTIONS

EF, JK, CB, and PB made substantial contributions to the writing, drafting, and revision of this manuscript. All authors approved the final published version of the manuscript.

FUNDING

EF is funded by the Medical Research Council. JK is funded in part by Innovate UK. PB is an NIHR Senior Investigator. This work was supported by the NIHR Great Ormond Street Hospital Biomedical Research Centre (GOSH BRC). The views expressed are those of the authors and not necessarily those of the NHS, the NIHR or the Department of Health.

REFERENCES

1. Forsythe E, Beales PL. Bardet-Biedl syndrome. In: Adam MP, Ardinger HH, Pagon RA, Wallace SE, Bean LJH, Mefford HC, Stephens K, Amemiya A, Ledbetter N, editors. *GeneReviews(R)*. Seattle, WA (2003).
2. Moore SJ, Green JS, Fan Y, Bhogal AK, Dicks E, Fernandez BA, et al. Clinical and genetic epidemiology of Bardet-Biedl syndrome in Newfoundland: a 22-year prospective, population-based, cohort study. *Am J Med Genet A* (2005) 132a(4):352–60. doi:10.1002/ajmg.a.30406
3. Farag TI, Teebi AS. High incidence of Bardet Biedl syndrome among the Bedouin. *Clin Genet* (1989) 36(6):463–4. doi:10.1111/j.1399-0004.1989.tb03378.x
4. Forsythe E, Beales PL. Bardet-Biedl syndrome. *Eur J Hum Genet* (2013) 21(1):8–13. doi:10.1038/ejhg.2012.115
5. Heon E, Kim G, Qin S, Garrison JE, Tavares E, Vincent A, et al. Mutations in C8ORF37 cause Bardet Biedl syndrome (BBS21). *Hum Mol Genet* (2016) 25(11):2283–94. doi:10.1093/hmg/ddw096
6. Khan AO, Decker E, Bachmann N, Bolz HJ, Bergmann C. C8orf37 is mutated in Bardet-Biedl syndrome and constitutes a locus allelic to non-syndromic retinal dystrophies. *Ophthalmic Genet* (2016) 37(3):290–3. doi:10.3109/13816810.2015.1066830
7. Schaefer E, Stoetzel C, Scheidecker S, Geoffroy V, Prasad MK, Redin C, et al. Identification of a novel mutation confirms the implication of IFT172 (BBS20) in Bardet-Biedl syndrome. *J Hum Genet* (2016) 61(5):447–50. doi:10.1038/jhg.2015.162
8. Mitchison HM, Valente EM. Motile and non-motile cilia in human pathology: from function to phenotypes. *J Pathol* (2017) 241(2):294–309. doi:10.1002/path.4843
9. Beales PL, Elcioglu N, Woolf AS, Parker D, Flinter FA. New criteria for improved diagnosis of Bardet-Biedl syndrome: results of a population survey. *J Med Genet* (1999) 36(6):437–46.
10. Samuel GN, Farsides B. Public trust and 'ethics review' as a commodity: the case of Genomics England Limited and the UK's 100,000 genomes project. *Med Health Care Philos* (2017). doi:10.1007/s11019-017-9810-1
11. Wright CF, Fitzgerald TW, Jones WD, Clayton S, McRae JF, van Kogelenberg M, et al. Genetic diagnosis of developmental disorders in the DDD study: a scalable analysis of genome-wide research data. *Lancet* (2015) 385(9975):1305–14. doi:10.1016/s0140-6736(14)61705-0
12. Vears DF, Senecal K, Borry P. Reporting practices for variants of uncertain significance from next generation sequencing technologies. *Eur J Med Genet* (2017) 60(10):553–8. doi:10.1016/j.ejmg.2017.07.016
13. Forsythe E, Sparks K, Best S, Borrows S, Hoskins B, Sabir A, et al. Risk factors for severe renal disease in Bardet-Biedl syndrome. *J Am Soc Nephrol* (2017) 28(3):963–70. doi:10.1681/ASN.2015091029
14. Daniels AB, Sandberg MA, Chen J, Weigel-DiFranco C, Fielding Hejtmancic J, Berson EL. Genotype-phenotype correlations in Bardet-Biedl syndrome.

Arch Ophthalmol (2012) 130(7):901–7. doi:10.1001/archophthalmol.2012.89
15. Feuillan PP, Ng D, Han JC, Sapp JC, Wetsch K, Spaulding E, et al. Patients with Bardet-Biedl syndrome have hyperleptinemia suggestive of leptin resistance. *J Clin Endocrinol Metab* (2011) 96(3):E528–35. doi:10.1210/jc.2010-2290
16. Imhoff O, Marion V, Stoetzel C, Durand M, Holder M, Sigaudy S, et al. Bardet-Biedl syndrome: a study of the renal and cardiovascular phenotypes in a French cohort. *Clin J Am Soc Nephrol* (2011) 6(1):22–9. doi:10.2215/CJN.03320410
17. Forsythe E, Sparks K, Hoskins BE, Bagkeris E, McGowan BM, Carroll PV, et al. Genetic predictors of cardiovascular morbidity in Bardet-Biedl syndrome. *Clin Genet* (2015) 87(4):343–9. doi:10.1111/cge.12373
18. Katsanis N, Eichers ER, Ansley SJ, Lewis RA, Kayserili H, Hoskins BE, et al. BBS4 is a minor contributor to Bardet-Biedl syndrome and may also participate in triallelic inheritance. *Am J Hum Genet* (2002) 71(1):22–9. doi:10.1086/341031
19. Hichri H, Stoetzel C, Laurier V, Caron S, Sigaudy S, Sarda P, et al. Testing for triallelism: analysis of six BBS genes in a Bardet-Biedl syndrome family cohort. *Eur J Hum Genet* (2005) 13(5):607–16. doi:10.1038/sj.ejhg.5201372
20. Abu-Safieh L, Al-Anazi S, Al-Abdi L, Hashem M, Alkuraya H, Alamr M, et al. In search of triallelism in Bardet-Biedl syndrome. *Eur J Hum Genet* (2012) 20(4):420–7. doi:10.1038/ejhg.2011.205
21. Topol EJ. Individualized medicine from prewomb to tomb. *Cell* (2014) 157(1):241–53. doi:10.1016/j.cell.2014.02.012
22. Hasin Y, Seldin M, Lusis A. Multi-omics approaches to disease. *Genome Biol* (2017) 18(1):83. doi:10.1186/s13059-017-1215-1
23. Tieder M, Levy M, Gubler MC, Gagnadoux MF, Broyer M. Renal abnormalities in the Bardet-Biedl syndrome. *Int J Pediatr Nephrol* (1982) 3(3):199–203.
24. Gourdol O, David L, Colon S, Bouvier R, Ayral A, Aguercif M, et al. [Renal involvement in the Laurence-Moon-Bardet-Biedl syndrome. Apropos of 3 cases]. *Pediatrie* (1984) 39(3):175–81.
25. Harnett JD, Green JS, Cramer BC, Johnson G, Chafe L, McManamon P, et al. The spectrum of renal disease in Laurence-Moon-Biedl syndrome. *N Engl J Med* (1988) 319(10):615–8. doi:10.1056/NEJM198809083191005
26. O'Dea D, Parfrey PS, Harnett JD, Hefferton D, Cramer BC, Green J. The importance of renal impairment in the natural history of Bardet-Biedl syndrome. *Am J Kidney Dis* (1996) 27(6):776–83. doi:10.1016/S0272-6386(96)90513-2
27. Putoux A, Mougou-Zerelli S, Thomas S, Elkhartoufi N, Audollent S, Le MM, et al. BBS10 mutations are common in 'Meckel'-type cystic kidneys. *J Med Genet* (2010) 47(12):848–52. doi:10.1136/jmg.2010.079392
28. Marion V, Schlicht D, Mockel A, Caillard S, Imhoff O, Stoetzel C, et al. Bardet-Biedl syndrome highlights the major role of the primary cilium in efficient water reabsorption. *Kidney Int* (2011) 79(9):1013–25. doi:10.1038/ki.2010.538
29. Putoux A, Attie-Bitach T, Martinovic J, Gubler MC. Phenotypic variability of Bardet-Biedl syndrome: focusing on the kidney. *Pediatr Nephrol* (2012) 27(1):7–15. doi:10.1007/s00467-010-1751-3
30. Tobin JL, Beales PL. Bardet-Biedl syndrome: beyond the cilium. *Pediatr Nephrol* (2007) 22(7):926–36.
31. Hamlington B, Ivey LE, Brenna E, Biesecker LG, Biesecker BB, Sapp JC. Characterization of courtesy stigma perceived by parents of overweight children with Bardet-Biedl syndrome. *PLoS One* (2015) 10(10):e0140705. doi:10.1371/journal.pone.0140705
32. Daskalakis M, Till H, Kiess W, Weiner RA. Roux-en-Y gastric bypass in an adolescent patient with Bardet-Biedl syndrome, a monogenic obesity disorder. *Obes Surg.* (2010) 20(1):121–5. doi:10.1007/s11695-009-9915-6
33. Mujahid S, Huda MS, Beales P, Carroll PV, McGowan BM. Adjustable gastric banding and sleeve gastrectomy in Bardet-Biedl syndrome. *Obes Surg* (2014) 24(10):1746–8. doi:10.1007/s11695-014-1379-7
34. Sahel JA, Marazova K, Audo I. Clinical characteristics and current therapies for inherited retinal degenerations. *Cold Spring Harb Perspect Med* (2014) 5(2):a017111. doi:10.1101/cshperspect.a017111
35. Estrada-Cuzcano A, Roepman R, Cremers FP, den Hollander AI, Mans DA. Non-syndromic retinal ciliopathies: translating gene discovery into therapy. *Hum Mol Genet* (2012) 21(R1):R111–24. doi:10.1093/hmg/dds298
36. Dias MF, Joo K, Kemp JA, Fialho SL, da Silva Cunha A Jr, Woo SJ, et al. Molecular genetics and emerging therapies for retinitis pigmentosa: basic research and clinical perspectives. *Prog Retin Eye Res* (2017). doi:10.1016/j.preteyeres.2017.10.004
37. Lee H, Lotery A. Gene therapy for RPE65-mediated inherited retinal dystrophy completes phase 3. *Lancet* (2017) 390(10097):823–4. doi:10.1016/s0140-6736(17)31622-7
38. Jin ZB, Okamoto S, Mandai M, Takahashi M. Induced pluripotent stem cells for retinal degenerative diseases: a new perspective on the challenges. *J Genet* (2009) 88(4):417–24. doi:10.1007/s12041-009-0063-5
39. Al-Shamekh S, Goldberg JL. Retinal repair with induced pluripotent stem cells. *Transl Res* (2014) 163(4):377–86. doi:10.1016/j.trsl.2013.11.002
40. Tucker BA, Mullins RF, Stone EM. Stem cells for investigation and treatment of inherited retinal disease. *Hum Mol Genet* (2014) 23(R1):R9–16. doi:10.1093/hmg/ddu124
41. Nguyen HV, Li Y, Tsang SH. Patient-specific iPSC-derived RPE for modeling of retinal diseases. *J Clin Med* (2015) 4(4):567–78. doi:10.3390/jcm4040567
42. Wiley LA, Burnight ER, Songstad AE, Drack AV, Mullins RF, Stone EM, et al. Patient-specific induced pluripotent stem cells (iPSCs) for the study and treatment of retinal degenerative diseases. *Prog Retin Eye Res* (2015) 44:15–35. doi:10.1016/j.preteyeres.2014.10.002
43. Zheng A, Li Y, Tsang SH. Personalized therapeutic strategies for patients with retinitis pigmentosa. *Expert Opin Biol Ther* (2015) 15(3):391–402. doi:10.1517/14712598.2015.1006192
44. Takahashi K, Tanabe K, Ohnuki M, Narita M, Ichisaka T, Tomoda K, et al. Induction of pluripotent stem cells from adult human fibroblasts by defined factors. *Cell* (2007) 131(5):861–72. doi:10.1016/j.cell.2007.11.019
45. Zhou T, Benda C, Dunzinger S, Huang Y, Ho JC, Yang J, et al. Generation of human induced pluripotent stem cells from urine samples. *Nat Protoc* (2012) 7(12):2080–9. doi:10.1038/nprot.2012.115
46. Aasen T, Raya A, Barrero MJ, Garreta E, Consiglio A, Gonzalez F, et al. Efficient and rapid generation of induced pluripotent stem cells from human keratinocytes. *Nat Biotechnol* (2008) 26(11):1276–84. doi:10.1038/nbt.1503
47. Staerk J, Dawlaty MM, Gao Q, Maetzel D, Hanna J, Sommer CA, et al. Reprogramming of human peripheral blood cells to induced pluripotent stem cells. *Cell Stem Cell* (2010) 7(1):20–4. doi:10.1016/j.stem.2010.06.002
48. Ajzenberg H, Slaats GG, Stokman MF, Arts HH, Logister I, Kroes HY, et al. Non-invasive sources of cells with primary cilia from pediatric and adult patients. *Cilia* (2015) 4:8. doi:10.1186/s13630-015-0017-x
49. Srivastava S, Ramsbottom SA, Molinari E, Alkanderi S, Filby A, White K, et al. A human patient-derived cellular model of Joubert syndrome reveals ciliary defects which can be rescued with targeted therapies. *Hum Mol Genet* (2017) 26(23):4657–67. doi:10.1093/hmg/ddx347
50. McIntyre JC, Williams CL, Martens JR. Smelling the roses and seeing the light: gene therapy for ciliopathies. *Trends Biotechnol* (2013) 31(6):355–63. doi:10.1016/j.tibtech.2013.03.005
51. Williams CL, Uytingco CR, Green WW, McIntyre JC, Ukhanov K, Zimmerman AD, et al. Gene therapeutic reversal of peripheral olfactory impairment in Bardet-Biedl syndrome. *Mol Ther* (2017) 25(4):904–16. doi:10.1016/j.ymthe.2017.02.006
52. Zhang W, Li L, Su Q, Gao G, Khanna H. Gene therapy using a miniCEP290 fragment delays photoreceptor degeneration in a mouse model of leber congenital amaurosis. *Hum Gene Ther* (2017) 29(1):42–50. doi:10.1089/hum.2017.049
53. Moore NA, Morral N, Ciulla TA, Bracha P. Gene therapy for inherited retinal and optic nerve degenerations. *Expert Opin Biol Ther* (2018) 18(1):37–49. doi:10.1080/14712598.2018.1389886
54. Bainbridge JW, Mehat MS, Sundaram V, Robbie SJ, Barker SE, Ripamonti C, et al. Long-term effect of gene therapy on Leber's congenital amaurosis. *N Engl J Med* (2015) 372(20):1887–97. doi:10.1056/NEJMoa1414221
55. Seo S, Mullins RF, Dumitrescu AV, Bhattarai S, Gratie D, Wang K, et al. Subretinal gene therapy of mice with Bardet-Biedl syndrome type 1. *Invest Ophthalmol Vis Sci* (2013) 54(9):6118–32. doi:10.1167/iovs.13-11673
56. Oren YS, Pranke IM, Kerem B, Sermet-Gaudelus I. The suppression of premature termination codons and the repair of splicing mutations in CFTR. *Curr Opin Pharmacol* (2017) 34:125–31. doi:10.1016/j.coph.2017.09.017
57. Lee HL, Dougherty JP. Pharmaceutical therapies to recode nonsense mutations in inherited diseases. *Pharmacol Ther* (2012) 136(2):227–66. doi:10.1016/j.pharmthera.2012.07.007

58. Richardson R, Smart M, Tracey-White D, Webster AR, Moosajee M. Mechanism and evidence of nonsense suppression therapy for genetic eye disorders. *Exp Eye Res* (2017) 155:24–37. doi:10.1016/j.exer.2017.01.001
59. Mutyam V, Du M, Xue X, Keeling KM, White EL, Bostwick JR, et al. Discovery of clinically approved agents that promote suppression of cystic fibrosis transmembrane conductance regulator nonsense mutations. *Am J Respir Crit Care Med* (2016) 194(9):1092–103. doi:10.1164/rccm.201601-0154OC
60. Mutyam V, Libby EF, Peng N, Hadjiliadis D, Bonk M, Solomon GM, et al. Therapeutic benefit observed with the CFTR potentiator, ivacaftor, in a CF patient homozygous for the W1282X CFTR nonsense mutation. *J Cyst Fibros* (2017) 16(1):24–9. doi:10.1016/j.jcf.2016.09.005
61. Xue X, Mutyam V, Thakerar A, Mobley J, Bridges RJ, Rowe SM, et al. Identification of the amino acids inserted during suppression of CFTR nonsense mutations and determination of their functional consequences. *Hum Mol Genet* (2017) 26(16):3116–29. doi:10.1093/hmg/ddx196
62. Finkel RS, Flanigan KM, Wong B, Bonnemann C, Sampson J, Sweeney HL, et al. Phase 2a study of ataluren-mediated dystrophin production in patients with nonsense mutation Duchenne muscular dystrophy. *PLoS One* (2013) 8(12):e81302. doi:10.1371/journal.pone.0081302
63. Reinig AM, Mirzaei S, Berlau DJ. Advances in the treatment of Duchenne muscular dystrophy: new and emerging pharmacotherapies. *Pharmacotherapy* (2017) 37(4):492–9. doi:10.1002/phar.1909
64. Bukowy-Bieryllo Z, Dabrowski M, Witt M, Zietkiewicz E. Aminoglycoside-stimulated readthrough of premature termination codons in selected genes involved in primary ciliary dyskinesia. *RNA Biol* (2016) 13(10):1041–50. doi:10.1080/15476286.2016.1219832
65. Goldmann T, Overlack N, Wolfrum U, Nagel-Wolfrum K. PTC124-mediated translational readthrough of a nonsense mutation causing Usher syndrome type 1C. *Hum Gene Ther* (2011) 22(5):537–47. doi:10.1089/hum.2010.067
66. Schwarz N, Carr AJ, Lane A, Moeller F, Chen LL, Aguila M, et al. Translational read-through of the RP2 Arg120stop mutation in patient iPSC-derived retinal pigment epithelium cells. *Hum Mol Genet* (2015) 24(4):972–86. doi:10.1093/hmg/ddu509
67. Garanto A, Chung DC, Duijkers L, Corral-Serrano JC, Messchaert M, Xiao R, et al. In vitro and in vivo rescue of aberrant splicing in CEP290-associated LCA by antisense oligonucleotide delivery. *Hum Mol Genet* (2016) 25(12):2552–63. doi:10.1093/hmg/ddw118
68. Garanto A, Collin RWJ. Design and in vitro use of antisense oligonucleotides to correct pre-mRNA splicing defects in inherited retinal dystrophies. *Methods Mol Biol* (2018) 1715:61–78. doi:10.1007/978-1-4939-7522-8_5
69. Goemans NM, Tulinius M, van den Akker JT, Burm BE, Ekhart PF, Heuvelmans N, et al. Systemic administration of PRO051 in Duchenne's muscular dystrophy. *N Engl J Med* (2011) 364(16):1513–22. doi:10.1056/NEJMoa1011367
70. Miller TM, Pestronk A, David W, Rothstein J, Simpson E, Appel SH, et al. An antisense oligonucleotide against SOD1 delivered intrathecally for patients with SOD1 familial amyotrophic lateral sclerosis: a phase 1, randomised, first-in-man study. *Lancet Neurol* (2013) 12(5):435–42. doi:10.1016/s1474-4422(13)70061-9
71. Slijkerman RW, Vache C, Dona M, Garcia-Garcia G, Claustres M, Hetterschijt L, et al. Antisense oligonucleotide-based splice correction for USH2A-associated retinal degeneration caused by a frequent deep-intronic mutation. *Mol Ther Nucleic Acids* (2016) 5(10):e381. doi:10.1038/mtna.2016.89
72. Lux CT, Scharenberg AM. Therapeutic gene editing safety and specificity. *Hematol Oncol Clin North Am* (2017) 31(5):787–95. doi:10.1016/j.hoc.2017.05.002
73. Lai M, Pifferi M, Bush A, Piras M, Michelucci A, Di Cicco M, et al. Gene editing of DNAH11 restores normal cilia motility in primary ciliary dyskinesia. *J Med Genet* (2016) 53(4):242–9. doi:10.1136/jmedgenet-2015-103539
74. Wu W, Lu Z, Li F, Wang W, Qian N, Duan J, et al. Efficient in vivo gene editing using ribonucleoproteins in skin stem cells of recessive dystrophic epidermolysis bullosa mouse model. *Proc Natl Acad Sci U S A* (2017) 114(7):1660–5. doi:10.1073/pnas.1614775114
75. Ma H, Marti-Gutierrez N, Park SW, Wu J, Lee Y, Suzuki K, et al. Correction of a pathogenic gene mutation in human embryos. *Nature* (2017) 548(7668):413–9. doi:10.1038/nature23305
76. Reardon S. *First CRISPR Clinical Trial Gets Green Light from US Panel* (2017). Available from: https://www.nature.com/news/first-crispr-clinical-trial-gets-green-light-from-us-panel-1.20137
77. Huai C, Jia C, Sun R, Xu P, Min T, Wang Q, et al. CRISPR/Cas9-mediated somatic and germline gene correction to restore hemostasis in hemophilia B mice. *Hum Genet* (2017) 136(7):875–83. doi:10.1007/s00439-017-1801-z
78. Seo S, Guo DF, Bugge K, Morgan DA, Rahmouni K, Sheffield VC. Requirement of Bardet-Biedl syndrome proteins for leptin receptor signaling. *Hum Mol Genet* (2009) 18(7):1323–31. doi:10.1093/hmg/ddp031
79. Mason K, Page L, Balikcioglu PG. Screening for hormonal, monogenic, and syndromic disorders in obese infants and children. *Pediatr Ann* (2014) 43(9):e218–24. doi:10.3928/00904481-20140825-08
80. Rhythm Pharmaceuticals. *Rhythm Expands Phase 2 Clinical Trials of Setmelanotide to the Treatment of Bardet-Biedl Syndrome Obesity*. Boston, MA: Rhythm Pharmaceuticals (2017).
81. Tobin JL, Beales PL. Restoration of renal function in zebrafish models of ciliopathies. *Pediatr Nephrol* (2008) 23(11):2095–9. doi:10.1007/s00467-008-0898-7
82. Armstrong S. Data, data everywhere: the challenges of personalised medicine. *BMJ* (2017) 359:j4546. doi:10.1136/bmj.j4546
83. Weinshilboum RM, Wang L. Pharmacogenomics: precision medicine and drug response. *Mayo Clin Proc* (2017) 92(11):1711–22. doi:10.1016/j.mayocp.2017.09.001

14

Experimental Models to Study Podocyte Biology: Stock-Taking the Toolbox of Glomerular Research

*Henning Hagmann and Paul T. Brinkkoetter**

Department II of Internal Medicine, Center for Molecular Medicine Cologne, University of Cologne, Cologne, Germany

Correspondence:
Paul T. Brinkkoetter
paul.brinkkoetter@uk-koeln.de

Diseases affecting the glomeruli of the kidney, the renal filtration units, are a leading cause of chronic kidney disease and end-stage renal failure. Despite recent advances in the understanding of glomerular biology, treatment of these disorders has remained extraordinarily challenging in many cases. The use of experimental models has proven invaluable to study renal, and in particular, glomerular biology and disease. Over the past 15 years, studies identified different and very distinct pathogenic mechanisms that result in damage, loss of glomerular visceral epithelial cells (podocytes) and progressive renal disease. However, animal studies and, in particular, mouse studies are often protracted and cumbersome due to the long reproductive cycle and high keeping costs. Transgenic and heterologous expression models have been speeded-up by novel gene editing techniques, yet they still take months. In addition, given the complex cellular biology of the filtration barrier, certain questions may not be directly addressed using mouse models due to the limited accessibility of podocytes for analysis and imaging. In this review, we will describe alternative models to study podocyte biology experimentally. We specifically discuss current podocyte cell culture models, their role in experimental strategies to analyze pathophysiologic mechanisms as well as limitations with regard to transferability of results. We introduce current models in *Caenorhabditis elegans, Drosophila melanogaster*, and *Danio rerio* that allow for analysis of protein interactions, and principle signaling pathways in functional biological structures, and enable high-throughput transgenic expression or compound screens in multicellular organisms.

Keywords: model organism, kidney diseases, podocyte, mechanosensation, glomerular filtration barrier

INTRODUCTION

Chronic kidney disease (CKD) is becoming an increasingly prevalent condition affecting almost 10% of the population in Western societies. The majority of kidney diseases that progress to end stage renal failure start in the glomerulus, the renal filtration unit, as a consequence of a very limited capacity of glomeruli for regeneration and the limited ability of terminally differentiated glomerular podocytes for self-renewal (1). The glomerular filtration barrier consists of three anatomic layers: fenestrated endothelial cells, the glomerular basement membrane and podocytes, post-mitotic epithelial cells located at the outer aspect of the capillary loops (**Figure 1B**). These cells enwrap the glomerular capillaries with their primary and secondary processes and form the outer layer of the filtration apparatus. All three layers contribute substantially to the glomerular filtration barrier and can be affected in human disease. Due to their exposed anatomic localization podocytes are constantly challenged not only by oxygen radicals, cytokines, immune complexes and inflammatory processes but also by mechanical forces. Podocyte damage plays a pivotal role in most, if not all, glomerular diseases that result in glomerulosclerosis (2). As podocyte loss cannot easily be compensated by cell proliferation the cells undergo hypertrophy, autophagy, and/or dedifferentiation depending on the injurious insult (3). Podocyte hypertrophy and the increase in cellular size and the covered area of the GBM represent protective measures to ascertain proper glomerular function. In contrast, dedifferentiation is considered to be maladaptive resulting in albuminuria and persistent podocyte loss. It has to be stressed, that the onset of albuminuria and even nephrotic range proteinuria does not require podocyte depletion. Mere cytoskeletal rearrangements, i.e., foot process effacement, are sufficient to cause massive albuminuria as often seen in patients with minimal change disease (MCD). A condition which lacks evidence of pathology in light microscopy but presents with vast foot-process effacement in electron microscopy. In the event of progressive or severe glomerular disease podocyte loss is the clue and patients develop massive albuminuria in combination with irreversible scarring, i.e., glomerulosclerosis (1, 4–7). Importantly, albuminuria and chronic kidney disease are independently associated with an increased risk for end stage renal failure and cardiovascular disease (8–10).

The finding that independent pathways and pathogenic principles contribute to the identical glomerular phenotype described as focal segmental glomerulosclerosis (FSGS) seems trivial but is of major importance. Podocytes are firmly attached to the underlying glomerular basement membrane and form a unique cell-cell contact to foot processes of neighboring podocytes, a cell junction called slit diaphragm. This specialized cell-cell contact is not only an integral part of the glomerular filtration barrier but also serves as signaling hub to regulate podocyte function (11). Over the past several years, various constituents of the podocyte slit diaphragm cell junction have been identified leading to the concept that the proteins at the slit diaphragm regulate podocyte biology through active signaling. The slit diaphragm bridges the distance between two adjacent foot processes, thus allowing formation of a filtration slit. In severe podocyte damage, the slit diaphragm disappears and podocytes simplify structure and shape due to cytoskeletal alterations, a process called foot process effacement (8, 10). Until recently, the function of the glomerular filtration barrier and the pathogenesis of proteinuria have not been well understood. This has changed with the identification of gene defects in (rare) human genetic diseases known to cause congenital or childhood steroid-resistant nephrotic syndrome and progressive glomerulosclerosis [for review see (9)]. These studies identified distinct deregulated pathways that independently contribute to podocyte injury and, potentially, loss of podocytes. Podocyte depletion has long been known to be the culprit of glomerulosclerosis and progressive loss of renal function (12–14). As multiple different pathogenic mechanisms result in proteinuria and FSGS lesions in kidney biopsies, it is not surprising that several clinical trials including all FSGS patients failed to provide new MCD/FSGS treatment options, e.g. the NIH has spent multimillion dollars on clinical trials that did not yield a single new drug for MCD/FSGS patients (15).

The advent of modern genetics with the development of animal models with cell specific gene manipulation including gene deletions and transgenic gene expression together with systems biology has deepened our understanding of the biology and physiology of the renal filtration barrier in states of health and disease. Despite our tremendous advances in understanding glomerular function and the contribution of the specific anatomic compartments to the renal filtration barrier, essential questions remain to be addressed as treatment of glomerular disorders is still unspecific and primarily based on various immunosuppressive regimens, including glucocorticoids or blockade of the renin-angiotensin-aldosterone system (15).

In the past, the use of experimental models has proven invaluable to study renal, and in particular, glomerular biology and disease. Even after the introduction of novel gene editing techniques, mouse models are time consuming. The relatively long reproductive cycle, high keeping cost, and not least the regulatory standards make these models less flexible. In this review, we will describe alternative models to study podocyte biology experimentally.

PODOCYTE CELL CULTURE

Podocyte cell culture models were the first models to study podocyte biology and are still widely used (16, 17) as gene and protein expression as well as environmental cues can be easily manipulated *in vitro* for mechanistic analyses (18, 19). Multiple human, mouse, and rat podocyte cell lines have been generated in the past (16, 17, 20–22). Most groups rely on immortalized mouse or human podocyte cell lines which are cultured under proliferative (33°C) and growth-restrictive (37°C) conditions. These studies promoted our understanding of glomerular diseases (19) as well as the cytoskeletal regulation (23), cell cycle control (24), cell death mechanisms (25), signaling pathways (26, 27) as well as protein degradation (28).

However, certain limitations apply and have to be taken into account when translating experimental findings from cultured podocyte cell lines; podocytes in culture are cultivated on petri-dishes as a monolayer in the absence of mesangial and endothelial cells in close proximity. Podocytes in culture do not encounter mechanical stretch nor the flow of primary urine filtrate (29). Hence, it is not surprising that podocyte cell lines do not form secondary processes with slit diaphragms in-between neighboring cells and show only a very limited expression of specific marker proteins including nephrin (30), podocin (31), or transient receptor potential cation channel 6 (26, 32, 33).

In an attempt to further characterize these widely used work horses of podocyte research our group recently applied modern MS/MS technologies and created a comprehensive map at a depth of more than 7,000 proteins expressed in proliferating and differentiated cultured podocytes *in vitro* (26). To this end, we examined an immortalized mouse podocyte cell line kindly provided by S. Shankland (Seattle, WA) as well as a conditionally immortalized human podocyte cell line obtained from M. Saleem (Bristol, UK), both are widely used cell-culture models generated by either isolation of primary podocytes from the immortomouse (34) or by retroviral transfection of primary human podocytes with a temperature-sensitive SV40 large T-cell antigen (35) (**Table 1**). The temperature shift from 33 to 37°C induces in both cell lines a proteostatic shift. Undifferentiated podocytes express high abundance of proteasomal proteins while differentiated podocytes express high abundance of lysosomal proteins. Additional studies using pulsed stable isotope labeling by amino acids in cell culture (pSILAC) and protein degradation assays determined protein dynamics and half-lives and revealed a globally increased stability of proteins in differentiated podocytes. Mitochondrial, cytoskeletal and membrane proteins were particularly stabilized in differentiated podocytes. However, the expression levels of so-called podocyte marker genes or podocytopathy gene products varied significantly as compared to primary cells. Highest levels were detected for Actin-regulating proteins comprising Myosin-9 (MYH9) (36), rho GDP-dissociation inhibitor 1 (ARHGDIA) (37) and alpha-actinin-4 (ACTN4) (5). Out of 15 podocytopathy-associated genes linked to cytoskeletal function 8 were expressed in the cultured cells (MYH9, ARHGDIA, ACTN4, anillin (ANLN), inverted formin-2 (INF2), unconventional myosin IE (MYO1E), synaptopodin (SYNPO), and podocalyxin (PODXL) (22, 38–41). With respect to basement membrane proteins 4 out of 8 were quantified in undifferentiated and differentiated human podocytes [CD151 antigen (CD151), integrin alpha-3 (ITGA3), integrin beta-4 (ITGB4), and laminin subunit beta-2 (LAMB2) (20, 42, 43). In contrast, only one out of six slit diaphragm proteins (CD2-associated protein (CD2AP) (44) could be detected.

TABLE 1 | Expression profiles of podocyte-specific marker proteins known as determinants of cell specificity as suggested by Shankland et al. (26).

Protein name	Gene name	Cultured Human Podocyte Proteome (45)		Cultured Mouse Podocyte Proteome (26)	
		33°C	37°C	33°C	37°C
CYTOSKELETAL PROTEINS					
Myosin-2	MYH2; MYHSA2	–	–	–	–
Podocalyxin	POD+L	+	+	+	+
Synaptopodin	SYNPO	+	+	+	+
Alpha-actinin-4	ACTN4	+	+	+	+
BASEMENT MEMBRANE PROTEINS					
Integrin alpha-3	ITGA3	+	+	+	+
Integrin beta-1	ITGB1	+	+	+	+
Integrin-linked protein kinase	HEL-S-28; ILK	+	+	+	+
SLIT DIAPHRAGM PROTEINS					
CD2-associated protein	CD2AP	+	+	+	+
Nephrin	NPHS1	–	–	–	–
Cytoplasmic protein NCK1	NCK1	+	+	+	+
Cytoplasmic protein NCK2	NCK2	+	+	+	+
Podocin	NPHS2	–	–	–	–
Short transient receptor potential cation channel 6	TRPC6	–	–	–	–
MEMBRANE PROTEINS					
Type-2 angiotensin II receptor	AGTR2	–	–	–	–
T-lymphocyte activation antigen CD80 (Activation B7-1 antigen)	CD80	–	–	–	–
P-Cadherin	CDH3	–	–	–	–
OTHER					
Transcription factor 21 (podocyte-expressed 1)	TCF21 (POD1)	–	–	–	–
Transforming growth factor beta-1/2	TGFB1/2	+	+	+	+
Vascular endothelial growth factor A	VEGFA	–	–	–	–
Wilms tumor protein 1	WT1	–	–	–	–

Respective proteins are either marked as expressed ("+") or not expressed ("–") in the two examined cell culture conditions (33°C = undifferentiated, and 37°C = differentiated cells). According to Schroeter et al. (45).

MODEL ORGANISMS TO STUDY PODOCYTE BIOLOGY

Caenorhabditis elegans with its short life cycle, completely established cell lineage including a neuronal map (connectome), compact and fully mapped genome, uncomplicated genetic modification by feeding of RNAi-expressing *E. coli*, and cost-effective keeping is a prime model for cell biology (46). In addition and in contrast to other multicellular model organisms, (genetically modified) individuals can be easily frozen, stored for the longer term, and revived with immediate capability to reproduce.

These characteristics make the nematode an ideal model to study signaling pathways and functionality of proteins in a multicellular organism and represent an advantage as compared to mammalian models.

Principle signaling pathways like e.g., the insulin/mTOR signaling cascade are generally well-conserved across species (47). Along this line, the observation that the insulin/mTOR pathway is induced and refers damage in podocytes with mitochondrial dysfunction due to the loss of Prohibitin-2 (PHB-2) was substantiated in *C. elegans* using worm strains expressing fluorescence labeled DAF-16 (48). After heat-shock DAF-16 is pooled in the nuclear compartment. Redistribution of DAF-16 to the cytoplasm depends on the activity of the insulin pathway. Consistently with data from podocyte-specific PHB-2 knockout mice, *phb-2*-deficient worms showed accelerated recovery of the DAF-2 (insulin receptor) mediated cytosolic redistribution of DAF-16.

However—with regard to glomerular research—*C. elegans* does not contain a filtering excretory organ homolog to the mammalian glomerulum. Nevertheless, ortholog genes in analogs structures can be studied in the nematode to understand principle mechanisms of podocyte morphogenesis and podocyte slit-diaphragm function.

The mammalian slit diaphragm is composed of the transmembranous immunoglobulin family proteins nephrin and Neph1. Nephrin and Neph1 are lipid raft associated proteins that refer outside-in signals by tyrosin phosphorylation. Mutations in the nephrin encoding gene NPHS1 or lack of NEPH1 lead to defective assembly of the foot processes and loss of the slit diaphragm which becomes evident as (congenital) nephrotic syndrome (49, 50). The adhesion molecules nephrin and Neph1 are well conserved across species. In *C. elegans* orthologs of Neph1 and Nephrin are SYG-1 and SYG-2, respectively. SYG-1 and SYG-2 refer cell-cell recognition in synapse development between the hermaphrodite specific neuron (HSN) and specialized epithelial guidepost cells adjacent to the nematode's vulva muscle cells medially in the hermaphrodites' soma. The two HSN (HSNL and HSNR) localize to the lateral aspects in the middle of the nematode and protrude their axonal processes ventrally, where they innervate the vulvar muscle cells and provide the neuronal circuit required for egg laying. Interaction of SYG-1 on the HSN axon with SYG-2 expressed on guidepost cells initiates intracellular signaling processes in HSN to trigger synapse formation and maintenance (51, 52). Mutations in either *syg-1* or *syg-2* fail to exhibit functional synapses due to aberrant placement of presynaptic sites (53, 54). Interestingly, heterologous expression of mammalian nephrin or Neph 1, −2 or −3 can rescue phenotypes of mutant *syg-1* or *syg-2* (55, 56). The cytoplasmic tail of SYG-2 is required for subcellular trafficking of SYG-2 itself, whereas the cytoplasmic domain of SYG-1 is required for synapse formation but dispensable in later stages (57). Although elegant ultrastructural analyses in mammalian and avian glomeruli have challenged the concept of heterophilic nephrin and Neph1 interaction at the slit diaphragm, synapse formation at the HSN in *C. elegans* may represent a suitable model to study signaling mechanisms at the cytoplasmic domains of nephrin and Neph1 by visualization of synaptic vesicles in SNB-1::YFP transgenic worms.

Another example for the utility of *C. elegans* in glomerular research is based on the homology of mammalian podocin and *C. elegans* MEC-2. Podocin is an essential constituent of the mammalian slit diaphragm complex, whereas MEC-2 is part of the mechanosensory complex of *C. elegans* sensing gentle touch. Both stomatin-like proteins share a central stretch of hydrophobic amino acids which refers membrane association while the amino and the carboxy terminal ends face the cytoplasm. The highly conserved PHB domain mediates homophilic interactions and lipid binding via palmitoylation, creating the microenvironment that regulates signaling via the associated ion channel proteins TRPC6 in mammals and the DEG/ENaC channel MEC-4/MEC-10 in *C. elegans* (58–60). This regulatory role of MEC-2 can not only be assessed by quantification of mechanoreceptor channel currents but also in functional *in vivo* assays measuring sensitivity to gentle touch in adult hermaphrodites (61). In addition, regular localization of MEC-2 and other components of the mechanosensory complex in a characteristic punctate pattern on the six mechanosensory neurons of *C. elegans* can be evaluated by staining with MEC-2 specific antibodies or employing MEC-4::YFP transgenic worms (28, 62). Identifying co-localization of the primarily mitochondrial protein Prohibitin 2 (PHB-2) and MEC-4 in mechanosensory punctae of touch receptor neurons in *C. elegans* as well as partial loss of touch sensitivity in PHB-2 knock down worms helped to establish the role of PHB-2 as a slit-diaphragm protein (63). In a recent paper, the ubiquitin ligase Ubr4 has been shown to control podocin protein stability and conservation of this molecular mechanism could be confirmed for MEC-2 in *C. elegans* assays, where the loss of the Ubr4 ortholog C44E4.1 (ubr-4) resulted in a more dispersed staining pattern of MEC-2 positive punctae (28).

With regard to glomerular research, studying *C. elegans* is instrumental as a functional read out for protein interactions, trafficking and protein turnover as well as signaling of conserved pathways in a multicellular organism. This holds true especially for mammalian podocin, nephrin, Neph 1, and their orthologs. A weakness of the nematode as a model of conserved principles in mammalian (patho-)physiology as well as for compound screens is the lack of organs homolog to heart, liver, central nervous systems, and of course filtering organs like the kidney.

Drosophila melanogaster evolved as another high-capacity model organism for glomerular research. Cell type specific gene inactivation and editing make the fly a versatile, adaptable, and expedite model. The reproductive cycle is around 12 days.

Similar to the nematode the Drosophila model allows to study protein interactions in functional biologic structures. In the fly adhesion molecules ortholog to mammalian nephrin and Neph proteins called sticks'n stones/hibris (sns/hbs) and kirre/dumbfounded (duf) are involved in cell-cell recognition, and cellular signaling events to control adhesion, cell shaping, and programmed cell death during eye development in the fly. During embryonal development Drosophila's facet eyes develop from a single layered epithelium and remain undifferentiated during almost the entirety of larval stages. In the final differentiation steps heterophilic interactions of sns/hbs and duf determine cell fate specification and are required for patterning and separation of ommatidea (64, 65).

During the last decade, research explored *Drosophila* nephrocytes as a novel tool of cell biology. The term was initially coined by Bruntz and Kowalsky, who discovered ammonia carmin absorbing cells around the heart, the digestive organs, and the nervous system in arthropods (66, 67). Nephrocytes are specialized filtrating cells with high endocytic activity, that may have detoxifying and sequestration function. In the adult fly there are two populations of nephrocytes. The Garland nephrocytes, which are assembled along the esophagus, and the pericardial nephrocytes, which palisade the heart tube. Nephrocytes are large cells with a surface laced by invaginations, so called labyrinthine channels, and covered by a continuous basement membrane. Near the apical surface the invaginations are abridged by a slit diaphragm (**Figure 1A**). Loss of the nephrin ortholog *sns* or the Neph ortholog *duf* results in loss of slit diaphragm structures, smaller lacunae and thickening of the basement membrane (68). Filtration across the pericardial nephrocyte slit diaphragm is limited to substances smaller than 70 kDa (69). Molecules that get filtered into the labyrinthine channels are taken up by the nephrocyte via endocytosis (70). In this regard the nephrocyte differs significantly from mammalian podocytes as to our current understanding. Filtration across the nephrocyte slit diaphragm as well as endocytosis can be assessed in assays on explanted nephrocytes employing different tracers, like e.g., GFP-, labeled albumin, horseradish peroxidase or dextrans of variable sizes (68, 69, 71, 72).

A novel transgenic fly model expressing secreted atrial natriuretic factor labeled with red fluorescent protein (ANF-RFP) from muscle cells and nephrocyte-specific green fluorescent protein (GFP) combined with the option of nephrocyte specific gene manipulation via a nephyrocyte specific Dot-Gal4 driver has implemented an expedite and reliable screening tool for genes associated with human disease (69). This model was employed to screen Drosophila orthologs of human monogenic nephrotic disease. Reassuringly, most of the pathogenic alterations were conserved in the fly (71, 73). Loss of Coq2 or Rab GTPases e.g., leads to loss of labyrinthine channels and loss of function in nephrocytes (71, 74).

In addition, rescue and overexpression studies with human orthologs are possible in Drosophila knockout models. Both eye and nephrocyte development were evaluated to identify a conserved amino acid motif in mammalian Neph1 to functionally replace Drosophila *duf*, whereas neither Neph2 nor Neph3 showed similar effects (75).

In general, the fly is an ideal model organism for high-throughput transgenic screens and rescue experiments, when variants of ortholog human genes are expressed in the respective drosophila knock out. The *in vivo* filtration assay or eye pattern formation serve as reliable and expedite readouts.

Danio rerio, the zebrafish, provides a third model organism of glomerular filtration. In striking contrast to the non-vertebrate *Drosophila* and *C. elegans models*, the zebrafish forms vascularized glomeruli in the pronephrons and the mesonephros during development with the mesonephros maintained in adult life. At the pronephros-stage the zebrafish kidney consists of two fused glomeruli with connection to the aorta draining primary urine into the pronephric tubuli followed by the pronephric ducts (76). The pronephros glomeruli already contain fenestrated endothelium, mesangial cells and podocytes that form a functional slit diaphragm (77). In addition, genome conservation of 70% between human and *Danio rerio* as well as versatile morphlino techniques, CRSPR/Cas-based gene editing and cross-species rescue models make the fish a primary model to study glomerular disease. Loss of zebrafish nephrin and podocin, which are specifically expressed in pronephric podocytes, leads to the loss of slit-diaphragms early in development (78). As in human nephrotic syndrome, pericardial edema, periocular edema, and general edema develops. Likewise disruption of zNeph1 or zNeph2 showed similar phenotypes (55). Besides structural analyses functional assays of glomerular filtration have emerged. Early on, the integrity of the filtration barrier was monitored qualitatively on fixed tissue after injections of large molecular weight dextran, which was detected in tubular epithelial cells in case of disruption of the glomerular filter (78). By now, several assays to quantify glomerular filtration have been established. Amongst these are *in vivo* fluorescence measurement in the eye or in large vessels in time-laps experiments after injection of fluorescence-labeled 10-, 70-, and/or 500-kDa dextrans (79). Another approach employs transgenic fish expressing eGFP-labeled vitamin D-binding protein (eGFPDBP) of a molecular weight of 78 kDa in the liver, which is repelled from glomerular filtration in healthy fish but leaks into urine in states of glomerular damage and can be quantified in the eye (accumulation in control) and—as excreted protein—in the water surrounding the fish (80).

ORGANOIDS

Generation of kidney organoids by differentiation of pluripotent stem cells (IPS cells) or re-aggregation of single cell suspensions of embryonic kidney cells in culture provided an important new tool for the study of kidney development and disease (81, 82).

However, the delicate morphology of the glomerular filter as well as the need for specific cellular interactions

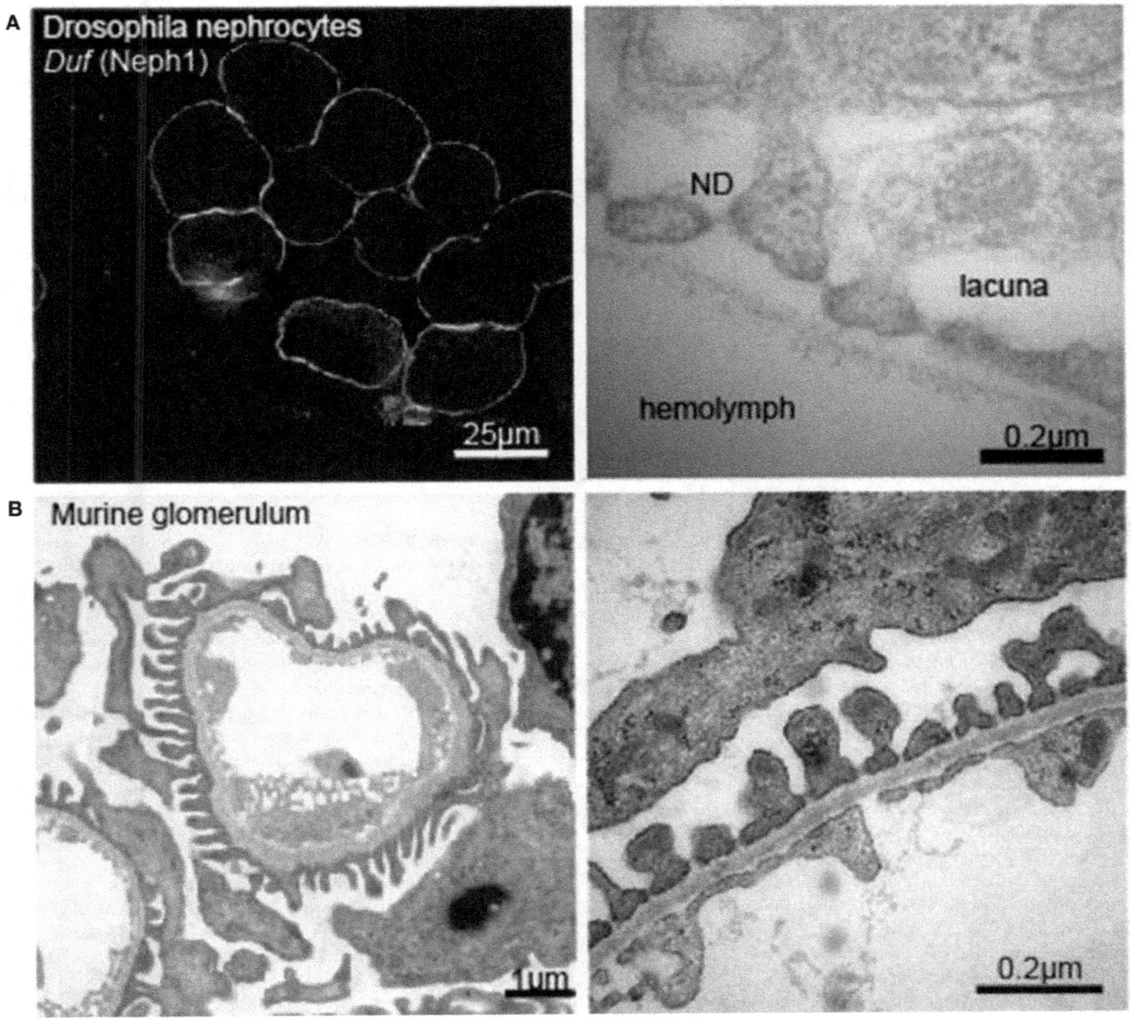

FIGURE 1 | (A) Immunofluorescence image of *Drosophila* nephrocytes stained with *Duf*(Neph1)-specific antibody (left tile) and electronmicrograph of the nephrocyte apical membrane showing lacunae, slit diaphragm and basement membrane (right tile). **(B)** Electron micrograph of a murine glomerular capillary (left tile) and higher magnification of the filtration barrier consisting of glomerular endothelium, basement membrane and podocyte foot processes (right tile).

and vascularization has hampered the study of glomerular biology on kidney organoids. In addition, recent single cell transcriptomic analysis of organoids has identified incomplete differentiation of all kidney organoid cell types, including podocyte progenitors (83).

In an elegant study, researchers generated organoids mixing murine embryonic kidney cells and implanted these organoids into nephrectomized athymic rats. They describe differentiation of morphologically and functionally intact glomeruli (84). In addition, the authors were able to integrate human amniotic fluid stem cells into chimeric organoids by mixing murine embryonic kidney cells and human amniotic fluid stem cells before *in vitro* organoid culture. Interestingly, also human amniotic fluid stem cells generated functional podocytes. Similar results were recently confirmed for human pluripotent stem cell derived organoids transplanted under the renal capsule of immunocompromised mice (85).

In conclusion, organoids will become a very important tool also in glomerular research. Again the complexity of glomerular structure and interaction of glomerular cell types is the major challenge to overcome.

CONCLUSION

Research of the last two decades has boosted our understanding of podocyte cell biology and genetics and provides growing understanding of the composition of the renal filtration barrier and cellular interactions needed to maintain its function. Experimental work in podocyte cell culture models informed on expression, trafficking, interaction and turnover of essential proteins of podocyte function. However, cell culture studies in podocytes are limited due to the fact that podocytes in culture lose their characteristic features. Cultured podocytes lack the intricate foot process morphology, cell polarity is incompletely preserved, and most importantly, intercellular contacts are neither structurally nor functionally close to the slit-diaphragm found *in vivo*. It is very clear that *in vivo* models are needed to understand glomerular physiology and to address podocyte diseases experimentally. Besides indispensable rodent models, model organisms like *C. elegans*, *Drosophila melanogaster*, and the zebrafish have entered the stage of glomerular research and allow unparalleled functional analyses of inter-cellular interactions and morphogenesis, signaling mechanisms, cell polarity, and filtration *in vivo*. Kidney organoids may become an additional important tool in the future.

AUTHOR CONTRIBUTIONS

All authors listed have made a substantial, direct and intellectual contribution to the work, and approved it for publication.

FUNDING

PB received grant support by the German Research Foundation (BR2955/6-1, KFO329 BR2955/8-1). HH was supported by the EKFS HH (2016-A62). HH and PB also received intramural funds from the Köln Fortune Program, University of Cologne.

ACKNOWLEDGMENTS

The authors thank S. Koehler for providing Drosophila images.

REFERENCES

1. Wanner N, Hartleben B, Herbach N, Goedel M, Stickel N, Zeiser R, et al. Unraveling the role of podocyte turnover in glomerular aging and injury. *J Am Soc Nephrol.* (2014) 25:707–16. doi: 10.1681/ASN.2013050452
2. Brinkkoetter PT, Ising C, Benzing T. The role of the podocyte in albumin filtration. *Nat Rev Nephrol.* (2013) 9:328–36. doi: 10.1038/nrneph.2013.78
3. Scott RP, Quaggin SE. Review series: the cell biology of renal filtration. *J Cell Biol.* (2015) 209:199–210. doi: 10.1083/jcb.201410017
4. Hodgin JB, Bitzer M, Wickman L, Afshinnia F, Wang SQ, O'Connor C, et al. Glomerular aging and focal global glomerulosclerosis: a podometric perspective. *J Am Soc Nephrol.* (2015) 26:3162–78. doi: 10.1681/ASN.2014080752
5. Kaplan JM, Kim SH, North KN, Rennke H, Correia LA, Tong HQ, et al. Mutations in ACTN4, encoding alpha-actinin-4, cause familial focal segmental glomerulosclerosis. *Nat Genet.* (2000) 24:251–6. doi: 10.1038/73456
6. Shi S, Yu L, Chiu C, Sun Y, Chen J, Khitrov G, et al. Podocyte-selective deletion of dicer induces proteinuria and glomerulosclerosis. *J Am Soc Nephrol.* (2008) 19:2159–69. doi: 10.1681/ASN.2008030312
7. Büscher AK, Beck BB, Melk A, Hoefele J, Kranz B, Bamborschke D, et al. Rapid response to Cyclosporin A and favorable renal outcome in nongenetic versus genetic steroid-resistant nephrotic syndrome. *Clin J Am Soc Nephrol.* (2016) 11:245–53. doi: 10.2215/CJN.07370715
8. Mundel P, Shankland SJ. Podocyte biology and response to injury. *J Am Soc Nephrol.* (2002) 13:3005–15. doi: 10.1097/01.ASN.0000039661.06947.FD
9. Pollak MR. Familial FSGS. *Adv Chronic Kidney Dis.* (2014) 21:422–5. doi: 10.1053/j.ackd.2014.06.001
10. Shankland SJ. The podocyte's response to injury: role in proteinuria and glomerulosclerosis. *Kidney Int.* (2006) 69:2131–47. doi: 10.1038/sj.ki.5000410
11. Benzing T. Signaling at the slit diaphragm. *J Am Soc Nephrol.* (2004) 15:1382–91. doi: 10.1097/01.ASN.0000130167.30769.55
12. Diamond JR, Karnovsky MJ. Focal and segmental glomerulosclerosis following a single intravenous dose of puromycin aminonucleoside. *Am J Pathol.* (1986) 122:481–7.
13. Kim YH, Goyal M, Kurnit D, Wharram B, Wiggins J, Holzman L, et al. Podocyte depletion and glomerulosclerosis have a direct relationship in the PAN-treated rat. *Kidney Int.* (2001) 60:957–68. doi: 10.1046/j.1523-1755.2001.060003957.x
14. Kriz W, Elger M, Nagata M, Kretzler M, Uiker S, Koeppen-Hageman I, et al. The role of podocytes in the development of glomerular sclerosis. *Kidney Int Suppl.* (1994) 45:S64–72.
15. Hogan J, Mohan P, Appel GB. Diagnostic tests and treatment options in glomerular disease: 2014 update. *Am J Kidney Dis.* (2014) 63:656–66. doi: 10.1053/j.ajkd.2013.09.019
16. Ni L, Saleem M, Mathieson PW. Podocyte culture: tricks of the trade. *Nephrology* (2012) 17:525–31. doi: 10.1111/j.1440–1797.2012.01619.x
17. Shankland SJ, Pippin JW, Reiser J, Mundel P. Podocytes in culture: past, present, and future. *Kidney Int.* (2007) 72:26–36. doi: 10.1038/sj.ki.5002291
18. Pereira EM, Labilloy A, Eshbach ML, Roy A, Subramanya AR, Monte S, et al. Characterization and phosphoproteomic analysis of a human immortalized podocyte model of Fabry disease generated using CRISPR/Cas9 technology. *Am J Physiol Renal Physiol.* (2016) 311:F1015–24. doi: 10.1152/ajprenal.00283.2016
19. Rinschen MM, Grahammer F, Hoppe A-K, Kohli P, Hagmann H, Kretz O, et al. YAP-mediated mechanotransduction determines the podocyte's response to damage. *Sci Signal.* (2017) 10:eaaf8165. doi: 10.1126/scisignal.aaf8165
20. Kambham N, Tanji N, Seigle RL, Markowitz GS, Pulkkinen L, Uitto J, et al. Congenital focal segmental glomerulosclerosis associated with beta4 integrin mutation and epidermolysis bullosa. *Am J Kidney Dis.* (2000) 36:190–6. doi: 10.1053/ajkd.2000.8293
21. Kohli P, Bartram MP, Habbig S, Pahmeyer C, Lamkemeyer T, Benzing T, et al. Label-free quantitative proteomic analysis of the YAP/TAZ interactome. *Am J Physiol Cell Physiol.* (2014) 306:C805–8. doi: 10.1152/ajpcell.00339.2013
22. Mele C, Iatropoulos P, Donadelli R, Calabria A, Maranta R, Cassis P, et al. MYO1E mutations and childhood familial focal segmental glomerulosclerosis. *N Engl J Med.* (2011) 365:295–306. doi: 10.1056/NEJMoa1101273
23. Jeruschke S, Jeruschke K, DiStasio A, Karaterzi S, Büscher AK, Nalbant P, et al. Everolimus stabilizes podocyte microtubules via enhancing TUBB2B and DCDC2 expression. *PLoS ONE* (2015) 10:e0137043. doi: 10.1371/journal.pone.0137043
24. Yang S, Liu L, Xu P, Yang Z. MKL1 inhibits cell cycle progression through p21 in podocytes. *BMC Mol Biol.* (2015) 16:1. doi: 10.1186/s12867-015-0029-5
25. Saurus P, Kuusela S, Dumont V, Lehtonen E, Fogarty CL, Lassenius MI, et al. Cyclin-dependent kinase 2 protects podocytes from apoptosis. *Sci Rep.* (2016) 6:21664. doi: 10.1038/srep21664
26. Rinschen MM, Schroeter CB, Koehler S, Ising C, Schermer B, Kann M, et al. Quantitative deep mapping of the cultured podocyte proteome uncovers shifts in proteostatic mechanisms during differentiation. *Am J Physiol Cell Physiol.* (2016) 311:C404–417. doi: 10.1152/ajpcell.00121.2016
27. Welsh GI, Hale LJ, Eremina V, Jeansson M, Maezawa Y, Lennon R, et al. Insulin signaling to the glomerular podocyte is critical for normal kidney function. *Cell Metab.* (2010) 12:329–40. doi: 10.1016/j.cmet.2010.08.015
28. Rinschen MM, Bharill P, Wu X, Kohli P, Reinert MJ, Kretz O, et al. The ubiquitin ligase Ubr4 controls stability of podocin/MEC-2 supercomplexes. *Hum Mol Genet.* (2016) 25:1328–44. doi: 10.1093/hmg/ddw016
29. Endlich K, Kliewe F, Endlich N. Stressed podocytes-mechanical forces, sensors, signaling and response. *Pflugers Arch.* (2017) 469:937–49. doi: 10.1007/s00424-017-2025-8
30. Garg P, Verma R, Nihalani D, Johnstone DB, Holzman LB. Neph1 cooperates with nephrin to transduce a signal that induces actin polymerization. *Mol Cell Biol.* (2007) 27:8698–712. doi: 10.1128/MCB.00948-07

31. Huber TB, Simons M, Hartleben B, Sernetz L, Schmidts M, Gundlach E, et al. Molecular basis of the functional podocin-nephrin complex: mutations in the NPHS2 gene disrupt nephrin targeting to lipid raft microdomains. *Hum Mol Genet.* (2003) 12:3397–405. doi: 10.1093/hmg/ddg360
32. Takano Y, Yamauchi K, Hiramatsu N, Kasai A, Hayakawa K, Yokouchi M, et al. Recovery and maintenance of nephrin expression in cultured podocytes and identification of HGF as a repressor of nephrin. *Am J Physiol Renal Physiol.* (2007) 292:F1573–82. doi: 10.1152/ajprenal.00423.2006
33. Reiser J, Polu KR, Möller CC, Kenlan P, Altintas MM, Wei C, et al. TRPC6 is a glomerular slit diaphragm-associated channel required for normal renal function. *Nat Genet.* (2005) 37:739–44. doi: 10.1038/ng1592
34. Griffin SV. Cyclin I protects podocytes from apoptosis. *J Biol Chem.* (2006) 281:28048–57. doi: 10.1074/jbc.M513336200
35. Saleem MA, O'Hare MJ, Reiser J, Coward RJ, Inward CD, Farren T, et al. A conditionally immortalized human podocyte cell line demonstrating nephrin and podocin expression. *J Am Soc Nephrol.* (2002) 13:630–8.
36. Kopp JB, Smith MW, Nelson GW, Johnson RC, Freedman BI, Bowden DW, et al. MYH9 is a major-effect risk gene for focal segmental glomerulosclerosis. *Nat Genet.* (2008) 40:1175–84. doi: 10.1038/ng.226
37. Gupta IR, Baldwin C, Auguste D, Ha KCH, El Andalousi J, Fahiminiya S, et al. ARHGDIA: a novel gene implicated in nephrotic syndrome. *J Med Genet.* (2013) 50:330–8. doi: 10.1136/jmedgenet-2012-101442
38. Barua M, Shieh E, Schlondorff J, Genovese G, Kaplan BS, Pollak MR. Exome sequencing and *in vitro* studies identified podocalyxin as a candidate gene for focal and segmental glomerulosclerosis. *Kidney Int.* (2014) 85:124–33. doi: 10.1038/ki.2013.354
39. Brown EJ, Schlöndorff JS, Becker DJ, Tsukaguchi H, Tonna SJ, Uscinski AL, et al. Mutations in the formin gene INF2 cause focal segmental glomerulosclerosis. *Nat Genet.* (2010) 42:72–6. doi: 10.1038/ng.505
40. Gbadegesin RA, Hall G, Adeyemo A, Hanke N, Tossidou I, Burchette J, et al. Mutations in the gene that encodes the F-actin binding protein anillin cause FSGS. *J Am Soc Nephrol.* (2014) 25:1991–2002. doi: 10.1681/ASN.2013090976
41. Tang VW, Brieher WM. FSGS3/CD2AP is a barbed-end capping protein that stabilizes actin and strengthens adherens junctions. *J Cell Biol.* (2013) 203:815–33. doi: 10.1083/jcb.201304143
42. Karamatic Crew V, Burton N, Kagan A, Green CA, Levene C, Flinter F, et al. CD151, the first member of the tetraspanin (TM4) superfamily detected on erythrocytes, is essential for the correct assembly of human basement membranes in kidney and skin. *Blood* (2004) 104:2217–23. doi: 10.1182/blood-2004-04-1512
43. Matejas V, Hinkes B, Alkandari F, Al-Gazali L, Annexstad E, Aytac MB, et al. Mutations in the human laminin beta2 (LAMB2) gene and the associated phenotypic spectrum. *Hum Mutat.* (2010) 31:992–1002. doi: 10.1002/humu.21304
44. Kim JM, Wu H, Green G, Winkler CA, Kopp JB, Miner JH, et al. CD2-associated protein haploinsufficiency is linked to glomerular disease susceptibility. *Science* (2003) 300:1298–300. doi: 10.1126/science.1081068
45. Schroeter C, Benzing T, Rinschen MM, Brinkkoetter P. *Deep Mapping of the Podocyte Proteome Unravels Altered Protein Dynamics During Differentiation.* New Orleans, LA: ASN Kidney Week (2017).
46. Brenner S. The genetics of caenorhabditis elegans. *Genetics* (1974) 77:71–94.
47. Papatheodorou I, Petrovs R, Thornton JM. Comparison of the mammalian insulin signalling pathway to invertebrates in the context of FOXO-mediated ageing. *Bioinformatics* (2014) 30:2999–3003. doi: 10.1093/bioinformatics/btu493
48. Ising C, Koehler S, Brähler S, Merkwirth C, Höhne M, Baris OR, et al. Inhibition of insulin/IGF-1 receptor signaling protects from mitochondria-mediated kidney failure. *EMBO Mol Med.* (2015) 7:275–87. doi: 10.15252/emmm.201404916
49. Kestilä M, Lenkkeri U, Männikkö M, Lamerdin J, McCready P, Putaala H, et al. Positionally cloned gene for a novel glomerular protein—nephrin—is mutated in congenital nephrotic syndrome. *Mol Cell* (1998) 1:575–82. doi: 10.1016/S1097-2765(00)80057-X
50. Donoviel DB, Freed DD, Vogel H, Potter DG, Hawkins E, Barrish JP, et al. Proteinuria and perinatal lethality in mice lacking NEPH1, a novel protein with homology to NEPHRIN. *Mol Cell Biol.* (2001) 21:4829–36. doi: 10.1128/MCB.21.14.4829-4836.2001
51. Ding M, Chao D, Wang G, Shen K. Spatial regulation of an E3 ubiquitin ligase directs selective synapse elimination. *Science* (2007) 317:947–51. doi: 10.1126/science.1145727
52. Patel MR, Lehrman EK, Poon VY, Crump JG, Zhen M, Bargmann CI, et al. Hierarchical assembly of presynaptic components in defined *C. elegans* synapses. *Nat Neurosci.* (2006) 9:1488–98. doi: 10.1038/nn1806
53. Shen K, Fetter RD, Bargmann CI. Synaptic specificity is generated by the synaptic guidepost protein SYG-2 and its receptor, SYG-1. *Cell* (2004) 116:869–81. doi: 10.1016/S0092-8674(04)00251-X
54. Shen K, Bargmann CI. The immunoglobulin superfamily protein SYG-1 determines the location of specific synapses in *C. elegans*. Cell (2003) 112:619–30. doi: 10.1016/S0092-8674(03)00113-2
55. Neumann-Haefelin E, Kramer-Zucker A, Slanchev K, Hartleben B, Noutsou F, Martin K, et al. A model organism approach: defining the role of Neph proteins as regulators of neuron and kidney morphogenesis. *Hum Mol Genet.* (2010) 19:2347–59. doi: 10.1093/hmg/ddq108
56. Wanner N, Noutsou F, Baumeister R, Walz G, Huber TB, Neumann-Haefelin E. Functional and spatial analysis of C. elegans SYG-1 and SYG-2, orthologs of the Neph/nephrin cell adhesion module directing selective synaptogenesis. *PLoS ONE* (2011) 6:e23598. doi: 10.1371/journal.pone.0023598
57. Chao DL, Shen K. Functional dissection of SYG-1 and SYG-2, cell adhesion molecules required for selective synaptogenesis in *C. elegans*. *Mol Cell Neurosci.* (2008) 39:248–57. doi: 10.1016/j.mcn.2008.07.001
58. Goodman MB, Ernstrom GG, Chelur DS, O'Hagan R, Yao CA, Chalfie M. MEC-2 regulates *C. elegans* DEG/ENaC channels needed for mechanosensation. *Nature* (2002) 415:1039–42. doi: 10.1038/4151039a
59. Huber TB, Schermer B, Müller RU, Höhne M, Bartram M, Calixto A, et al. Podocin and MEC-2 bind cholesterol to regulate the activity of associated ion channels. *Proc Natl Acad Sci USA.* (2006) 103:17079–86. doi: 10.1073/pnas.0607465103
60. Anderson M, Kim EY, Hagmann H, Benzing T, Dryer SE. Opposing effects of podocin on the gating of podocyte TRPC6 channels evoked by membrane stretch or diacylglycerol. *Am J Physiol Cell Physiol.* (2013) 305:C276–289. doi: 10.1152/ajpcell.00095.2013
61. O'Hagan R, Chalfie M, Goodman MB. The MEC-4 DEG/ENaC channel of *Caenorhabditis elegans* touch receptor neurons transduces mechanical signals. *Nat Neurosci.* (2005) 8:43–50. doi: 10.1038/nn1362
62. Zhang S, Arnadottir J, Keller C, Caldwell GA, Yao CA, Chalfie M. MEC-2 is recruited to the putative mechanosensory complex in *C. elegans* touch receptor neurons through its stomatin-like domain. *Curr Biol.* (2004) 14:1888–96. doi: 10.1016/j.cub.2004.10.030
63. Ising C, Bharill P, Brinkkoetter S, Brähler S, Schroeter C, Koehler S, et al. Prohibitin-2 depletion unravels extra-mitochondrial functions at the kidney filtration barrier. *Am J Pathol.* (2016) 186:1128–39. doi: 10.1016/j.ajpath.2015.12.018
64. Cagan R. *Chapter 5 Principles of Drosophila Eye Differentiation. Current Topics in Developmental Biology [Internet].* Elsevier (2009) [cited 2018 Feb 13]. p. 115–35. Available online http://linkinghub.elsevier.com/retrieve/pii/S0070215309890054
65. Bao S, Fischbach K-F, Corbin V, Cagan RL. Preferential adhesion maintains separation of ommatidia in the Drosophila eye. *Devel Biol.* (2010) 344:948–56. doi: 10.1016/j.ydbio.2010.06.013
66. Bruntz L. Contribution à l'étude de l'excrétion chez les Arthropodes. *Arch Biol.* (1903) 20:217–22.
67. Kowalevsky A. *Ein Beitrag zur Kenntnis der Exkretionsorgane.* Leipzig:Biologisches Zentralblatt. (1889) p. 9.
68. Weavers H, Prieto-Sánchez S, Grawe F, Garcia-López A, Artero R, Wilsch-Bräuninger M, et al. The insect nephrocyte is a podocyte-like cell with a filtration slit diaphragm. *Nature* (2009) 457:322–6. doi: 10.1038/nature07526
69. Zhang F, Zhao Y, Han Z. An *in vivo* functional analysis system for renal gene discovery in drosophila pericardial nephrocytes. *J Am Soc Nephrol.* (2013) 24:191–7. doi: 10.1681/ASN.2012080769
70. Kosaka T. Reversible blockage of membrane retrieval and endocytosis in the garland cell of the temperature-sensitive mutant of *Drosophila melanogaster*, shibirets1. *J Cell Biol.* (1983) 97:499–507. doi: 10.1083/jcb.97.2.499
71. Hermle T, Braun DA, Helmstädter M, Huber TB, Hildebrandt F. Modeling monogenic human nephrotic syndrome in the *Drosophila*

garland cell nephrocyte. *J Am Soc Nephrol.* (2017) 28:1521–33. doi: 10.1681/ASN.2016050517

72. Crossley AC. The ultrastructure and function of pericardial cells and other nephrocytes in an insect: *Calliphora erythrocephala*. *Tissue Cell.* (1972) 4:529–60. doi: 10.1016/S0040-8166(72)80029-6
73. Fu Y, Zhu J-Y, Richman A, Zhao Z, Zhang F, Ray PE, et al. A Drosophila model system to assess the function of human monogenic podocyte mutations that cause nephrotic syndrome. *Hum Mol Genet.* (2017) 26:768–80. doi: 10.1093/hmg/ddw428
74. Fu Y, Zhu J-Y, Zhang F, Richman A, Zhao Z, Han Z. Comprehensive functional analysis of Rab GTPases in Drosophila nephrocytes. *Cell Tissue Res.* (2017) 368:615–27. doi: 10.1007/s00441-017-2575-2
75. Helmstädter M, Lüthy K, Gödel M, Simons M, Ashish null, Nihalani D, et al. Functional study of mammalian Neph proteins in *Drosophila melanogaster*. *PLoS ONE* (2012) 7:e40300. doi: 10.1371/journal.pone.0040300
76. Wingert RA, Davidson AJ. The zebrafish pronephros: a model to study nephron segmentation. *Kidney Int.* (2008) 73:1120–7. doi: 10.1038/ki.2008.37
77. Ebarasi L, Oddsson A, Hultenby K, Betsholtz C, Tryggvason K. Zebrafish: a model system for the study of vertebrate renal development, function, and pathophysiology. *Curr Opin Nephrol Hypertens.* (2011) 20:416–24. doi: 10.1097/MNH.0b013e3283477797
78. Kramer-Zucker AG, Wiessner S, Jensen AM, Drummond IA. Organization of the pronephric filtration apparatus in zebrafish requires Nephrin, Podocin and the FERM domain protein Mosaic eyes. *Dev Biol.* (2005) 285:316–29. doi: 10.1016/j.ydbio.2005.06.038
79. Kotb AM, Müller T, Xie J, Anand-Apte B, Endlich K, Endlich N. Simultaneous assessment of glomerular filtration and barrier function in live zebrafish. *Am J Physiol Renal Physiol.* (2014) 307:F1427–34. doi: 10.1152/ajprenal.00029.2014
80. Hanke N, Staggs L, Schroder P, Litteral J, Fleig S, Kaufeld J, et al. "Zebrafishing" for novel genes relevant to the glomerular filtration barrier. *Biomed Res Int.* (2013) 2013:658270. doi: 10.1155/2013/658270
81. Takasato M, Er PX, Chiu HS, Maier B, Baillie GJ, Ferguson C, et al. Kidney organoids from human iPS cells contain multiple lineages and model human nephrogenesis. *Nature* (2015) 526:564–8. doi: 10.1038/nature15695
82. Morizane R, Lam AQ, Freedman BS, Kishi S, Valerius MT, Bonventre JV. Nephron organoids derived from human pluripotent stem cells model kidney development and injury. *Nat Biotechnol.* (2015) 33:1193–200. doi: 10.1038/nbt.3392
83. Wu H, Uchimura K, Donnelly E, Kirita Y, Morris SA, Humphreys BD. Comparative analysis of kidney organoid and adult human kidney single cell and single nucleus transcriptomes (2017). [cited 23 Apr 2018] Available from: http://biorxiv.org/lookup/doi/10.1101/232561
84. Xinaris C, Benedetti V, Novelli R, Abbate M, Rizzo P, Conti S, et al. Functional human podocytes generated in organoids from amniotic fluid stem cells. *J Am Soc Nephrol.* (2016) 27:1400–11. doi: 10.1681/ASN.2015030316
85. van den Berg CW, Ritsma L, Avramut MC, Wiersma LE, van den Berg BM, Leuning DG, et al. Renal subcapsular transplantation of PSC-derived kidney organoids induces neo-vasculogenesis and significant glomerular and tubular maturation *in vivo*. *Stem Cell Rep.* (2018) 10:751–65. doi: 10.1016/j.stemcr.2018.01.041

15

Update on Hereditary Kidney Stone Disease and Introduction of a New Clinical Patient Registry in Germany

Jan Halbritter[1]*, Anna Seidel[1], Luise Müller[1], Ria Schönauer[1] and Bernd Hoppe[2]

[1] Division of Nephrology, Department of Internal Medicine, University of Leipzig, Leipzig, Germany, [2] Division of Pediatric Nephrology, University Children's Hospital, Bonn, Germany

****Correspondence:***
Jan Halbritter
jan.halbritter@medizin.uni-leipzig.de

Kidney stone disease is an increasingly prevalent condition with remarkable clinical heterogeneity, with regards to stone composition, age of manifestation, rate of recurrence, and impairment of kidney function. Calcium-based kidney stones account for the vast majority of cases, but their etiology is poorly understood, notably their genetic drivers. As recent studies indicate, hereditary conditions are most likely underestimated in prevalence, and new disease genes are constantly being identified. As a consequence, there is an urgent need of a more efficient documentation and collection of cases with underlying hereditary conditions, to better understand shared phenotypic presentation and common molecular mechanisms. By implementation of a centralized patient registry on hereditary kidney stone disease in Germany, we aim to help closing the vast knowledge gap on genetics of kidney stone disease. In this context, clinical registries are indispensable for several reasons: first, delineating better phenotype–genotype associations will allow more precise patient stratification in future clinical research studies. Second, identifying new disease genes and new mechanisms will further reduce the rate of unknown nephrolithiasis/nephrocalcinosis etiology; and third, deciphering new molecular targets will pave the way to develop drugs for recurrence prevention in severely affected families.

Keywords: nephrolithiasis, hereditary, nephrocalcinosis, kidney stone disease, monogenic, registry

Incidence and prevalence of kidney stone disease continues to rise in the general population. With a lifetime prevalence of up to 10%, nephrolithiasis (NL) and nephrocalcinosis (NC) are therefore major health burdens, especially in the Western World (1). NL and NC are associated with significant morbidity and progression to chronic kidney disease due to recurrence, repetitive surgical/endoscopic intervention, and concomitant inflammation. On a simplified level, kidney stone formation results from an imbalance of urinary inhibitors (e.g., citrate, magnesium, uromoduline, and pyrophosphate) and promoters (e.g., oxalate, calcium, phosphate, urate, and cystine) of crystallization, exceeding supersaturation with consecutive aggregation, nucleation, and stone growth at Randall's plaque (**Figure 1**). This imbalance can be due to altered enteral and/or renal handling of either promotors or inhibitors, such as enteral malsecretion of oxalate or renal malreabsorption of calcium (**Figure 1**).

The underlying etiology of NL is thought to be multifactorial with an environmental, notable dietary, hormonal, and genetic component. In twin studies, the heritability of kidney stones has been estimated at 56% (3), and up to two-thirds of hypercalciuric stone formers have relatives with NL (4). Although calcium-containing kidney stones account for more than 80% of all, the genetic basis of such stones remains largely unknown (5). Except for variants in *CLDN14*, *TRPV5*, *SLC34A1*, *ALPL*, *CASR*, and *UMOD*, genome-wide association studies have yet to yield substantial genetic factors (6–8). However, risk alleles have been identified within genes that were also found to transmit

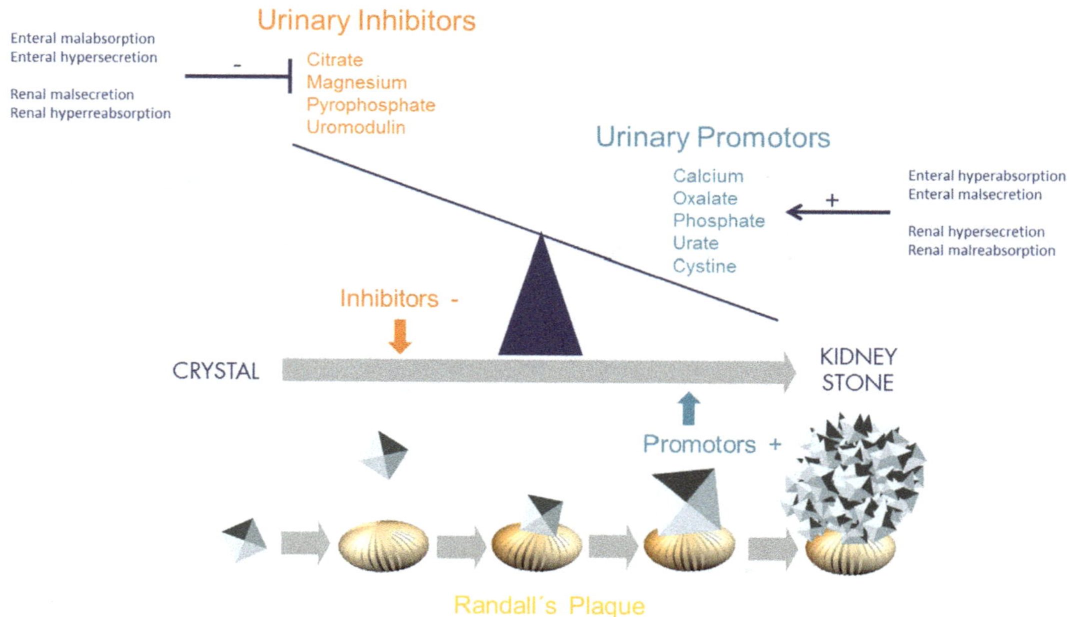

FIGURE 1 | Imbalance of urinary inhibitors and promotors of crystallization leading to kidney stone formation. Concentration of urinary inhibitors and promotors is influenced and controlled by both intestinal and renal transporters (GI–kidney axis). These transporters and exchangers, such as SLC26A1, are responsible for secretion and absorption. With regards to oxalate, enteral hyperabsorption but malsecretion, and/or renal hypersecretion but malabsorption leads to urinary oxalate levels exceeding supersaturation and thereby promoting crystallization and consecutive stone formation [adapted from Ref. (2)].

the disease on a Mendelian basis, such as *CASR*, *SLC34A1*, and *SLC2A9* (9, 10). To date, more than 30 single genes with an Online Mendelian Inheritance in Man-defined phenotype have been identified to be implicated in NL/NC, if mutated (**Table 1**).

Modes of inheritance in monogenic forms include autosomal-dominant, autosomal-recessive, and X-linked transmission. Interestingly, in several of these genes, both recessive and dominant modes of inheritance have been reported: *SLC7A9*, *SLC34A1*, *SLC34A3*, *SLC2A9*, *SLC22A12*, and *SLC4A1*. While most of the syndromic and severe congenital disorders exhibit a recessive inheritance pattern (Bartter, Lowe, Dent, FHHNC, and distal renal tubular acidosis with sensorineural deafness), milder conditions are rather associated with mutations in dominant genes. The majority of encoded proteins constitute renal solute transporters (e.g., SLC34A1, SLC34A3, and SLC9A3R1), but also chloride channels (CLCN5), tight-junction proteins (e.g., CLDN16/CLDN19), and metabolizing enzymes (e.g., AGXT, APRT, and CYP24A1) have been found defective in patients with NL/NC. Hence, the underlying defect is mostly located in the tubular system of the kidney itself and can therefore be attributed as tubulopathy. Conversely, *a priori* extrarenal conditions, as in primary hyperoxaluria (PH) where dysfunction of liver enzymes (AGXT, GRHPR, and HOGA1) cause oxalate accumulation with secondary renal affection, are conceivable causes of NL/NC. Although each disease phenotype is thought to represent a relatively rare entity, single-gene causes may account for a significant number of patients by their broad genetic heterogeneity (42). Apart from genetic heterogeneity, there is also an allelic variation, where truncating variants rather result in a loss of function and missense variants (hypomorphs) may cause rather subtle defects, which can be clinically overseen, especially in adult stone formers. Another recently appreciated phenomenon is about gene dosage effects in several of the aforementioned kidney stone genes. In *SLC34A3* for instance, encoding one of the main phosphate transporters in the proximal tubule (NaPiIIc), it was shown that heterozygous individuals can no longer be merely regarded as healthy carriers, as they display renal calcifications and/or bone manifestation significantly more frequent than wild-type individuals; but still to a lesser degree than biallelic (homozygous and compound heterozygous) individuals (43). Similar observations were reported for families with mutations in *CYP24A1* (44). The contribution of monogenic disorders to the overall prevalence of kidney stone disease has not been studied comprehensively in the past. Especially, genetic evidence based on broad screenings of a multitude of causative genes in large patient cohorts is lacking. Comprehensive genetic testing has been too costly and inefficient in the past. For most individuals with NL/NC, mutation analysis for a causative genetic defect has therefore not been accessible, despite the fact that knowledge of the molecular cause of NL/NC may have important consequences for prognosis, prophylaxis and/or treatment. Only rough estimates have been derived from clinical observation studies: based on a huge data collection of stone composition analysis, it was concluded that monogenic causes do not exceed 9.6% in children and 1.6% in adults (45). In the last decade, however, this situation has begun to change, with the advent of high-throughput sequencing techniques.

TABLE 1 | Genes, known to cause monogenic forms of NL/NC.

Gene symbol[a]	Gene name	Disease entity	MIM phenotype #	Mode	Reference
ADCY10	Adenylate cyclase 10	Idiopathic (absorptive) hypercalciuria, susceptibility	143870	AD	(11)
AGXT	Alanine-glyoxylate aminotransferase	Primary hyperoxaluria (PH), type 1, PH1	259900	AR	(12)
APRT	Adenine phosphoribosyltransferase	Adenine phosphoribosyltransferase deficiency, APRT	614723	AR	(13)
ATP6V0A4	ATPase, H+ transporting, lysosomal V0 subunit a4	dRTA	602722	AR	(14)
ATP6V1B1	ATPase, H+ transporting, lysosomal, V1 subunit B1	dRTA with deafness	267300	AR	(15)
CA2	Carbonic anhydrase II	Osteopetrosis + d/pRTA	259730	AR	(16)
CASR	Calcium-sensing receptor	Hypocalcemia with Bartter syndrome/hypocalcemia, AD	601198	AD	(17)
CLCN5	Chloride channel, voltage-sensitive 5	Dent disease/NL, type 1	300009/310468	XR	(18)
CLCNKB	Chloride channel, voltage-sensitive Kb	Bartter syndrome, type 3	607364	AR	(19)
CLDN16	Claudin 16	Familial hypomagnesemia with hypercalciuria and NC, FHHNC	248250	AR	(20)
CLDN19	Claudin 19	Familial hypomagnesemia with hypercalciuria and NC with ocular abnormalities	248190	AR	(21)
CYP24A1	Cytochrome P450, family 24, subfamily A, polypeptide 1	1,25-(OH) D-24 hydroxylase deficiency, infantile hypercalcemia	143880	AR	(22)
FAM20A	Family with sequence similarity 20, member A	Enamel renal syndrome, amelogenesis imperfect, and NC	204690	AR	(23)
GRHPR	Glyoxylate reductase/hydroxypyruvate reductase	PH, type 2, PH2	260000	AR	(24)
HNF4A	Hepatocyte nuclear factor 4, alpha	MODY + Fanconi syndrome + NC (p.R76W)	125850	AD	(25)
HOGA1	4-Hydroxy-2-oxoglutarate aldolase 1	PH, type 3, PH3	613616	AR	(26)
HPRT1	Hypoxanthine phosphoribosyltransferase 1	Kelley–Seegmiller syndrome, partial HPRT deficiency, HPRT-related gout	300323	XR	(27)
KCNJ1	Potassium inwardly rectifying channel, subfamily J, member 1	Bartter syndrome, type 2	241200	AR	(28)
MAGED2	Melanoma antigen, family D, 2	Bartter syndrome, type 5	300971	XR	(29)
OCRL	Oculocerebrorenal syndrome of Lowe	Lowe syndrome/Dent disease 2	309000/300555	XR	(30)
SLC12A1	Solute carrier family 12, member 1	Bartter syndrome, type 1	601678	AR	(31)
SLC26A1	Solute carrier family 26 (sulfate transporter), member 1	Ca-oxalate-NL	167030	AR	(32)
SLC22A12	Solute carrier family 22 (organic anion/urate transporter), member 12	Renal hypouricemia, RHUC1	220150	AD/AR	(33)
SLC2A9	Solute carrier family 2 (facilitated glucose transporter), member 9	Renal hypouricemia, RHUC2	612076	AD/AR	(10)
SLC34A1	Solute carrier family 34 (sodium phosphate), member 1	Hypophosphatemic NL, osteoporosis-1, NPHLOP1/Fanconi renotubular syndrome 2	612286/613388	AD/AR	(34)
SLC34A3	Solute carrier family 34 (sodium phosphate), member 3	Hypophosphatemic rickets with hypercalciuria	241530	AR	(35)
SLC3A1	Solute carrier family 3 (cystine, dibasic and neutral amino acid transporters, activator of cystine, dibasic and neutral amino acid transport), member 1	Cystinuria, type A	220100	AR	(36)
SLC4A1	Solute carrier family 4, anion exchanger, member 1	Primary dRTA, dominant/recessive	179800/611590	AD/AR	(37)
SLC7A9	Solute carrier family 7 (glycoprotein-associated amino acid transporter light chain, bo, +system), member 9	Cystinuria, type B	220100	AD/AR	(38)
SLC9A3R1	Solute carrier family 9, subfamily A (NHE3, cation proton antiporter 3), member 3 regulator 1	Hypophosphatemic NL, osteoporosis-2, NPHLOP2	612287	AD	(39)
VDR	Vitamin D (1,25-dihydroxyvitamin D3) receptor	Idiopathic hypercalciuria	277440	AD	(40)
XDH	Xanthine dehydrogenase	Xanthinuria, type 1	278300	AR	(41)

[a]*For HNF4A the MIM-phenotype number denotes MODY type 1, as occurrence of Fanconi syndrome and NC has only been shown in the presence of a specific allele: p.R76W.*

AD, autosomal dominant; AR, autosomal recessive; dRTA, distal renal tubular acidosis; MODY, maturity onset diabetes of the young; NC, nephrocalcinosis; NL, nephrolithiasis; pRTA, proximal renal tubular acidosis; XR, X-chromosomal recessive.

HIGH-THROUGHPUT MUTATION ANALYSIS IN PATIENTS WITH NL/NC

To investigate patients with kidney stone disease for the presence of pathogenic mutations in known disease genes, we established a gene panel based on microfluidic multiplex-PCR and consecutive NextGen sequencing (Fluidigm™/NGS) (46, 47).

In a "pilot-study," we consecutively recruited 268 genetically unresolved individuals from typical kidney stone clinics; 102 pediatric and 166 adult probands. As a result, we identified 50 deleterious variants in 14 out of 30 analyzed genes, leading to a molecular diagnosis in 15% of all cases. In the pediatric subgroup, we detected a causative mutation in 21%, while among adults, deleterious variants were present in 11% (**Figure 2A**) (48). Mutations in the cystinuria-gene *SLC7A9* were found most frequently in the adult cohort (**Figure 2B**). Two follow-up studies were able to confirm these results. First, in an exclusively pediatric cohort of 143 NL/NC patients, 17% of cases were explained by mutations in 14 different genes (49). Second, in a cohort of 51 families with age of NL/NC manifestation before 25 years, targeted WES was used to detect a genetic cause in almost 30% (50). Not surprisingly, recessive mutations were more frequently found among neonates and in cases of congenital disease, whereas dominant conditions usually manifested later in life. These data indicate that genetic kidney stone disease is an underdiagnosed condition, despite the fact that the molecular diagnosis will potentially influence prognosis, prophylaxis, and/or treatment. A limitation worth mentioning, however, is a potential selection bias due to recruitment from specialist kidney stone clinics in all of the three aforementioned studies.

IDENTIFICATION OF NOVEL HUMAN DISEASE GENES BY CANDIDATE-GENE APPROACH

High-throughput mutation analysis is also used to screen for pathogenic variants in various candidate genes. One of the most interesting recent findings was the discovery of human mutations in *SLC26A1* (32). Since the first description of Ca-oxalate (CaOx) kidney stone formation and NC in Slc26a1 (Sat1)-knockout mice by Dawson et al. in 2010, *SLC26A1* has been a bona fide NL-candidate gene (51). SLC26A1 encodes an anion exchanger expressed at the basolateral membrane of proximal renal tubules, ileum, and jejunum. Consequently, by using a candidate-gene approach, pathogenic variants were identified in humans with a history of early onset CaOx-NL, namely, two unrelated individuals with biallelic missense variants (32). Functionally, pathogenicity of the identified variants was demonstrated *in vitro*, leading to intracellular mis-trafficking and impaired transport activity (32). Defective SLC26A1 therefore constitutes a new cause of CaOx-NL and should be considered when testing individuals for causes of recurrent CaOx-stone formation.

NEW CLINICAL PATIENT REGISTRY FOR HEREDITARY KIDNEY STONE DISEASE

Most epidemiological data on increasing prevalence in Western countries are derived from US databases. Although urgently needed, centralized European databases are not available at the time. As aforementioned genetic studies on prevalence of hereditary kidney stone disease were executed with small cohorts from specialized centers in both Europe and the US, a translation to the general situation in Europe is not valid. While in the US, the *Rare Kidney Stone Consortium* constitutes a platform that integrates and coordinates registry, basic science, and clinical research activities for rare conditions such as cystinuria, PH, APRT deficiency, Dent and Lowe disease, no comparable data collection on patients with hereditary kidney stone disease has been implemented neither in Europe nor in Germany today. In collaboration with the existing European PH registry, *OxalEurope* (Prof. Bernd Hoppe, University of Bonn), and through funding by *Deutsche Forschungsgemeinschaft* and *Else Kröner-Fresenius Stiftung*, we recently established a clinical

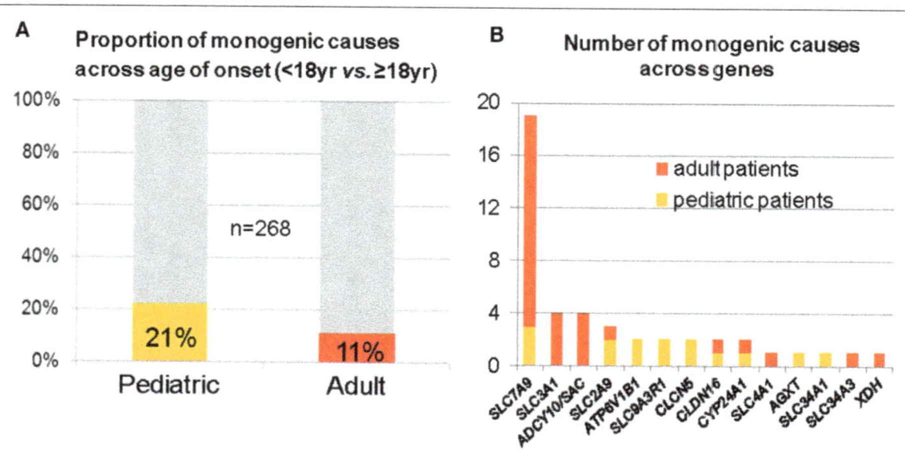

FIGURE 2 | Mutation analysis of 30 known monogenic nephrolithiasis (NL)/nephrocalcinosis (NC) genes in 268 patients with NL/NC. **(A)** Fraction of monogenic causes in pediatric and adult subcohort. **(B)** Number of monogenic causes across genes (red denotes adults; orange denotes pediatric patients). Of note, *SLC7A9* was found most frequently mutated, especially in young adults.

TABLE 2 | Inclusion criteria for mutation analysis in clinical patient registry.

Clinical criteria
Pediatric age of onset or onset during early adulthood (<40 years) plus
Positive family history or
Recurrence (>3x) or
Indicative phenotype (e.g., RTA, cystinuria, and NC) or
Established molecular genetic diagnosis

patient "Registry for hereditary kidney stone disease" at the University of Leipzig. The registry is nationally supported by the German Societies of Adult Nephrology (DGfN) and Pediatric Nephrology (GPN). It is further enrolled at the German Clinical Trials Register (DRKS-ID: DRKS00012891). As a fundamental part of study recruitment, high-throughput mutation analysis for known and novel kidney stone genes is offered on a research basis for patients without an established molecular diagnosis but with a clinical picture that points to an underlying genetic susceptibility: e.g., early age of onset (<40 years), positive family history, indicative phenotypes such as NC, cystinuria, or RTA, and severely recurrent NL (>3×) (**Table 2**). While patients with an already established genetic diagnosis are generally enrolled, cases with secondary NL/NC causes, such as malignancy, sarcoidosis, and primary hyperparathyroidism, do not get included in genetic analysis. To actively enroll patients, a clinical center will usually need approval by the local Institutional Review Board; a process for which we offer our help and assistance by providing respective templates. Upon ethics approval, consent form and clinical data sheets (e.g., clinical questionnaire) can be downloaded from our registry website (http://www.mks-registry.net). To ensure thorough clinical phenotyping, we will be asking for substantial patient information such as ethnicity, consanguinity, family history, age of onset, recurrence (defined as every putatively new kidney stone event), daily fluid intake, surgical interventions, and extrarenal involvement among others. The documents can be filled in by the patient with the help of the enrolling physician. In addition, biochemical serum parameters, including creatinine, eGFR, PTH, vitamin D, electrolytes, uric acid, and urinalysis (pH, calcium, phosphate, magnesium, uric acid, citrate, oxalate, and cystine, preferably from 24-h urine, if not spot urine), as well as data on stone composition analysis will be requested upon enrollment. Taking into account that 24-h urine collection and stone composition analysis is not routinely performed at all institutions, we include these parameters upon availability. 2-yearly clinical follow-up visits of enrolled patients are desirable but not mandatory. After registration, recruiting clinical centers will be provided with a personalized login to enter patient data *via* our registry website (http://www.mks-registry.net). Alternatively, we offer entering the data electronically when sent to us on paper. Entered data will be stored on a secured server and can be accessed by participating clinical centers to view their own patient data. The following websites provide further information:

https://www.dgfn.eu/hereditaere-nierensteinleiden.html
https://www.drks.de/drks_web/navigate.do?navigationId=trial.HTML&TRIAL_ID=DRKS00012891

In summary, kidney stone disease is an increasingly prevalent condition which is clinically heterogeneous and poorly understood, notably its genetic drivers. As a series of recent studies indicated, monogenic conditions are most likely underestimated in prevalence. By implementation of a centralized patient registry on hereditary kidney stone disease, we will contribute to overcome, at least in part, the vast knowledge gap on genetics of kidney stone disease. In this context, clinical registries are valuable sources for several reasons: first, delineating better phenotype–genotype associations will be crucial for more precise patient stratification in future clinical research studies. Second, identifying new disease genes with new disease mechanisms will diminish the gap of unknown NL/NC etiology; and third, deciphering new molecular targets helps to pave the way for developing drugs of recurrence prevention in severely affected families.

ETHICS STATEMENT

This study was carried out in accordance with the recommendations of "Ethikkommission an der Medizinischen Fakultät der Universität Leipzig" with written informed consent from all subjects. All subjects gave written informed consent in accordance with the Declaration of Helsinki. The protocol was approved by the "Ethikkommission an der Medizinischen Fakultät der Universität Leipzig."

AUTHOR CONTRIBUTIONS

JH conceived and wrote the manuscript. BH, AS, LM, and RS edited the manuscript and built up the registry's infrastructure that is introduced to the reader.

FUNDING

The research is funded by project grants from DFG (HA 6908/2-1) and EKFS (2016_A52) to JH. This work was further supported by the Federal Ministry of Education and Research (BMBF), Germany, FKZ: 01EO1501 to JH.

REFERENCES

1. Scales CD, Jr., Smith AC, Hanley JM, Saigal CS. Prevalence of kidney stones in the United States. *Eur Urol* (2012) 62:160–5.
2. Pfau A, Knauf F. Update on nephrolithiasis: core curriculum 2016. *Am J Kidney Dis* (2016) 68:973–85. doi:10.1053/j.ajkd.2016.05.016
3. Goldfarb DS, Fischer ME, Keich Y, Goldberg J. A twin study of genetic and dietary influences on nephrolithiasis: a report from the Vietnam Era Twin (VET) Registry. *Kidney Int* (2005) 67:1053–61. doi:10.1111/j.1523-1755.2005.00170.x
4. Stechman MJ, Loh NY, Thakker RV. Genetics of hypercalciuric nephrolithiasis: renal stone disease. *Ann N Y Acad Sci* (2007) 1116:461–84. doi:10.1196/annals.1402.030
5. Sayer JA. Progress in understanding the genetics of calcium-containing nephrolithiasis. *J Am Soc Nephrol* (2017) 28:748–59. doi:10.1681/ASN.2016050576
6. Thorleifsson G, Holm H, Edvardsson V, Walters GB, Styrkarsdottir U, Gudbjartsson DF, et al. Sequence variants in the CLDN14 gene associate

with kidney stones and bone mineral density. *Nat Genet* (2009) 41:926–30. doi:10.1038/ng.404
7. Gudbjartsson DF, Holm H, Indridason OS, Thorleifsson G, Edvardsson V, Sulem P, et al. Association of variants at UMOD with chronic kidney disease and kidney stones-role of age and comorbid diseases. *PLoS Genet* (2010) 6:e1001039. doi:10.1371/journal.pgen.1001039
8. Oddsson A, Sulem P, Helgason H, Edvardsson VO, Thorleifsson G, Sveinbjörnsson G, et al. Common and rare variants associated with kidney stones and biochemical traits. *Nat Commun* (2015) 6:7975. doi:10.1038/ncomms8975
9. Döring A, Gieger C, Mehta D, Gohlke H, Prokisch H, Coassin S, et al. SLC2A9 influences uric acid concentrations with pronounced sex-specific effects. *Nat Genet* (2008) 40:430–6. doi:10.1038/ng.107
10. Matsuo H, Chiba T, Nagamori S, Nakayama A, Domoto H, Phetdee K, et al. Mutations in glucose transporter 9 gene SLC2A9 cause renal hypouricemia. *Am J Hum Genet* (2008) 83:744–51. doi:10.1016/j.ajhg.2008.11.001
11. Reed BY, Gitomer WL, Heller HJ, Hsu MC, Lemke M, Padalino P, et al. Identification and characterization of a gene with base substitutions associated with the absorptive hypercalciuria phenotype and low spinal bone density. *J Clin Endocrinol Metab* (2002) 87:1476–85. doi:10.1210/jcem.87.4.8300
12. Purdue PE, Allsop J, Isaya G, Rosenberg LE, Danpure CJ. Mistargeting of peroxisomal L-alanine:glyoxylate aminotransferase to mitochondria in primary hyperoxaluria patients depends upon activation of a cryptic mitochondrial targeting sequence by a point mutation. *Proc Natl Acad Sci U S A* (1991) 88:10900–4. doi:10.1073/pnas.88.23.10900
13. Hidaka Y, Palella TD, O'Toole TE, Tarlé SA, Kelley WN. Human adenine phosphoribosyltransferase. Identification of allelic mutations at the nucleotide level as a cause of complete deficiency of the enzyme. *J Clin Invest* (1987) 80:1409–15. doi:10.1172/JCI113219
14. Smith AN, Skaug J, Choate KA, Nayir A, Bakkaloglu A, Ozen S, et al. Mutations in ATP6N1B, encoding a new kidney vacuolar proton pump 116-kD subunit, cause recessive distal renal tubular acidosis with preserved hearing. *Nat Genet* (2000) 26:71–5. doi:10.1038/79208
15. Karet FE, Finberg KE, Nelson RD, Nayir A, Mocan H, Sanjad SA, et al. Mutations in the gene encoding B1 subunit of H+-ATPase cause renal tubular acidosis with sensorineural deafness. *Nat Genet* (1999) 21:84–90. doi:10.1038/5022
16. Venta PJ, Welty RJ, Johnson TM, Sly WS, Tashian RE. Carbonic anhydrase II deficiency syndrome in a Belgian family is caused by a point mutation at an invariant histidine residue (107 His→Tyr): complete structure of the normal human CA II gene. *Am J Hum Genet* (1991) 49:1082–90.
17. Pearce SH, Williamson C, Kifor O, Bai M, Coulthard MG, Davies M, et al. A familial syndrome of hypocalcemia with hypercalciuria due to mutations in the calcium-sensing receptor. *N Engl J Med* (1996) 335:1115–22. doi:10.1056/NEJM199610103351505
18. Lloyd SE, Pearce SH, Fisher SE, Steinmeyer K, Schwappach B, Scheinman SJ, et al. A common molecular basis for three inherited kidney stone diseases. *Nature* (1996) 379:445–9. doi:10.1038/379445a0
19. Simon DB, Bindra RS, Mansfield TA, Nelson-Williams C, Mendonca E, Stone R, et al. Mutations in the chloride channel gene, CLCNKB, cause Bartter's syndrome type III. *Nat Genet* (1997) 17:171–8. doi:10.1038/ng1097-171
20. Simon DB, Lu Y, Choate KA, Velazquez H, Al-Sabban E, Praga M, et al. Paracellin-1, a renal tight junction protein required for paracellular Mg2+ resorption. *Science* (1999) 285:103–6. doi:10.1126/science.285.5424.103
21. Konrad M, Schaller A, Seelow D, Pandey AV, Waldegger S, Lesslauer A, et al. Mutations in the tight-junction gene claudin 19 (CLDN19) are associated with renal magnesium wasting, renal failure, and severe ocular involvement. *Am J Hum Genet* (2006) 79:949–57. doi:10.1086/508617
22. Schlingmann KP, Kaufmann M, Weber S, Irwin A, Goos C, John U, et al. Mutations in CYP24A1 and idiopathic infantile hypercalcemia. *N Engl J Med* (2011) 365:410–21. doi:10.1056/NEJMoa1103864
23. Jaureguiberry G, De la Dure-Molla M, Parry D, Quentric M, Himmerkus N, Koike T, et al. Nephrocalcinosis (enamel renal syndrome) caused by autosomal recessive FAM20A mutations. *Nephron Physiol* (2012) 122:1–6. doi:10.1159/000349989
24. Cramer SD, Ferree PM, Lin K, Milliner DS, Holmes RP. The gene encoding hydroxypyruvate reductase (GRHPR) is mutated in patients with primary hyperoxaluria type II. *Hum Mol Genet* (1999) 8:2063–9. doi:10.1093/hmg/8.11.2063
25. Hamilton AJ, Bingham C, McDonald TJ, Cook PR, Caswell RC, Weedon MN, et al. The HNF4A R76W mutation causes atypical dominant Fanconi syndrome in addition to a β cell phenotype. *J Med Genet* (2014) 51:165–9. doi:10.1136/jmedgenet-2013-102066
26. Belostotsky R, Seboun E, Idelson GH, Milliner DS, Becker-Cohen R, Rinat C, et al. Mutations in DHDPSL are responsible for primary hyperoxaluria type III. *Am J Hum Genet* (2010) 87:392–9. doi:10.1016/j.ajhg.2010.07.023
27. Davidson BL, Tarlé SA, van Antwerp M, Gibbs DA, Watts RW, Kelley WN, et al. Identification of 17 independent mutations responsible for human hypoxanthine-guanine phosphoribosyltransferase (HPRT) deficiency. *Am J Hum Genet* (1991) 48:951–8.
28. Simon DB, Karet FE, Rodriguez-Soriano J, Hamdan JH, DiPietro A, Trachtman H, et al. Genetic heterogeneity of Bartter's syndrome revealed by mutations in the K+ channel, ROMK. *Nat Genet* (1996) 14:152–6. doi:10.1038/ng1096-152
29. Laghmani K, Beck BB, Yang S-S, Seaayfan E, Wenzel A, Reusch B, et al. Polyhydramnios, transient antenatal Bartter's syndrome, and MAGED2 mutations. *N Engl J Med* (2016) 374:1853–63. doi:10.1056/NEJMoa1507629
30. Reilly DS, Lewis RA, Ledbetter DH, Nussbaum RL. Tightly linked flanking markers for the Lowe oculocerebrorenal syndrome, with application to carrier assessment. *Am J Hum Genet* (1988) 42:748–55.
31. Simon DB, Karet FE, Hamdan JM, DiPietro A, Sanjad SA, Lifton RP. Bartter's syndrome, hypokalaemic alkalosis with hypercalciuria, is caused by mutations in the Na-K-2Cl cotransporter NKCC2. *Nat Genet* (1996) 13:183–8. doi:10.1038/ng0696-183
32. Gee HY, Jun I, Braun DA, Lawson JA, Halbritter J, Shril S, et al. Mutations in SLC26A1 cause nephrolithiasis. *Am J Hum Genet* (2016) 98:1228–34. doi:10.1016/j.ajhg.2016.03.026
33. Enomoto A, Kimura H, Chairoungdua A, Shigeta Y, Jutabha P, Cha SH, et al. Molecular identification of a renal urate anion exchanger that regulates blood urate levels. *Nature* (2002) 417:447–52. doi:10.1038/nature742
34. Prié D, Huart V, Bakouh N, Planelles G, Dellis O, Gérard B, et al. Nephrolithiasis and osteoporosis associated with hypophosphatemia caused by mutations in the type 2a sodium-phosphate cotransporter. *N Engl J Med* (2002) 347:983–91. doi:10.1056/NEJMoa020028
35. Lorenz-Depiereux B, Benet-Pages A, Eckstein G, Tenenbaum-Rakover Y, Wagenstaller J, Tiosano D, et al. Hereditary hypophosphatemic rickets with hypercalciuria is caused by mutations in the sodium-phosphate cotransporter gene SLC34A3. *Am J Hum Genet* (2006) 78:193–201. doi:10.1086/499410
36. Calonge MJ, Gasparini P, Chillarón J, Chillón M, Gallucci M, Rousaud F, et al. Cystinuria caused by mutations in rBAT, a gene involved in the transport of cystine. *Nat Genet* (1994) 6:420–5. doi:10.1038/ng0494-420
37. Bruce LJ, Cope DL, Jones GK, Schofield AE, Burley M, Povey S, et al. Familial distal renal tubular acidosis is associated with mutations in the red cell anion exchanger (Band 3, AE1) gene. *J Clin Invest* (1997) 100:1693–707. doi:10.1172/JCI119694
38. Feliubadaló L, Font M, Purroy J, Rousaud F, Estivill X, Nunes V, et al. Non-type I cystinuria caused by mutations in SLC7A9, encoding a subunit (bo,+AT) of rBAT. *Nat Genet* (1999) 23:52–7. doi:10.1038/12652
39. Karim Z, Gérard B, Bakouh N, Alili R, Leroy C, Beck L, et al. NHERF1 mutations and responsiveness of renal parathyroid hormone. *N Engl J Med* (2008) 359:1128–35. doi:10.1056/NEJMoa0802836
40. Scott P, Ouimet D, Valiquette L, Guay G, Proulx Y, Trouvé ML, et al. Suggestive evidence for a susceptibility gene near the vitamin D receptor locus in idiopathic calcium stone formation. *J Am Soc Nephrol* (1999) 10:1007–13.
41. Ichida K, Amaya Y, Kamatani N, Nishino T, Hosoya T, Sakai O. Identification of two mutations in human xanthine dehydrogenase gene responsible for classical type I xanthinuria. *J Clin Invest* (1997) 99:2391–7. doi:10.1172/JCI119421
42. Hildebrandt F. Genetic kidney diseases. *Lancet* (2010) 375:1287–95. doi:10.1016/S0140-6736(10)60236-X
43. Dasgupta D, Wee MJ, Reyes M, Li Y, Simm PJ, Sharma A, et al. Mutations in SLC34A3/NPT2c are associated with kidney stones and nephrocalcinosis. *J Am Soc Nephrol* (2014) 25:2366–75. doi:10.1681/ASN.2013101085
44. O'Keeffe DT, Tebben PJ, Kumar R, Singh RJ, Wu Y, Wermers RA. Clinical and biochemical phenotypes of adults with monoallelic and biallelic CYP24A1 mutations: evidence of gene dose effect. *Osteoporos Int* (2016) 27:3121–5. doi:10.1007/s00198-016-3615-6
45. Jungers P, Joly D, Blanchard A, Courbebaisse M, Knebelmann B, Daudon M. Lithiases rénales héréditaires monogéniques. Récents acquis

diagnostiques et thérapeutiques. *Nephrol Ther* (2008) 4:231–55. doi:10.1016/j.nephro.2007.12.005

46. Halbritter J, Diaz K, Chaki M, Porath JD, Tarrier B, Fu C, et al. High-throughput mutation analysis in patients with a nephronophthisis-associated ciliopathy applying multiplexed barcoded array-based PCR amplification and next-generation sequencing. *J Med Genet* (2012) 49:756–67. doi:10.1136/jmedgenet-2012-100973
47. Halbritter J, Porath JD, Diaz KA, Braun DA, Kohl S, Chaki M, et al. Identification of 99 novel mutations in a worldwide cohort of 1,056 patients with a nephronophthisis-related ciliopathy. *Hum Genet* (2013) 132:865–84. doi:10.1007/s00439-013-1297-0
48. Halbritter J, Baum M, Hynes AM, Rice SJ, Thwaites DT, Gucev ZS, et al. Fourteen monogenic genes account for 15% of nephrolithiasis/nephrocalcinosis. *J Am Soc Nephrol* (2015) 26:543–51. doi:10.1681/ASN.2014040388
49. Braun DA, Lawson JA, Gee HY, Halbritter J, Shril S, Tan W, et al. Prevalence of monogenic causes in pediatric patients with nephrolithiasis or nephrocalcinosis. *Clin J Am Soc Nephrol* (2016) 11:664–72. doi:10.2215/CJN.07540715
50. Daga A, Majmundar AJ, Braun DA, Gee HY, Lawson JA, Shril S, et al. Whole exome sequencing frequently detects a monogenic cause in early onset nephrolithiasis and nephrocalcinosis. *Kidney Int* (2018) 93:204–13. doi:10.1016/j.kint.2017.06.025
51. Dawson PA, Russell CS, Lee S, McLeay SC, van Dongen JM, Cowley DM, et al. Urolithiasis and hepatotoxicity are linked to the anion transporter Sat1 in mice. *J Clin Invest* (2010) 120:706–12. doi:10.1172/JCI31474

16

Renal Cell Carcinoma in von Hippel–Lindau Disease—From Tumor Genetics to Novel Therapeutic Strategies

Emily Kim[1,2] *and Stefan Zschiedrich*[3]*

[1] *Department of Radiation Oncology, Faculty of Medicine, Albert Ludwigs University of Freiburg, Freiburg, Germany,* [2] *German Cancer Consortium (DKTK), Partner Site Freiburg, Freiburg, Germany,* [3] *Renal Division, Department of Medicine IV, Faculty of Medicine, Albert Ludwigs University of Freiburg, Freiburg, Germany*

***Correspondence:**
Stefan Zschiedrich
stefan.zschiedrich@uniklinik-freiburg.de

von Hippel–Lindau (VHL) disease is an autosomal dominant syndrome caused by mutations in the VHL tumor-suppressor gene, leading to the dysregulation of many hypoxia-induced genes. Affected individuals are at increased risk of developing recurrent and bilateral kidney cysts and dysplastic lesions which may progress to clear cell renal cell carcinoma (ccRCC). Following the eponymous *VHL* gene inactivation, ccRCCs evolve through additional genetic alterations, resulting in both intratumor and intertumor heterogeneity. Genomic studies have identified frequent mutations in genes involved in epigenetic regulation and phosphoinositide 3-kinase–AKT–mechanistic target of rapamycin (mTOR) pathway activation. Currently, local therapeutic options include nephron-sparing surgery and alternative ablative procedures. For advanced metastatic disease, systemic treatment, including inhibition of vascular endothelial growth factor pathways and mTOR pathways, as well as immunotherapy are available. Multimodal therapy, targeting multiple signaling pathways and/or enhancing the immune response, is currently being investigated. A deeper understanding of the fundamental biology of ccRCC development and progression, as well as the development of novel and targeted therapies will be accelerated by new preclinical models, which will greatly inform the search for clinical biomarkers for diagnosis, prognosis, and response to treatment.

Keywords: von Hippel–Lindau disease, renal cell carcinoma, cancer genetics, predictive biomarkers, preclinical models, new therapeutic targets

INTRODUCTION

von Hippel–Lindau (VHL) disease is an autosomal dominant, multiorgan visceral cysts and tumor syndrome. The disease name derives from the German ophthalmologist Eugen von Hippel who studied two cases of striking retinal angiomas and the Swedish pathologist Arvid Lindau who detected a connection between cerebellar hemangioblastomas, retinal angiomas, and other visceral tumors (1, 2). The first report of VHL dates from 1894, when Collins described vascular intraocular tumors in two siblings (3). VHL manifestations can be found in retinal hemangioblastoma, cerebellar and spinal hemangioblastoma, renal cysts and clear cell renal cell carcinoma (ccRCC), liver hemangioma, pancreatic cysts, pancreatic microcystic serous adenoma and pancreatic neuroendocrine tumors, pheochromocytoma (PCC), epididymal and broad ligament cystadenoma, and endolymphatic sac tumors. In 1964, Melmon and Rosen suggested clinical diagnostic criteria that are still valid today. VHL disease has been classified depending on the presence of PCC in VHL type 1 (without PCC) and type 2 (with PCC). VHL type 2 is further subclassified in type 2A (with PCC but without ccRCC), type 2B (with PCC and ccRCC), and type 2C (PCC only) (4–6). Practically, however, practitioners do not rely on this classification because families can move between clinical subtypes.

von Hippel–Lindau disease is caused by mutations in the *VHL* tumor-suppressor gene, located on chromosome 3p25-26. *VHL* was mapped to chromosome 3 in 1988 and cloned in 1993 (7, 8). The incidence of VHL disease is approximately 1:36,000 (9). Although VHL disease typically presents in early adulthood, manifestation of retinal angiomas, PCCs, and ccRCCs has been reported earlier; therefore, guidelines recommend starting surveillance programs for eye examination at 2–5 years and abdominal imaging at 6–10 years (10–12).

Most patients develop ccRCCs that arise from microscopic precursor lesions present in both kidneys. The number of nonmalignant cysts lined with clear cells in an average VHL kidney was estimated to be 1,100, and the number of clear cell renal neoplasms (solid and cystic) to be 600 (13). Optimally, early RCC can be detected, observed, and surgically removed before progression to metastatic disease (14). However, repeated surgery for multifocal bilateral disease is followed by increased risk of end-stage renal disease (ESRD) requiring renal transplantation or dialysis.

THE ROLE OF VHL

Whether hereditary or sporadic, ccRCC is characterized by mutations in the VHL tumor-suppressor gene on chromosome 3 (3p25-26) and a subsequent loss of heterozygosity. VHL, Elongin B (encoded by *TCEB1*), and Elongin C form a stable complex that targets hypoxia-inducible factor α (HIFα) subunits for proteolytic degradation under normoxic conditions (15). In the presence of hypoxia or in the absence of functional VHL tumor-suppressor protein, HIFα subunits HIF1α and HIF2α are stabilized, binding together with ARNT (HIF1β) to hypoxia-response elements to activate genes involved in angiogenesis, cell cycle, cell proliferation, glucose, and lipid metabolism, among others. Mutations of *TCEB1* that abrogate binding of Elongin B to VHL can also increase HIFα expression in ccRCCs with intact *VHL* (16). Mutations in *VHL* and *TCEB1* were mutually exclusive, supporting a permissive role for VHL complex degradation and HIFα stabilization in tumorigenesis.

ADDITIONAL GENE MUTATIONS

Approximately 15 years after *VHL* was identified as the genetic basis for VHL, further driver mutations for ccRCC were identified, summarized in **Table 1**. Exome sequencing of tumors identified additional inactivating mutations on chromosome 3 in tumor suppressors polybromo-1 (*PBRM1*), SET domain-containing 2 (*SETD2*), and BRCA1-associated protein-1 (*BAP1*), which are chromatin and histone regulators located at 3p21 (17–19). *PBRM1* and *BAP1* mutations are mutually exclusive, with *BAP1* mutations correlating with higher grade disease (19, 20). Large-scale genomic sequencing showed that these three tumor-suppressor genes, located near *VHL* at 3p21, are the most frequently mutated genes in ccRCC after *VHL* (16, 21). Other significantly mutated genes included histone-modifiers *KDM5C* and *KDM6A*, previously implicated in ccRCC (17–19, 22), genes in the phosphoinositide 3-kinase (PI3K)/AKT pathway, such as mechanistic target of rapamycin (*mTOR*), *PIK3CA*, and *PTEN*, as well as *TCEB1* (Elongin C) (16, 21). The tumor-suppressor gene *TP53* is infrequently mutated, playing a lesser role than in many other solid tumors.

TUMOR HETEROGENEITY

Clear cell renal cell carcinoma has a moderate somatic mutation frequency compared with other solid tumors and these mutations progress in a branched evolutionary manner (24, 25). The evolutionary history of sporadic ccRCC in 10 individuals was investigated by exome sequencing of multiregion samples from primary ccRCCs and metastases (26). Intratumor heterogeneity was present in all tumors, indicating that a single biopsy underestimates the genomic complexity of a tumor. Tumor phylogeny, similar to an evolutionary tree, showed that inactivation of *VHL* and loss of chromosome 3p were ubiquitous early truncal events. *PBRM1* inactivation was a frequent mutation, occurring early as a truncal mutation in three tumors and as a later event in three

TABLE 1 | Frequently mutated genes in clear cell renal cell carcinoma (16, 21, 23).

Gene	Chromosome	Protein	Function	Mutation (%)
VHL	3p25.3	von Hippel–Lindau (VHL) disease	VHL, Elongin B and C complex	49–82
PBRM1	3p21.1	Polybromo 1	SWI-SNF complex chromatin remodeling	29–41
SETD2	3p21.31	SET domain-containing 2	Histone H3K36 methyltransferase	8–12
BAP1	3p21.1	BRCA1-associated protein 1	Histone deubiquitinase	6–10
KDM5C	Xp11.22	Lysine demethylase 5C (JARID1C)	H3K4 demethylase	4–8
mTOR	1p36.22	Mechanistic target of rapamycin kinase	Phosphoinositide 3-kinase (PI3K)–AKT–mechanistic target of rapamycin (mTOR) pathway	5–6
PTEN	10q23.31	Phosphatase and tensin homolog	PI3K–AKT–mTOR pathway	4
PIK3CA	3q26.32	PI3K catalytic subunit α	PI3K–AKT–mTOR pathway	3–5
TP53	17p13.1	Tumor protein P53	Cell cycle	2–3
TCEB1 (ELOB)	16p13.3	Elongin B	VHL, Elongin B and C complex	1–3

Loss of heterozygosity at 3p was reported in over 90% of cases, and mutations in components of the PI3K–AKT–mTOR pathway in 28–76%.

others. Distinct subclones, spatially separated within a single tumor, contained mutations that appeared in a branched rather than linear manner. Subclonal driver mutations were similar to those identified by earlier studies, such as chromatin modifiers, regulators of mTORC1 pathway, and tumor-suppressor *TP53*. Parallel evolution was observed in certain genes, in which different evolutionary paths or branches in a tumor resulted in inactivation of the same gene by separate mechanisms. Recurrent mutations in *PBRM1*, *SETD2*, *BAP1*, and *KDM5C* suggest an evolutionary selection for epigenetic dysregulation in tumorigenesis. Branched subclonal mutations were highly variable and contained more C>T transitions than truncal mutations, potentially useful as prognostic and predictive biomarkers.

Genomic analysis of ccRCC has established the fundamental role for VHL inactivation and HIF dysregulation, the importance of chromatin regulation and histone modification, and the involvement of the mTORC1 pathway. The central role of chromosome remodeling in the development and the progression of ccRCC implicates epigenetic dysregulation as a permissive factor in tumorigenesis and a novel target for therapeutic agents and candidate biomarkers. However, the molecular mechanisms whereby epigenetic alterations result in transcriptional dysregulation is currently unclear. Mutations and copy number alterations were detected in *mTOR* (mammalian target of rapamycin), *PIK3CA* (PI3K catalytic subunit-α), TSC1, and *PTEN* (16, 21). Mutually exclusive gene alterations of the PI3K/Akt/mTOR pathway were detected in approximately 28% of tumors (21). Activation of the PI3K/Akt/mTOR pathway may underlie the efficacy of mTOR inhibitors, such as everolimus and temsirolimus.

In kidneys of individuals with VHL disease, VHL-deficient lesions with constitutive HIF activation were detectable by carbonic anhydrase IX staining, allowing the progression from single cells to ccRCC to be easily observed (27). HIF activation occurs extremely early in the disease. Most lesions are single cells, with very few multicellular dysplastic lesions and cystic lesions, showing that loss of VHL function alone is insufficient for ccRCC formation (27). Renal cysts are classified as benign, atypical, and malignant. HIF-1α is expressed in all VHL-deficient renal cells, whereas HIF-2α is highly expressed in renal tubular cysts and ccRCC (27).

Multiregion whole exome sequencing of four tumors from one individual with VHL disease delineated multifocal tumors of independent clonal origins (28). Each tumor exhibited a loss of chromosome 3p, each with a distinctly different breakpoint. Tumor evolution was more linear than branching compared with sporadic ccRCC, with markedly less intratumor heterogeneity. Convergent mTOR pathway activation was observed in all tumors through distinct gene mutations. The evolutionary history of 40 tumors from 6 individuals with VHL was examined by whole-genome sequencing (29). Tumors showed more genetic homogeneity than sporadically occurring tumors, which are generally removed at a later stage. However, the lack of overlapping sets of single-nucleotide variants as well as copy number variants between tumors indicated that ccRCCs evolved independently. A similar approach with different *VHL* subtypes could elucidate the effect of genetic background on the disease. For example, type 1 VHL disease (without PCC) is associated with truncation or exon deletion of germline VHL, whereas missense mutation is associated with type 2 disease (with PCC) (30). ccRCC occurs in Types 1 and 2B, which poorly downregulate HIF-1α but not 2A and 2C (6, 31).

PRECLINICAL MODELS

Tumor xenografts using human ccRCC cell lines or tissue have been extensively used in mice to evaluate potential therapies. Likewise, injecting zebrafish with patient-derived xenografts and human cell lines is a rapid, low-cost preclinical model system of cancer (32, 33). Genetically engineered animal models of biallelic mutation of *VHL* alone in both mouse and zebrafish recapitulate features of early human disease, but not the formation of ccRCC. HIF activation appears to be necessary, but not sufficient for tumor formation in animal models of ccRCC.

Initial animal models were developed by genetically modifying levels of VHL and HIFα. Homozygous deletion of *Vhl* is embryonic lethal at 10.5–12.5 days in mice due to defective placental vasculogenesis; heterozygous mice fail to develop kidney tumors (34). Kidney-specific inactivation of *Vhl* is insufficient for ccRCC development, but results in multiple cysts with constitutive HIF-α expression and metabolic alterations marked by lipid and glycogen accumulation similar to early human disease (35). Transgenic overexpression of HIF-1α or HIF-2α resulted in simple cysts (36, 37). Likewise in zebrafish embryos, homozygous inactivation of *VHL* (*vhl*$^{-/-}$) results in a kidney with enlarged proximal pronephric tubules, disorganized cilia, accumulated lipid and glycogen, cell proliferation, and apoptosis. This phenotype was rescued by a specific HIF2α inhibitor, showing that the zebrafish model system could be used to facilitate rapid screening of candidate drugs (38).

The identification of additional mutations underlying ccRCC has informed the development of genetically engineered mouse models that are more analogous to human disease. After *VHL*, the most frequently mutated genes in ccRCC were chromosome and histone regulators *PBRM1*, *SETD2*, and *BAP1* (16, 21). Epigenetic genes were targeted in recent studies. Kidney-specific dual inactivation of *Vhl* and *Bap1* or *Pbrm1* using *Pax8-Cre* in mice recapitulated human ccRCC with cytoplasmic accumulation of glycogen and lipids (39). Bap1-deficient cystic tumors were high grade, whereas Pbrm1-deficient solid tumors showed a longer latency. Pbrm1-deficient tumors were converted from low to high grade by disruption of one *Tsc1* allele, resulting in mTORC1 activation. Intriguingly, ccRCC appeared to arise from Bowman capsule cells rather than the proximal tubule based on gene inactivation using more specific *Pax8-Cre* drivers.

Kidney-specific inactivation of *Vhl* and *Pbrm1* using *Ksp-Cre* model the histopathological and molecular features, and gradual onset of human ccRCC (40). *Ksp-Cre* is expressed both in renal tubular cells and the Bowman capsule. Bilateral, multifocal tumors were marked by the clear cytoplasm, high glycogen, and carbonic anhydrase IX staining similar to human ccRCC. A stepwise progression was observed from normal to cystic lesions over 6 months, developing into multifocal ccRCC at ~10 months. Loss of PBRM1 further amplified the activation of HIF1 (hetereodimer

HIF-1α and HIF-1β) and STAT3 pathways caused by loss of *Vhl*. Activation of mTORC1 was implicated as the third event leading to ccRCC.

Inactivation of *Vhl*, *Rb1*, and *Trp53* in mice induced precursor cysts and gradually developing ccRCC tumors (41). Mutations were observed in genes involved in the primary cilium, *Kif3a* and *Kif3b*. Transcriptional analysis showed a gene expression profile similar to that observed in human ccRCC, with upregulation of HIF-1α and HIF-2α, mTOR activity. Mouse tumors showed variable response to anti-angiogenic therapy, and partial response to acriflavine, which interferes with the dimerization of HIF-1α and HIF-2α.

Zebrafish with multiple mutations of VHL disease-related genes are another potential preclinical model for exploring the progression and metastasis of ccRCC with the advantage of live imaging.

CURRENT TREATMENT STRATEGIES

Active Surveillance

Clear cell renal cell carcinomas grow slowly and small tumors <3 cm are at low risk to metastasize in VHL (42, 43). Currently, active surveillance until a threshold size of 3–4 cm is recommended for surgical intervention (43–46), resulting in a recurrence-free survival rate of 76% at 5 years and 20% at 8 years (47).

Regular screening is advised to detect RCC at an early stage and small tumors are followed with serial imaging. To improve the quality of life and survival of these patients, a balance between two goals is paramount: preventing metastases and preserving renal function. The goal is to treat before the tumor metastasizes, but to minimize consequences of the treatment such as compromised renal function. Through better surveillance by regularly scheduled imaging, individuals are living longer; however, a longer lifespan increases the probability of developing multiple RCCs and other sequelae of the disease.

Treatment of Localized Disease

Surgery

Early RCC can be detected, observed, and surgically removed before progression to metastatic disease (14, 48). However, repeated surgery for multicentric bilateral disease is followed by increased risk of ESRD requiring renal replacement therapy. Nephron-sparing surgery at a tumor size of 3–4 cm is the current treatment standard, replacing radical nephrectomy which compromised renal function and resulted in early dialysis. However, repeated partial nephrectomy reduces renal function, eventually causing ESRD. Delaying the interval to kidney surgery without increasing the risk of metastases prolongs sufficient renal function and delays dialysis. Independently of VHL disease, chronic kidney disease is associated with increased risk of death, cardiovascular events, and hospitalization (49). Progression to ESRD not only impacts quality of life but further increases morbidity—the yearly mortality rate of patients receiving long-term dialysis is 15–20% (50).

Locally recurrent disease is not uncommon after both partial nephrectomy and ablative therapy. Therapy options include observation, initial or repeat ablation, initial or repeat partial nephrectomy, radical nephrectomy, or systemic therapy (51). Salvage operation has a high major complication rate approaching 20% (52).

As renal surveillance of VHL patients has shifted surgical treatment from the resection of large tumors to the management of multiple small asymptomatic tumors, nephron-sparing therapeutic options are increasingly used. These minimally invasive procedures include percutaneous radiofrequency ablation (RFA), microwave ablation (MWA), cryoablation, and stereotactic body radiotherapy (SBRT) which are compared with surgery in **Table 2**.

Radiofrequency Ablation

Initially a treatment for non-surgical candidates, RFA has been used as a first-line procedure used to treat smaller and less numerous stage T1a lesions, and for renal salvage (46). Tumor necrosis is achieved with the heat of 50–100°C of radiofrequency energy transmitted by one or multiple needles in the tumor tissue. Placement of these needles can be achieved both laparoscopically or percutaneous (51).

Short-term local recurrence rates of RFA compare favorably with partial nephrectomy. A study of RFA treated T1 RCC reported a 13% retreatment rate for residual disease, a recurrence-free survival of 94%, and disease-free survival of 88% at 5 years (53). A study of T1a tumors treated with RFA versus partial nephrectomy reported a recurrence-free survival of 91.7 versus 94.6%, and an identical disease-free survival of 89% at 5 years (54). A recent study of 20 RCCs of 1–4 cm diameter in 9 VHL patients treated with RFA showed no recurrence and preserved

TABLE 2 | Local treatment modalities for clear cell renal cell carcinoma, including indication, frequent complications and limitations of surgery, and ablation techniques.

Treatment	Indication	Frequent complications	Limitations
Nephron-sparing surgery	Gold standard procedure	Bleeding, urinary fistula	Renal insufficiency (especially with repeated interventions)
Radiofrequency ablation	Tumor diameter <4 cm	Perirenal hematoma, postoperative fever, gross hematuria, seldom intraabdominal fistula, bowel injury	Large vessels draw in thermal energy. Large tumors
Microwave ablation	Tumor diameter <4 cm, possible in centrally located tumors	Hematuria, numbness, flank pain, thermal injury, urine fistula, subcapsular renal hemorrhage, seldom urinoma, abscess	Large tumors
Cryoablation	Tumor diameter <4 cm	Bleeding, cardiopulmonary decompensation, myocardial infarct, utero-pelvic junction obstruction	Centrally located tumors
Stereotactic body radiation	Tumor diameter 2–3 cm, not limited by tumor proximity to vessel or collecting system	Nausea, fatigue, skin rash, local pain	Nearby organs of risk (intestine, stomach) require careful planning

kidney function with a median follow-up of 102 months (55). Zagoria and colleagues concluded that long-term tumor control could be achieved in lesions treated smaller than 4 cm diameter (56). Another group reported increased risk of residual tumor for lesions >3.5 cm diameter (57). Clearly, there is a decrease of disease-free survival with every centimeter increase of the lesion (56). Although RFA is performed in many centers, conclusions about long-term efficacy are limited by the relatively short follow-up interval and small study sizes.

Microwave Ablation

Electromagnetic microwaves, transmitted from one or multiple antennas placed in the tumor can create a thermal field that causes tumor tissue necrosis (58). The antennas can be placed percutaneously, laparoscopically, or less often in an open approach. The potential benefit of Microwave Ablation (MWA) compared with RFA is that intratumoral temperatures with MWA are less affected by the heat sink effect, since MWA is less dependent on the electrical conductivity of the tissue. Larger tumors can be ablated with MWA compared to RFA; therefore, a maximum diameter of 4 cm was recommended in most studies (59–62). Several authors suggest MWA can be performed in tumors close to renal sinus or collecting system—a clear advantage over the other ablation techniques (62, 63).

Cryoablation

Cryoablation either laparoscopic or percutaneous, is a minimally invasive procedure that freezes and destroys small tumors (64–67). The cryoprobe is cooled down to −185 to −195°C by a nitrogen-based liquid guided through the tip of the probe. Cryoablation is less precise than RFA as it requires three applicators and a tumor margin of 10 mm. Thus, RFA of a 2-cm mass ablates approximately 10 cm^3 of normal tissue, whereas cryoablation treatment ablates 30 cm^3 of normal tissue (68). The location of the tumor within the kidney plays a critical role in treatment success, as centrally located tumors more frequently fail effective tumor cell destruction (69–71). Treatment failure is also significantly associated with tumor size >4 cm (72).

Stereotactic Body Radiotherapy

Stereotactic body radiotherapy (SBRT) is a method of external beam radiotherapy that precisely targets tumors with high individual doses. Multiple 3D conformal beams or intensity-modulated RT ensure the delivery of highly conformal dose distribution with a steep gradient falloff at the tumor margin to minimize injury of surrounding normal tissue (73, 74). SBRT provides superior renal tumor control compared with conventional radiation therapy, both *in vitro* and *in vivo* (75–77). Despite concerns that radiation may accelerate mutational events, stereotactic treatment of VHL tumors (primary and metastatic RCC, as well as hemangioblastomas) showed no increase in tumor formation of surrounding tissue after doses of 30–40 Gy (78–81). Two reviews reported a local control rate of over 90% for large primary RCCs and up to 98% for small tumors (82, 83). The treatment is non-invasive, with a low toxicity and mild deterioration of renal function (84). Lesions close to collecting vessels are also amenable to therapy (85). Mild side effects included nausea, fatigue, skin rash, and local pain. Similar to other ablative therapies, assessment of the long-term efficacy is limited by the short follow-up interval and small study size.

In summary, because of the lack of comparing long-term studies, partial nephrectomy for tumors of 3–4 cm diameter is still the standard of care. However, minimal-invasive physically treatment with RFA, MWA, cryoablation, and SBRT carries certain treatment advantages. The choice of resection versus ablative treatment is dependent upon the tumor localization, treatment availability, and experience of the VHL center.

Treatment of Advanced ccRCC

Advances in imaging and localized therapy have greatly improved detection and survival rates for VHL patients with early ccRCC. Currently, metastatic ccRCC is difficult to cure despite the availability of multiple systemic therapies. Before 2005, systemic therapy consisted of cytokine therapy with interleukin-2 and interferon-alpha, which was marked by severe toxicity and low response rates. Drugs that target the VHL–HIF–vascular endothelial growth factor (VEGF) pathway such as VEGF receptor inhibitors (sunitinib, sorafenib, pazopanib, and axitinib) significantly improved outcome (86–89). Bevacizumab, an anti-VEGF monoclonal antibody, was the first recombinant human monoclonal antibody that showed clinical efficacy in advanced disease (90). Today, sunitinib and pazopanib are approved first-line tyrosine kinase inhibitors for metastatic ccRCC.

Mechanistic target of rapamycin inhibitors like everolimus and temsirolimus aim at the "mechanistic target of rapamycin" complex mTORC1 which controls fundamental cellular functions such as growth, proliferation, and apoptosis. Intravenous temsirolimus was approved in 2007 following a study showing improved progressive free survival (PFS) compared with interferon alone or combination therapy with interferon and temsirolimus (91). For oral everolimus, PFS was longer in the treated group versus placebo group (92).

In 2016, cabozantinib was approved as a second-line inhibitor of VEGF receptor and a broad range of type III receptor tyrosine kinases. Both PFS and median overal survival were longer for cabozantinib treated patients versus everolimus treatment (93, 94). Levantinib, an oral multityrosine kinase, showed a synergistic effect with everolimus in patients previously pretreated for advanced ccRCC (95, 96).

Checkpoint inhibitors target "programmed cell death 1" (PD1), PD1-ligand, and cytotoxic T lymphocyte-associated protein 4 (CTLA-4) to activate T cell function. Nivolumab is a fully humanized IgG4 antibody against PD1, a negative regulator of T cell function, which improved survival in a subset of patients (97). Regardless of the targeted pathway, single agent treatment shows limited efficacy, with eventual treatment failure. Building on clinical experience favoring multiagent therapy (98), ongoing clinical trials are investigating combinations of kinase inhibitor treatments with immunotherapy, as well as combinations of immune modulators nivolumab and ipilimumab, an inhibitor of CTLA-4. A regression of metastases was observed after stereotactic radiotherapy in 4 of 28 renal cell carcinoma patients (99), suggesting that radiotherapy could enhance an immune response (98). Clinical trials testing the combination of radiotherapy with immunotherapy or targeted therapy are in progress (NCT02781506, NCT02019576, and NCT02978404).

Therapeutic options of advanced ccRCC have rapidly advanced over the past decade. Effective agents in advanced ccRCC have now been tested in earlier ccRCC stages and become appropriate first-line therapy drugs (100). Ideally, these drugs could serve as candidate perioperative agents with the potential to optimize postoperative outcome (101). In terms of precision medicine, the challenge now is to match a given patient with the optimal therapeutic agents with the help of robust molecular biomarkers.

THERAPEUTIC TARGETS AND FUTURE TRIALS

Traditional chemotherapy and conventional radiotherapy, unspecifically directed against highly proliferative cells, is poorly effective in ccRCC. Multiple dysregulated signaling pathways have recently been identified and therapies that target these pathways have shown clinical efficacy in a subset of patients. ccRCCs are highly vascular and treated by currently approved anti-angiogenic agents. Downstream components of the VHL–HIF–VEGF pathway are modulated by receptor tyrosine kinase inhibitors (axitinib, cabozantinib, levantinib, pazopanib, sorafenib, and sunitinib), as well as anti-VEGF monoclonal antibodies (bevacizumab). The PI3K/Akt/mTOR pathway is targetable by mTOR inhibitors (everolimus, temsirolimus), which reduces the accumulation of HIF protein.

Genomic profiling is a potential guide for treatment and prognosis. No predictive biomarkers have been validated for selecting treatment, but several candidate biomarkers for treatment response have been identified through retrospective patient studies using tumor DNA. For example, mutations in *MTOR*, *TSC1*, or *TSC2* were associated with response to mTOR inhibitors, 21% in responders versus 11% in non-responders (102). But many responders (56%) had no mTOR pathway mutation. A positive response to first-line everolimus was associated with *PBRM1* mutations, and a negative response with *BAP1* mutations. In addition, *KDM5* mutations were associated with better response with first-line sunitinib than with everolimus (103). These genomic biomarkers are currently being evaluated in prospective studies. Other potential biomarkers include RNA sequencing to detect structural rearrangement and transcription levels, microRNA sequencing, DNA methylation profiling, and metabolomics.

Given the inherent intratumor heterogeneity of ccRCC, therapy that targets truncal events involving *VHL* or chromosome 3p may be more effective than targeting subclonal pathways. *VHL* and *TCEB1* are mutually exclusive mutations in ccRCC, resulting in VHL complex degradation and HIFα stabilization. HIF-2α, constitutively activated in ccRCC, is mainly expressed in renal, lung, hepatic, and endothelial cells. Although transcription factors are difficult to target, a novel HIF-2α inhibitor PT2399 was recently developed which prevents binding of HIF-2α to ARNT/HIF-1β to activate a HIF-responsive promoter. Treatment with a HIF-2α inhibitor was investigated by grafting human ccRCC cell lines or patient tumor cells into nude mice, and by inactivating *vhl* in a zebrafish model.

Specific HIF-2α inhibition resulted in tumor regression in a subset of ccRCC cell line xenografts in mouse models of primary and metastatic ccRCC, in 10 of 18 patient-derived RCC xenografts in mice, and a patient with extensively pretreated metastatic ccRCC, who remained progression free for 11 months. Sensitivity to PT2399 correlated with a higher level of HIF-2α expression, and the presence of p53 (104, 105). Clinical trials with the HIF-2α inhibitor PT2385 are currently in progress (NCT02293980 and NCT03108066). Given the diversity of response, predictive biomarkers, such as HIF-2α and p53, may be useful for effective, targeted treatment. In zebrafish, treatment of $vhl^{-/-}$ embryos with a specific HIF2α inhibitor rescued pronephric abnormalities similar to human precancerous disease (38).

CONCLUSION

Genomic sequencing has revolutionized the understanding of ccRCC by identifying multiple driver genes beyond *VHL*. Genetically engineered animal models to investigate combinations of *VHL*, epigenetic, and other genes provide a powerful preclinical model for elucidating the biology of ccRCC, developing novel combinatorial therapies, and identifying candidate biomarkers for clinical validation. In particular, uncovering the molecular basis driving tumor heterogeneity and the role of epigenetic genes will identify new pathways for intervention. Insights from these model systems will be clinically applicable to both hereditary and sporadic ccRCCs.

Surveillance and surgery remain standard of care in early ccRCC, while ablative therapies provide options for alternative treatment. For early ccRCC, current recommendations for intervention based solely on size could be better informed by prognostic tumor markers indicating a potential for aggressive growth, progression, and metastasis. Non-invasive biomarkers in blood or urine would be ideal for surveillance to avoid tissue biopsy. For advanced disease, a multiagent approach is supported by both clinical and preclinical observations, and ongoing clinical trials are currently in progress to evaluate treatment regimens and prognostic genomic biomarkers. In the future, genomic profiling is likely to be augmented by transcriptional and metabolomics analysis, as well as DNA methylation status. The efficacy of targeted therapy informed by tumor profiling may be limited by intratumor and intertumor heterogeneity. Immunotherapy has the potential to circumvent the high mutational load; clinical trials are in progress with single agent and multimodal therapy, targeting multiple signaling pathways or enhancing the immune response with stereotactic radiation.

AUTHOR CONTRIBUTIONS

Both authors made substantial contribution to the work and approved the final version for publication.

FUNDING

The article processing charge was funded by the German Research Foundation (DFG) and the University of Freiburg in the funding programme Open Access Publishing.

REFERENCES

1. von Hippel E. Über eine sehr seltene Erkrankung der Netzhaut. *Graefe Arch Opthalmol* (1904) 59:83–106. doi:10.1007/BF01994821
2. Lindau A. Zur Frage der Angiomatosis Retinae und Ihrer Hirncomplikation. *Acta Ophthalmol* (1927) 4:193–226. doi:10.1111/j.1755-3768.1926.tb07786.x
3. Collins E. Intra-ocular growths. *Trans Ophthalmol Soc U K* (1894) 14:141–9.
4. Neumann HP, Wiestler OD. Clustering of features of von Hippel-Lindau syndrome: evidence for a complex genetic locus. *Lancet* (1991) 337:1052–4. doi:10.1016/0140-6736(91)91705-Y
5. Chen F, Kishida T, Yao M, Hustad T, Glavac D, Dean M, et al. Germline mutations in the von Hippel-Lindau disease tumor suppressor gene: correlations with phenotype. *Hum Mutat* (1995) 5:66–75. doi:10.1002/humu.1380050109
6. Hoffman MA, Ohh M, Yang H, Klco JM, Ivan M, Kaelin WG Jr. von Hippel-Lindau protein mutants linked to type 2C VHL disease preserve the ability to downregulate HIF. *Hum Mol Genet* (2001) 10:1019–27. doi:10.1093/hmg/10.10.1019
7. Seizinger BR, Rouleau GA, Ozelius LJ, Lane AH, Farmer GE, Lamiell JM, et al. Von Hippel-Lindau disease maps to the region of chromosome 3 associated with renal cell carcinoma. *Nature* (1988) 332:268–9. doi:10.1038/332268a0
8. Latif F, Tory K, Gnarra J, Yao M, Duh FM, Orcutt ML, et al. Identification of the von Hippel-Lindau disease tumor suppressor gene. *Science* (1993) 260:1317–20. doi:10.1126/science.8493574
9. Maher ER, Iselius L, Yates JR, Littler M, Benjamin C, Harris R, et al. Von Hippel-Lindau disease: a genetic study. *J Med Genet* (1991) 28:443–7. doi:10.1136/jmg.28.7.443
10. Binderup ML, Bisgaard ML, Harbud V, Moller HU, Gimsing S, Friis-Hansen L, et al. Von Hippel-Lindau disease (vHL). National clinical guideline for diagnosis and surveillance in Denmark. 3rd edition. *Dan Med J* (2013) 60:B4763.
11. Verein_Vhl-Betroffener_Familien_E.V. (2017). Available: http://www.hippel-lindau.de/
12. VHLAlliance. (2017). Available: www.vhl.org
13. Walther MM, Lubensky IA, Venzon D, Zbar B, Linehan WM. Prevalence of microscopic lesions in grossly normal renal parenchyma from patients with von Hippel-Lindau disease, sporadic renal cell carcinoma and no renal disease: clinical implications. *J Urol* (1995) 154:2010–4; discussion 2014–5. doi:10.1097/00005392-199512000-00007
14. Jilg CA, Neumann HP, Glasker S, Schafer O, Ardelt PU, Schwardt M, et al. Growth kinetics in von Hippel-Lindau-associated renal cell carcinoma. *Urol Int* (2012) 88:71–8. doi:10.1159/000333348
15. Schoenfeld AR, Davidowitz EJ, Burk RD. Elongin BC complex prevents degradation of von Hippel-Lindau tumor suppressor gene products. *Proc Natl Acad Sci U S A* (2000) 97:8507–12. doi:10.1073/pnas.97.15.8507
16. Sato Y, Yoshizato T, Shiraishi Y, Maekawa S, Okuno Y, Kamura T, et al. Integrated molecular analysis of clear-cell renal cell carcinoma. *Nat Genet* (2013) 45:860–7. doi:10.1038/ng.2699
17. Dalgliesh GL, Furge K, Greenman C, Chen L, Bignell G, Butler A, et al. Systematic sequencing of renal carcinoma reveals inactivation of histone modifying genes. *Nature* (2010) 463:360–3. doi:10.1038/nature08672
18. Guo G, Gui Y, Gao S, Tang A, Hu X, Huang Y, et al. Frequent mutations of genes encoding ubiquitin-mediated proteolysis pathway components in clear cell renal cell carcinoma. *Nat Genet* (2011) 44:17–9. doi:10.1038/ng.1014
19. Varela I, Tarpey P, Raine K, Huang D, Ong CK, Stephens P, et al. Exome sequencing identifies frequent mutation of the SWI/SNF complex gene PBRM1 in renal carcinoma. *Nature* (2011) 469:539–42. doi:10.1038/nature09639
20. Pena-Llopis S, Vega-Rubin-De-Celis S, Liao A, Leng N, Pavia-Jimenez A, Wang S, et al. BAP1 loss defines a new class of renal cell carcinoma. *Nat Genet* (2012) 44:751–9. doi:10.1038/ng.2323
21. Cancer Genome Atlas Research Network. Comprehensive molecular characterization of clear cell renal cell carcinoma. *Nature* (2013) 499:43–9. doi:10.1038/nature12222
22. van Haaften G, Dalgliesh GL, Davies H, Chen L, Bignell G, Greenman C, et al. Somatic mutations of the histone H3K27 demethylase gene UTX in human cancer. *Nat Genet* (2009) 41:521–3. doi:10.1038/ng.349
23. Hakimi AA, Chen YB, Wren J, Gonen M, Abdel-Wahab O, Heguy A, et al. Clinical and pathologic impact of select chromatin-modulating tumor suppressors in clear cell renal cell carcinoma. *Eur Urol* (2013) 63:848–54. doi:10.1016/j.eururo.2012.09.005
24. Gerlinger M, Rowan AJ, Horswell S, Math M, Larkin J, Endesfelder D, et al. Intratumor heterogeneity and branched evolution revealed by multiregion sequencing. *N Engl J Med* (2012) 366:883–92. doi:10.1056/NEJMoa1113205
25. Lawrence MS, Stojanov P, Polak P, Kryukov GV, Cibulskis K, Sivachenko A, et al. Mutational heterogeneity in cancer and the search for new cancer-associated genes. *Nature* (2013) 499:214–8. doi:10.1038/nature12213
26. Gerlinger M, Horswell S, Larkin J, Rowan AJ, Salm MP, Varela I, et al. Genomic architecture and evolution of clear cell renal cell carcinomas defined by multiregion sequencing. *Nat Genet* (2014) 46:225–33. doi:10.1038/ng.2891
27. Mandriota SJ, Turner KJ, Davies DR, Murray PG, Morgan NV, Sowter HM, et al. HIF activation identifies early lesions in VHL kidneys: evidence for site-specific tumor suppressor function in the nephron. *Cancer Cell* (2002) 1:459–68. doi:10.1016/S1535-6108(02)00071-5
28. Fisher R, Horswell S, Rowan A, Salm MP, De Bruin EC, Gulati S, et al. Development of synchronous VHL syndrome tumors reveals contingencies and constraints to tumor evolution. *Genome Biol* (2014) 15:433. doi:10.1186/s13059-014-0433-z
29. Fei SS, Mitchell AD, Heskett MB, Vocke CD, Ricketts CJ, Peto M, et al. Patient-specific factors influence somatic variation patterns in von Hippel-Lindau disease renal tumours. *Nat Commun* (2016) 7:11588. doi:10.1038/ncomms11588
30. Crossey PA, Richards FM, Foster K, Green JS, Prowse A, Latif F, et al. Identification of intragenic mutations in the von Hippel-Lindau disease tumour suppressor gene and correlation with disease phenotype. *Hum Mol Genet* (1994) 3:1303–8. doi:10.1093/hmg/3.8.1303
31. Clifford SC, Cockman ME, Smallwood AC, Mole DR, Woodward ER, Maxwell PH, et al. Contrasting effects on HIF-1alpha regulation by disease-causing pVHL mutations correlate with patterns of tumourigenesis in von Hippel-Lindau disease. *Hum Mol Genet* (2001) 10:1029–38. doi:10.1093/hmg/10.10.1029
32. Stoletov K, Klemke R. Catch of the day: zebrafish as a human cancer model. *Oncogene* (2008) 27:4509–20. doi:10.1038/onc.2008.95
33. Konantz M, Balci TB, Hartwig UF, Dellaire G, Andre MC, Berman JN, et al. Zebrafish xenografts as a tool for in vivo studies on human cancer. *Ann N Y Acad Sci* (2012) 1266:124–37. doi:10.1111/j.1749-6632.2012.06575.x
34. Gnarra JR, Ward JM, Porter FD, Wagner JR, Devor DE, Grinberg A, et al. Defective placental vasculogenesis causes embryonic lethality in VHL-deficient mice. *Proc Natl Acad Sci U S A* (1997) 94:9102–7. doi:10.1073/pnas.94.17.9102
35. Rankin EB, Tomaszewski JE, Haase VH. Rend cyst development in mice with conditional inactivation of the von Hippel-Lindau tumor suppressor. *Cancer Res* (2006) 66:2576–83. doi:10.1158/0008-5472.CAN-05-3241
36. Fu L, Wang G, Shevchuk MM, Nanus DM, Gudas LJ. Generation of a mouse model of von Hippel-Lindau kidney disease leading to renal cancers by expression of a constitutively active mutant of HIF1alpha. *Cancer Res* (2011) 71:6848–56. doi:10.1158/0008-5472.CAN-11-1745
37. Fu L, Wang G, Shevchuk MM, Nanus DM, Gudas LJ. Activation of HIF2alpha in kidney proximal tubule cells causes abnormal glycogen deposition but not tumorigenesis. *Cancer Res* (2013) 73:2916–25. doi:10.1158/0008-5472.CAN-12-3983
38. Noonan HR, Metelo AM, Kamei CN, Peterson RT, Drummond IA, Iliopoulos O. Loss of vhl in the zebrafish pronephros recapitulates early stages of human clear cell renal cell carcinoma. *Dis Model Mech* (2016) 9:873–84. doi:10.1242/dmm.024380
39. Gu YF, Cohn S, Christie A, Mckenzie T, Wolff N, Do QN, et al. Modeling renal cell carcinoma in mice: Bap1 and Pbrm1 inactivation drive tumor grade. *Cancer Discov* (2017) 7:900–17. doi:10.1158/2159-8290.CD-17-0292
40. Nargund AM, Pham CG, Dong Y, Wang PI, Osmangeyoglu HU, Xie Y, et al. The SWI/SNF protein PBRM1 restrains VHL-loss-driven clear cell renal cell carcinoma. *Cell Rep* (2017) 18:2893–906. doi:10.1016/j.celrep.2017.02.074
41. Harlander S, Schonenberger D, Toussaint NC, Prummer M, Catalano A, Brandt L, et al. Combined mutation in Vhl, Trp53 and Rb1 causes clear cell renal cell carcinoma in mice. *Nat Med* (2017) 23:869–77. doi:10.1038/nm.4343
42. Duffey BG, Choyke PL, Glenn G, Grubb RL, Venzon D, Linehan WM, et al. The relationship between renal tumor size and metastases in patients

with von Hippel-Lindau disease. *J Urol* (2004) 172:63–5. doi:10.1097/01.ju.0000132127.79974.3f
43. Jilg CA, Neumann HP, Glasker S, Schafer O, Leiber C, Ardelt PU, et al. Nephron sparing surgery in von Hippel-Lindau associated renal cell carcinoma; clinicopathological long-term follow-up. *Fam Cancer* (2012) 11:387–94. doi:10.1007/s10689-012-9525-7
44. Ploussard G, Droupy S, Ferlicot S, Ples R, Rocher L, Richard S, et al. Local recurrence after nephron-sparing surgery in von Hippel-Lindau disease. *Urology* (2007) 70:435–9. doi:10.1016/j.urology.2007.04.040
45. Matin SF, Ahrar K, Wood CG, Daniels M, Jonasch E. Patterns of intervention for renal lesions in von Hippel-Lindau disease. *BJU Int* (2008) 102:940–5. doi:10.1111/j.1464-410X.2008.07718.x
46. Joly D, Mejean A, Correas JM, Timsit MO, Verkarre V, Deveaux S, et al. Progress in nephron sparing therapy for renal cell carcinoma and von Hippel-Lindau disease. *J Urol* (2011) 185:2056–60. doi:10.1016/j.juro.2011.02.007
47. Roupret M, Hopirtean V, Mejean A, Thiounn N, Dufour B, Chretien Y, et al. Nephron sparing surgery for renal cell carcinoma and von Hippel-Lindau's disease: a single center experience. *J Urol* (2003) 170:1752–5. doi:10.1097/01.ju.0000092780.85876.de
48. Chittiboina P, Lonser RR. Von Hippel-Lindau disease. *Handb Clin Neurol* (2015) 132:139–56. doi:10.1016/B978-0-444-62702-5.00010-X
49. Go AS, Chertow GM, Fan D, Mcculloch CE, Hsu CY. Chronic kidney disease and the risks of death, cardiovascular events, and hospitalization. *N Engl J Med* (2004) 351:1296–305. doi:10.1056/NEJMoa041031
50. Rocco MV, Frankenfield DL, Hopson SD, Mcclellan WM. Relationship between clinical performance measures and outcomes among patients receiving long-term hemodialysis. *Ann Intern Med* (2006) 145:512–9. doi:10.7326/0003-4819-145-7-200610030-00009
51. Ljungberg B, Bensalah K, Canfield S, Dabestani S, Hofmann F, Hora M, et al. EAU guidelines on renal cell carcinoma: 2014 update. *Eur Urol* (2015) 67:913–24. doi:10.1016/j.eururo.2015.01.005
52. Johnson A, Sudarshan S, Liu J, Linehan WM, Pinto PA, Bratslavsky G. Feasibility and outcomes of repeat partial nephrectomy. *J Urol* (2008) 180:89–93; discussion 93. doi:10.1016/j.juro.2008.03.030
53. Psutka SP, Feldman AS, Mcdougal WS, Mcgovern FJ, Mueller P, Gervais DA. Long-term oncologic outcomes after radiofrequency ablation for T1 renal cell carcinoma. *Eur Urol* (2013) 63:486–92. doi:10.1016/j.eururo.2012.08.062
54. Olweny EO, Park SK, Tan YK, Best SL, Trimmer C, Cadeddu JA. Radiofrequency ablation versus partial nephrectomy in patients with solitary clinical T1a renal cell carcinoma: comparable oncologic outcomes at a minimum of 5 years of follow-up. *Eur Urol* (2012) 61:1156–61. doi:10.1016/j.eururo.2012.01.001
55. Allasia M, Soria F, Battaglia A, Gazzera C, Calandri M, Caprino MP, et al. Radiofrequency ablation for renal cancer in von Hippel-Lindau syndrome patients: a prospective cohort analysis. *Clin Genitourin Cancer* (2017). doi:10.1016/j.clgc.2017.07.027
56. Zagoria RJ, Pettus JA, Rogers M, Werle DM, Childs D, Leyendecker JR. Long-term outcomes after percutaneous radiofrequency ablation for renal cell carcinoma. *Urology* (2011) 77:1393–7. doi:10.1016/j.urology.2010.12.077
57. Iannuccilli JD, Dupuy DE, Beland MD, Machan JT, Golijanin DJ, Mayo-Smith WW. Effectiveness and safety of computed tomography-guided radiofrequency ablation of renal cancer: a 14-year single institution experience in 203 patients. *Eur Radiol* (2016) 26:1656–64. doi:10.1007/s00330-015-4006-7
58. Goldberg SN, Gazelle GS, Mueller PR. Thermal ablation therapy for focal malignancy: a unified approach to underlying principles, techniques, and diagnostic imaging guidance. *AJR Am J Roentgenol* (2000) 174:323–31. doi:10.2214/ajr.174.2.1740323
59. Li X, Liang P, Yu J, Yu XL, Liu FY, Cheng ZG, et al. Role of contrast-enhanced ultrasound in evaluating the efficiency of ultrasound guided percutaneous microwave ablation in patients with renal cell carcinoma. *Radiol Oncol* (2013) 47:398–404. doi:10.2478/raon-2013-0038
60. Moreland AJ, Ziemlewicz TJ, Best SL, Hinshaw JL, Lubner MG, Alexander ML, et al. High-powered microwave ablation of t1a renal cell carcinoma: safety and initial clinical evaluation. *J Endourol* (2014) 28:1046–52. doi:10.1089/end.2014.0190
61. Yu J, Zhang G, Liang P, Yu XL, Cheng ZG, Han ZY, et al. Midterm results of percutaneous microwave ablation under ultrasound guidance versus retroperitoneal laparoscopic radial nephrectomy for small renal cell carcinoma. *Abdom Imaging* (2015) 40:3248–56. doi:10.1007/s00261-015-0500-2
62. Gao Y, Liang P, Yu X, Yu J, Cheng Z, Han Z, et al. Microwave treatment of renal cell carcinoma adjacent to renal sinus. *Eur J Radiol* (2016) 85:2083–9. doi:10.1016/j.ejrad.2016.09.018
63. Castle SM, Salas N, Leveillee RJ. Initial experience using microwave ablation therapy for renal tumor treatment: 18-month follow-up. *Urology* (2011) 77:792–7. doi:10.1016/j.urology.2010.12.028
64. Uchida M, Imaide Y, Sugimoto K, Uehara H, Watanabe H. Percutaneous cryosurgery for renal tumours. *Br J Urol* (1995) 75:132–6; discussion 136–7. doi:10.1111/j.1464-410X.1995.tb07297.x
65. Ko YH, Choi H, Kang SG, Park HS, Lee JG, Kim JJ, et al. Efficacy of laparoscopic renal cryoablation as an alternative treatment for small renal mass in patients with poor operability: experience from the Korean single center. *J Laparoendosc Adv Surg Tech A* (2010) 20:339–45. doi:10.1089/lap.2009.0431
66. Tanagho YS, Bhayani SB, Kim EH, Figenshau RS. Renal cryoablation versus robot-assisted partial nephrectomy: Washington University long-term experience. *J Endourol* (2013) 27:1477–86. doi:10.1089/end.2013.0192
67. Georgiades CS, Rodriguez R. Efficacy and safety of percutaneous cryoablation for stage 1A/B renal cell carcinoma: results of a prospective, single-arm, 5-year study. *Cardiovasc Intervent Radiol* (2014) 37:1494–9. doi:10.1007/s00270-013-0831-8
68. Park BK, Kim CK, Park SY, Shen SH. Percutaneous radiofrequency ablation of renal cell carcinomas in patients with von Hippel Lindau disease: indications, techniques, complications, and outcomes. *Acta Radiol* (2013) 54:418–27. doi:10.1177/0284185113475441
69. Yoost TR, Clarke HS, Savage SJ. Laparoscopic cryoablation of renal masses: which lesions fail? *Urology* (2010) 75:311–4. doi:10.1016/j.urology.2009.09.038
70. Breen DJ, Bryant TJ, Abbas A, Shepherd B, Mcgill N, Anderson JA, et al. Percutaneous cryoablation of renal tumours: outcomes from 171 tumours in 147 patients. *BJU Int* (2013) 112:758–65. doi:10.1111/bju.12122
71. Yamanaka T, Yamakado K, Yamada T, Fujimori M, Takaki H, Nakatsuka A, et al. CT-guided percutaneous cryoablation in renal cell carcinoma: factors affecting local tumor control. *J Vasc Interv Radiol* (2015) 26:1147–53. doi:10.1016/j.jvir.2015.04.031
72. Kim HK, Pyun JH, Kim JY, Kim SB, Cho S, Kang SG, et al. Renal cryoablation of small renal masses: a Korea University experience. *Korean J Urol* (2015) 56:117–24. doi:10.4111/kju.2015.56.2.117
73. Lax I, Blomgren H, Naslund I, Svanstrom R. Stereotactic radiotherapy of malignancies in the abdomen. Methodological aspects. *Acta Oncol* (1994) 33:677–83. doi:10.3109/02841869409121782
74. Lo SS, Fakiris AJ, Chang EL, Mayr NA, Wang JZ, Papiez L, et al. Stereotactic body radiation therapy: a novel treatment modality. *Nat Rev Clin Oncol* (2010) 7:44–54. doi:10.1038/nrclinonc.2009.188
75. Onufrey V, Mohiuddin M. Radiation therapy in the treatment of metastatic renal cell carcinoma. *Int J Radiat Oncol Biol Phys* (1985) 11:2007–9. doi:10.1016/0360-3016(85)90285-8
76. Deschavanne PJ, Fertil B. A review of human cell radiosensitivity in vitro. *Int J Radiat Oncol Biol Phys* (1996) 34:251–66. doi:10.1016/0360-3016(95)02029-2
77. DiBiase SJ, Valicenti RK, Schultz D, Xie Y, Gomella LG, Corn BW. Palliative irradiation for focally symptomatic metastatic renal cell carcinoma: support for dose escalation based on a biological model. *J Urol* (1997) 158:746–9. doi:10.1097/00005392-199709000-00013
78. Beitler JJ, Makara D, Silverman P, Lederman G. Definitive, high-dose-per-fraction, conformal, stereotactic external radiation for renal cell carcinoma. *Am J Clin Oncol* (2004) 27:646–8. doi:10.1097/01.coc.0000145289.57705.07
79. Wersall PJ, Blomgren H, Lax I, Kalkner KM, Linder C, Lundell G, et al. Extracranial stereotactic radiotherapy for primary and metastatic renal cell carcinoma. *Radiother Oncol* (2005) 77:88–95. doi:10.1016/j.radonc.2005.03.022
80. Svedman C, Karlsson K, Rutkowska E, Sandstrom P, Blomgren H, Lax I, et al. Stereotactic body radiotherapy of primary and metastatic renal lesions for patients with only one functioning kidney. *Acta Oncol* (2008) 47:1578–83. doi:10.1080/02841860802123196
81. Asthagiri AR, Mehta GU, Zach L, Li X, Butman JA, Camphausen KA, et al. Prospective evaluation of radiosurgery for hemangioblastomas in von Hippel-Lindau disease. *Neuro Oncol* (2010) 12:80–6. doi:10.1093/neuonc/nop018

82. Siva S, Pham D, Gill S, Corcoran NM, Foroudi F. A systematic review of stereotactic radiotherapy ablation for primary renal cell carcinoma. *BJU Int* (2012) 110:E737–43. doi:10.1111/j.1464-410X.2012.11550.x
83. De Meerleer G, Khoo V, Escudier B, Joniau S, Bossi A, Ost P, et al. Radiotherapy for renal-cell carcinoma. *Lancet Oncol* (2014) 15:e170–7. doi:10.1016/S1470-2045(13)70569-2
84. Siva S, Jackson P, Kron T, Bressel M, Lau E, Hofman M, et al. Impact of stereotactic radiotherapy on kidney function in primary renal cell carcinoma: establishing a dose-response relationship. *Radiother Oncol* (2016) 118:540–6. doi:10.1016/j.radonc.2016.01.027
85. Staehler M, Bader M, Schlenker B, Casuscelli J, Karl A, Roosen A, et al. Single fraction radiosurgery for the treatment of renal tumors. *J Urol* (2015) 193:771–5. doi:10.1016/j.juro.2014.08.044
86. Escudier B, Eisen T, Stadler WM, Szczylik C, Oudard S, Siebels M, et al. Sorafenib in advanced clear-cell renal-cell carcinoma. *N Engl J Med* (2007) 356:125–34. doi:10.1056/NEJMoa060655
87. Motzer RJ, Hutson TE, Tomczak P, Michaelson MD, Bukowski RM, Rixe O, et al. Sunitinib versus interferon alfa in metastatic renal-cell carcinoma. *N Engl J Med* (2007) 356:115–24. doi:10.1056/NEJMoa065044
88. Sternberg CN, Davis ID, Mardiak J, Szczylik C, Lee E, Wagstaff J, et al. Pazopanib in locally advanced or metastatic renal cell carcinoma: results of a randomized phase III trial. *J Clin Oncol* (2010) 28:1061–8. doi:10.1200/JCO.2009.23.9764
89. Rini BI, Escudier B, Tomczak P, Kaprin A, Szczylik C, Hutson TE, et al. Comparative effectiveness of axitinib versus sorafenib in advanced renal cell carcinoma (AXIS): a randomised phase 3 trial. *Lancet* (2011) 378:1931–9. doi:10.1016/S0140-6736(11)61613-9
90. Yang JC, Haworth L, Sherry RM, Hwu P, Schwartzentruber DJ, Topalian SL, et al. A randomized trial of bevacizumab, an anti-vascular endothelial growth factor antibody, for metastatic renal cancer. *N Engl J Med* (2003) 349:427–34. doi:10.1056/NEJMoa021491
91. Hudes G, Carducci M, Tomczak P, Dutcher J, Figlin R, Kapoor, et al. Temsirolimus, Interferon alfa, or both for advanced renal-cell carcinoma. *N Engl J Med* (2007) 356:2271–81. doi:10.1056/NEJMoa066838
92. Motzer RJ, Escudier B, Oudard S, Hutson TE, Porta C, Bracarda S, et al. Phase 3 trial of everolimus for metastatic renal cell carcinoma: final results and analysis of prognostic factors. *Cancer* (2010) 116:4256–65. doi:10.1002/cncr.25219
93. Choueiri TK, Escudier B, Powles T, Mainwaring PN, Rini BI, Donskov F, et al. Cabozantinib versus everolimus in advanced renal-cell carcinoma. *N Engl J Med* (2015) 373:1814–23. doi:10.1056/NEJMoa1510016
94. Choueiri TK, Escudier B, Powles T, Tannir NM, Mainwaring PN, Rini BI, et al. Cabozantinib versus everolimus in advanced renal cell carcinoma (METEOR): final results from a randomised, open-label, phase 3 trial. *Lancet Oncol* (2016) 17:917–27. doi:10.1016/S1470-2045(16)30107-3
95. Motzer RJ, Hutson TE, Glen H, Michaelson MD, Molina A, Eisen T, et al. Lenvatinib, everolimus, and the combination in patients with metastatic renal cell carcinoma: a randomised, phase 2, open-label, multicentre trial. *Lancet Oncol* (2015) 16:1473–82. doi:10.1016/S1470-2045(15)00290-9
96. Motzer RJ, Hutson TE, Ren M, Dutcus C, Larkin J. Independent assessment of lenvatinib plus everolimus in patients with metastatic renal cell carcinoma. *Lancet Oncol* (2016) 17:e4–5. doi:10.1016/S1470-2045(15)00543-4
97. Motzer RJ, Escudier B, Mcdermott DF, George S, Hammers HJ, Srinivas S, et al. Nivolumab versus everolimus in advanced renal-cell carcinoma. *N Engl J Med* (2015) 373:1803–13. doi:10.1056/NEJMoa1510665
98. Twyman-Saint Victor C, Rech AJ, Maity A, Rengan R, Pauken KE, Stelekati E, et al. Radiation and dual checkpoint blockade activate non-redundant immune mechanisms in cancer. *Nature* (2015) 520:373–7. doi:10.1038/nature14292
99. Wersall PJ, Blomgren H, Pisa P, Lax I, Kalkner KM, Svedman C. Regression of non-irradiated metastases after extracranial stereotactic radiotherapy in metastatic renal cell carcinoma. *Acta Oncol* (2006) 45:493–7. doi:10.1080/02841860600604611
100. Choueiri TK, Halabi S, Sanford BL, Hahn O, Michaelson MD, Walsh MK, et al. Cabozantinib versus sunitinib as initial targeted therapy for patients with metastatic renal cell carcinoma of poor or intermediate risk: the alliance A031203 CABOSUN trial. *J Clin Oncol* (2017) 35:591–7. doi:10.1200/JCO.2016.70.7398
101. Ravaud A, Motzer RJ, Pandha HS, George DJ, Pantuck AJ, Patel A, et al. Adjuvant sunitinib in high-risk renal-cell carcinoma after nephrectomy. *N Engl J Med* (2016) 375:2246–54. doi:10.1056/NEJMoa1611406
102. Kwiatkowski DJ, Choueiri TK, Fay AP, Rini BI, Thorner AR, De Velasco G, et al. Mutations in TSC1, TSC2, and mTOR are associated with response to rapalogs in patients with metastatic renal cell carcinoma. *Clin Cancer Res* (2016) 22:2445–52. doi:10.1158/1078-0432.CCR-15-2631
103. Hsieh JJ, Chen D, Wang PI, Marker M, Redzematovic A, Chen YB, et al. Genomic biomarkers of a randomized trial comparing first-line everolimus and sunitinib in patients with metastatic renal cell carcinoma. *Eur Urol* (2017) 71:405–14. doi:10.1016/j.eururo.2016.10.007
104. Chen W, Hill H, Christie A, Kim MS, Holloman E, Pavia-Jimenez A, et al. Targeting renal cell carcinoma with a HIF-2 antagonist. *Nature* (2016) 539:112–7. doi:10.1038/nature19796
105. Cho H, Du X, Rizzi JP, Liberzon E, Chakraborty AA, Gao W, et al. On-target efficacy of a HIF-2alpha antagonist in preclinical kidney cancer models. *Nature* (2016) 539:107–11. doi:10.1038/nature19795

17

Treatment of Genetic Forms of Nephrotic Syndrome

Markus J. Kemper[1] *and Anja Lemke*[2*]

[1] *AK Nord Heidberg, Asklepios Medical School GmbH, Hamburg, Germany,* [2] *Universitätsklinikum Hamburg-Eppendorf, Hamburg, Germany*

Correspondence:
Anja Lemke
lemke_anja@gmx.de

Idiopathic steroid-resistant nephrotic syndrome (SRNS) is most frequently characterized by focal segmental glomerulosclerosis (FSGS) but also other histological lesions, such as diffuse mesangial sclerosis. In the past two decades, a multitude of genetic causes of SRNS have been discovered raising the question of effective treatment in this cohort. Although no controlled studies are available, this review will discuss treatment options including pharmacologic interventions aiming at the attenuation of proteinuria in genetic causes of SRNS, such as inhibitors of the renin–angiotensin–aldosterone system and indomethacin. Also, the potential impact of other interventions to improve podocyte stability will be addressed. In this respect, the treatment with cyclosporine A (CsA) is of interest, since a podocyte stabilizing effect has been demonstrated in various experimental models. Although clinical response to CsA in children with genetic forms of SRNS is inferior to sporadic SRNS, some recent studies show that partial and even complete response can be achieved even in individual patients inherited forms of nephrotic syndrome. Ideally, improved pharmacologic and molecular approaches to induce partial or even complete remission will be available in the future, thus slowing or even preventing the progression toward end-stage renal disease.

Keywords: steroid-resistiant nephrotic syndrome, mutations, cyclosporine, treatment, congenital nephrotic syndrome, Wilms tumor suppressor Gene 1, NPHS1, podocytes

INTRODUCTION

For many years, steroid-resistant nephrotic syndrome (SRNS), especially focal segmental glomerulosclerosis (FSGS) was thought to be an immunological disorder. This concept was supported by the response to immunosuppression in many patients and by the fact that recurrence after renal transplantation occurred, possibly due to the presence of a humoral factor, e.g., produced by the immune system (1) However, it is now known that a significant proportion of patients with SRNS [FSGS, but also diffuse mesangial sclerosis (DMS)] have an inherited cause of the nephrotic syndrome (NS), e.g., affecting structural proteins such as nephrin or podocin (2). At first sight, immunosuppression in such patients with inherited structural defects of the podocytes makes no sense. Yet, clinical observations, typically made in patients who were treated with immunosuppression as the genetic result was not yet available, show that a subset of patients does achieve partial or complete remission associated with such treatment. This raises the issue of optimal treatment in this cohort. Should all patients receive immunosuppressive treatment and if so, for how long and in what form? Are their clinical characteristics that can guide treatment? In general, prospective studies addressing this issue have never been performed and evidence pro -and contra- have been generated by retrospective series. Also, treatment options beyond immunosuppression (supportive and pharmacologic) have never been addressed prospectively, which is not surprising due to the rarity, severity, and heterogeneity of the diseases involved.

General Considerations

Several factors have to be considered before choosing treatment for genetic causes of SRNS. First, the age of presentation and severity of initial symptoms is of utmost importance. In this respect, patients with congenital and infantile NS are probably the most problematic group, because children often present with severe symptoms, sometimes antenatally (3). Historically, the so called "Finnish" type of NS is a good example and aggressive treatment led to a dramatic improvement of survival and long-term-outcome (4). Although patients presenting with infantile NS (onset in the first year of life) have a high risk of carrying a monogenic mutation (5), it should be noted that some patients can have a good prognosis reaching remission with supportive treatment alone (6); individual patients may in fact have minimal change disease responding to steroids. Thus, not only genetic testing but also renal biopsy should be considered in this group.

Second, genetic testing results need to be considered for treatment. Although only mutations in few genes are frequent, there are now panels available testing for 30 or more genes and it can be assumed that there will be new genetic causes in the future. This implies a clinical heterogeneity, not only among identical but also between different genotypes. In this respect, it needs to be at least mentioned that there is often a delay in getting results of genetic testing, which often takes weeks, sometimes months (and sometimes years because new variants are to be detected). Some patients with a negative initial test result may have a yet undiscovered monogenetic cause, and this has implications in choosing a therapeutic approach.

The last problem arises from the fact that there is no universal consensus regarding the definition of treatment response. A (rapid) complete remission of proteinuria is the ideal situation and will generally be accepted without any discussion. However, the definition of partial remission is much more problematic. Fluctuations of proteinuria are difficult to evaluate as they can occur with and without treatment. Most authors would agree that a reduction of proteinuria, for instance, by 50% can be regarded as partial remission, others would demand a concomitant increase of serum-albumin with cessation of edema, which obviously is of greater clinical relevance. There is also no consensus on how to exactly assess the impact of treatment on glomerular filtration rate (GFR) and renal survival.

Supportive and Non-Immunologic Treatment for Genetic Causes of NS

Congenital and Infantile NS

The prognosis of congenital NS has improved substantially in recent years. No differences in mortality and transplant outcome between Finnish and non-Finnish patients with *NPHS1* mutations was noted in a recent registry report on 170 patients (4). Finnish patients started dialysis much earlier because of early bilateral nephrectomy, while in non-Finnish, many other interventions were performed (but not reported on in detail). Despite this, outcome of *NPHS1* patients on renal replacement therapy in fact compared to patients with congenital anomalies of the kidney and urinary tract (CAKUT). No details of treatment approaches and mortality prior end-stage renal disease are presented however. These may influence morbidity and mortality in patients with *NPHS1* and other genetic causes, however and include the following options.

Albumin Infusions

In severe forms of congenital but also infantile NS regular (mostly daily) albumin infusions have been recommended to decrease edema, increase urine output, and enhance nutrition (7). This strategy requires sufficient renal function; otherwise, fluid overload may occur with potentially severe consequences, such as cardiac failure or pulmonary edema. Since infusions have to be performed regularly, often daily, a central venous access is usually necessary with the associated risks of infection, thrombosis, and hospitalization. Of interest, a recent report by Reynolds et al. (7) showed that after adequate training, administration of albumin can be performed at home, which has an important impact on quality of life. Unfortunately, in reports on regular albumin infusions, other treatments have been used as well (see below). In a yet unpublished French study, 96% of patients received albumin infusions initially daily, with a subsequent reduction in frequency in many patients. It was even discontinued in 10 patients. However, in this report, data about concomitant drug treatment are not available (Berody et al. accepted by NDT, complete citation expected to be available in February).

Nephrectomy

Unilateral or even bilateral nephrectomy has been used as therapeutic option to decrease or stop proteinuria. Bilateral nephrectomy is probably the most aggressive approach, which will on the one hand completely stop proteinuria, normalize protein and lipid status, and improve nutritional state, but on the other, make (peritoneal) dialysis treatment inevitable (3). Unilateral nephrectomy has been advocated by some authors to reduce proteinuria in children with congenital NS, again often in addition with medical treatment (indomethacin and captopril). In one study (8), serum albumin (sAlb) increased from 11 to 18 g/l after 6–12 months and the number of albumin infusions could be reduced later. This series of five patients also documented an increase in height standard deviation score.

Renin–Angiotensin–Aldosterone System (RAAS) Inhibitors (With/Without Indomethacin)

A further more conservative approach is drug treatment in order to reduce GFR and thus decrease proteinuria. The value of inhibiting the RAAS by ACE inhibitors (ACEI) and angiotensin receptor blockers (ARBS) in proteinuric renal diseases has been established for many years (9), starting from studies of IgA nephritis. Therefore, in clinical practice, RAAS inhibitors are widely used frequently even in the absence of hypertension. The mechanisms of action relate to decreasing intraglomerular pressure as well as anti-TGFβ properties leading to deceleration of the progression of renal insufficiency. The Cochrane group (9) included RAAS inhibitors in their recommendations for treatment of SRNS but no large studies concerning their use in congenital or infantile NS are available. In one (8), RAAS inhibitors were combined with indomethacin and unilateral nephrectomy. Licht et al. (10) used a stepwise approach: five patients with different causes of congenital NS were treated with captopril and indomethacin serum protein and growth improved in four children. Unilateral nephrectomy was only deemed necessary in two patients during the subsequent course.

Although published evidence is limited, these studies support a stepwise approach in a clinically stable patient with congenital/infantile NS starting with the use of RAAS inhibitors. In neonates and infants, captopril has been most frequently used and can be titrated best. In severe cases, a combination with indomethacin seems justified; if edema are controlled by this approach (unilateral), nephrectomy can be avoided.

Non-Immunologic Treatment in Pediatric and Adolescent Genetic SRNS

Presentation of SRNS after the neonatal period usually leads to a different approach, because the underlying genotype and histological lesions are typically different; *NPHS2* mutations are probably the most frequent single genetic cause (2). Bilateral or unilateral nephrectomy is only practiced in individual severe cases. Treatment with steroids usually has been initiated prior diagnosis and—per definition—failed. Since results of genetic testing are not available immediately in many patients, further treatment, e.g., with calcineurin-inhibitors will be considered and initiated, except maybe in syndromic SRNS. In most published registries (11–13), patients with genetic nephrotic syndrome had received immunosuppressive treatment.

As in congenital and infantile NS, treatment with RAAS inhibitors are a possibility to decrease proteinuria, slow progression of chronic kidney disease, and treat hypertension. RAAS inhibitors are often used in combination with immunosuppressants in glomerulonephrits and NS, although few systematic studies are available evaluating the isolated or combined treatment. As mentioned before, RAAS inhibitors are recommended by the Cochrane group (9) because of two studies. Yi et al. (14) treated SRNS patients with fosinopril and prednisone and compared to a group receiving prednisone alone. Proteinuria decreased significantly in both groups but more in the fosinopril-treated patients. Bagga et al. (15) studied the effect of enalapril at high and low doses showing that there is a dose-related reduction in proteinuria. The benefits of a combined treatment of ACEI and ARBS was suggested by small prospective study in eight patients with SRNS (16). One case report documented complete remission with captopril; regular albumin infusions could be stopped at the age of 15 months (17). Combined antiproteinuric therapy with RAAS inhibitors was also able to induce complete remission in a patient with Nail–Patella syndrome and NS (18). Although all these studies are small and data on genetic causes are not always provided, the long experience with RAAS inhibitors in children would probably be in favor for early use of these drugs in pediatric patients, especially since they are tolerated well and can also be used for associated hypertension. Nevertheless, more controlled data are desirable. Of interest, a current controlled study comparing sparsetan (a dual acting angiotensin receptor blocker and highly selective endotheline Type A receptor antagonist) with irbesartan has been initiated in FSGS to assess the impact also in genetic forms of NS (19).

OTHER OPTIONS

In individual patients with FSGS (mainly with permeability factor associated NS), treatment with galactose had been reported to be beneficial. Trachtman et al. (20) evaluated treatment of FSGS with a TNF- α inhibiting antibody adalimumab and galactose, the latter being an intersting non-immunologic treatment option also for genetic forms of FSGS. In the cited study, 2 out of 7 patients with FSGS had a 50% reduction in proteinuria after galactose, confirming previous case reports. Data on genetic testing in patients are not available, so no definite conclusion about the utility of galactose in genetic SRNS can be drawn. Unfortunately, a controlled trial with a monoclonal anti-TGF-β antibody (fresolimumab) in SRNS did not lead to a significant reduction in proteinuria (21).

Similarly, the use of vitamin D analogs and stimulation of the calcium-sensing receptor has been assessed. Experimental studies have shown that stimulation of the calcium-sensing-receptor enhances podocyte stability and thus cinacalcet (or vitamin D) may be an option to improve proteinuria in NS (22). So far, data on cinacalcet are not available, but a recent meta-analysis in IgA nephropathy suggested an effect of vitamin D supplementation (23). However, a recent randomized controlled trial of vitamin D supplementation in steroid-sensitive NS did not reduce relapse rate, arguing against a direct podocyte stabilizing effect of vitamin D (24). Although definitive conclusions of these alternative approaches cannot be drawn, future studies into the field of podocyte stabilization by non-immunosuppressive drugs are warranted and could have an important impact on treatment in genetic SRNS.

Immunosuppression in Hereditary SRNS

Evidence from Experimental Studies

Several experimental studies have suggested that immunosuppressants have a direct glomerular effect leading to podocyte stabilization and thus have efficacy beyond their immunological actions. Some agents, such as cyclosporine also have a hemodynamic (nephrotoxic) effect leading, e.g., to reduction of GFR, thereby reducing proteinuria (25).

The initial studies confirming a stabilization of the glomerular cytoskeleton by cyclosporine independent of the immunosuppressive action was provided by Faul et al. (26) and confirmed by various other studies that will not be described in detail (27). Also, steroids, levamisole, mechanistic target of Rapamycin (mTOR) inhibitors, and even Rituximab have received attention in experimental studies although clinical data are virtually non-existent. For instance, glucocorticoids have been shown to protect and enhance recovery of cultured murine podocytes *via* actin filament stabilization (28, 29). Levamisole, a drug that has never been used in SRNS, was able to induce expression of glucocorticoid receptor (GR) and to activate GR signaling and also protected against podocyte injury in a cell model (30). Also, low-dose rapamycin, an inhibitor of the mTOR, diminished disease progression in an experimental model of FSGS (31). Finally, rituximab, a B-cell-depleting antibody, may bind directly on sphingomyelin phosphodiesterase acid-like 3b protein (SMPDL3b), and thus could have an effect at the cellular level (32).

In summary, there is now emerging evidence that immunosuppressants, especially cyclosporine A (CsA), have a stabilizing effect at the podocyte levels aside from their immunological actions in experimental models and thus may be valuable therapeutic options in the treatment also of genetic forms of SRNS.

CLINICAL DATA ON IMMUNOSUPPRESSANTS IN GENETIC NS

Most authors would agree that children with *NPHS2* mutations do not respond to treatment with steroids (33). However, in their first report on mutations in the *Plectin1 (PLEC1) gene*, the authors mention two patients who responded to prednisolone treatment (34). This could not be confirmed from a French series (35); interestingly, the authors report on three unaffected and unrelated patients with homozygous PLCE1 mutations but without clinical disease. Thus, the natural history of SRNS with PLEC1 mutations may be different and modifier genes and environmental factors may play a role. There are no data, whether patients with SRNS and other mutations have a documented partial or complete remission after initial steroid treatment.

To our knowledge, no data on treatment with mycophenolate mofetil (MMF) are available in genetic NS. Unfortunately, in a randomized US study comparing MMF with cyclosporine, genetic testing was not performed (36). In contrast, data on treatment with calcineurin inhibitors (mainly CsA) in cohorts with genetic SRNS have been published; in most of these studies, genetic diagnosis was confirmed *post hoc*, sometimes after years. Unfortunately, response to treatment interventions is often not detailed and sometimes interpretations are superficial.

In two studies from Buscher et al. (12, 13), the vast majority of patients with genetic FSGS did not achieve remission with cyclosporine. In the first study on 91 patients, mutation in 1 of 6 genes studied were detected in 52% of patients. None of the patients with mutations showed a complete response to CsA, but two patients with Wilms tumor suppressor gene 1 (*WT1*) mutation showed partial remission. The response rate of CSA was significantly better without mutations in podocyte genes (68 vs. 17%, $p < 0.005$). In the second, larger retrospective multicenter study by Buscher et al., 131/231 patients with SRNS had an identified genetic diagnosis, including 60 patients with congenital NS; of these, 63 (48%) patients had received CSA. 2 patients (1 with congenital NS, CNS) entered complete and 5 partial remission (none with CNS). In summary, this series documents a partial or complete response to CSA in 19% of hereditary SRNS (with no details on genotype stated) and 1.7% of congenital NS.

In a recent report from the Podonet consortium, 906/1,354 patients with SRNS were treated with immunosuppressants (380 with one, 173 with two, and 59 with three or more different, respectively) (11). Among 74 patients with documented genetic diagnosis, two patients had complete and 8 partial remission, respectively. Another four patients entered partial remission with a combination of CSA and RAAS inhibitor. Thus, in this series, a total of 14/74 (19%) patients with genetic SRNS seemed to have a response to immunosuppression.

In our own retrospective single center study (37) of nine SRNS patients with an identified genetic diagnosis (excluding patients with CNS, *WT1* mutations, and syndromic NS), we observed a partial (2 patients with *NPHS2* mutations) or complete (one patient with compound heterozygous *NPHS1* and one with a dominant *ACTN4* mutation, respectively) remission. Thus 4/9 (44%) showed some response to CSA; **Figure 1** demonstrates evolution of serum-albumin levels in two patients with a complete and partial response, respectively.

Currently, no controlled data are available as to how long CSA treatment in genetic forms of SRNS should be continued, if no response is documented. The series by Klaassen et al. (12, 13, 37), however, show that most patients with complete remission responded after a median of 2 months, so that this treatment period seems to be a minimum. It is currently unknown, whether patients with distinct mutation, e.g., in *WT1* or *NPHS2* show a differential response.

EXPERIENCES IN SPECIFIC GENETIC DISORDERS

WT1-Mutations

The Wilms Tumor Suppressor Gene 1 (WT1) is a transcription factor with many functions, among them transcriptional as well as tumor-suppressor activities. WT1 plays a pivotal role in early urogenital and kidney development (38), in adults, it continues to be a key regulator of podocyte function (39). Mutations in *WT1* mostly occur as spontaneous heterozygous germline mutations, but familiar cases are also described. Type and location of specific mutations allow for limited prediction of clinical course, histology, and comorbidities (40). By far, not all patients show all symptoms of the classical syndromal descriptions associated with *WT1* mutation: Denys–Drash syndrome described in patients with missense mutations, it includes DMS, SRNS rapidly progressing to end-stage renal disease, XY disorder in sex development with complete gonadal dysgenesis, and a high risk of developing Wilms' tumor. Frazier Syndrome is typically caused by mutations affecting the canonic donor splice site of intron 9, patients present with streak gonads, and are at high risk of developing gonadoblastoma.

There is evidence from studies with small patient numbers that early initiation of treatment with CsA in combination with RAAS inhibitors can lead to favorable response of NS in patients with *WT1* mutations (41). Gellermann et al. report on three children with WT1 mutations and FSGS in whom long-term reduction of proteinuria could be achieved through treatment with CSA in combination with steroids and RAAS inhibitors while maintaining normal renal function (42). Wasilewska et al. describe a patient with *WT1* mutation and DMS on histology in whom nephrotic range proteinuria resolved after initiation of treatment with CSA and enalapril (43). Buscher et al. report two patients affected by NS due to mutations in *WT1* showing a partial response to CsA with a reduction of proteinuria and normalization of sAlb (13). Unfortunately, in their 2016 study, Buscher et al. do not give details on their patients with *WT1* mutations treated with CSA (12). Further studies are needed to define in more detail which patients with *WT1* mutations (type of mutation and histological changes) can benefit from immunosuppressive treatment with

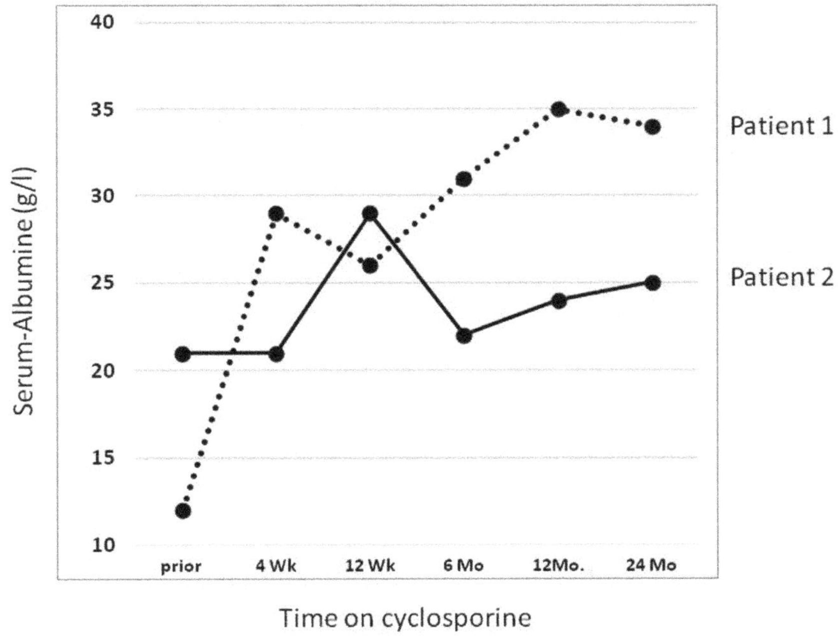

FIGURE 1 | Effect of cyclosporine treatment on evolution of serum albumin (sAlb) levels. Detailed data on two patients reported by Klaassen et al. (37). Dashed line: Patient 1 with compound heterozygous *NPHS1* mutation (c.928G > A, p.Asp310Asn; c.2816-3T > G, p.?) rapidly showed complete remission with concomitant normalization of sAlb. Solid line: Patient 2 with a homozygous *NPHS2* mutation (NPHS2: c.467dupT, p.Leu156Phefs*11) achieved partial remission and albumin infusions were discontinued. He reached ESRD after 5.0 years.

CSA. Mechanisms mediating the benefits of CSA, other than stabilizing podocyte cytoskeleton, in patients with disturbed WT1 expression also need further elucidation (41). Collection of patients with *WT1*-mutations in a prospective registry has been initiated by the German Society of Pediatric Nephrology (GPN).

Coenzyme Q_{10} (CoQ_{10})-Deficiency

CoQ_{10}, also known as ubiquinone, is involved in many essential cellular processes, especially in the mitochondria. Its biosynthesis requires at least 15 genes. So far, mutations in eight of these genes have been found to cause primary CoQ_{10} deficiency, which results in diseases with variable age of onset. Associated clinical phenotypes are ranging from a multisystem disease to nephropathy or isolated central nervous system disease (myopathy or cerebellar ataxia) (44). Nephropathy can result in steroid resistant NS and loss of renal function in an isolated form (45) or in combination with sensorineural deafness (46) or other neurological symptoms (47).

In contrast to most mitochondrial respiratory chain disorders, for which there is no effective treatment, patients with primary CoQ_{10} deficiency partially respond to oral CoQ_{10} supplementation (48). *In vitro* data and first clinical experiences suggest that high-dose oral treatment with CoQ_{10} has the potential to stop the progression of encephalopathy, muscular symptoms, and NS and even induce remission, if initiated early enough. Heeringa et al. (46) describe proteinuria and hearing loss in patients with coenzyme Q_{10} biosynthesis monooxygenase (*COQ6*)-mutations. *In vitro*, apoptosis caused by *COQ6*-knockdown was partially reversed by CoQ_{10} treatment. The authors report a positive response to treatment with CoQ_{10} and RAAS inhibitors in two children with mild disease. Ashraf et al. (49) describe that mutations in the aarF domain containing kinase 4 gene (ADCK4) leads to CoQ_{10} deficiency causing SRNS. Knockdown of *ADCK4* in podocytes resulted in decreased migration, which was reversed by CoQ10 addition. Indeed, one individual with *ADCK4*-mutation was successfully treated with CoQ_{10} supplementation. Once severe kidney or neurological damage is established, this cannot be reversed (47, 48).

Gene Therapy in Genetic Forms of SRNS

So far, no successful gene therapeutic approaches have been reported for hereditary forms of SRNS. However, a mouse model for NPHS2 has recently been reported (50) and may have important consequences also for the development of specific molecular treatment approaches. Other investigations have indicated a role of specific miRNAs in the etiology of FSGS, which may be amenable to specific treatment (51). Taken together, studies into the molecular biology of SRNS have a yet undiscovered potential to develop new treatment modalities and potentially a cure for certain genetic forms of SRNS.

SUMMARY

Although no adequate systematic treatment studies have been performed in patients with genetic forms of NS, choice of treatment needs to consider clinical factors (e.g., severity of clinical presentation and age of presentation). In a clinically stable patient with congenital/infantile NS, use of an RAAS inhibitor could be

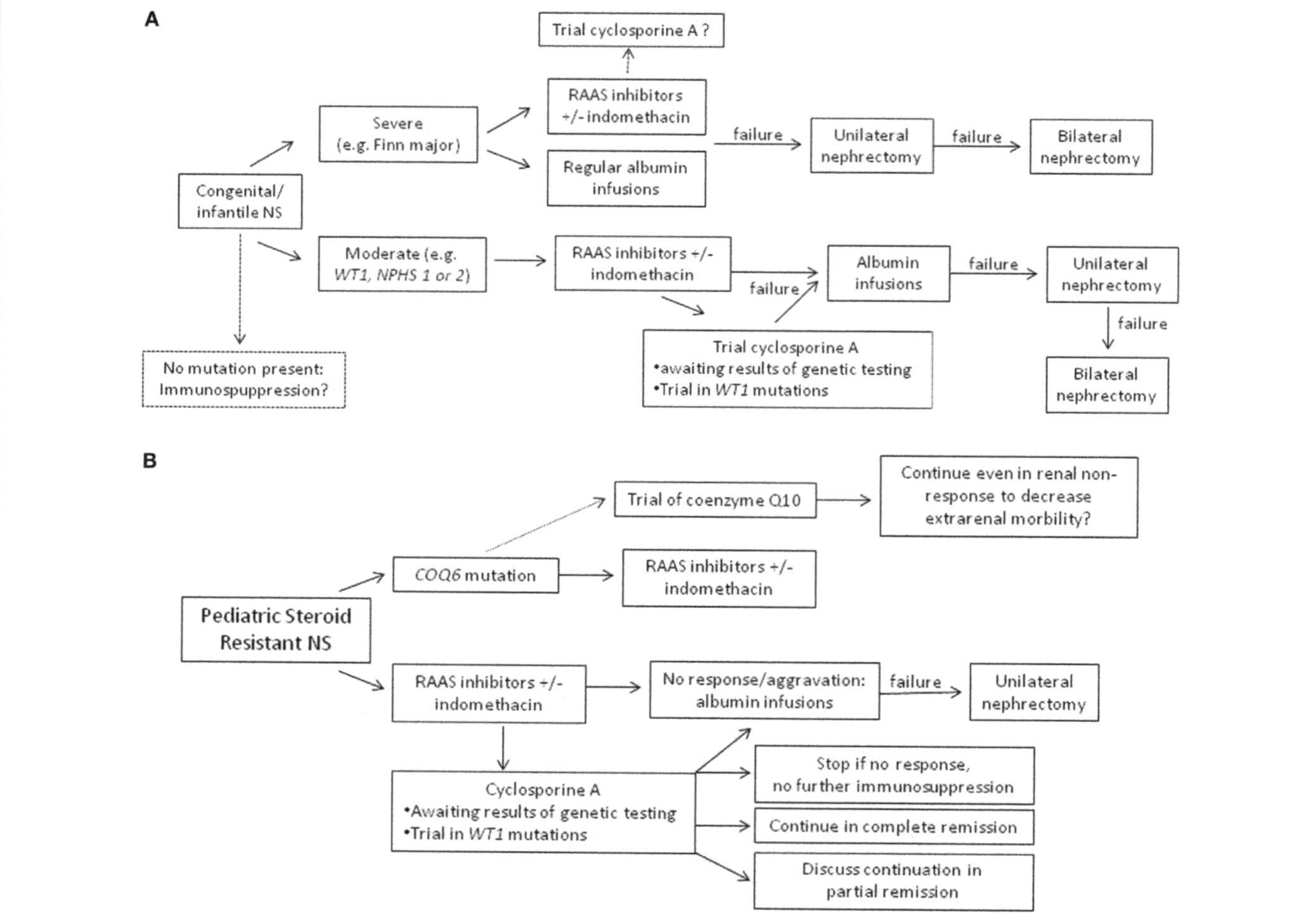

FIGURE 2 | Suggestion of an algorithm for treatment in genetic nephrotic syndrome (NS). **(A)** Congenital and infantile NS with positive testing results. **(B)** Pediatric steroid-resistant nephrotic syndrome, where often, results of genetic testing are not available immediately.

first choice. In neonates and infants, captopril has been most frequently used and can be titrated best. In severe cases, a combination of RAAS inhibitor with indomethacin seems appropriate in order to avoid (unilateral or even bilateral) nephrectomy, which is an effective option in severely affected individuals. In steroid-resistant NS patients, most patients with Mendelian forms seem resistant to immunosuppressive treatment. Yet, several studies have shown that in some patients, a complete or partial remission with CSA can be achieved also in hereditary SRNS, including patients with infantile nephrotic syndrome (**Figure 2**). Therefore, in our opinion, a therapeutic trial with CSA in genetic SRNS is justified, since especially CSA has been shown to exert a relevant podocyte stabilizing effect, which may reduce proteinuria in some patients. In the future, more clinical studies of optimal treatment of genetic SRNS are necessary, also evaluating the impact of confounding factors, such as genotype/phenotype correlations, impact of attenuation of proteinuria on rate of progression into ESRD, and others. Ultimately, gene therapy will hopefully be available in the future offering a specific cure of (some) genetic causes of steroid resistant NS.

AUTHOR CONTRIBUTIONS

MK wrote the first draft of the manuscript; AL wrote sections of the manuscript. Both authors contributed to manuscript revision, read, and approved the submitted version.

REFERENCES

1. Kemper MJ, Valentin L, van Husen M. Difficult-to-treat idiopathic nephrotic syndrome: established drugs, open questions and future options. *Pediatr Nephrol* (2017). doi:10.1007/s00467-017-3780-7
2. Sadowski CE, Lovric S, Ashraf S, Pabst WL, Gee HY, Kohl S, et al. A single-gene cause in 29.5% of cases of steroid-resistant nephrotic syndrome. *J Am Soc Nephrol* (2015) 26(6):1279–89. doi:10.1681/ASN.2014050489
3. Holmberg C, Antikainen M, Ronnholm K, Ala Houhala M, Jalanko H. Management of congenital nephrotic syndrome of the Finnish type. *Pediatr Nephrol* (1995) 9(1):87–93. doi:10.1007/BF00858984
4. Holtta T, Bonthuis M, Van Stralen KJ, Bjerre A, Topaloglu R, Ozaltin F, et al. Timing of renal replacement therapy does not influence survival and growth in children with congenital nephrotic syndrome caused by mutations in NPHS1: data from the ESPN/ERA-EDTA Registry. *Pediatr Nephrol* (2016) 31(12):2317–25. doi:10.1007/s00467-016-3517-z

5. Hinkes BG, Mucha B, Vlangos CN, Gbadegesin R, Liu J, Hasselbacher K, et al. Nephrotic syndrome in the first year of life: two thirds of cases are caused by mutations in 4 genes (NPHS1, NPHS2, WT1, and LAMB2). *Pediatrics* (2007) 119(4):e907–19. doi:10.1542/peds.2006-2164
6. Kim JJ, Clothier J, Sebire NJ, Milford DV, Moghal N, Trompeter RS. Nephrotic syndrome in infancy can spontaneously resolve. *Pediatr Nephrol* (2011) 26(10):1897–901. doi:10.1007/s00467-011-1911-0
7. Reynolds BC, Pickles CW, Lambert HJ, Ognjanovic M, Crosier J, Johnson SA, et al. Domiciliary administration of intravenous albumin in congenital nephrotic syndrome. *Pediatr Nephrol* (2015) 30(11):2045–50. doi:10.1007/s00467-015-3177-4
8. Kovacevic L, Reid CJ, Rigden SP. Management of congenital nephrotic syndrome. *Pediatr Nephrol* (2003) 18(5):426–30. doi:10.1007/s00467-003-1131-3
9. Hodson EM, Wong SC, Willis NS, Craig JC. Interventions for idiopathic steroid-resistant nephrotic syndrome in children. *Cochrane Database Syst Rev* (2016) 10:CD003594. doi:10.1002/14651858.CD003594.pub5
10. Licht C, Eifinger F, Gharib M, Offner G, Michalk DV, Querfeld U. A stepwise approach to the treatment of early onset nephrotic syndrome. *Pediatr Nephrol* (2000) 14(12):1077–82. doi:10.1007/s004670000386
11. Trautmann A, Schnaidt S, Lipska-Zietkiewicz BS, Bodria M, Ozaltin F, Emma F, et al. Long-term outcome of steroid-resistant nephrotic syndrome in children. *J Am Soc Nephrol* (2017) 28(10):3055–65. doi:10.1681/ASN.2016101121
12. Buscher AK, Beck BB, Melk A, Hoefele J, Kranz B, Bamborschke D, et al. Rapid response to cyclosporin A and favorable renal outcome in nongenetic versus genetic steroid-resistant nephrotic syndrome. *Clin J Am Soc Nephrol* (2016) 11(2):245–53. doi:10.2215/CJN.07370715
13. Buscher AK, Kranz B, Buscher R, Hildebrandt F, Dworniczak B, Pennekamp P, et al. Immunosuppression and renal outcome in congenital and pediatric steroid-resistant nephrotic syndrome. *Clin J Am Soc Nephrol* (2010) 5(11): 2075–84. doi:10.2215/CJN.01190210
14. Yi Z, Li Z, Wu XC, He QN, Dang XQ, He XJ. Effect of fosinopril in children with steroid-resistant idiopathic nephrotic syndrome. *Pediatr Nephrol* (2006) 21(7):967–72. doi:10.1007/s00467-006-0096-4
15. Bagga A, Mudigoudar BD, Hari P, Vasudev V. Enalapril dosage in steroid-resistant nephrotic syndrome. *Pediatr Nephrol* (2004) 19(1):45–50. doi:10.1007/s00467-003-1314-y
16. Supavekin S, Surapaitoolkorn W, Tancharoen W, Pattaragarn A, Sumboonnanonda A. Combined renin angiotensin blockade in childhood steroid-resistant nephrotic syndrome. *Pediatr Int* (2012) 54(6):793–7. doi:10.1111/j.1442-200X.2012.03668.x
17. Soliman NA, Francis M, Heeringa SF, Chernin G. Complete remission of nephrotic syndrome in an infant with focal segmental glomerulosclerosis: is it renin-angiotensin blockade? *Pediatr Nephrol* (2009) 24(5):1065–70. doi:10.1007/s00467-008-1026-4
18. Proesmans W, Van Dyck M, Devriendt K. Nail-patella syndrome, infantile nephrotic syndrome: complete remission with antiproteinuric treatment. *Nephrol Dial Transplant* (2009) 24(4):1335–8. doi:10.1093/ndt/gfn725
19. Komers R, Gipson DS, Nelson P, Adler S, Srivastava T, Derebail VK, et al. Efficacy and safety of Sparsentan compared with Irbesartan in patients with primary focal segmental glomerulosclerosis: randomized, controlled trial design (DUET). *Kidney Int Rep* (2017) 2(4):654–64. doi:10.1016/j.ekir.2017.02.019
20. Trachtman H, Fervenza FC, Gipson DS, Heering P, Jayne DR, Peters H, et al. A phase 1, single-dose study of fresolimumab, an anti-TGF-beta antibody, in treatment-resistant primary focal segmental glomerulosclerosis. *Kidney Int* (2011) 79(11):1236–43. doi:10.1038/ki.2011.33
21. Vincenti F, Fervenza FC, Campbell KN, Diaz M, Gesualdo L, Nelson P, et al. A phase 2, double-blind, placebo-controlled, randomized study of fresolimumab in patients with steroid-resistant primary focal segmental glomerulosclerosis. *Kidney Int Rep* (2017) 2(5):800–10. doi:10.1016/j.ekir.2017.03.011
22. Oh J, Beckmann J, Bloch J, Hettgen V, Mueller J, Li L, et al. Stimulation of the calcium-sensing receptor stabilizes the podocyte cytoskeleton, improves cell survival, and reduces toxin-induced glomerulosclerosis. *Kidney Int* (2011) 80(5):483–92. doi:10.1038/ki.2011.105
23. Deng J, Zheng X, Xie H, Chen L. Calcitriol in the treatment of IgA nephropathy with non-nephrotic range proteinuria: a meta-analysis of randomized controlled trials. *Clin Nephrol* (2017) 87(1):21–7. doi:10.5414/CN108915
24. Banerjee S, Basu S, Sengupta J. Vitamin D in nephrotic syndrome remission: a case-control study. *Pediatr Nephrol* (2013) 28(10):1983–9. doi:10.1007/s00467-013-2511-y
25. Bensman A, Niaudet P. Non-immunologic mechanisms of calcineurin inhibitors explain its antiproteinuric effects in genetic glomerulopathies. *Pediatr Nephrol* (2010) 25(7):1197–9. doi:10.1007/s00467-010-1469-2
26. Faul C, Donnelly M, Merscher-Gomez S, Chang YH, Franz S, Delfgaauw J, et al. The actin cytoskeleton of kidney podocytes is a direct target of the antiproteinuric effect of cyclosporine A. *Nat Med* (2008) 14(9):931–8. doi:10.1038/nm.1857
27. Wakamatsu A, Fukusumi Y, Hasegawa E, Tomita M, Watanabe T, Narita I, et al. Role of calcineurin (CN) in kidney glomerular podocyte: CN inhibitor ameliorated proteinuria by inhibiting the redistribution of CN at the slit diaphragm. *Physiol Rep* (2016) 4(6). doi:10.14814/phy2.12679
28. Ransom RF, Lam NG, Hallett MA, Atkinson SJ, Smoyer WE. Glucocorticoids protect and enhance recovery of cultured murine podocytes via actin filament stabilization. *Kidney Int* (2005) 68(6):2473–83. doi:10.1111/j.1523-1755.2005.00723.x
29. Mallipattu SK, Guo Y, Revelo MP, Roa-Pena L, Miller T, Ling J, et al. Kruppel-like factor 15 mediates glucocorticoid-induced restoration of podocyte differentiation markers. *J Am Soc Nephrol* (2017) 28(1):166–84. doi:10.1681/ASN.2015060672
30. Jiang L, Dasgupta I, Hurcombe JA, Colyer HF, Mathieson PW, Welsh GI. Levamisole in steroid-sensitive nephrotic syndrome: usefulness in adult patients and laboratory insights into mechanisms of action via direct action on the kidney podocyte. *Clin Sci (Lond)* (2015) 128(12):883–93. doi:10.1042/CS20140749
31. Zschiedrich S, Bork T, Liang W, Wanner N, Eulenbruch K, Munder S, et al. Targeting mTOR signaling can prevent the progression of FSGS. *J Am Soc Nephrol* (2017) 28(7):2144–57. doi:10.1681/ASN.2016050519
32. Fornoni A, Sageshima J, Wei C, Merscher-Gomez S, Aguillon-Prada R, Jauregui AN, et al. Rituximab targets podocytes in recurrent focal segmental glomerulosclerosis. *Sci Transl Med* (2011) 3(85):85ra46. doi:10.1126/scitranslmed.3002231
33. Ruf RG, Lichtenberger A, Karle SM, Haas JP, Anacleto FE, Schultheiss M, et al. Patients with mutations in NPHS2 (podocin) do not respond to standard steroid treatment of nephrotic syndrome. *J Am Soc Nephrol* (2004) 15(3):722–32. doi:10.1097/01.ASN.0000113552.59155.72
34. Hinkes B, Wiggins RC, Gbadegesin R, Vlangos CN, Seelow D, Nurnberg G, et al. Positional cloning uncovers mutations in PLCE1 responsible for a nephrotic syndrome variant that may be reversible. *Nat Genet* (2006) 38(12):1397–405. doi:10.1038/ng1918
35. Boyer O, Benoit G, Gribouval O, Nevo F, Pawtowski A, Bilge I, et al. Mutational analysis of the PLCE1 gene in steroid resistant nephrotic syndrome. *J Med Genet* (2010) 47(7):445–52. doi:10.1136/jmg.2009.076166
36. Gipson DS, Trachtman H, Kaskel FJ, Greene TH, Radeva MK, Gassman JJ, et al. Clinical trial of focal segmental glomerulosclerosis in children and young adults. *Kidney Int* (2011) 80(8):868–78. doi:10.1038/ki.2011.195
37. Klaassen I, Ozgoren B, Sadowski CE, Moller K, van Husen M, Lehnhardt A, et al. Response to cyclosporine in steroid-resistant nephrotic syndrome: discontinuation is possible. *Pediatr Nephrol* (2015) 30(9):1477–83. doi:10.1007/s00467-015-3109-3
38. Pritchard-Jones K, Fleming S, Davidson D, Bickmore W, Porteous D, Gosden C, et al. The candidate Wilms' tumour gene is involved in genitourinary development. *Nature* (1990) 346(6280):194–7. doi:10.1038/346194a0
39. Guo JK, Menke AL, Gubler MC, Clarke AR, Harrison D, Hammes A, et al. WT1 is a key regulator of podocyte function: reduced expression levels cause crescentic glomerulonephritis and mesangial sclerosis. *Hum Mol Genet* (2002) 11(6):651–9. doi:10.1093/hmg/11.6.651
40. Lehnhardt A, Karnatz C, Ahlenstiel-Grunow T, Benz K, Benz MR, Budde K, et al. Clinical and molecular characterization of patients with heterozygous mutations in wilms tumor suppressor gene 1. *Clin J Am Soc Nephrol* (2015) 10(5):825–31. doi:10.2215/CJN.10141014
41. Stefanidis CJ, Querfeld U. The podocyte as a target: cyclosporin A in the management of the nephrotic syndrome caused by WT1 mutations. *Eur J Pediatr* (2011) 170(11):1377–83. doi:10.1007/s00431-011-1397-6
42. Gellermann J, Stefanidis CJ, Mitsioni A, Querfeld U. Successful treatment of steroid-resistant nephrotic syndrome associated with WT1 mutations. *Pediatr Nephrol* (2010) 25(7):1285–9. doi:10.1007/s00467-010-1468-3

43. Wasilewska AM, Kuroczycka-Saniutycz E, Zoch-Zwierz W. Effect of cyclosporin A on proteinuria in the course of glomerulopathy associated with WT1 mutations. *Eur J Pediatr* (2011) 170(3):389–91. doi:10.1007/s00431-010-1278-4
44. Desbats MA, Lunardi G, Doimo M, Trevisson E, Salviati L. Genetic bases and clinical manifestations of coenzyme Q10 (CoQ 10) deficiency. *J Inherit Metab Dis* (2015) 38(1):145–56. doi:10.1007/s10545-014-9749-9
45. Diomedi-Camassei F, Di Giandomenico S, Santorelli FM, Caridi G, Piemonte F, Montini G, et al. COQ2 nephropathy: a newly described inherited mitochondriopathy with primary renal involvement. *J Am Soc Nephrol* (2007) 18(10):2773–80. doi:10.1681/ASN.2006080833
46. Heeringa SF, Chernin G, Chaki M, Zhou W, Sloan AJ, Ji Z, et al. COQ6 mutations in human patients produce nephrotic syndrome with sensorineural deafness. *J Clin Invest* (2011) 121(5):2013–24. doi:10.1172/JCI45693
47. Salviati L, Sacconi S, Murer L, Zacchello G, Franceschini L, Laverda AM, et al. Infantile encephalomyopathy and nephropathy with CoQ10 deficiency: a CoQ10-responsive condition. *Neurology* (2005) 65(4):606–8. doi:10.1212/01.wnl.0000172859.55579.a7
48. Montini G, Malaventura C, Salviati L. Early coenzyme Q10 supplementation in primary coenzyme Q10 deficiency. *N Engl J Med* (2008) 358(26):2849–50. doi:10.1056/NEJMc0800582
49. Ashraf S, Gee HY, Woerner S, Xie LX, Vega-Warner V, Lovric S, et al. ADCK4 mutations promote steroid-resistant nephrotic syndrome through CoQ10 biosynthesis disruption. *J Clin Invest* (2013) 123(12):5179–89. doi:10.1172/JCI69000
50. Tabatabaeifar M, Wlodkowski T, Simic I, Denc H, Mollet G, Weber S, et al. An inducible mouse model of podocin-mutation-related nephrotic syndrome. *PLoS One* (2017) 12(10):e0186574. doi:10.1371/journal.pone.0186574
51. Leierer J, Mayer G, Kronbichler A. Primary focal segmental glomerulosclerosis: miRNAs and targeted therapies. *Eur J Clin Invest* (2016) 46(11):954–64. doi:10.1111/eci.12676

18

Identification of a Novel Heterozygous *De Novo* 7-bp Frameshift Deletion in *PBX1* by Whole-Exome Sequencing Causing a Multi-Organ Syndrome Including Bilateral Dysplastic Kidneys and Hypoplastic Clavicles

Korbinian Maria Riedhammer[1,2], Corinna Siegel[2], Bader Alhaddad[2], Carmen Montoya[3], Reka Kovacs-Nagy[2], Matias Wagner[2,4,5], Thomas Meitinger[2,4] and Julia Hoefele[2]*

[1] Department of Nephrology, Klinikum rechts der Isar, Technical University of Munich, Munich, Germany, [2] Institute of Human Genetics, Klinikum rechts der Isar, Technical University of Munich, Munich, Germany, [3] KfH Center of Pediatric Nephrology, Children's Hospital Munich Schwabing, Munich, Germany, [4] Institute of Human Genetics, Helmholtz Zentrum Munich, Neuherberg, Germany, [5] Institute of Neurogenomics, Helmholtz Zentrum Munich, Neuherberg, Germany

***Correspondence:**
Julia Hoefele
julia.hoefele@tum.de

Introduction: Congenital anomalies of the kidney and urinary tract (CAKUT) represent the primary cause of chronic kidney disease in children. Many genes have been attributed to the genesis of this disorder. Recently, haploinsufficiency of *PBX1* caused by microdeletions has been shown to result in bilateral renal hypoplasia and other organ malformations.

Materials and methods: Here, we report on a 14-year-old male patient with congenital bilateral dysplastic kidneys, cryptorchidism, hypoplastic clavicles, developmental delay, impaired intelligence, and minor dysmorphic features. Presuming a syndromic origin, we performed SNP array analysis to scan for large copy number variations (CNVs) followed by whole-exome sequencing (WES). Sanger sequencing was done to confirm the variant's *de novo* status.

Results: SNP array analysis did not reveal any microdeletions or -duplications larger than 50 or 100 kb, respectively. WES identified a novel heterozygous 7-bp frameshift deletion in *PBX1* (c.413_419del, p.Gly138Valfs*40) resulting in a loss-of-function. The *de novo* status could be confirmed by Sanger sequencing.

Discussion: By WES, we identified a novel heterozygous *de novo* 7-bp frameshift deletion in *PBX1*. Our findings expand the spectrum of causative variants in *PBX1*-related CAKUT. In this case, WES proved to be the apt technique to detect the variant responsible for the patient's phenotype, as single gene testing is not feasible given the multitude of genes involved in CAKUT and SNP array analysis misses rare single-nucleotide variants and small Indels.

Keywords: CAKUT, *PBX1*, dysplastic kidneys, hypoplastic clavicles, developmental delay

INTRODUCTION

Congenital anomalies of the kidney and urinary tract (CAKUT) represent the primary cause of chronic kidney disease in children. CAKUT is the collective term for many different renal and urinary tract malformations. In recent years, a multitude of monogenic disease-causing genes has been discovered (1). Disruption of the normal nephrogenesis by pathogenic variants in genes involved in kidney development is a basic principle of CAKUT (2).

When it comes to heterogeneous diseases like CAKUT, with many different genes involved, large-scale next-generation sequencing has become an extremely useful tool for the unbiased detection of pathogenic variants (3). In whole-exome sequencing (WES), the coding regions (the exome) of the human genome are enriched and sequenced. This has proven to be both an economic, as the exome only comprises 1% of the genome, and a pragmatic approach, as about 85% of disease-related variants can be found in the exome (4).

PBX1 encodes a transcription factor that has already been linked to nephrogenesis as shown by *Pbx1*-deficient mice (5). Additionally, earlier mouse models revealed its role in bone formation (6). In 2017, microdeletions comprising *PBX1* as a minimal common region could be identified by microarray analysis in eight patients with syndromic CAKUT with predominantly renal hypoplasia. In the same publication, it was shown that *PBX1* was strongly expressed in the fetal kidney and brain (7). Here, we report on a 14-year-old male patient presenting to the pediatric nephrology department with the predominant clinical features of bilateral dysplastic kidneys, hypoplastic clavicles, and developmental delay.

MATERIALS AND METHODS

This study was approved by the local Ethics Committee of the Technical University of Munich and performed according to the standard of the Helsinki Declaration of 1975. Written informed consent was obtained from the parents of the participant for publication of this case report. Blood samples were collected after written informed consent.

DNA was extracted from peripheral blood using the Gentra Puregene Blood Kit (Qiagen, Hilden, Germany) according to the manufacturer's instructions. The DNA sample of the patient was analyzed by using the SNP Array Affymetrix® CytoScanTM 750 K Array (Affymetrix® Inc., Santa Clara, CA, USA) with an average space between two oligonucleotides of 4 kb. Scanning was performed by the Affymetrix® GeneChip Scanner 3000 7G (resolution 0.51–2.5 µm). The data analysis was conducted using the Affymetrix® Chromosome Analysis Suite Software (ChAS), version 3.0, hg19.

Exome sequencing was performed using a Sure Select Human All Exon 60 Mb V6 Kit (Agilent) and a HiSeq4000 (Illumina) as previously described (8, 9). Reads were aligned to the UCSC human reference assembly (hg19) with BWA v.0.5.8. More than 98% of the exome was covered at least 20×. *PBX1* was covered >20× to 100%. Single-nucleotide variants and small insertions and deletions were detected with SAMtools v.0.1.7. Variant prioritization was performed based on an autosomal recessive pattern of inheritance (homozygous or putative compound heterozygous variants with a minor allele frequency <0.1%) as well as an autosomal dominant pattern of inheritance (heterozygous variants with a minor allele frequency <0.001%).

Sanger sequencing was used to confirm the identified variant and to test the patient's parents. Oligonucleotide primer sequences are available upon request.

CASE REPORT AND RESULTS

The 14-year-old boy is the first child of healthy parents (**Figure 1**). He has one younger healthy brother and one younger healthy half-brother. The patient was born at a gestational age of 38 weeks [birth weight: 2,840 g (25th–50th percentile), birth length: 48 cm (10th–25th percentile)]. There were no obvious malformations noted at birth. During the neonatal period, a slender thorax and short clavicles were identified clinically. Body height was on the third percentile during infancy and early childhood (**Figure 2**) and a global developmental delay (including motor and speech delay) was diagnosed on regular pediatric screening examinations.

An ultrasound of the kidneys at 3 months of age revealed small kidneys with hyperechogenic parenchyma. The boy was then regularly seen by a pediatric nephrologist. By the age of six, the right kidney had a length of 6.2 cm (<1st percentile, see **Figure 3**), the left kidney had a length of 5.8 cm (<1st percentile, see **Figure 4**). Kidney function ranged between eGFR 59 mL/min/1.73 m^2 at 4 years of age, 90 mL/min/1.73 m^2 at 8 years of age, and 69 mL/min/1.73 m^2 at 13 years of age (Schwartz estimate, CKD II). Moreover, the patient had bilateral cryptorchidism for which he received hormonal therapy by the age of 2 years.

Psychological intelligence testing by the age of 13 revealed a below average speech comprehension (IQ 81), a reduced information processing speed (IQ 74) and an impaired auditory working memory (IQ 77).

On orthopedic examination the patient had a slim shoulder profile, impaired abduction of the arms, and a hunched back. Thoracic X-ray revealed hypoplastic clavicles (**Figure 5**, only left clavicle visible). He also had some dysmorphic features (wide nasal bridge, short neck, bilateral overfolding of the helix, and bilateral clinodactyly).

In this child, we presumed a syndromic origin and initially performed SNP array analysis. However, no microdeletions or

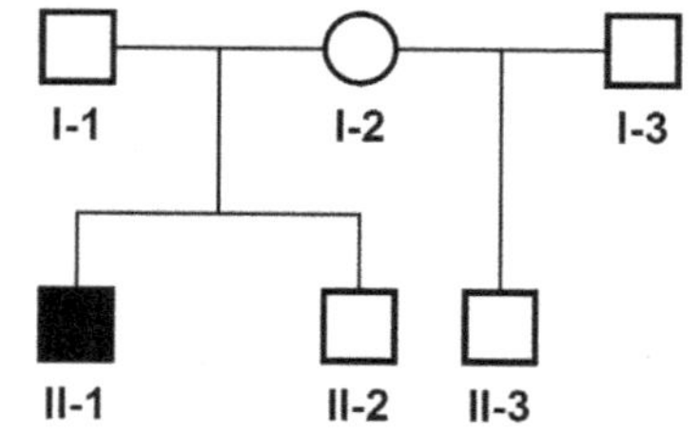

FIGURE 1 | Pedigree of the family. Solid symbol, affected individual; circles, females; squares, males.

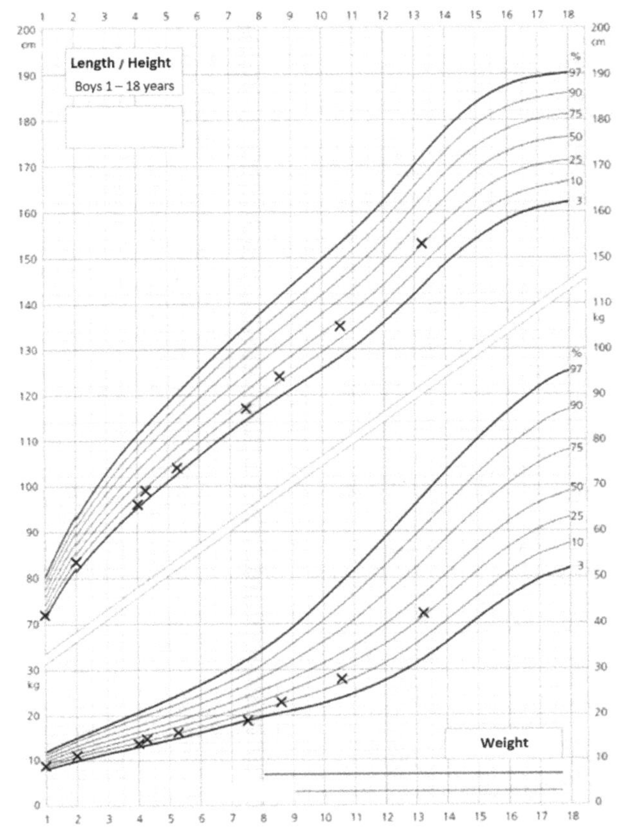

FIGURE 2 | Growth and weight charts of the patient. These charts are gender specific and refer to boys. *x*-axis, age (years); *y*-axis, height (centimeter, upper part of the figure) and weight (kilograms, lower part of the figure).

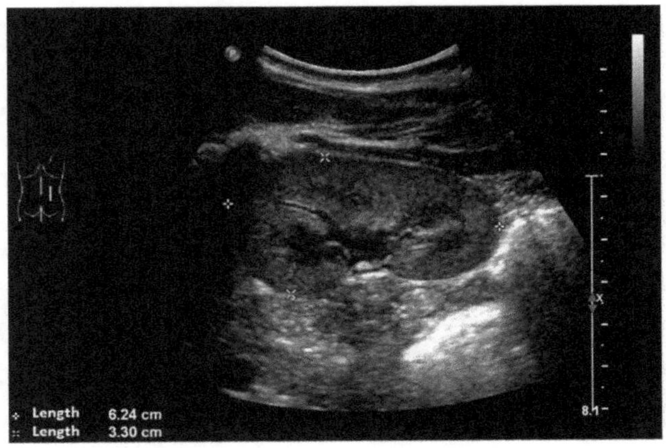

FIGURE 3 | Ultrasound of the right kidney with a length of 6.2 cm (<1st percentile).

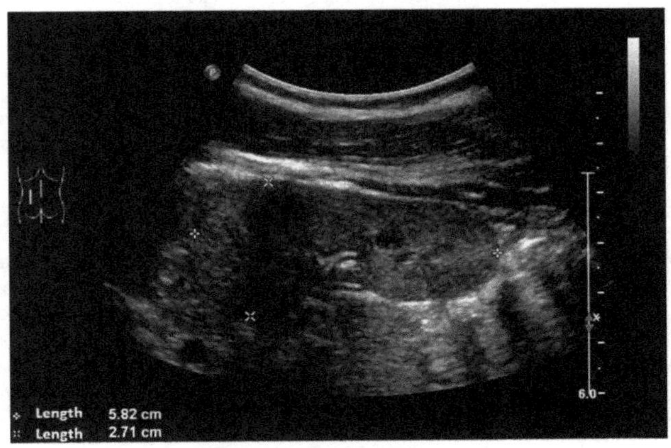

FIGURE 4 | Ultrasound of the left kidney with a length of 5.8 cm (<1st percentile).

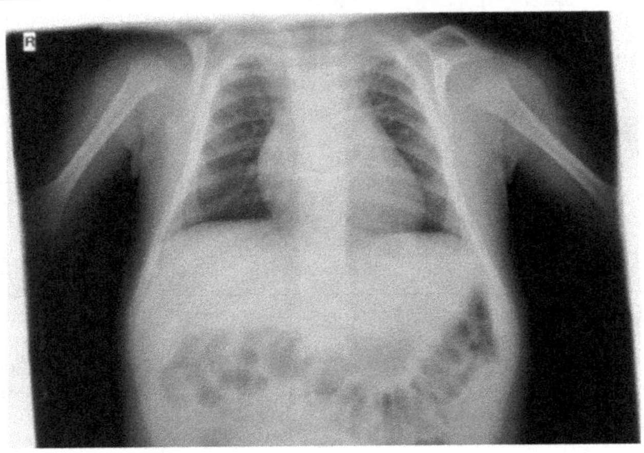

FIGURE 5 | X-ray (detail of a babygram) of the patient at the age of 7 months showing a hook-shaped hypoplastic left clavicle.

duplications (copy number variations, CNVs) larger than 50 or 100 kb, respectively, could be detected. As CAKUT have been associated with a large number of genes, we then performed WES. By WES, we could identify a novel heterozygous 7-bp deletion in *PBX1* leading to a frameshift (c.413_419delGGGCAGG, p.Gly138Valfs*40), resulting in either nonsense-mediated decay of the mRNA or a truncated protein lacking the DNA-binding domain. The variant is not listed in 60,000 control individuals of the Exome Aggregation Consortium (ExAC) browser. The ExAC browser does not list any high-confidence loss-of-function variants in *PBX1* indicating that *PBX1* is intolerant to loss-of-function variants. To verify the *de novo* status of the variant, we performed Sanger sequencing in the patient and his parents. The variant could not be detected in the blood DNA of both parents (**Figure 6**).

DISCUSSION

CAKUT represent the primary cause of chronic kidney disease in children and many genes have been attributed to the genesis of this disorder with both dominant and recessive modes of inheritance.

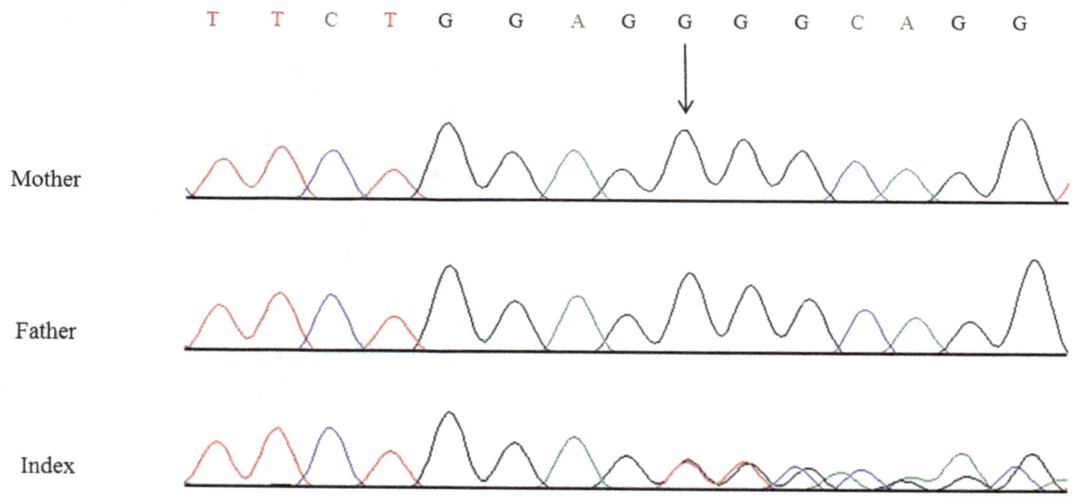

FIGURE 6 | Partial nucleotide sequence of exon 3 of *PBX1* of the patient and his parents showing the heterozygous *de novo* variant c.413_419delGGGCAGG, p.Gly138Valfs*40. Shown reference sequence: TTCTGGAGGGGCAGG. Genomic position of the variant: chr1:164761876–164761882 (hg19, transcript NM_002585.3).

TABLE 1 | Summary of genetic changes in *PBX1* and clinical features reported so far.

Patient	Kidney/urinary tract phenotype	Kidney function	Extrarenal phenotype	Genetic change	Protein change	Mode of inheritance
This report	Bilateral dysplasia, hyperechogenicity	eGFR = 59–90 mL/min/1.73 m²	Bilateral cryptorchidism, hypoplastic clavicles, postnatal growth retardation (height third percentile), global developmental delay (including motor and speech delay), impaired intelligence, dysmorphic features (wide nasal bridge, short neck, bilateral overfolding of the helix, bilateral clinodactyly)	c.[413_419delGGGCAGG];[=]	p.[Gly138Valfs*40];[=]	*de novo*
K175	Bilateral hypoplasia	eGFR = 40 mL/min/1.73 m² (at 21 years)	Deafness, scoliosis	c.[428delA];[=]	p.[Asn143Thrfs*37];[=]	*de novo*
K179	Bilateral cystic hypodysplasia	eGFR = 51 mL/min/1.73 m² (at 11 years)	Dysmorphic features, developmental delay	c.[550C>T];[=]	p.[Arg184*];[=]	*de novo*
K186	Bilateral hypoplasia with oligonephronia	Oligohydramnios	No	c.[511-2A>G];[=] (exon 4, splice acceptor site variant)		*de novo*
K181	Hypoplastic horseshoe kidney, absence of corticomedullar differentiation	eGFR = 40 mL/min/1.73 m² (at 39 years)	Deafness	2.5-Mb deletion (encompassing 8 genes)		*de novo*
K136	Unilateral agenesis/small hyperechogenic kidney	Normal renal function (at 18 months)	Dysmorphic features, impaired intelligence	9.1-Mb deletion (encompassing 131 genes)		*de novo*
PT1	Normal kidney phenotype, bifid right ureter, bilateral pelvis dilatation, bilateral VUR, small urethral valve	Not available	Sacral pit, postnatal growth retardation (weight and height < 3rd percentile), severe global developmental delay, neonatal hypotonia, bilateral perceptive hearing loss, dysmorphic features (low-set ears, anteverted nares, prominent philtrum, thick lips, uvula bifida), seizures in infancy	6.0-Mb deletion (chr1:161650414–167622545, encompassing 36 genes)		*de novo*

(*Continued*)

TABLE 1 | Continued

Patient	Kidney/urinary tract phenotype	Kidney function	Extrarenal phenotype	Genetic change	Protein change	Mode of inheritance
PT2	Bilateral renal hypoplasia, nephrocalcinosis	eGFR = 40 mL/ min/1.73 m^2 (at 1.5 months)	VSD, ductus arteriosus, severe kyphoscoliosis, postnatal growth retardation (weight and height < 3rd percentile), microcephaly (<3rd percentile), global developmental delay (including motor delay), deep sound hearing loss, dysmorphic features (antimongoloid eyesplit, frontal bossing, anterior fontanelle closed prematurely, low-set, pointed ears), hypermetropism	9.2-Mb deletion (chr1:162703368–171908659, encompassing 62 genes)		*de novo*
PT3	Bilateral renal hypodysplasia, right renal ectopia, hyperechogenicity, dedifferentiation	eGFR = 66 mL/ min/1.73 m^2 (at 5 years)	VSD, ductus arteriosus, sacral pit, mild global developmental delay (including motor and speech delay), dysmorphic features (hypoplastic lobes, left-sided ear pit, long, narrow face, wide nasal bridge, broad nasal tip, mild retrognatia)	2.8-Mb deletion (chr1:163193466 –166058476, encompassing 11 genes)		*de novo*
PT4	Bilateral renal hypoplasia, hyperechogenicity	Normal, eGFR = 106 mL/ min/1.73 m^2 (at 2 years)	Bilateral cryptorchidism, multiple skeletal malformations (shoulder blade, acromioclavicular joint, skull basis, vertebral defects, hip dislocation), postnatal growth retardation (weight 3rd to 10th percentile), motor delay, hypotonia, dysmorphic features (small, low-set, posteriorly rotated ears, abnormal folding of the helix, divergent strabismus, short nose, anteverted nares, prominent philtrum, short neck)	1.5-Mb deletion (chr1:163574086–165092429, only encompassing *PBX1*)		*de novo*
PT5	Bilateral renal hypoplasia	CKD stage 3 (at 3 years)	Corpus callosum hyoplasia, sacral pit, anal malposistion, difficult neonatal adaptation, unilateral vocal fold paralysis, postnatal growth retardation (weight 3rd to 10th, height <3rd percentile), global developmental delay, neonatal hypotonia, hearing loss, dysmorphic features (prominent metopic ridge, broad nasal bridge, abnormally hemmed ears, hypertelorism, epicanthus, divergent strabismus, thin upper lip, long hands and feet, unilateral fifth finger clinodactyly), encopresia, enuresia	3.6-Mb deletion (chr1:163811431–167385298, encompassing 16 genes)		*de novo*
PT6	Bilateral renal hypodysplasia	CKD stage 5 (transplant at 10 months)	Unilateral cryptorchidism, mitral regurgitation, left ventricular hypertrophy, spina bifida occulta, unilateral inguinal hernia, mild global developmental delay (including motor and speech delay), autism spectrum disorder	0.9-Mb deletion (chr1:164330973–165207097, encompassing 2 genes)		unknown
PT7	Horseshoe kidney	Not available	VSD, ASD, ductus arteriosus, cleft of the posterior arch of L5, anal malposition, postnatal growth retardation (weight 3rd, height 3rd—10th percentile), microcephaly (<3rd percentile), global developmental delay (including motor and speech delay), hearing loss, dysmorphic features (thin, low-set hair, anteverted, low-set ears, crumpled, thick helix, thick lower lip, prognathism, mandibular hypermobility, dental malocclusion, bilateral clinodactyly), wide-based gait	6.9-Mb deletion (chr1:164501003–171424595, encompassing 51 genes)		*de novo*
PT8	Bilateral renal hypoplasia, right renal ectopia, right renal dysplasia	Normal, eGFR = 130 mL/ min/1.73 m^2 (at 4.2 years)	Right cryptorchidism, mild global developmental delay (including motor and speech delay), autism spectrum disorder, bilateral conductive hearing loss, dysmorphic features (bilateral ear dysplasia), joint laxity	0.3-Mb deletion (chr1:164523918–164799811, only encompassing *PBX1*)		unknown

Patients K175, K179, K186, K181, K136 see Ref. (11); patients PT1-8 see Ref. (7). Reference genome for deletion coordinates: hg19; ASD, atrial septal defect; eGFR, estimated glomerular filtration rate; VSD, ventricular septal defects.

CAKUT mainly occur as part of (multi-organ) syndromes but there are also isolated cases described in the literature (1, 2, 10). Just recently, haploinsufficiency of *PBX1* caused by microdeletions was shown to result in bilateral renal hypoplasia and other organ malformations (7). Furthermore, a targeted exome sequencing of 330 genes in 204 unrelated CAKUT patients could identify five novel *de novo* heterozygous loss-of-function variants/deletions in *PBX1* (11).

PBX1 encodes a transcription factor which promotes protein–protein interaction and is important for organogenesis (12). *Pbx1*$^{-/-}$ mice die at an embryonic age and show extensive organ malformations including hypoplastic kidneys with unilateral agenesis (5). In a further publication, *Pbx1*-deficient mice exhibited—besides multiple organ malformations—a pronounced skeletal phenotype with a slender thorax, hunched posture, and axial malformations. *PBX1* is highly expressed in proliferating chondrocytes (6). Additionally, there is strong *PBX1* expression in the fetal brain (7), and it regulates patterning of the cerebral cortex in progenitor neurons in mice (13). To date, two publications reported CAKUT phenotypes related to pathogenic *PBX1* variants/microdeletions; however, only two of the eight patients published by Le Tanno et al. had heterozygous microdeletions only encompassing *PBX1* (7). The phenotype of these patients involved, among other things, bilateral renal hypoplasia with hyperechogenic parenchyma, cryptorchidism, skeletal malformations, and developmental delay. The other patients in this publication had larger deletions involving a more extensive set of genes contributing to the phenotype. The five patients with novel loss-of-function variants/deletions in *PBX1* identified in a targeted exome sequencing study (11) lacked a detailed genotype–phenotype correlation, as only limited information on the extrarenal phenotype was provided. See **Table 1** for a detailed summary of the genetic changes in *PBX1* and clinical features described so far.

The patient in our report displayed a complex clinical picture with kidney and skeletal malformations and a neuronal phenotype with developmental delay and impairment of intelligence. In addition to the previously published data from *PBX1* mouse models, microdeletions and loss-of-function variants/deletions mentioned above, we provide a detailed description of the phenotype and make the case for an improved diagnostic approach in CAKUT: in this patient our diagnostic algorithm involved SNP array analysis which did not yield a positive result. We then performed WES and identified a novel heterozygous *de novo* 7-bp frameshift deletion in *PBX1* (c.413_419del, p.Gly138Valfs*40). For future CAKUT cases, we recommend directly employing whole-exome or whole-genome sequencing, as these are the apt techniques to identify new pathogenic variants/CNVs in this genetically heterogeneous syndrome. This is especially true for syndromal and familial CAKUT. In patients with isolated CAKUT, however, diagnostic yield is probably rather low, as less than 10% carry variants in 20 known CAKUT genes (2).

ETHICS STATEMENT

This study was carried out in accordance with the recommendations of the Ethics Committee of the Technical University of Munich with written informed consent from all subjects. All subjects gave written informed consent in accordance with the Declaration of Helsinki. The protocol was approved by the Ethics Committee of the Technical University of Munich.

AUTHOR CONTRIBUTIONS

KR, MW, TM, and JH were responsible for writing and revision of the manuscript. CS and CM cared for the patient and provided the clinical data. KR, BA, RK-N, and MW did the exome analysis.

ACKNOWLEDGMENTS

The authors would like to thank the family for participation and Dr. M. Steinborn from the Department of Diagnostic and Pediatric Radiology, Schwabing Hospital, Munich, Germany, for permission to use the X-ray. This work was supported by the German Research Foundation (DFG) and the Technical University of Munich (TUM) in the framework of the Open Access Publishing Program.

REFERENCES

1. Vivante A, Kohl S, Hwang DY, Dworschak GC, Hildebrandt F. Single-gene causes of congenital anomalies of the kidney and urinary tract (CAKUT) in humans. *Pediatr Nephrol* (2014) 29:695–704. doi:10.1007/s00467-013-2684-4
2. Capone VP, Morello W, Taroni F, Montini G. Genetics of congenital anomalies of the kidney and urinary tract: the current state of play. *Int J Mol Sci* (2017) 18. doi:10.3390/ijms18040796
3. Petersen BS, Fredrich B, Hoeppner MP, Ellinghaus D, Franke A. Opportunities and challenges of whole-genome and -exome sequencing. *BMC Genet* (2017) 18:14. doi:10.1186/s12863-017-0479-5
4. Majewski J, Schwartzentruber J, Lalonde E, Montpetit A, Jabado N. What can exome sequencing do for you? *J Med Genet* (2011) 48:580–9. doi:10.1136/jmedgenet-2011-100223
5. Schnabel CA, Godin RE, Cleary ML. Pbx1 regulates nephrogenesis and ureteric branching in the developing kidney. *Dev Biol* (2003) 254:262–76. doi:10.1016/S0012-1606(02)00038-6
6. Selleri L, Depew MJ, Jacobs Y, Chanda SK, Tsang KY, Cheah KS, et al. Requirement for Pbx1 in skeletal patterning and programming chondrocyte proliferation and differentiation. *Development* (2001) 128:3543–57.
7. Le Tanno P, Breton J, Bidart M, Satre V, Harbuz R, Ray PF, et al. PBX1 haploinsufficiency leads to syndromic congenital anomalies of the kidney and urinary tract (CAKUT) in humans. *J Med Genet* (2017) 54:502–10. doi:10.1136/jmedgenet-2016-104435
8. Haack TB, Gorza M, Danhauser K, Mayr JA, Haberberger B, Wieland T, et al. Phenotypic spectrum of eleven patients and five novel MTFMT mutations identified by exome sequencing and candidate gene screening. *Mol Genet Metab* (2014) 111:342–52. doi:10.1016/j.ymgme.2013.12.010
9. Wortmann SB, Zietkiewicz S, Kousi M, Szklarczyk R, Haack TB, Gersting SW, et al. CLPB mutations cause 3-methylglutaconic aciduria, progressive brain atrophy, intellectual disability, congenital neutropenia, cataracts, movement disorder. *Am J Hum Genet* (2015) 96:245–57. doi:10.1016/j.ajhg.2014.12.013
10. Weber S. Novel genetic aspects of congenital anomalies of kidney and urinary tract. *Curr Opin Pediatr* (2012) 24:212–8. doi:10.1097/MOP.0b013e32834fdbd4

11. Heidet L, Moriniere V, Henry C, De Tomasi L, Reilly ML, Humbert C, et al. Targeted exome sequencing identifies PBX1 as involved in monogenic congenital anomalies of the kidney and urinary tract. *J Am Soc Nephrol* (2017) 28:2901–14. doi:10.1681/ASN.2017010043
12. Yu J, Mcmahon AP, Valerius MT. Recent genetic studies of mouse kidney development. *Curr Opin Genet Dev* (2004) 14:550–7. doi:10.1016/j.gde.2004.07.009
13. Golonzhka O, Nord A, Tang PL, Lindtner S, Ypsilanti AR, Ferretti E, et al. Pbx regulates patterning of the cerebral cortex in progenitors and postmitotic neurons. *Neuron* (2015) 88:1192–207. doi:10.1016/j.neuron.2015.10.045

19

Gastrostomy Tube Insertion in Pediatric Patients with Autosomal Recessive Polycystic Kidney Disease (ARPKD)

Kathrin Burgmaier[1], Joy Brandt[1], Rukshana Shroff[2], Peter Witters[3], Lutz T. Weber[1], Jörg Dötsch[1], Franz Schaefer[4], Djalila Mekahli[5,6] and Max C. Liebau[1,7]*

[1] Department of Pediatrics, University Hospital of Cologne, Cologne, Germany, [2] Great Ormond Street Hospital for Children NHS Foundation Trust, London, United Kingdom, [3] Department of Pediatric Gastroenterology and Hepatology, University Hospitals Leuven, Leuven, Belgium, [4] Division of Pediatric Nephrology, Center for Pediatric and Adolescent Medicine, University of Heidelberg, Heidelberg, Germany, [5] Department of Pediatric Nephrology, University Hospitals Leuven, Leuven, Belgium, [6] PKD Research Group, Department of Development and Regeneration, KU Leuven, University of Leuven, Leuven, Belgium, [7] Center for Molecular Medicine, University Hospital of Cologne, Cologne, Germany

***Correspondence:**
Max C. Liebau
max.liebau@uk-koeln.de

Introduction: Autosomal recessive polycystic kidney disease (ARPKD) is a severe hepatorenal disorder of childhood. Early renal disease in ARPKD may require renal replacement therapy and is associated with failure to thrive resulting in a need for nasogastric tube feeding or gastrostomy. In ARPKD patients, the benefit of a gastrostomy in nutrition and growth needs to be weighed against the potential risk of complications of congenital hepatic fibrosis (CHF) and portal hypertension like variceal bleeding. CHF in ARPKD has thus been considered as a relative contraindication for gastrostomy insertion. Yet, data on gastrostomies in pediatric patients with ARPKD is lacking.

Methods: We conducted a web-based survey study among pediatric nephrologists, pediatric hepatologists and pediatric gastroenterologists on their opinions on and experiences with gastrostomy insertion in ARPKD patients.

Results: 196 participants from 39 countries shared their opinion. 45% of participants support gastrostomy insertion in all ARPKD patients, but portal hypertension is considered to be a contraindication by a subgroup of participants. Patient-specific data was provided for 38 patients indicating complications of gastrostomy that were in principal comparable to non-ARPKD patients. Bleeding episodes were reported in 3/38 patients (7.9%). Two patients developed additional severe complications. Gastrostomy was retrospectively considered as the right decision for the patient in 35/38 (92.1%) of the cases.

Conclusions: This report on the results of an online survey gives first insights into the clinical practice of gastrostomy insertion in ARPKD patients. For the majority of participating physicians benefits of gastrostomy insertion retrospectively outweigh complications and risks. More data will be required to lay the foundation for clinical recommendations.

Keywords: ARPKD, congenital hepatic fibrosis, portal hypertension, peritoneal dialysis, *PKHD1*, pediatric polycystic kidney disease

INTRODUCTION

Autosomal recessive polycystic kidney disease (ARPKD) is a rare but severe disorder mainly affecting the liver and the kidneys. The disorder represents one of the leading reasons for pediatric dialysis and kidney-, liver- or combined liver and kidney transplantation. Renal involvement may present very early in life with massively enlarged polycystic kidneys and end stage kidney disease (ESKD), requiring renal replacement therapy (1, 2). Liver involvement due to congenital hepatic fibrosis (CHF) tends to present later in life and is associated with portal hypertension in up to 60% of patients with subsequent development of splenomegaly and collateral circulation (1–3). Esophageal varices have been reported in up to 56% of ARPKD patients with the risk of variceal bleeding (1–3).

Chronic kidney disease (CKD) is associated with growth failure and it has been suggested that ARPKD patients are at a particularly high risk (3, 4). Immaturity and early uremia may affect enteral feeding. Severe ARPKD is also accompanied by massive kidney enlargement and pulmonary hypoplasia. Abdominal distension and ventilation may complicate nutrition resulting in a need for persistent nasogastric feeding.

Concerns have been raised concerning gastrostomy in ARPKD patients. Infection risk is an issue in patients on peritoneal dialysis (PD) (5, 6). If possible, gastrostomy insertion in PD patients should take place prior to or at the same time of PD catheter placement. If gastrostomy insertion becomes necessary after onset of PD, an open surgical procedure with protective sutures is recommended as opposed to the endoscopic technique (7). An increased risk of variceal bleeding in patients with portal hypertension and an increased risk of spleen injury in case of splenomegaly have been suggested for endoscopic gastrostomy insertion in patients with cystic fibrosis associated liver disease and portal hypertension (8) and patients with liver cirrhosis (9). Furthermore, the development of stomal varices after gastrostomy has been discussed (8, 10). ARPKD with accompanying portal hypertension and possible future liver transplantation has been classified as a relative contraindication for gastrostomy insertion in children by the French society of gastrointestinal endoscopy (11) and within the position paper of the European Society for Paediatric Gastroenterology, Hepatology, and Nutrition (ESPGHAN) on management of percutaneous endoscopic gastrostomy in children and adolescents (12).

To the best of our knowledge there are no previous studies addressing clinical approaches towards gastrostomy insertion and complications of gastrostomy in pediatric ARPKD patients. In order to gain insight into current practice, we conducted an anonymous web-based survey among pediatric nephrologists, pediatric hepatologists and pediatric gastroenterologists on their opinion and experiences concerning benefits, risks, and methods of gastrostomy insertion in ARPKD patients.

Abbreviations: ARPKD, autosomal recessive polycystic kidney disease; CHF, congenital hepatic fibrosis; CKD, chronic kidney disease; ESKD, end-stage kidney disease; GI, gastrointestinal; HD, hemodialysis; HTN, hypertension; n.s., not significant; PD, peritoneal dialysis; PEG, percutaneous endoscopic gastrostomy.

METHODS

Study Design, Survey Development, Survey Content, and Administration

Questionnaires on the current clinical practice in gastrostomy insertion in patients with ARPKD (Supplementary data 1) were designed and validated by an expert group of pediatric nephrologists, hepatologists, and gastroenterologists. The survey was conducted in two steps: the first part was designed to assess general data on the background of participants as well as opinions regarding gastrostomy in patients suffering from CKD in general and ARPKD patients in particular. An additional aim was to identify specific conditions regarded as contraindications. The second part of the survey was designed to address gastrostomy insertion in ARPKD more specifically with respect to age at insertion, technique of insertion, periinterventional antibiotic and antifungal prophylaxis, signs of hepatic ARPKD involvement and conduction of dialysis at time of insertion. We specifically asked for observed complications after gastrostomy insertion in patients and for management of gastrostomy in case of subsequent transplantation. The survey ended with a personal evaluation of the risk-benefit analysis and the management of gastrostomy in non-ARPKD patients prior to transplantation.

The survey was an anonymous, web-based, cross-sectional study on a voluntary basis. Invitation to participate in the survey was sent to members of the European Society of Pediatric Nephrology (ESPN) study group, the International Pediatric Peritoneal Dialysis Network (IPDN) study group, the ARegPKD Consortium, the European Society for Paediatric Gastroenterology, Hepatology and Nutrition (ESPGHAN) Hepatology Interest Group, and the Pediatric Gastroenterology Internet Bulletin Board (PEDGI). The participants were asked to avoid duplicate entries in case of repeated invitation for the first part of the survey and to coordinate patient-specific entries within the own center in order to avoid multiple replies from a single center for the second part of the survey. The study was approved by the Ethics Committee of the Medical Faculty of the University of Cologne, Germany.

We received responses from 196 participants out of 39 countries with the largest groups of participants deriving from Germany (26), Poland (19), the United States of America (18), Belgium (17), the United Kingdom (14), France and Spain (each 11). Five or less participants each came from Argentinia, Australia, Austria, Brazil, Chile, China, Croatia, Denmark, Estonia, Georgia, Greece, Hungary, India, Iran, Kuwait, Lithuania, Macedonia, Netherlands, New Zealand, Oman, Pakistan, Peru, Portugal, Russia, Saudi Arabia, South Africa, South Korea, Sweden, Switzerland, and the United Arab Emirates. The profession of the participants was indicated as pediatric nephrologists (n = 141, 74.2%), pediatric hepatologists and/or gastroenterologists (n = 39, 20.5%), pediatrician (n = 3, 1.6%), pedatric nephrology/dialysis nurse (educator) (n = 2, 1.0%), dietitian (n = 2, 1.0%), and pediatric intensivist, adult nephrologist and trainee pediatric nephrology (each 1, each 0.5%). There were no replies by pediatric surgeons. 161/166 (97.0%) participants indicated that they took care of ARPKD patients in follow-up with a median number of 6 ARPKD patients (minimum one patient, maximum 60 patients). 152/164 (92.7%) participants performed pediatric PD and 145/164 (88.4%) performed hemodialysis (HD) at their institution. 118/162 (72.8%) participants performed kidney transplantation at their center, 65/159 (40.9%) performed liver transplantation, and 53/158 (33.5%) performed combined liver and kidney transplantation. 99/158 (60.7%) participants indicated that they had experience with management of variceal/portal hypertensive bleeding at their institution.

Patient-specific data was entered by 21 participants for a total of 38 patients. Most patients were from Germany, the United States of America, Denmark, and Iran. All patients showed specific characteristics in terms of country of origin, age, gender, and treatment modalities making duplicate entries of a single patient unlikely. Information regarding 32/38 (84.2%) patients was entered by pediatric nephrologists, for 3 (7.9%) patients information was given by pediatric hepatologists, information regarding one patient (2.6%) was entered by a pediatric gastroenterologist, pediatrician in training, and a nurse, respectively.

Statistical Analysis

Age at insertion of gastrostomy is given as median with interquartile range. All other variables were categorical and evaluated using descriptive statistics. Differences between nominal variables were calculated using Chi-Square test, significance was considered for $p < 0.05$. Data analysis was performed using IBM SPSS Statistics 22 for Windows.

RESULTS

General Attitude Toward Gastrostomy Insertion in CKD and ARPKD

In principle, 121/166 (72.9%) participants supported gastrostomy insertion in patients with CKD and ESKD (**Figure 1**). Regarding gastrostomy insertion in ARPKD patients, participants showed more detailed answers: while 71/158 (44.9%) supported insertion in all ARPKD patients, 15/158 (9.5%) did not support gastrostomy insertion in ARPKD patients. 23/158 (14.6%) participants supported gastrostomy insertion only in ARPKD patients without signs of portal hypertension, 10/158 (6.3%) only in patients without PD and 9/158 (5.7%) only in patients without signs of portal hypertension and/or without PD (**Figure 1**). There were significantly more nephrologists [61/117 (52.1%)] supporting gastrostomy in all ARPKD patients compared to gastroenterologists/hepatologists [7/28 (25.0%), $p = 0.01$]. There was a trend to a more restrictive support of gastrostomy insertion in patients with signs of portal hypertension and/or PD in pediatric gastroenterologists/hepatologists compared to pediatric nephrologists (n.s., **Figure 1**). A substantial number of participants (28/158, 17.7%) raised other or additional concerns, that encompassed general factors ("precise case-by-case-decision," "only in failure of all other techniques of feeding," "fear of increased risk of severe local infections after transplantation," "reluctance of surgeons or gastroenterologists to perform procedure"), PD-associated factors ("more strict indication in PD patients," "only surgical procedure in case of PD") and factors associated with portal hypertension ("more strict indication in case of portal hypertension," "future liver transplantation as contraindication") (**Figure 1**).

Indications for Gastrostomy Insertion and Hepatic Involvement Prior to Insertion in ARPKD Patients

Indications for gastrostomy insertion are shown in **Figure 2A**. Median age at insertion was 1.41 years (interquartile range 0.50–2.00 years). The youngest patient was 0.08 years, the oldest patient was 11.00 years old at gastrostomy insertion.

Prior to gastrostomy insertion more than half of the centers screened for varices in ARPKD patients (12/22, 54.5%). Most centers used esophagogastroduodenoscopy and/or ultrasound. Evaluation of the hepatic phenotype in specific patients indicated splenomegaly in 19/38 (50%) patients at time of gastrostomy insertion and evidence of collateral circulation (e.g., oesophageal varices) in 7/38 (18.4%) of patients (**Figure 2B**).

Method of Gastrostomy Insertion in ARPKD Patients

In the identified 38 patients, gastrostomy was inserted via endoscopy in 21/38 (55.3%), laparoscopically in 4/38 (10.5%), and in an open surgical approach in 9/38 (23.7%) patients. This differs from the opinion indicated in the first part of the survey, in which participants reported to favor insertion via endoscopy (60/130, 46.2%) or laparoscopic (37/130, 28.5%), while open insertion was preferred by only 4/130 (3.1%) participants with 29/130 (22.3%) participants being unsure about their preference in ARPKD patients (**Figure 3A**). The preference of different methods of insertion did not differ between pediatric gastroenterologists/hepatologists and nephrologists. In general CKD/ESKD patients, 72/117 (61.5%) participants favored endoscopic insertion, 25/117 (21.4%) laparoscopic, and 2/117 (1.7%) open insertion, while 18/117 (15.4%) were unsure about their preferred method.

Complications of Gastrostomy in ARPKD Patients

Reported complications of gastrostomy insertion encompassed excessive granulation tissue (7/38, 18.4%) and wound infection (5/38, 13.2%). In 3/38 (7.9%) patients each leakage of PD fluid or stomach fluid through gastrostomy was reported. One patient each (2.6% each) developed stomal varices, bleeding episodes due to variceal bleeding and excessive bleeding from gastrostomy exit site 9 months after insertion (**Figure 3B**). Other complications encompassed buried bumper, hernia, requirement of surgical closure after gastrostomy removal and a suspected association with a recurrent *Clostridium difficile* infection. One patient was reported to have suffered from preinterventional hypotension during anesthetic induction with subsequent cerebral infarction. 5/38 (13.2%) patients required

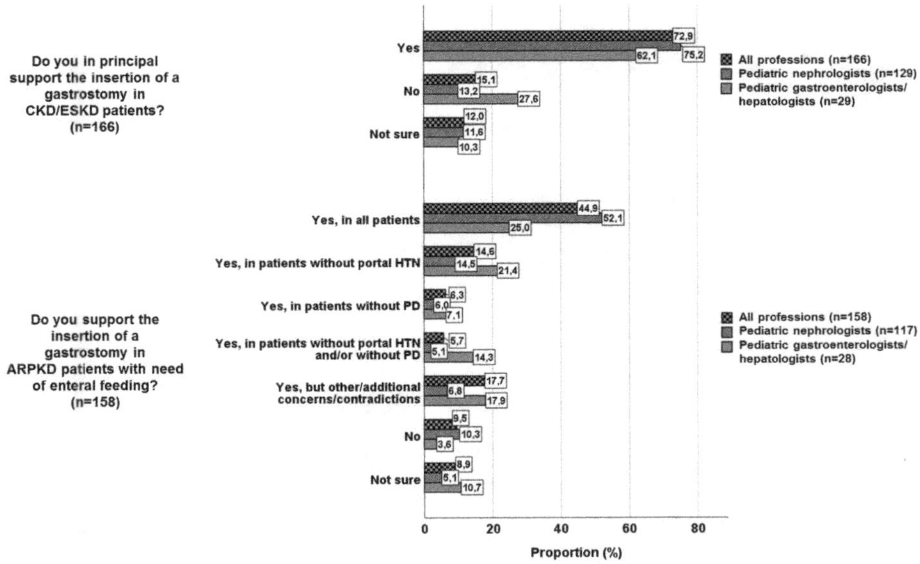

FIGURE 1 | Support of gastrostomy insertion in CKD/ESKD patients and in ARPKD patients (HTN, hypertension; PD, peritoneal dialysis).

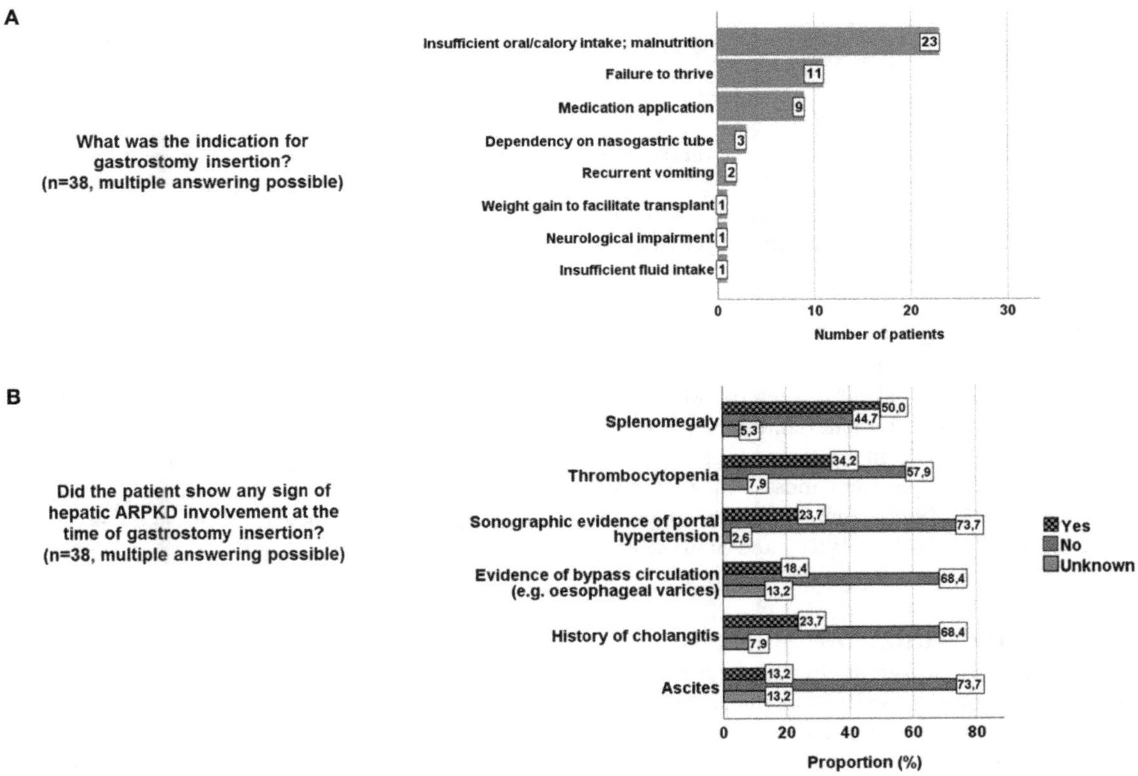

FIGURE 2 | (A) Indications for gastrostomy insertion in 38 ARPKD patients. **(B)** Hepatic phenotype at time of gastrostomy insertion in 38 ARPKD patients.

surgical revision (change to button, herniotomy, surgical closure, due to infection), including one patient who was reported to have developed fulminant sepsis with subsequent death. Detailed information regarding causality and temporal connection of gastrostomy with fulminant sepsis was not available due to the anonymous setting of the survey. 7/52 (13.5%) colleagues

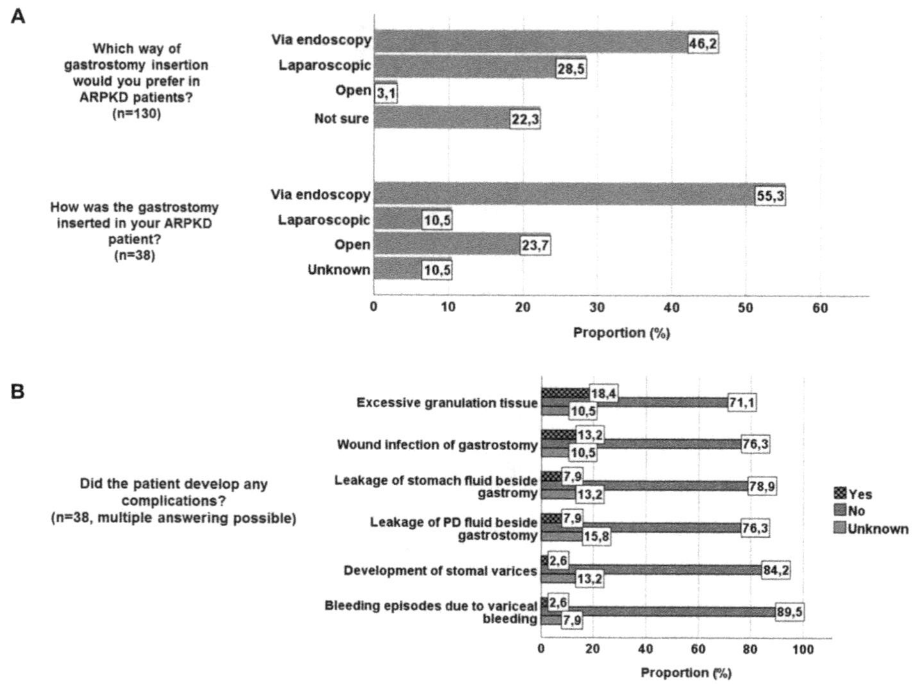

FIGURE 3 | (A) Opinion regarding way of gastrostomy insertion in ARPKD patients and way of gastrostomy insertion in 38 ARPKD patients. **(B)** Reported complications of gastrostomy in 38 ARPKD patients.

who responded to the general questionnaire indicated the requirement for gastrostomy removal in ARPKD patients for various reasons (gastrocutaneous fistula, infection, discomfort of patient resp. parents'refusal of continuation, pretransplant removal due to sufficient weight gain).

Antiinfectious Prophylaxis

Prophylactic antibiotics were applied to all patients undergoing gastrostomy insertion in 8/22 (36.4%) centers, while 3/22 (13.6%) centers indicated prophylactic antibiotics only in ARPKD patients. No prophylactic antibiotics were given in 7/22 (31.8%) centers. Cephalosporines were most frequently used [8/10 (80.0%) centers]. 2/22 (9.1%) centers used prophylactic antifungals (fluconazole) in both ARPKD and non-ARPKD patients.

Dialysis and Transplantation

10/38 (26.3%) patients with gastrostomy already performed PD at time of gastrostomy insertion. 4/38 (10.5%) patients performed HD at time of gastrostomy insertion. 13/38 patients (34.2%) started PD after gastrostomy insertion, 2/38 (5.3%) patients started HD after gastrostomy insertion.

18/38 (47.4%) patients underwent transplantation with inserted gastrostomy (10 kidney transplantations, 8 combined liver and kidney transplantations). Gastrostomy was removed at timepoint of transplantation in 3 cases (one patient with kidney transplantation from one center in Iran, two patients with combined liver and kidney transplantation from one German center) and was kept in all other patients. In non-ARPKD patients gastrostomy was removed in 6/64 (9.4%) centers prior to transplantation. One colleague reported that gastrostomy is removed in non-ARPKD patients in case of liver, but not in case of kidney transplantation.

General Evaluation of Gastrostomy in ARPKD Patients

63/158 (39.9%) participants indicated at least one ARPKD patient who had undergone gastrostomy insertion at their center with 7/65 (10.8%) colleagues recalling significant complications. Yet, in summary, 58/64 (90.6%) participants retrospectively summarized that gastrostomy insertion was the right decision for their patients, including 12/15 (80.0%) pediatric gastroenterologists/hepatologists, and 42/45 (93.3%) pediatric nephrologists ($p = 0.14$).

In summary 34/38 (89.5%) patients were considered to benefit from gastrostomy with respect to development and growth. Gastrostomy insertion was evaluated as right decision for the patient in 35/38 (92.1%) patients. In two cases gastrostomy insertion was interpreted as not beneficial for the patient, with one patient developing preinterventional hypotension with neurological sequelae and one patient dying from fulminant sepsis with unclear causality or temporal connection to gastrostomy insertion.

DISCUSSION

Based on an online survey we report on the first data on current practice of gastrostomy insertion in patients with ARPKD. To the best of our knowledge, this pediatric ARPKD cohort is the first to be reported with details on method of insertion and associated complications.

When evaluating the opinion in a first survey with 196 participants, ARPKD was considered to be a special condition in comparison to other CKD/ESKD causes. Both portal hypertension and PD were mentioned as (relative) contraindications for gastrostomy in ARPKD patients. This reflects the presumption of these two conditions as precautions for gastrostomy insertion in ARPKD patients (5, 7, 11, 12). Interestingly, pediatric gastroenterologists/hepatologists seemed to be more cautious in inserting gastrostomy in comparison to pediatric nephrologists. These differences in opinions may point out the need of a multidisciplinary discussion of both indications and contraindications between pediatric nephrologists and gastroenterologists/hepatologists to offer a uniform concept to affected patients and their families.

The common indications of insertion in 38 ARPKD patients encompassed malnutrition, failure to thrive and safe medication administration. Weight gain can be a major challenge in CKD and ARPKD (6, 13), but is substantial for achievement of a sufficient body weight for transplantation (about 10 kg in many centers). After kidney transplantation, a safe way of medication and fluid application via gastrostomy can facilitate management. Importantly, the indication for gastrostomy tube insertion in a specific ARPKD patient needs to be assessed on a case-by-case basis implementing the aspects of malnutrition as well as the renal, hepatic and neurological phenotype of an individual patient.

Our series does not report greatly increased proportions of complications in ARPKD patients compared to other pediatric patients. The most frequent reported complications were excessive granulation tissue and wound infection not exceeding complication rates in larger series of children with percutaneous endoscopic or laparoscopic gastrostomy (12, 14–16). Two cases reported in our study deserve a closer look: in one patient who had undergone bilateral nephrectomy and who suffered from severe blood pressure variations, arterial hypotension developed during anesthetic induction for gastrostomy insertion. This lead to sequelae of neurological impairment and the attending physician's assessment that the gastrostomy insertion was the wrong decision for this specific patient. However, the reported complication may appear to be related rather to the general risks of anesthesia after bilateral nephrectomy than to the specific intervention of gastrostomy insertion. In another case, a colleague reported fulminant sepsis with death in an APRKD patient. From our data, we cannot specify whether this event was directly linked to gastrostomy insertion, as detailed information on this case was not available in our anonymous study.

Regarding the hepatic phenotype of patients requiring gastrostomy, conditions of portal hypertension and/or possible future liver transplantation are considered as relative contraindications for percutaneous endoscopic gastrostomy (PEG) insertion by the ESPGHAN (12). The position paper mentions the risk of *de novo* portosystemic shunts and peristomal varices which could cause severe bleeding and pose major challenges for future liver transplantation. Very limited evidence of similar scenarios dealing with portal hypertension in patients with PEG are cited from the literature (12) in form of only two studies with 2 respectively 5 patients suffering from portal hypertension receiving PEG (17, 18). The authors underline that careful preparation and adequate expertise are mandatory requirements for PEG insertions in these specific patients. In our survey, surprisingly, half of the 38 ARPKD patients showed some form of hepatic involvement/phenotype at the time of gastrostomy insertion. Apparently, the benefits of gastrostomy insertion were considered to outweigh potential complications in these patients. Bleeding-related complications were reported in 3 of 38 patients (7.9%): one patient each was reported to suffer from stomal varices respectively bleeding episodes due to variceal bleeding summing up to two patients (5.3%) with portal hypertension related bleeding complications. The third patient (1 of 38, 2.6%) was reported to suffer from excessive bleeding from gastrostomy exit site 9 months after insertion. It remained unclear whether this bleeding episode was related to portal hypertension or rather to gastrostomy tube induced mucosal irritation. In the literature, data are very limited regarding bleeding complications in pediatric patients with portal hypertension and gastrostomy. First data exist for children with cystic fibrosis associated liver disease: two case series with 7 and 37 patients report no bleeding episodes attributable to varices or development of stomal varices, minor complications in common frequency and no procedure-related mortality (8, 10). Compared to this, the rate of complications related to portal hypertension in our series may seem to be relevant and needs to be taken into consideration in the decision process prior to gastrostomy insertion. Assuming that the patient with excessive bleeding from gastrostomy exit site 9 months after insertion suffered from tube induced mucosal irritation, this rate seems to be within the same range of a single center experience from South Korea (19). In this study on 236 pediatric non-ARPKD patients undergoing gastrostomy insertion due to poor nutrition, swallowing difficulty, and upper gastrointestinal obstruction gastrointestinal (GI) bleeding due to gastrostomy irritation was reported in up to 5.4% of their cohort (19).

The ESPGHAN position paper on management of PEG insertion in children and adolescents does not indicate any evidence regarding the management of gastrostomy tubes in patients with potential upcoming liver transplantations (12). Almost half of the patients (18/38) with inserted gastrostomy in our dataset underwent transplantation with a gastrostomy in situ. Ten patients received isolated kidney transplantation and 8 patients received combined liver and kidney transplantation. In three patients (two with combined liver and kidney transplantation, one with isolated kidney transplantation), gastrostomy was removed at the timepoint of transplantation. No adverse events or severe complications were reported in the courses after transplantation. As there is no recommendation regarding timepoint of gastrostomy removal in children after transplantation, risks and benefits need to be outweighed in every single patient (20, 21). Our data without severe complications in the post-transplant courses in 15 ARPKD patients with gastrostomy in situ (9 patients with isolated kidney transplantation, 6 patients with combined liver and kidney transplantation) may set a basis for discussing the timepoint of gastrostomy removal.

Limitations of our survey include the anonymous questionnaire which does not allow queries for both participants and survey organizers in case of uncertainties. The set-up of the survey may result in a selection bias of centers. We can neither exclude a bias in participation due to personal experiences nor a bias in reporting in both positive and negative aspects. Due to pre-determined answer possibilities, specifications were not possible in all questions. Answers of questions might be biased to a nephrologic point of view, since three quarter of all participants indicated to be pediatric nephrologists and only 20% indicated to be pediatric gastroenterologists/hepatologists. We did not receive replies from pediatric surgeons potentially precluding addition of information from a surgical point of view. On the other hand, regular patient care and follow-up is provided by pediatric nephrologists and gastroenterologists/hepatologists in most pediatric ARPKD patients. Furthermore, pediatric gastroenterologists/hepatologists take care of gastrostomy insertion and follow-up in the first place in many centers consulting pediatric surgeons only in case of uncertainties or contraindications for non-surgical insertion. As further limitation, patient-specific data did not encompass a longitudinal follow-up of data on growth and development.

The choice of insertion method in complex patients—such as children with ARPKD—is subject to local habits and experiences at specific centers. Since the cohort of pediatric ARPKD patients displays major phenotypic variability with respect to growth and development as well as renal and hepatic phenotype, the results of our survey can neither be extrapolated to daily clinical practice without critical case-by-case discussion in a multidisciplinary team nor replace future clinical practice recommendations or guidelines.

Despite these limitations, this study sets a first basis of reporting encouraging international experiences with gastrostomy insertion in pediatric ARPKD patients. In summary, gastrostomy insertion was evaluated as a correct decision for the patient and outweighing developing complications in most cases. Due to the concomitant hepatorenal affection, children with ARPKD rely on a multidisciplinary collaboration of both pediatric nephrologists and gastroenterologists/hepatologists (22). In order to set a basis for development of management recommendations in a multidisciplinary approach, international initiatives like the recently established ARPKD registry Study ARegPKD will further help to define indications and contraindications of gastrostomy insertion in ARPKD patients (23' 24).

AUTHOR CONTRIBUTIONS

KB, JB, RS, PW, LW, JD, FS, DM, and ML drafted the manuscript. KB, JB, RS, PW, FS, DM, and ML designed the questionnaire. All authors reviewed and approved the final manuscript.

ACKNOWLEDGMENTS

We thank all participating members of the mentioned societies for their input and support. ML was supported by grants of the GPN, the European Society for Paediatric Nephrology, the German PKD foundation, the Koeln Fortune program, the GEROK program of the Medical Faculty of University of Cologne, and the Marga and Walter Boll-Foundation. ML and FS are supported by the the German Federal Ministry of Research and Education (BMBF grant 01GM1515). The Pediatric Study Center Cologne was supported by the German Federal Ministry of Research and Education (BMBF grant 01KN1106). KB was supported by the Koeln Fortune program of the Medical Faculty of University of Cologne.

REFERENCES

1. Adeva M, El-Youssef M, Rossetti S, Kamath PS, Kubly V, Consugar MB, et al. Clinical and molecular characterization defines a broadened spectrum of autosomal recessive polycystic kidney disease (ARPKD). *Medicine* (2006) **85**:1–21. doi: 10.1097/01.md.0000200165.90373.9a
2. Bergmann C, Senderek J, Windelen E, Küpper F, Middeldorf I, Schneider F, et al. Clinical consequences of PKHD1 mutations in 164 patients with autosomal-recessive polycystic kidney disease (ARPKD). *Kidney Int.* (2005) **67**:829–48. doi: 10.1111/j.1523-1755.2005.00148.x
3. Guay-Woodford LM, Desmond RA. Autosomal recessive polycystic kidney disease: the clinical experience in North America. *Pediatrics* (2003) **111**(5 Pt 1):1072–80. doi: 10.1542/peds.111.5.1072
4. Lilova M, Kaplan BS, Meyers KEC. Recombinant human growth hormone therapy in autosomal recessive polycystic kidney disease. *Pediatr Nephrol Berl Ger.* (2003) **18**:57–61. doi: 10.1007/s00467-002-0986-z
5. von Schnakenburg C, Feneberg R, Plank C, Zimmering M, Arbeiter K, Bald M, et al. Percutaneous endoscopic gastrostomy in children on peritoneal dialysis. *Perit Dial Int J Int Soc Perit Dial.* (2006) **26**:69–77.
6. Zurowska AM, Fischbach M, Watson AR, Edefonti A, Stefanidis CJ, European Paediatric Dialysis Working Group. Clinical practice recommendations for the care of infants with stage 5 chronic kidney disease (CKD5). *Pediatr Nephrol Berl Ger.* (2013) **28**:1739–48. doi: 10.1007/s00467-012-2300-z
7. Warady BA, Bakkaloglu S, Newland J, Cantwell M, Verrina E, Neu A, et al. Consensus Guidelines for the prevention and treatment of Catheter-related Infections and peritonitis in pediatric patients receiving peritoneal dialysis:

2012 update. *Perit Dial Int J Int Soc Perit Dial.* (2012) **32**(Suppl. 2):S32–86. doi: 10.3747/pdi.2011.00091

8. Vandeleur M, Massie J, Oliver M. Gastrostomy in children with cystic fibrosis and portal hypertension. *J Pediatr Gastroenterol Nutr.* (2013) **57**:245–7. doi: 10.1097/MPG.0b013e3182952e39
9. Baltz JG, Argo CK, Al-Osaimi AMS, Northup PG. Mortality after percutaneous endoscopic gastrostomy in patients with cirrhosis: a case series. *Gastrointest Endosc.* (2010) **72**:1072–5. doi: 10.1016/j.gie.2010.06.043
10. Oliver MR, Heine RG, Ng CH, Volders E, Olinsky A. Factors affecting clinical outcome in gastrostomy-fed children with cystic fibrosis. *Pediatr Pulmonol.* (2004) **37**:324–9. doi: 10.1002/ppul.10321
11. Le Sidaner A, Bouteloup C, Cano N, Schneider S, Lachaux A, Michaud L, et al. *Consensus en Endoscopie Digestive (CED) Gastrostomie et Jéjunostomie Percutanées Endoscopiques.* (2007) Available online at: http://www.sfed.org/files/documents_sfed/files/recommandations/GastrostomieJejunostomie.pdf (Accessed October 2017, 24).
12. Heuschkel RB, Gottrand F, Devarajan K, Poole H, Callan J, Dias JA, et al. ESPGHAN position paper on management of percutaneous endoscopic gastrostomy in children and adolescents. *J Pediatr Gastroenterol Nutr.* (2015) **60**:131–41. doi: 10.1097/MPG.0000000000000501
13. Rees L, Azocar M, Borzych D, Watson AR, Büscher A, Edefonti A, et al. Growth in very young children undergoing chronic peritoneal dialysis. *J Am Soc Nephrol.* (2011) **22**:2303–12. doi: 10.1681/ASN.2010020192
14. McSweeney ME, Kerr J, Jiang H, Lightdale JR. Risk factors for complications in infants and children with percutaneous endoscopic gastrostomy tubes. *J Pediatr.* (2015) **166**:1514–9.e1. doi: 10.1016/j.jpeds.2015.03.009
15. Merli L, De Marco EA, Fedele C, Mason EJ, Taddei A, Paradiso FV, et al. Gastrostomy placement in children: percutaneous endoscopic gastrostomy or laparoscopic gastrostomy? *Surg Laparosc Endosc Percutan Tech.* (2016) **26**:381–4. doi: 10.1097/SLE.0000000000000310
16. Hansen E, Qvist N, Rasmussen L, Ellebaek MB. Postoperative complications following percutaneous endoscopic gastrostomy are common in children. *Acta Paediatr.* (2017) **106**:1165–9. doi: 10.1111/apa.13865
17. Duché M, Habès D, Lababidi A, Chardot C, Wenz J, Bernard O. Percutaneous endoscopic gastrostomy for continuous feeding in children with chronic cholestasis. *J Pediatr Gastroenterol Nutr.* (1999) **29**:42–5. doi: 10.1097/00005176-199907000-00012
18. Sawyerr AM, Ghosh S, Eastwood MA. Satisfactory outcome of percutaneous endoscopic gastrostomy in two patients with cirrhosis and portal hypertension. *Am J Gastroenterol.* (1995) **90**:826–8.
19. Kim J, Koh H, Chang EY, Park SY, Kim S. Single center experience with gastrostomy insertion in pediatric patients: a 10-year review. *Pediatr Gastroenterol Hepatol Nutr.* (2017) **20**:34–40. doi: 10.5223/pghn.2017.20.1.34
20. Wong H, Mylrea K, Cameron A, Manion I, Bass J, Feber J, et al. Caregiver attitudes towards gastrostomy removal after renal transplantation. *Pediatr Transplant.* (2005) **9**:574–8. doi: 10.1111/j.1399-3046.2005.00341.x
21. Ledermann S. When should gastrostomy tubes be removed following successful renal transplantation? *Pediatr Transplant.* (2005) **9**:553–4. doi: 10.1111/j.1399-3046.2005.00355.x
22. Van Hoeve K, Mekahli D, Morava E, Levtchenko E, Witters P. Liver involvement in kidney disease and vice versa. *Pediatr Nephrol Berl Ger.* (2018) **33**:957–71. doi: 10.1007/s00467-017-3715-3
23. Ebner K, Feldkoetter M, Ariceta G, Bergmann C, Buettner R, Doyon A, et al. Rationale, design and objectives of ARegPKD, a European ARPKD registry study. *BMC Nephrol.* (2015) **16**:22. doi: 10.1186/s12882-015-0002-z
24. Ebner K, Schaefer F, Liebau MC, ARegPKD Consortium. Recent progress of the ARegPKD registry study on autosomal recessive polycystic kidney disease. *Front Pediatr.* (2017) **5**:18. doi: 10.3389/fped.2017.00018

20

Exploring the Clinical and Genetic Spectrum of Steroid Resistant Nephrotic Syndrome: The PodoNet Registry

Agnes Trautmann[1*], *Beata S. Lipska-Ziętkiewicz*[2] *and Franz Schaefer*[1]
on behalf of the PodoNet Consortium

[1] *Division of Pediatric Nephrology, University Center for Pediatrics and Adolescent Medicine, Heidelberg, Germany,* [2] *Clinical Genetics Unit, Department of Biology and Medical Genetics, Medical University of Gdańsk, Gdańsk, Poland*

***Correspondence:**
Agnes Trautmann
agnes.trautmann@med.uni-heidelberg.de

Background: Steroid resistant nephrotic syndrome (SRNS) is a rare condition, accounting for 10–15% of all children with idiopathic nephrotic syndrome. SRNS can be caused by genetic abnormalities or immune system dysfunction. The prognosis of SRNS varies from permanent remission to progression to end-stage kidney disease, and post-transplant recurrence is common.

Objectives: The PodoNet registry project aims to explore the demographics and phenotypes of immune-mediated and genetic forms of childhood SRNS, to assess genotype-phenotype correlations, to evaluate clinical management and long-term outcomes, and to search for novel genetic entities and diagnostic and prognostic biomarkers in SRNS.

Methods: In 2009, an international registry for SRNS was established to collect retro- and prospective information on renal and extrarenal disease manifestations, histopathological and genetic findings and information on family history, pharmacotherapy responsiveness and long-term outcomes. To date, more than 2,000 patients have been enrolled at 72 pediatric nephrology centers, constituting the largest pediatric SRNS cohort assembled to date.

Results: In the course of the project, traditional Sanger sequencing was replaced by NGS-based gene panel screening covering over 30 podocyte-related genes complemented by whole exome sequencing. These approaches allowed to establish genetic diagnoses in 24% of the patients screened, widened the spectrum of genetic disease entities presenting with SRNS phenotype (*COL4A3-5, CLCN5*), and contributed to the discovery of new disease causing genes (*MYOE1, PTPRO*). Forty two percent of patients responded to intensified immunosuppression with complete or partial remission of proteinuria, whereas 58% turned out multi-drug resistant. Medication responsiveness was highly predictive of a favorable long-term outcome, whereas the diagnosis of genetic disease was associated with a high risk to develop end-stage renal disease during childhood. Genetic SRNS forms were generally resistant to immunosuppressive treatment, justifying to avoid such pharmacotherapies altogether once a genetic diagnosis is established. Even symptomatic anti-proteinuric treatment with RAS antagonists seems to be challenging and of limited efficacy in genetic forms of SRNS. The risk of post-transplant disease recurrence was around 30% in non-genetic SRNS whereas it is negligible in genetic cases.

Conclusion: In summary, the PodoNet Registry has collected detailed clinical and genetic information in a large SRNS cohort and continues to generate fundamental insights regarding demographic and etiological disease aspects, genotype-phenotype associations, the efficacy of therapeutic strategies, and long-term patient and renal outcomes including post-transplant disease recurrence.

Keywords: SRNS, nephrotic syndrome, NPHS2, WT1, steroid resistant nephrotic syndrome

INTRODUCING THE PODONET REGISTRY STUDY FOR STEROID RESISTANT NEPHROTIC SYNDROME

While most children with idiopathic nephrotic syndrome respond to oral glucocorticoid therapy and have a favorable long-term prognosis, ~10–15% of children do not respond and are classified as steroid resistant nephrotic syndrome (SRNS). SRNS is a rare (incidence 3–4 per million person-years) and challenging clinical condition with heterogeneous etiology and highly variable disease courses and outcomes.

Whereas, a relevant fraction of SRNS children respond to intensified immunosuppressive therapy with temporary or persistent proteinuria remission, others exhibit primary multidrug resistance. Traditionally, the diagnostic and prognostic assessment of SRNS has been based on histopathological categorization. In recent years however, the understanding of SRNS pathophysiology has transformed fundamentally with the discovery of a rapidly growing number of genetic disorders of the podocytes. These novel insights have created a need to redefine diagnostic assessment, prognostic classification and therapeutic approaches in childhood-onset SRNS. However, clinical research in SRNS is compromised by the low incidence and heterogeneity of the disorder. To overcome the limitations related to the rarity of the disorder, the PodoNet Consortium set up an international web-based registry for childhood SRNS and CNS (www.podonet.org).

The objectives of the PodoNet registry project are to explore the demographics and phenotypes of immune-mediated and genetic forms of childhood SRNS, to evaluate genotype-phenotype correlations, to evaluate clinical management and long-term outcomes, and to search for genetic entities and novel diagnostic and prognostic biomarkers of SRNS. Data collection is focused on the characteristics at first disease manifestation, genetic and histopathological findings, the responsiveness to pharmacological therapies, long-term renal survival, and post-transplant disease recurrence.

This manuscript reviews the accomplishments of the international PodoNet project since 2009, focusing on both genetic and clinical aspects of SRNS. The international PodoNet registry study with retro- and prospective data of currently more than 2,000 patients provides extended knowledge about SRNS demographics, SRNS genotype-phenotype correlations, therapeutic and prognostic outcomes and has discovered new genetic disorders. These results contribute to an improved understanding of the different SRNS entities and to a re-classification of SRNS based on molecular etiology and responsiveness to second-line treatment.

PODONET STUDY COHORT: METHODS AND DEFINITIONS

The PodoNet registry is a web-based clinical database (www.podonet.org) for primary steroid resistant (SRNS) and congenital nephrotic syndrome (CNS). The registry follows patients with childhood-onset (age < 20 years) primary SRNS, CNS or persistent subnephrotic proteinuria with likely genetic disease, but not patients with secondary SRNS. Since August 2009, investigators from 72 clinical units in 28 countries have enrolled 2041 patients (**Figure 1**). The patients derive mainly from European countries (~85%) but also from the Middle East and Latin America (15%) (1). Consanguinity and familial disease occurrence were most common in the Middle Eastern countries (**Figure 2**). Details on the structure of the PodoNet study cohort along with the registry study protocol and description were recently published (1).

Genetic screening was initially performed using Sanger sequencing of individual genes following a diagnostic screening algorithm based on age at presentation and extrarenal symptoms. From 2013 onward, next generation panel sequencing (NGS) of more than 30 podocytopathy-associated genes was systematically applied. Details of the diagnostic genetic screening studies and their completeness are described below.

Intensified immunosuppressive (IIS) therapies applied after confirmation of steroid resistance (persistent nephrotic-range proteinuria after 4 weeks oral prednisone at 60 mg/m^2 per day), included intravenous steroid pulses, calcineurin inhibitors (CNI), mycophenolate-mofetil (MMF), the combination of CNI and MMF, oral and intravenous cyclophosphamide (CPH), and rituximab.

The response to IIS (complete, partial, no remission) was assessed using a standardized set of criteria using changes in proteinuria and serum albumin, as previously defined (1, 2).

To categorize IIS responsiveness as a basis for predicting long-term outcomes, the evaluation period was restricted to the first year of IIS treatment and disease. Patients with CNS were excluded. If patients were treated with more than one intensified immunosuppressive treatment in the first year, the most efficacious treatment and the best antiproteinuric response was identified. Patients who were unresponsive to any IIS applied were classified as multi-drug resistant.

End-stage kidney disease (ESKD) was defined by attainment of CKD stage 5 and/or start of renal replacement therapy.

All statistical analyses of the reported individual studies of the PodoNet registry were performed using SAS® Version 9.4 (Cary, USA). Statistical details can be obtained from the original articles (1–5).

CLINICAL AND GENETIC SPECTRUM OF THE PODONET COHORT STUDY—RESULTS AND DISCUSSION

Clinical Aspects of SRNS

First Manifestation

Among all patients reported to the PodoNet Registry, 6% presented with congenital nephrotic syndrome, 7% manifested as early infantile nephrotic syndrome (onset age 3–11 months), 51% at 1–5 years, 23% at 6–11 years, and 13% at age 12 years and older (**Figure 3**).

Hypoalbuminemia was most pronounced in congenital nephrotic syndrome (mean serum albumin 17 g/L) and least marked in adolescent-onset disease (26 g/L). Likewise, hypertension at diagnosis was most prevalent in adolescents (28%) as compared to 14% in infants. A small fraction of patients (8.7%) were diagnosed with non-nephrotic proteinuria, but progressed to full nephrotic syndrome during follow-up (1).

63.5% of children had a normal renal function (CKD stage 1), 23.5% a mildly impaired renal function at first presentation. Chronic kidney disease (CKD stage 3 and 4) was present in 13% (1). 7.4% of patients progressed to ESKD in the first year, whereas the median time to ESKD was 2.8 years.

Extrarenal disease manifestations pointing to a syndromic disorder most commonly included neurological symptoms (5.3% including brain anomalies, microcephaly and/or mental retardation), short stature (5.1%) and facial dysmorphism (2.2%).

Histopathological Findings

The predominant histopathological diagnosis was FSGS in 56% of all PodoNet patients, followed by minimal-change nephropathy (MCN) with 20% and mesangioproliferative GN (MesPGN) with 11% (**Figure 4**). The predominance of FSGS was also found in other SRNS populations (6–9), albeit with some variability likely related to variations of ethnic composition, biopsy indication policies, and disease duration at time of biopsy.

Twelve percent of the PodoNet patients received a second renal biopsy during the course of the disease. Two thirds of the re-biopsied patients previously diagnosed with MCN or MesGN showed FSGS in the second biopsy, and 10% of those with FSGS progressed to global glomerulosclerosis (GGS).

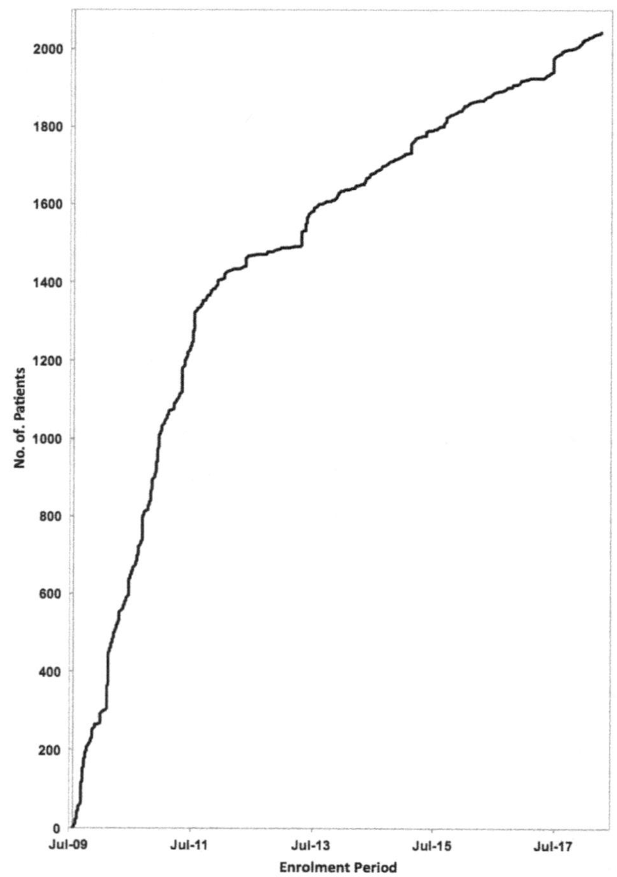

FIGURE 1 | Patient enrolment to the PodoNet Registry. 2,041 children with SRNS have been registered at 72 clinical pediatric nephrology centers in 28 countries since August 2009.

The children in our cohort who initially presented with FSGS, MCN, or MesPGN displayed similar severity of hypoalbuminemia (25–27 g/dl) and comparable prevalence of hypertension (15–18%). Patients with FSGS were on average slightly older (6 years vs. 4 years for MCN/MesPGN) and presented with a slightly lower eGFR than patients with MCN/MesPGN.

The other histopathological entities found in children with SRNS - diffuse mesangial sclerosis (DMS, 3%), membranoproliferative glomerulopathy (MPGN, 2%), membranous nephropathy (MN, 2%)—were much less common. Typically, patients with these diagnoses manifested with milder initial hypoalbuminemia but slightly higher prevalence of hypertension (23–26%) than patients with FSGS, MCN and MesPGN. Patients with DMS usually presented at earlier age (median age of 1.3 years), similar to the observations of the SRNS Study Group where DMS was found in 27% of infants (10) with established renal failure and an identified genetic cause in almost two thirds of cases (1). In patients with FSGS, the detection rate of genetic disease was lower with 22% and lowest with 12% in children with MCN (1).

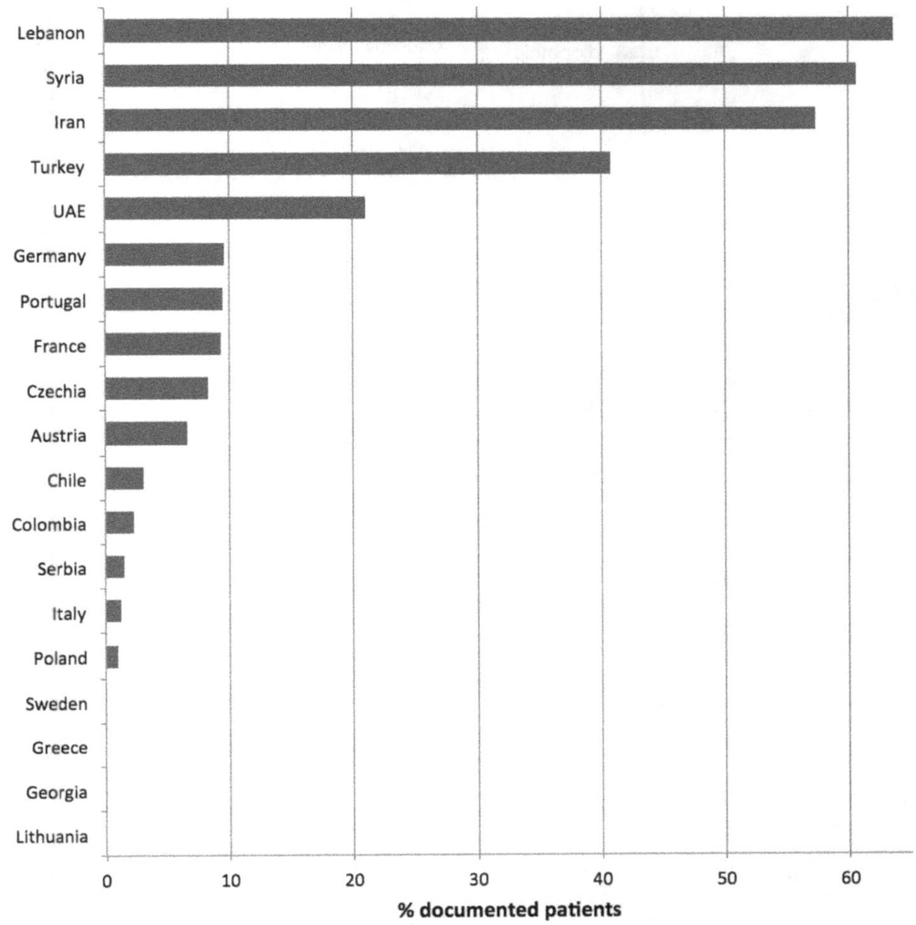

FIGURE 2 | Documented parental consanguinity per country. Only countries with more than 10 registered patients were considered.

Genetic Aspects of SRNS

Diagnostic Screening Studies

To date, a total of 1,554 individual PodoNet patients were genetically screened for hereditary podocytopathies. Initially, the most commonly screened genes were *NPHS2* and *WT1* performed by Sanger sequencing whereas other podocyte genes were screened more selectively guided by age, histopathology, and/or syndromic features. These included *WT1* disease (sex reversal/urogenital abnormalities and malignancies), mitochondrial dysfunction (myopathy, cardiomyopathy, impaired hearing), Pierson syndrome (impaired vision), and Schimke syndrome (osteodysplasia) (1).

Since 2014, next generation sequencing (NGS) gene panels were used to systematically screen for all known podocytopathy genes as part of the EURenOmics project (www.eurenomics.org). Identified mutations in the panel sequencing were confirmed by Sanger sequencing. To date, 539 unrelated patients with documented multi-drug resistance or unknown responsiveness to intensified immunosuppressive therapy were screened by NGS panel including more than 30 podocyte specific genes. These included 214 novel consecutively enrolled cases and 315 previously tested negative by conventional screening of *NPHS2* and exons 8–9 of *WT1*.

Overall, since the beginning of the PodoNet Registry genetic diagnoses were established in 373 SRNS patients (24% of those tested; 19% of the entire cohort). This mutation detection rate is slightly lower compared to that recently reported in a study of 1783 SRNS families (29.5%) (10).

In line with other SRNS studies (9, 10), mutations in *NPHS2*, *WT1* and *NPHS1* represented the most common genetic SRNS causes, accounting for 42, 16, and 13% of cases, respectively (**Table 1**). Using the NGS gene panel, mutations were identified in 27% of novel consecutive patients and in 17% of patients previously found negative for *NPHS2* and exons 8–9 of *WT1* mutations. Hence, almost half of all genetic SRNS patients carry a mutation in *NPHS2* or the zinc finger domains of *WT1*, which could provide a rationale for a cost-effective two-step mutational screening algorithm.

The mutation detection rate was highest in children with CNS and significantly lower with increasing age at first manifestation during the first 6 years of life (**Figure 3**), in

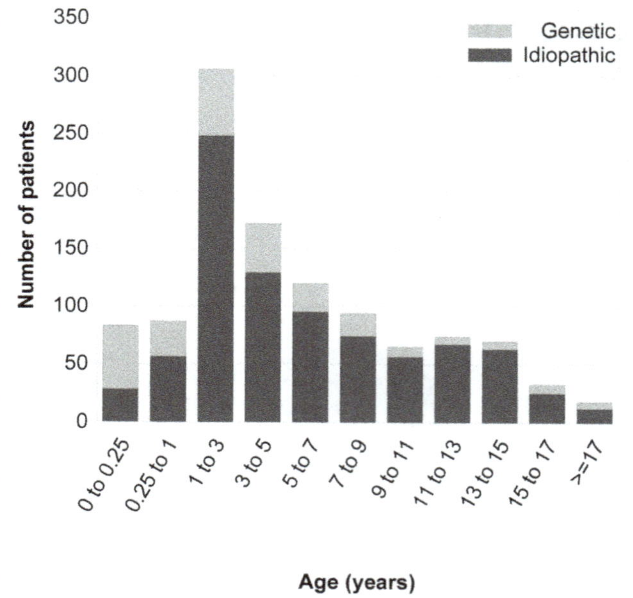

FIGURE 3 | Age at first disease manifestation in children with and without an identified genetic cause of steroid-resistant nephrotic syndrome.

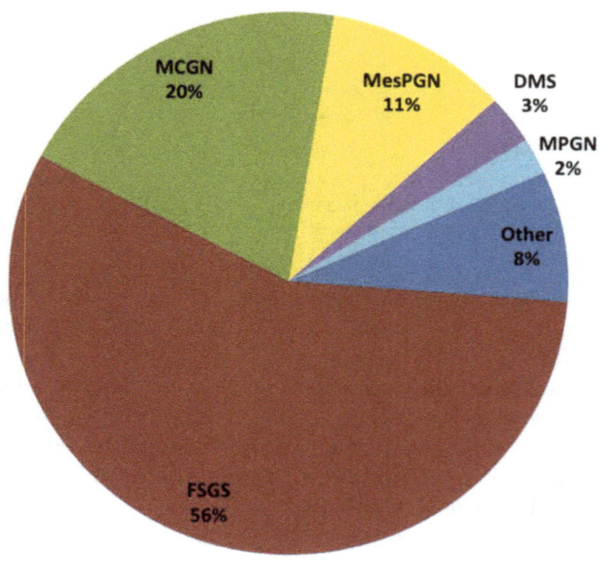

FIGURE 4 | Distribution of underlying histopathologic diagnosis in the first renal biopsy performed in 1,651 children with SRNS from the PodoNet cohort.

keeping with observations by the SRNS Study Group (10) and the German Pediatric Nephrology Society (9). While genetic screening strategies for diagnosing childhood-onset nephrotic syndrome were generally established when the PodoNet registry was founded, screening strategies for adolescent-onset disease were not well-established. Utilizing our PodoNet cohort, 297 patients with non-syndromic SRNS and disease onset in the

TABLE 1 | Mutation screening results.

Causative gene	N	%
NPHS2	156	41.8
WT1	59	15.8
NPHS1	47	12.6
SMARCAL1	20	5.4
PLCE1	14	3.8
ADCK4	13	3.5
COL4A5	11	1.3
LMX1B	10	2.7
INF2	8	2.1
LAMB2	8	2.1
COQ6	6	1.6
MYO1E	6	1.6
PTPRO	5	1.3
TRPC6	3	0.8
CLCN5	2	0.5
COQ2	2	0.5
PAX2	2	0.5
ACTN4	1	0.3
COL4A3	1	0.3
Others	4	1.1
All	373	100

Genetic diagnoses in 373 of 1,554 genetically screened children with hereditary SRNS (24%).

second decade of life were screened for mutations in *NPHS2*, *WT1*, *TRPC6*, *ACTN4*, and *INF2* (3). Seventy-nine percent of adolescents had a sporadic disease occurrence, 21% familial disease occurrence (17% autosomal-recessive, 4% autosomal-dominant forms). The overall mutation rate in the adolescent age group in those five genes was 11%, separated into 30% in the autosomal-dominant cases, 13% in the autosomal-recessive and 10% of the sporadic cases. *NPHS2* mutations accounted for 7% of all adolescent cases. Based on the common involvement of p.R229Q in late-onset SRNS, an approach of a two-step screening algorithm (limiting full sequencing of the *NPHS2* gene to carriers of the p.R229Q polymorphism) was suggested in previous studies (11, 12). As only 56% of adolescents with *NPHS2*-associated disease were compound-heterozygous for a mutation combined with the p.R229Q polymorphism in the PodoNet cohort, we suggested to rather screen the entire coding sequence of *NPHS2* in all sporadic and autosomal-recessive cases of juvenile SRNS. The considerations of selective and limited genetic screening in adolescents subsequently became largely obsolete with the advent of next generation sequencing.

Gene Exploration Studies

One of the aims of the PodoNet Network is to foster the identification of new SRNS causing genes. Registered PodoNet patients were evaluated regarding familial disease occurrence and negative screening in the known SRNS genes and biomaterial was collected. This allows to contribute and to perform whole-genome linkage analysis and high-throughput sequencing in affected families. PodoNet Consortium partners have identified two new SRNS causing genes participation of SRNS families of the PodoNet cohort in 2011: *PTPRO* (13) and *MYO1E* (14).

PTPRO-associated SRNS

The role of the protein tyrosine phosphatase receptor type O (*PTPRO*) gene, also known as *GLEPP1* (glomerular epithelial protein 1) gene, is the regulation of glomerular pressure and permselectivity. The protein PTPRO is a tyrosine phosphatase expressed at the apical membrane of the podocyte foot processes. Thyrosine phosphorylation of tight junction proteins plays a major role in controlling paracellular permeability, cell signaling and actin cytoskeleton remodeling.

PTPRO mutations were identified in 5 of 29 affected children from two of 17 tested families with so far unknown genetic disease. The disease onset varied between 5 and 14 years, the initial serum albumin varied between 19 and 40 g/L at first manifestation. Apart from one affected child, none of the children had progressed to ESKD 2–5 years after first manifestation. Renal biopsy, performed in 2 children, revealed MCN as well as FSGS (13) and electron microscopy showed diffuse podocyte foot process fusion and extensive microvillus transformation of podocytes. The subsequent testing of almost 2000 SRNS cases of all age groups performed within the frames of the EuRenOmics project did not identify any further individuals with pathogenic biallelic *PTPRO* mutations, demonstrating its extremely rare character.

MYO1E-associated SRNS

MYO1E encodes a non-muscle class I myosin (Myo1E) which is expressed mainly at the podocyte plasma membrane in the glomerulus. The role of Myo1E is maintaining the function of the glomerular filtration barrier and promoting the podocyte motility. Two mutations in *MYO1E* were identified in two families (3 siblings, 1 other child), which are closely associated with autosomal recessive SRNS/FSGS (14).

The age at disease onset of the index patient was 9 years; the siblings and the fourth child were diagnosed earlier (between age of 1–4 years). The histopathological diagnosis was FSGS in all children, electron microscopy showed thickening and disorganization of the glomerular basement membrane.

All four patients showed generally non-responsiveness to intensified immunosuppression. Cyclosporine A therapy was associated with a transient proteinuria reduction in 2 of 4 children, possibly related to a direct podocyte cytoskeleton stabilizing effect of calcineurin inhibition. One affected member progressed to ESKD at age of 13 years; the other affected siblings had milder disease courses, possibly related to earlier diagnosis and/or to effective antiproteinuric treatment. Three further unrelated individuals with *MYO1E* biallelic mutations were subsequently identified through NGS gene panel screening, all of them presented in early infancy.

Genotype-Phenotype Association Studies

WT1-associated SRNS

WT1 mutations are associated with a wide range of clinical phenotypes. The PodoNet consortium explored the phenotypic spectrum and analyzed potential genotype-phenotype correlations in 61 patients with *WT1*-associated SRNS, the largest cohort studied to date (4). Both renal and extrarenal phenotypes were found to be clearly associated with the type and location of the causative *WT1* mutation.

55 of 61 patients (90%) carried mutations in the *hot spot region* (exons 8 and 9 and their intronic junctions). The mutations were categorized as exonic mutations (40/61 patients) including truncating mutations, DNA-binding-site mutations and other missense mutation and as intronic mutations (21/61 patients, KTS intron 9 and other intronic mutations). The two largest subgroups (70%) are exonic mutations affecting the nucleotides coding for DNA-binding residues and intronic (9) KTS mutations, the latter are classically associated with Denys-Drash- and Frasier-syndrome.

Patients with exonic mutations were significantly younger at diagnosis (1.1 vs. 4.5 years), presented with more severe proteinuria, edema, and hypertension and progressed more rapidly to ESKD (5-year renal survival from diagnosis 36 vs. 85%) and had a higher risk for nephroblastoma (73 vs. 19%) than patients with intronic mutations. Gonadoblastoma occurs less frequently than Wilms tumors and are more likely to develop in patients with sex reversal commonly associated with intronic mutation.

Missense mutations affecting the DNA-binding site were associated with diffuse mesangial sclerosis (74%), early steroid-resistant nephrotic syndrome onset [0.9 (0.2–1.6) years] and rapid progression to ESKD. Truncating mutations implicated the highest Wilms tumor risk (78%) but had typically late-onset SRNS [12.3 (0.6–15.3) years]. Intronic (KTS) mutations were most likely to present as isolated SRNS (37%) with a median onset at the age of 4.5 (3.1–8.1) years, FSGS (67%) and slow progression (median ESKD age 13.6 years). All patients with isolated SRNS were genotypic and phenotypic females.

In contrast to the consistent associations of mutation type and clinical disease manifestation, histopathology showed high diagnostic and prognostic variability. Furthermore, genital and urinary tract abnormalities varied widely, from hypospadias and unilateral cryptorchidism to global penoscrotal hypoplasia. Genital malformations were detected in 50% of all patients. Male-to female sex reversal occurred exclusively in patients with intronic KTS mutation and exonic DNA-binding site mutation.

We concluded that establishing the genetic diagnosis and identifying the mutation type and localization is important to assess the associated features and complications. The important impact for the clinical decision is the consideration when is the appropriate timing to perform bilateral nephrectomy or gonadectomy to prevent the development of malignancies.

SMARCAL1-associated SRNS

Schimke immuno-osseous dysplasia (SIOD), caused by mutations in *SMARCAL1*, is a rare multisystem disorder characterized by the combination of progressive proteinuric glomerulopathy with spondyloepiphyseal dysplasia, growth retardation, dysmorphic features, episodic neutro-/lymphopenia and thrombocytopenia, defective T-cellular immunity, autoimmune disorders, abnormal skin pigmentation, and cerebral infarcts. Early mortality due to severe opportunistic infections or cerebral events is common.

The PodoNet consortium analyzed the renal and extrarenal phenotypic spectrum and genotype-phenotype associations in 34 PodoNet patients from 28 families—the largest *SMARCAL1*-associated nephropathy cohort to date (5). The diagnosis of *SMARCAL1*-associated disease was made either by the presence of typical syndromic feature or unexpectedly by NGS panel screening (11/34 children). All patients diagnosed incidentally through NGS screening were short in stature (height SDS −3.2 ± 1.5) but these patients developed a milder if any extrarenal phenotype during follow-up, with 88% 10-year patient survival as compared to 40% in the patients diagnosed by typical SIOD features.

The timing of proteinuria onset (median age 4.5 (IQR 3.2–7.2) years, nephrotic-range in 69% of children) and the rate of progression to ESKD were similar in all patients. Median age at ESKD was 8.7 (IQR 5.6–10) years. Renal biopsy showed FSGS in 81.5% and MCN in the remaining patients. The extrarenal symptoms, but not the renal phenotype, correlated with the type of *SMARCAL1* genetic mutation.

Since the study demonstrated that in a substantial number of patients SIOD initially presents as isolated SRNS with short stature, it was concluded that *SMARCAL1* screening should be performed routinely also in non-syndromic SRNS and should be included into the SRNS gene panels.

ADCK4-associated SRNS

Mutations in *ADCK4* (also known as *COQ8*) were recently identified as a novel autosomal-recessive cause of adolescent-onset SRNS caused by defective Coenzyme Q_{10} biosynthesis in podocytes. Hereditary defects of CoQ_{10} biosynthesis can cause SRNS as part of multiorgan involvement or as isolated SRNS.

Systematic *ADCK4* screening was performed in large cohort of 534 SRNS patients, including 202 patients of the PodoNet cohort (15). *ADCK4* mutations were identified in 26 patients from 12 families with a mutation detection rate of 1.9%. The disease almost exclusively manifested during adolescence, typically with subnephrotic to nephrotic-range proteinuria with no or mild edema but with advanced CKD in 46% of patients progressing to ESKD within a median of 9 months after diagnosis. Renal biopsies revealed FSGS in all biopsied patients. *ADCK4* mutations showed a mainly renal-limited phenotype, with mild neurological features in 5 of 26 patients (occasional seizures, mild mental retardation, retinitis pigmentosa).

ADCK4-associated glomerulopathy is the first hereditary form of SRNS with a potentially causative molecular therapy. Oral supplementation of CoQ_{10} reduces proteinuria and stabilizes renal function when applied early in the course of disease (16). Therefore, *ADCK4* mutation screening should be included into NGS screening of all patients with adolescent-onset proteinuric kidney disease.

COL4A3-5-associated SRNS

There is increasing evidence for overlapping phenotypes caused by abnormalities in the *COL4* genes and those primarily associated with SRNS/FSGS (17–20).

Among 481 patients of the PodoNet Cohort screened in *COL4A3-5*, 11 carried pathogenic mutations in *COL4A5*, and one was homozygous for a mutation in *COL4A3*.

The detection rate of 2.5% is identical to a recent pediatric study from the UK, where disease-causing mutations in *COL4A3-5* genes were identified in six out of 255 individuals with an SRNS phenotype (19). Other studies found even higher rates of *COL4* mutations particularly in adult SRNS cohorts, but these included heterozygous variants in *COL4A3/4* which are unlikely to cause severe and progressive proteinuric kidney disease (17, 18). In line with other recent studies, all patients with *COL4* gene mutations in our cohort showed FSGS on biopsy and no extrarenal disease manifestations were reported (17–19). These findings support the notion that genetic abnormalities collagen type IV formation may result in a phenotype of isolated nephrotic range proteinuria.

CLCN5-associated nephropathy

A novel mutation in the *CLCN5* gene (c.2000delC) was detected by exome sequencing in a family from the PodoNet cohort with apparently isolated nephrotic range proteinuria that had been classified as familial SRNS on clinical grounds. Both affected children were screened negative in 31 glomerulopathy-related genes. Mutations in *CLCN5*, which encodes a voltage-gated chloride ion channel expressed selectively in the renal tubule, are the major cause of Dent disease. Dent disease is an X-linked proximal renal tubular disorder; the key features include low-molecular weight proteinuria, hypercalciuria, nephrocalcinosis, and/or nephrolithiasis.

The genetic finding triggered clinical investigation for a putative tubular defect, which revealed asymptomatic hypercalciuria in only one of two children studied. In the absence of nephrocalcinosis and nephrolithiasis, Dent disease was not considered as a potential differential diagnosis of nephrotic-range proteinuria before. The genetic classification of the disease has important therapeutic and prognostic implications for the affected children. The children had been (mis)-classified as familial SRNS based on the observed nephrotic range proteinuria (>1 g/m^2 per day). Our case illustrates the genetic and phenotypic heterogeneity of proteinuric kidney diseases. The remarkable phenotypic variability of mutations in *CLCN5* suggests that this gene should be included in NGS panel screening for hereditary proteinuric disorders.

TREATMENT AND LONG-TERM OUTCOME OF SRNS

Responsiveness of SRNS Patients to Intensified Immunosuppression

Whereas, the initial treatment of idiopathic nephrotic syndrome with oral glucocorticoids is well-established, we observed a large variety of the intensified immunosuppressive protocols and algorithms applied following the diagnosis of primary steroid resistance (**Figure 5**). In an analysis of immunosuppressive therapies applied in 612 SRNS patients in the first year after diagnosis of steroid resistance (2), 62% of children were treated with a single treatment protocol, 28% with two, and 10% with three or more different immunosuppressive drug combinations as a polypragmatic therapeutic approach. While approximately three quarters of patients received Calcineurin inhibitors as first line therapy, others were administered intravenous steroid pulses, mycophenolate mofetil, oral or intravenous cyclophoshamide, or Rituximab (**Figure 5**). More than 80% of patients were co-treated with oral steroids initially, and more than 70% with renin angiotensin aldosterone system (RAS) antagonists.

Applying a standardized set of criteria to define treatment response and remission, we observed only 41% of included 612 SRNS patients to respond to any intensified immunosuppression with a relevant proteinuria reduction to IIS (24% with complete, 17% with partial remission), whereas 59% of patients remained unresponsive—often to several therapeutic interventions (**Figure 6**). The highest rates of complete (30%) or partial (19%) remission were achieved with CNI based protocols. These response rates are in the lower range of previously reported treatment experience, where complete remission was observed in 31% to 89% and partial remission in 19 to 38% of patients (9, 21–25). The variation of the response rates may be related to the selection and composition of the individual study cohorts and the chosen set of response criteria.

The efficacy of CNI-based therapies in the PodoNet cohort was by far superior to steroid pulses, cyclophosphamide, and MMF monotherapy, all of which did not show any therapeutic effect in around 85% of patients as first line therapy (**Figure 6**) and were completely non-efficacious as second- or third-line therapies in CNI resistant patients. These findings confirm previous studies (26–31) and provide strong evidence against the use of these therapeutics in SRNS. Notably, B-cell depleting therapy with Rituximab induced complete remission in 44%, and partial remission in 15% of patients (1).

RAS inhibition has been demonstrated to lower proteinuria by 40–50% in patients with SRNS (32, 33). In the PodoNet cohort, RAS inhibition alone was associated with partial proteinuria remission in 21% and even maintained complete remission in 27% of patients (1). Hence, the frequent co-administration of RAS antagonists with immunosuppressive agents is a major confounder to the efficacy analysis of the latter.

Among the 602 cohort patients available for pharmacotherapy analysis 82% had sporadic disease, 74 (12%) confirmed genetic disease and 36 (6%) familial disease with negative genetic screening in all known podocytopathy genes.

Do Patients With Genetic SRNS Respond to Immunosuppression?

Anecdotal clinical observations in previous case series and small retrospective studies suggested that individual patients with pathogenic mutations in podocytopathy genes might show some responsiveness to intensified immunosuppression. In total, 11 hereditary SRNS patients reported in literature developed complete remission and 17 partial remission of proteinuria while on calcineurin inhibitor and usually concomitant RAS antagonist therapy (4, 34–38). A non-immunological antiproteinuric action

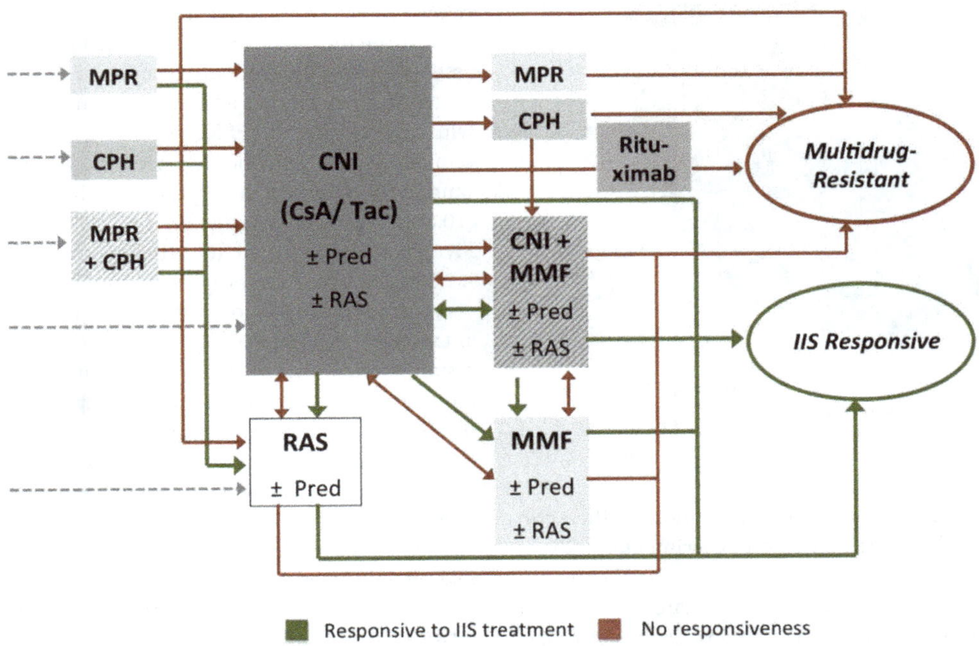

FIGURE 5 | Immunosuppressive treatments applied following diagnosis of primary steroid resistance: oral prednisolone (Pred), methylprednisolone pulses (MPR), calcineurin inhibitors (CNI), mycophenolate-mofetil (MMF), cyclophosphamide (CPH). Approximately 50% of children were co-treated with renin-angiotensin-aldosterone-system inhibitors (RAS). Patients responding to the intensified immunosuppressive (IIS) treatment were classified as IIS responsive (green), others as multi-drug resistant (red).

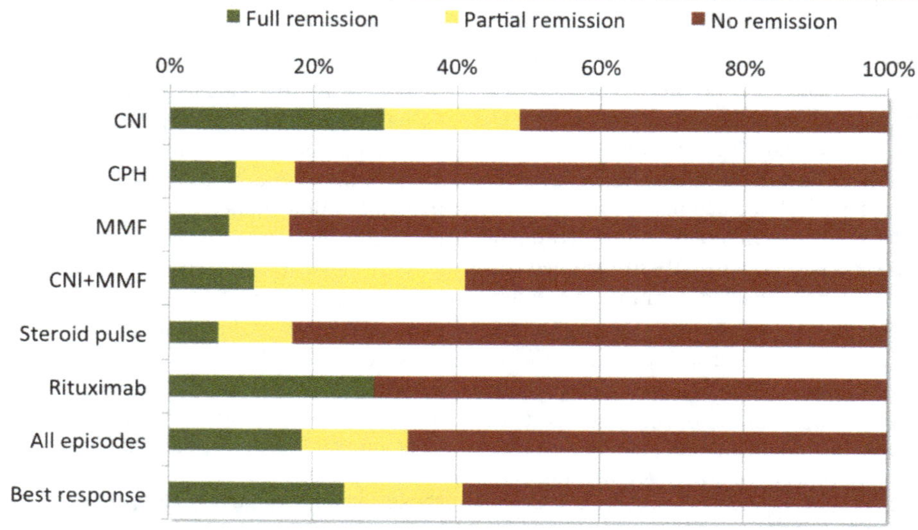

FIGURE 6 | Response to IIS treatment episodes during first year after disease onset in 612 children with SRNS. In total, 232 (38%) patients were treated with more than one treatment protocol during the first year after disease onset. Most efficacious treatment (=best response) was used to classify patients [adapted from Table 2, (2)].

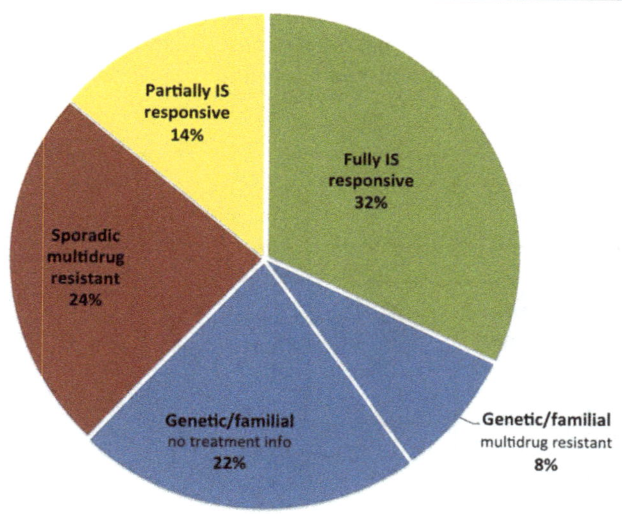

FIGURE 7 | Distribution of SRNS subtypes in the PodoNet cohort according to etiology and treatment responsiveness.

of Ciclosporin A (CsA) mediated by stabilization of the actin cytoskeleton has been suggested based on experimental findings (39).

The PodoNet registry allowed to evaluate the largest cohort of children with hereditary podocytopathies to date exposed to calcineurin inhibitor and other immunosuppressive therapy. Complete or partial proteinuria responsiveness to pharmacotherapy was observed in 45% of children with sporadic disease and in 47% of those with familial, gene screening negative disease, whereas only 13% of patients with hereditary podocytopathies displayed any, mostly transient responsiveness to pharmacotherapy (2).

Transient complete remission was documented in only two out of 74 patients (2.7%) diagnosed with genetic disease in whom extended treatment and response data were available: one child with a *WT1* mutation reportedly achieved complete remission for 2 weeks after start of CsA, followed by subnephrotic range proteinuria for > 11 years. Another child with *NPHS2*-associated disease achieved complete remission for 4–6 weeks, followed by a relapse and subsequently persistent proteinuria with progression to ESKD within 4 years. Transient partial remission with reduction of proteinuria to the non-nephrotic range was observed in response to CsA in another 8 patients (10.8%) with genetic disease (4 *NPHS2*, 3 *WT1*, 1 *COQ6*). Five of these returned to nephrotic-range proteinuria within <2.5 years, and four progressed to CKD stage 3–5 within <5 years. Importantly, 4 of 8 patients were co-treated with RAS antagonists. It is impossible to differentiate whether the transient responsiveness was related to calcineurin inhibition, supportive antiproteinuric RAS antagonist therapy or the natural course of disease with diminishing proteinuria due to worsening renal function. Notably, almost all patients with genetic disease and apparent CsA responsiveness progressed to ESKD soon despite ongoing therapy.

Hence, the findings in the PodoNet cohort argue against a relevant nephroprotective effect of calcineurin inhibition—or other immunosuppressive therapies—in children with genetic forms of SRNS and support the notion that such patients should be spared immunosuppressant side effects. On the other hand, the knowledge about the heterogeneity of underlying genetic disease mechanisms might help to develop specific podocyte-protecting treatment strategies in order to minimize proteinuria. A promising example of an innovative gene specific treatment option is successful use of CoQ10 in children with SRNS due to genetic defects leading to CoQ10 deficiency (15, 16, 40). In the light of these findings and given the progress in the speed, comprehensiveness and cost efficacy brought about by next-generation sequencing, genetic screening should be considered in all SRNS patients at the time of diagnosis of steroid resistance prior to starting intensified immunosuppressive treatment.

Finally, the efficacy of other supportive and/or preventive treatment strategies including antiproteinuric therapies and treatment of hyperlipidemia have not yet been studied in detail in the PodoNet or other cohorts and await exploration in future studies.

Long-Term Outcome and Risk Factors for ESKD

Historically, the prognosis of SRNS was mainly staged according to histopathologic findings, with limited predictability of medium- and long-term disease outcomes (41–46). Providing comprehensive clinical and biochemical information with up to 15 years of follow-up, the PodoNet database allows to assess the prognostic effect of early treatment responsiveness in the context of genetic and histopathologic findings, which provide a rationale for a evidence-based reclassification of SRNS into sporadic immunosuppression-responsive (32%), sporadic multidrug-resistant (24%), genetic, and familial SRNS (30%)(**Figure 7**).

The average overall ESKD-free survival of patients with primary SRNS in the PodoNet cohort was 74% at 5 years, 58% at 10 years and 48% at 15 years, in keeping with previous cohort studies in which 5-year renal survival ranged from 65 to 92% and 15-year survival from 34 to 72% (43, 45, 47–49).

Responsiveness to intensified immunosuppression was highly predictive of long-term outcomes: Whereas complete remission during the first treatment year was associated with 94% 15-year renal survival, only 37% of the multidrug resistant patients were not in end-stage disease 15 years after disease onset (2). A fraction of patients achieved partial remission; it is controversial whether such intermediate response patterns reflect pharmacological effects on the immune system or non-specific proteinuria-lowering effects of RAS antagonists and possibly calcineurin inhibitors. Notably, partial proteinuria reduction was associated with superior long-term renal survival compared to patients with multidrug resistant proteinuria. The other key determinant of long-term renal outcome was the identification a genetic disease cause (2): Three quarters of patients diagnosed with a hereditary podocytopathy progressed to end-stage kidney disease within 15 years, as compared to only 4% of SRNS patients with sporadic disease and responsiveness to immunosuppressive

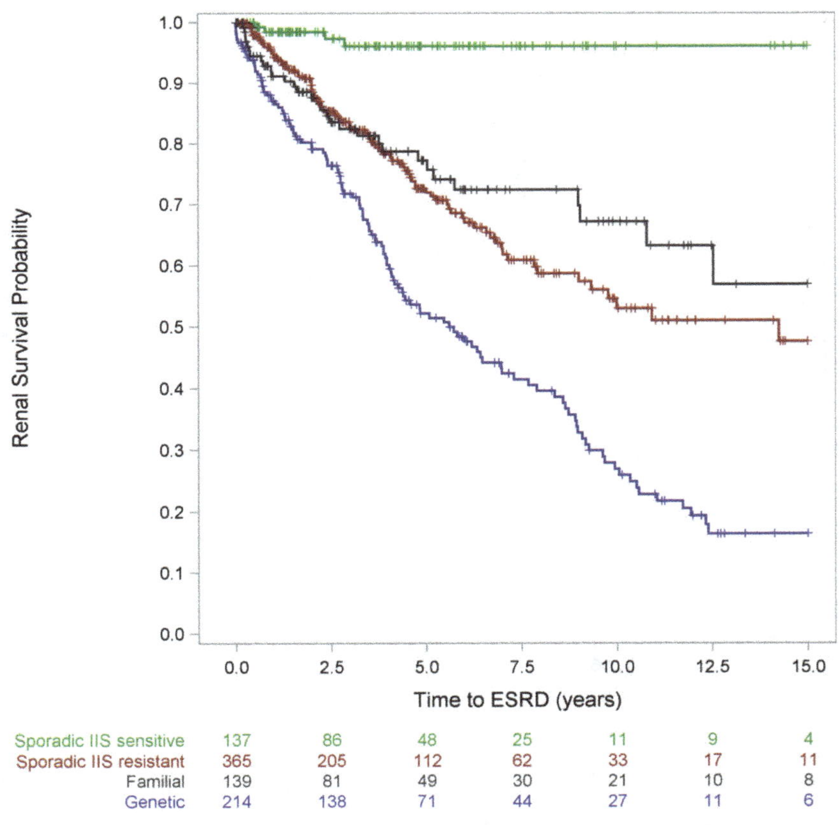

FIGURE 8 | Renal survival by disease category. Patients with partial responsiveness to intensified immunosuppressive (IIS) therapy were classified IIS resistant for this analysis.

therapy (**Figure 8**). Long-term renal outcomes were remarkably similar in children with different genetic disease entities. The 10-year renal survival rate was 72% for *NPHS2*-associated nephropathy, 77% for *WT1*-associated disease and 71% for the less common podocytopathies (2).

Remarkably, the outcome of children with proven genetic disease was also inferior compared to patients with multidrug-resistant disease in whom no genetic diagnosis could be established. The prognostic values of genetic diagnosis and immunosuppression responsiveness were found to be independent by multivariate analysis: ESKD risk was increased by 150% in patients in whom a genetic diagnosis was established whereas complete remission reduced renal risk by 87% in patients who achieved complete remission and by 50% in those who responded partially to immunosuppressive therapy (2).

Traditionally, the diagnostic categorization and prognostic evaluation in SRNS was based on histopathologic diagnosis. As expected, we found strong associations between histopathologic findings at time of diagnosis and long-term renal survival: ESKD-free survival was significantly higher for MCN than FSGS (79% v. 37% at 15 years) (**Figure 9**), and the overall ESKD risk of children diagnosed with FSGS was 4-fold higher compared to MCN (2). Children diagnosed with DMS showed the poorest outcomes, with a 20-fold increase of ESKD risk relative to MCN with progression to ESKD in 80% within 5 years after initial SRNS manifestation. Importantly, the prognostic value of FSGS and DMS prevailed even when adjusting for CKD stage at diagnosis, responsiveness to intensified immunosuppression, and the presence or absence of a genetic diagnosis (2). For instance, a patient with a genetic podocyte disorder, multidrug resistance, and a given eGFR will still have a nearly threefold higher ESKD risk with the diagnosis of FSGS compared with MCN. Hence, the independence of genetic and histopathological findings in the multivariate risk analysis suggests that histopathological assessment is still relevant in the genetic era.

Additional independent risk factors of progression to ESKD were identified as age <1 year and older than 5 years at disease onset and advanced CKD at initial presentation (2).

Which Lessons Have We Learned From the Podonet Registry So Far?

The understanding of the underlying molecular, genetic and pathophysiological mechanisms of SRNS has profoundly advanced during the past decade. Established in 2009, the PodoNet registry has grown to one of the largest pediatric SRNS cohorts with more than 2000 children feeding clinical and genetic research. While the large size of the cohort is a major asset, the incompleteness of data reporting and biosample availability has been a limitation to data analysis and interpretation. Also, in the early years of the Network technological limitations

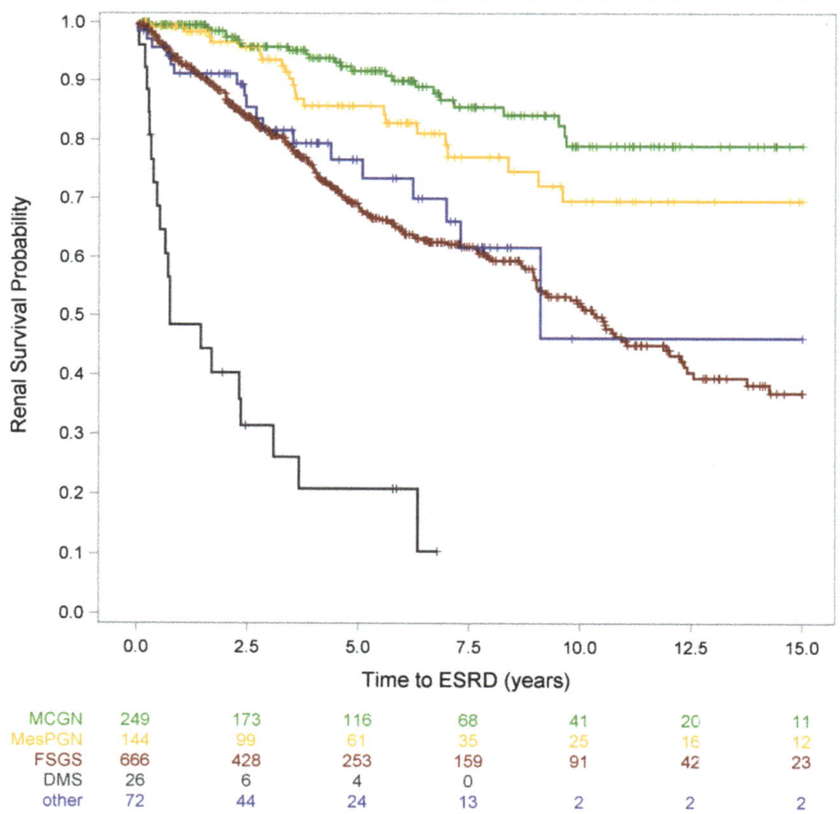

FIGURE 9 | Renal survival by histopathological diagnosis [from Trautmann et al. (2).

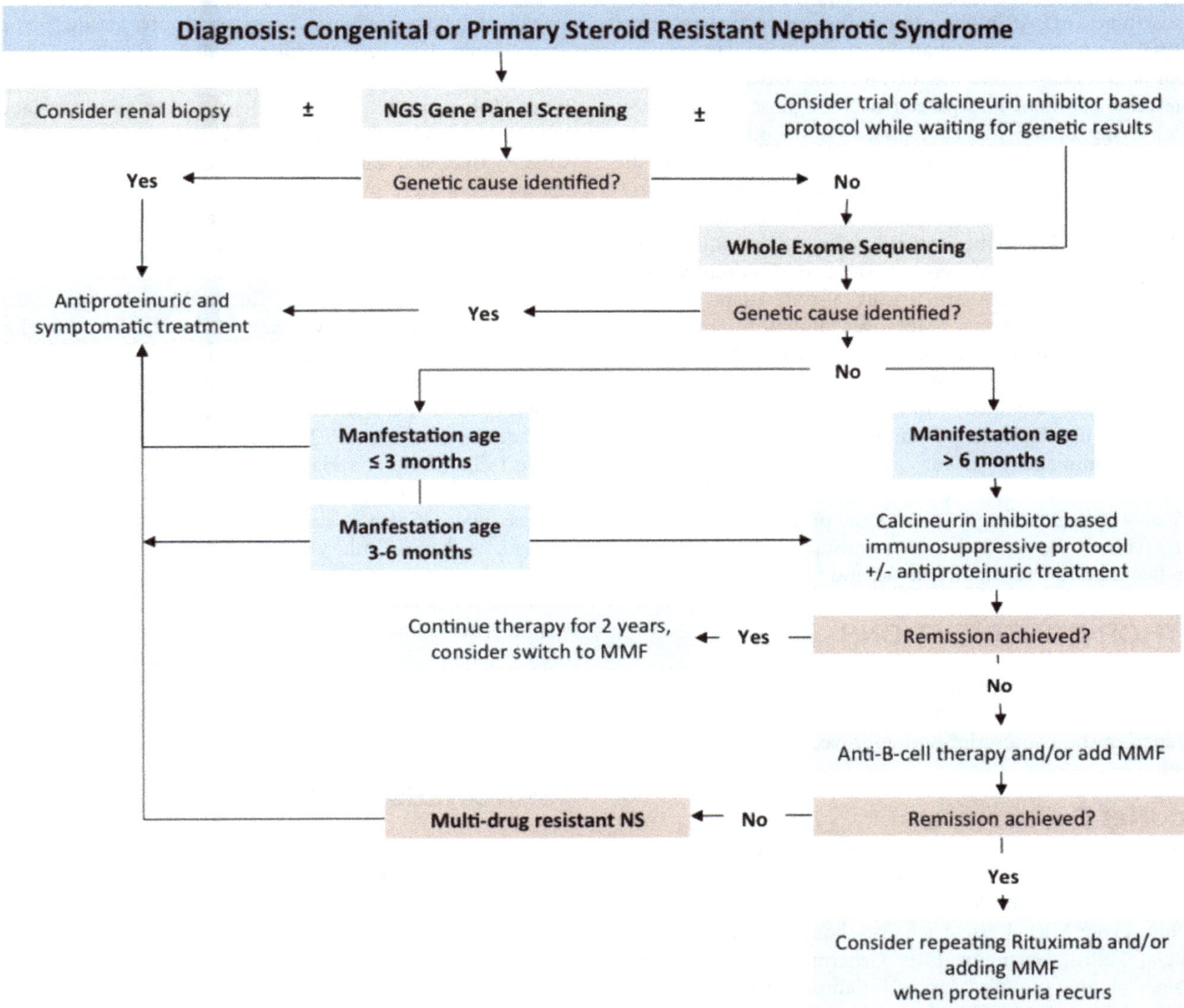

FIGURE 10 | Proposed diagnostic and therapeutic algorithm for children with CNS/SRNS.

and restricted resources hampered genetic screening. These limitations were partially overcome in later years thanks to improved funding and the central implementation of podocyte gene panel sequencing.

The discovery of numerous novel genetic podocytopathies and the progress in diagnostic screening technology have already changed clinical practice during the time span of the PodoNet project. Initially, children underwent a diagnostic algorithm and were selectively screened for individual SRNS genes by means of Sanger sequencing based on clinical criteria and depending on age at disease onset. With the advent of NGS technologies genetic screening has become much more rapid, comprehensive and cost-effective and consequently rapidly transgressed from an optional adjunct to a key component of the diagnostic workup in SRNS. This transformation is well-reflected in the output of PodoNet as well as other study consortia (10).

The PodoNet network has been an active player in this field by contributing to gene discoveries, developing and systematically applying podocytopathy gene panels, and analyzing phenotypes and outcomes by comprehensive assessment of clinical, genetic, and histopathological findings as well as responsiveness to pharmacotherapies.

Our studies allow concluding that genetic screening should be initiated as soon as the diagnosis of steroid resistance has been made, in parallel to renal biopsy (**Figure 10**).

We obtained evidence that genetic forms of SRNS are largely non-responsive to intensified immunosuppressive therapy, which, in consequence, should be avoided in patients with genetic disease. Future research will address in detail the short- and long-term usefulness of RAS inhibition and other supportive treatment strategies in genetic podocytopathies.

Our studies also have highlighted the lacking specificity of the most common histopathological diagnoses with respect to identifying underlying etiologies. On the other hand, the histopathological diagnosis was found to retain some prognostic value even when the genetic status of a patient is known.

In immune-mediated forms of SRNS, calcineurin inhibition was demonstrated to be the most efficacious second-line therapy following the diagnosis of steroid resistance. Children resistant to calcineurin inhibitors are usually also resistant to other immunosuppressive agents. Moreover, initial responsiveness to calcineurin inhibitors is uniquely predictive of long-term preservation of kidney function.

The insights obtained from the PodoNet cohort will facilitate the development of rational evidence based clinical practice recommendations for SRNS. In view of the major prognostic differences associated with genetic findings and pharmacotherapeutic responsiveness, we propose to sub-classify SRNS patients as sporadic immunosuppression-responsive, sporadic multidrug-resistant, genetic, and familial SRNS.

AUTHOR CONTRIBUTIONS

AT, BL-Z, FS contributed substantially to the acquisition, analysis, and/or interpretation of the data, participated actively in preparing the manuscript and approved the submitted final version.

PodoNet Collaborators

Austria: Dagmar Csaicsich; Chile: Marta Azocar, Santiago; Lily Quiroz, Santiago; **Colombia**: Lina Maria Serna Higuita, Medellín; **Czech Republic**: Jirí Dušek, Prague; **France**: Bruno Ranchin, Lyon; Michel Fischbach, Strasbourg; **Georgia**: Tinatin Davitaia, Tbilisi; **Germany**: Jutta Gellermann, Berlin; Sandra Habbig, Cologne; Jun Oh, Markus J. Kemper, Hamburg; Anette Melk, Hannover; Agnes Trautmann, Franz Schaefer, Heidelberg; Hagen Staude, Rostock; **Greece:** Nikoleta Printza, Thessaloniki; **Hungary**: Peter Sallay, Budapest; **Iran:** Alaleh Gheissari, Isfahan; **Italy**: Marina Noris, Bergamo; Andrea Pasini, Bologna; Gian Marco Ghiggeri, Monica Bodria, Genova; Gianluigi Ardissino, Milano; Elisa Benetti, Padova; Francesco Emma, Rome; **Lebanon**: Bilal Aoun, Beirut; Pauline Abou-Jaoudé, Byblos; **Lithuania**: Augustina Jankauskiene, Vilnius; **Poland**: Anna Wasilewska, Białystok; Ewa Gacka, Chorzow; Beata S. Lipska-Ziętkiewicz, Aleksandra Zurowska, Gdansk; Dorota Drozdz, Krakow; Marcin Tkaczyk, Małgorzata Stanczyk, Lodz; Halina Borzecka, Lublin; Magdalena Silska, Poznan; Tomasz Jarmolinski, Szczecin; Agnieszka Firszt-Adamczyk, Torun; Mieczyslaw Litwin, Elzbieta Kuzma-Mroczkowska, Hanna Szymanik-Grzelak, Warsaw; Anna Medynska, Wroclaw; Maria Szczepanska, Zabrze; **Portugal**: Alberto Caldas Afonso, Porto; Helena Jardim, Porto; **Romania**: Adrian Lungu, Bucharest; **Serbia:** Amira Peco-Antic Belgrade; Radovan Bogdanovic, Belgrade; **Sweden:** Rafael T. Krmar, Stockholm; **Switzerland**: Sybille Tschumi, Bern; **Syria:** Bassam Saeed, Damascus; **Turkey:** Ali Anarat, Adana; Ayse Balat, Gaziantep; Z. Esra Baskin, Ankara; Nilgun Cakar, Ankara; Ozlem Erdogan, Ankara; Birsin Özcakar, Ankara; Fatih Ozaltin, Ankara; Onur Sakallioglu, Ankara; Oguz Soylemezoglu, Ankara; Sema Akman, Antalya; Faysal Gok, Gulhane; Salim Caliskan, Istanbul; Cengiz Candan, Istanbul; Alev Yilmaz, Istanbul; Sevgi Mir, Izmir; Ipek Akil, Pelin Ertan, Manisa; Ozan Özkaya, Samsun; Mukaddes Kalyoncu, Trabzon; **United Arab Emirates:** Eva Simkova, Loai Akram Eid, Dubai; **Ukraine:** Svetlana Fomina, Kiev; Roman Sobko, Lviv.

ACKNOWLEDGMENTS

The PodoNet project has been made possible by support received from E-Rare (German Ministry of Education and Research), the EU 7th Framework Programme (EURenOmics, grant 2012-305608), the Polish Ministry of Science and Education (grant N402631840), the German Research Foundation (Scha 477/11-1), and the Scientific and Technological Research Council of Turkey (TUBITAK) (grant 108S417).

REFERENCES

1. Trautmann A, Bodria M, Ozaltin F, Gheisari A, Melk A, Azocar M, et al. Spectrum of steroid-resistant and congenital nephrotic syndrome in children: the PodoNet registry cohort. *Clin J Am Soc Nephrol.* (2015) 10:592–600. doi: 10.2215/cjn.06260614
2. Trautmann A, Schnaidt S, Lipska-Zietkiewicz BS, Bodria M, Ozaltin F, Emma F, et al. Long-Term outcome of steroid-resistant nephrotic syndrome in children. *J Am Soc Nephrol.* (2017) 28:3055–65. doi: 10.1681/asn.2016101121
3. Lipska BS, Iatropoulos P, Maranta R, Caridi G, Ozaltin F, Anarat A, et al. Genetic screening in adolescents with steroid-resistant nephrotic syndrome. *Kidney Int.* (2013) 84:206–13. doi: 10.1038/ki.2013.93
4. Lipska BS, Ranchin B, Iatropoulos P, Gellermann J, Melk A, Ozaltin F, et al. Genotype-phenotype associations in WT1 glomerulopathy. *Kidney Int.* (2014) 85:1169–78. doi: 10.1038/ki.2013.519
5. Lipska-Zietkiewicz BS, Gellermann J, Boyer O, Gribouval O, Zietkiewicz S, Kari JA, et al. Low renal but high extrarenal phenotype variability in Schimke immuno-osseous dysplasia. *PLoS ONE* (2017) 12:e0180926. doi: 10.1371/journal.pone.0180926
6. Srivastava T, Simon SD, Alon US. High incidence of focal segmental glomerulosclerosis in nephrotic syndrome of childhood. *Pediatr Nephrol.* (1999) 13:13–8. doi: 10.1007/s004670050555
7. Bonilla-Felix M, Parra C, Dajani T, Ferris M, Swinford RD, Portman RJ, et al. Changing patterns in the histopathology of idiopathic nephrotic syndrome in children. *Kidney Int.* (1999) 55:1885–90. doi: 10.1046/j.1523-1755.1999.00408.x
8. Banaszak B, Banaszak P. The increasing incidence of initial steroid resistance in childhood nephrotic syndrome. *Pediatr Nephrol.* (2012) 27:927–32. doi: 10.1007/s00467-011-2083-7
9. Buscher AK, Beck BB, Melk A, Hoefele J, Kranz B, Bamborschke D, et al. Rapid response to cyclosporin a and favorable renal outcome in nongenetic versus genetic steroid-resistant nephrotic syndrome. *Clin J Am Soc Nephrol.* (2016) 11:245–53. doi: 10.2215/cjn.07370715

10. Sadowski CE, Lovric S, Ashraf S, Pabst WL, Gee HY, Kohl S, et al. A single-gene cause in 29.5% of cases of steroid-resistant nephrotic syndrome. *J Am Soc Nephrol.* (2015) 26:1279–89. doi: 10.1172/jci79504
11. Machuca E, Hummel A, Nevo F, Dantal J, Martinez F, Al-Sabban E, et al. Clinical and epidemiological assessment of steroid-resistant nephrotic syndrome associated with the NPHS2 R229Q variant. *Pediatr Nephrol.* (2009) 75:727–35. doi: 10.1038/ki.2008.650
12. Santin S, Bullich G, Tazon-Vega B, Garcia-Maset R, Gimenez I, Silva I, et al. Clinical utility of genetic testing in children and adults with steroid-resistant nephrotic syndrome. *Clin J Am Soc Nephrol.* (2011) 6:1139–48. doi: 10.2215/cjn.05260610
13. Ozaltin F, Ibsirlioglu T, Taskiran EZ, Baydar DE, Kaymaz F, Buyukcelik M, et al. Disruption of PTPRO causes childhood-onset nephrotic syndrome. *Am J Hum Genet.* (2011) 89:139–47. doi: 10.1016/j.ajhg.2011.05.026
14. Mele C, Iatropoulos P, Donadelli R, Calabria A, Maranta R, Cassis P, et al. MYO1E mutations and childhood familial focal segmental glomerulosclerosis. *New England J Med.* (2011) 365:295–306. doi: 10.1056/NEJMoa1101273
15. Korkmaz E, Lipska-Zietkiewicz BS, Boyer O, Gribouval O, Fourrage C, Tabatabaei M, et al. ADCK4-Associated glomerulopathy causes adolescence-Onset FSGS. *J Am Soc Nephrol.* (2015) 27:63–8. doi: 10.1681/asn.2014121240
16. Atmaca M, Gulhan B, Korkmaz E, Inozu M, Soylemezoglu O, Candan C, et al. Follow-up results of patients with ADCK4 mutations and the efficacy of CoQ10 treatment. (2017) 32:1369–75. doi: 10.1007/s00467-017-3634-3
17. Malone AF, Phelan PJ, Hall G, Cetincelik U, Homstad A, Alonso AS, et al. Rare hereditary COL4A3/COL4A4 variants may be mistaken for familial focal segmental glomerulosclerosis. *Kidney Int.* (2014) 86:1253–9. doi: 10.1038/ki.2014.305
18. Gast C, Pengelly RJ, Lyon M, Bunyan DJ, Seaby EG, Graham N, et al. Collagen (COL4A) mutations are the most frequent mutations underlying adult focal segmental glomerulosclerosis. *Nephrol Dialysis, Transpl.* (2016) 31:961–70. doi: 10.1093/ndt/gfv325
19. Sen ES, Dean P, Yarram-Smith L, Bierzynska A, Woodward G, Buxton C, et al. Clinical genetic testing using a custom-designed steroid-resistant nephrotic syndrome gene panel: analysis and recommendations. *J Med Genet.* (2017) 54:795–804. doi: 10.1136/jmedgenet-2017-104811
20. McCarthy HJ, Bierzynska A, Wherlock M, Ognjanovic M, Kerecuk L, Hegde S, et al. Simultaneous sequencing of 24 genes associated with steroid-resistant nephrotic syndrome. *Clin J Am Soc Nephrol.* (2013) 8:637–48. doi: 10.2215/cjn.07200712
21. Niaudet P. Treatment of childhood steroid-resistant idiopathic nephrosis with a combination of cyclosporine and prednisone. French society of pediatric nephrology. *J Pediatr.* (1994) 125(6 Pt 1):981–6.
22. Cattran DC, Appel GB, Hebert LA, Hunsicker LG, Pohl MA, Hoy WE, et al. A randomized trial of cyclosporine in patients with steroid-resistant focal segmental glomerulosclerosis. North America Nephrotic Syndrome Study Group. *Kidney Int.* (1999) 56:2220–6. doi: 10.1046/j.1523-1755.1999.00778.x
23. El-Husseini A, El-Basuony F, Mahmoud I, Sheashaa H, Sabry A, Hassan R, et al. Long-term effects of cyclosporine in children with idiopathic nephrotic syndrome: a single-centre experience. *Nephrol Dialysis Transpl.* (2005) 20:2433–8. doi: 10.1093/ndt/gfi059
24. Ghiggeri GM, Catarsi P, Scolari F, Caridi G, Bertelli R, Carrea A, et al. Cyclosporine in patients with steroid-resistant nephrotic syndrome: an open-label, nonrandomized, retrospective study. *Clin Ther.* (2004) 26:1411–8. doi: 10.1016/j.clinthera.2004.09.012
25. Hino S, Takemura T, Okada M, Murakami K, Yagi K, Fukushima K, et al. Follow-up study of children with nephrotic syndrome treated with a long-term moderate dose of cyclosporine. *Am J Kidney Dis.* (1998) 31:932–9. doi: 10.1053/ajkd.1998.v31.pm9631836
26. Inaba A, Hamasaki Y, Ishikura K, Hamada R, Sakai T, Hataya H, et al. Long-term outcome of idiopathic steroid-resistant nephrotic syndrome in children. *Pediatr Nephrol.* (2016) 31:425–34. doi: 10.1007/s00467-015-3174-7.
27. Plank C, Kalb V, Hinkes B, Hildebrandt F, Gefeller O, Rascher W. Cyclosporin A is superior to cyclophosphamide in children with steroid-resistant nephrotic syndrome-a randomized controlled multicentre trial by the Arbeitsgemeinschaft fur Padiatrische Nephrologie. *Pediatr Nephrol.* (2008) 23:1483–93. doi: 10.1007/s00467-008-0794-1
28. Tarshish P, Tobin JN, Bernstein J, Edelmann CM, Jr. Cyclophosphamide does not benefit patients with focal segmental glomerulosclerosis. a report of the International Study of Kidney Disease in Children. *Pediatr Nephrol.* (1996) 10:590–3.
29. Bajpai A, Bagga A, Hari P, Dinda A, Srivastava RN. Intravenous cyclophosphamide in steroid-resistant nephrotic syndrome. *Pediatr Nephrol.* (2003) 18:351–6. doi: 10.1007/s00467-003-1095-3
30. Hinkes B, Vlangos C, Heeringa S, Mucha B, Gbadegesin R, Liu J, et al. Specific podocin mutations correlate with age of onset in steroid-resistant nephrotic syndrome. *J Am Soc Nephrol.* (2008) 19:365–71. doi: 10.1681/asn.2007040452
31. Latta K, von Schnakenburg C, Ehrich JH. A meta-analysis of cytotoxic treatment for frequently relapsing nephrotic syndrome in children. *Pediatr Nephrol.* (2001) 16:271–82.
32. Bagga A, Mudigoudar BD, Hari P, Vasudev V. Enalapril dosage in steroid-resistant nephrotic syndrome. *Pediatr Nephrol.* (2004) 19:45–50. doi: 10.1007/s00467-003-1314-y
33. Li Z, Duan C, He J, Wu T, Xun M, Zhang Y, et al. Mycophenolate mofetil therapy for children with steroid-resistant nephrotic syndrome. *Pediatr Nephrol.* (2010) 25:883–8. doi: 10.1007/s00467-009-1375-7
34. Ruf RG, Lichtenberger A, Karle SM, Haas JP, Anacleto FE, Schultheiss M, et al. Patients with mutations in NPHS2 (podocin) do not respond to standard steroid treatment of nephrotic syndrome. *J Am Soc Nephrol.* (2004) 15:722–32. doi: 10.1097/01.ASN.0000113552.59155.72
35. Frishberg Y, Rinat C, Megged O, Shapira E, Feinstein S, Raas-Rothschild A. Mutations in NPHS2 encoding podocin are a prevalent cause of steroid-resistant nephrotic syndrome among Israeli-Arab children. *J Am Soc Nephrol.* (2002) 13:400–5.
36. Caridi G, Bertelli R, Di Duca M, Dagnino M, Emma F, Onetti Muda A, et al. Broadening the spectrum of diseases related to podocin mutations. *J. Am. Soc. Nephrol.* (2003) 14:1278–86. doi: 10.1097/01.ASN.0000060578.79050.E0
37. Buscher AK, Kranz B, Buscher R, Hildebrandt F, Dworniczak B, Pennekamp P, et al. Immunosuppression and renal outcome in congenital and pediatric steroid-resistant nephrotic syndrome. *Clin J Am Soc Nephrol.* 2010) 5:2075–84. doi: 10.2215/cjn.01190210
38. Weber S, Gribouval O, Esquivel EL, Moriniere V, Tete MJ, Legendre C, et al. NPHS2 mutation analysis shows genetic heterogeneity of steroid-resistant nephrotic syndrome and low post-transplant recurrence. *Kidney Int.* (2004) 66:571–9. doi: 10.1111/j.1523-1755.2004.00776.x
39. Faul C, Donnelly M, Merscher-Gomez S, Chang YH, Franz S, Delfgaauw J, et al. The actin cytoskeleton of kidney podocytes is a direct target of the antiproteinuric effect of cyclosporine A. *Nat Med.* (2008) 14:931–8. doi: 10.1038/nm.1857
40. Montini G, Malaventura C, Salviati L. Early coenzyme Q10 supplementation in primary coenzyme Q10 deficiency. *New England J Med.* (2008) 358:2849–50. doi: 10.1056/NEJMc0800582
41. Cattran DC, Rao P. Long-term outcome in children and adults with classic focal segmental glomerulosclerosis. *Am J Kidney Dis.* (1998) 32:72–9.
42. Gipson DS, Chin H, Presler TP, Jennette C, Ferris ME, Massengill S, et al. Differential risk of remission and ESRD in childhood FSGS. *Pediatr Nephrol.* (2006) 21:344–9. doi: 10.1007/s00467-005-2097-0
43. Paik KH, Lee BH, Cho HY, Kang HG, Ha IS, Cheong HI, et al. Primary focal segmental glomerular sclerosis in children: clinical course and prognosis. *Pediatr Nephrol.* (2007) 22:389–95. doi: 10.1007/s00467-006-0301-5
44. Abrantes MM, Cardoso LS, Lima EM, Penido Silva JM, Diniz JS, Bambirra EA, et al. Predictive factors of chronic kidney disease in primary focal segmental glomerulosclerosis. *Pediatr Nephrol.* (2006) 21:1003–12. doi: 10.1007/s00467-006-0138-y
45. Martinelli R, Okumura AS, Pereira LJ, Rocha H. Primary focal segmental glomerulosclerosis in children: prognostic factors. *Pediatr Nephrol.* (2001) 16:658–61. doi: 10.1007/s004670100639

46. Abeyagunawardena AS, Sebire NJ, Risdon RA, Dillon MJ, Rees L, Van't Hoff W, et al. Predictors of long-term outcome of children with idiopathic focal segmental glomerulosclerosis. *Pediatr Nephrol.* (2007) 22:215–21. doi: 10.1007/s00467-006-0264-6
47. Gipson DS, Troost JP, Lafayette RA, Hladunewich MA, Trachtman H, Gadegbeku CA, et al. Complete remission in the nephrotic syndrome study network. *Clin J Am Soc Nephrol.* (2016) 11:81–9. doi: 10.2215/cjn.02560315
48. Mekahli D, Liutkus A, Ranchin B, Yu A, Bessenay L, Girardin E, et al. Long-term outcome of idiopathic steroid-resistant nephrotic syndrome: a multicenter study. *Pediatr Nephrol.* (2009) 24:1525–32. doi: 10.1007/s00467-009-1138-5
49. Niaudet P. *Pediatric Nephrology*. 5th ed. Philadelphia, PA: Lippincott Williams and Wilkins (2004).

21

Update on Genetic Conditions Affecting the Skin and the Kidneys

*Antonia Reimer[1,2], Yinghong He[1] and Cristina Has[1]**

[1] *Department of Dermatology, Faculty of Medicine, Medical Center, University of Freiburg, Freiburg, Germany,*
[2] *Berta-Ottenstein-Programme, Faculty of Medicine, University of Freiburg, Freiburg, Germany*

Correspondence:
Cristina Has
cristina.has@uniklinik-freiburg.de

Genetic conditions affecting the skin and kidney are clinically and genetically heterogeneous, and target molecular components present in both organs. The molecular pathology involves defects of cell–matrix adhesion, metabolic or signaling pathways, as well as tumor suppressor genes. This article gives a clinically oriented overview of this group of disorders, highlighting entities which have been recently described, as well as the progress made in understanding well-known entities. The genetic bases as well as molecular cell biological mechanisms are described, with therapeutic applications.

Keywords: epidermolysis bullosa, mosaicism, genodermatosis, kidney, mutation, RASopathy, nevus, renal anomaly

INTRODUCTION

Anomalies of both skin and kidney occur in a vast number of genetic conditions. There are two major reasons for this concomitant occurrence of clinical manifestations. First, skin and kidney share a common embryological background represented by mesoderm for dermal connective tissue and kidneys. Second, various molecules involved in adhesion (e.g., integrin α3, CD151), cholesterol biosynthesis (e.g., NSDHL), or signaling pathways [e.g., Wnt, hedgehog (Hh), Ras/MAPK] are highly relevant for the development, structure, and function of both organs. In some syndromes, cutaneous and renal involvements are among the striking, pathognomonic features. Many of these disorders are recognizable at birth or early childhood.

Renal anomalies include congenital abnormalities of the kidney and urinary tract (CAKUT) (e.g., renal hypoplasia or aplasia, horseshoe deformations, anomalies of the urine collection system), malfunctioning of glomerular filtration, and the predisposition for tumors. The spectrum of skin anomalies is wide including pigmentation anomalies, skin dryness and ichthyosis, vascular anomalies (e.g., nevi flammei and hemangiomas), benign and malign skin tumors, abnormal hair, and nail dystrophy.

In this overview, genetic conditions affecting the skin and the kidneys are divided into three main groups:

1. Monogenic disorders with skin and renal involvement
2. Disorders due to postzygotic mosaicism
3. Chromosomal aberrations.

Abbreviations: CAKUT, congenital abnormalities of the kidney and urinary tract; EB, epidermolysis bullosa; Hh, hedgehog; HLRCC, hereditary leiomyomatosis and renal cell cancer; LEOPARD, Lentigines, Electrocardiographic abnormalities, Ocular hypertelorism, Pulmonary stenosis, Abnormalities of genitalia, Retardation of growth and Deafness; NF1, neurofibromatosis type 1; NS, Noonan syndrome; TSC, tuberous sclerosis complex.

MONOGENIC DISORDERS WITH SKIN AND RENAL INVOLVEMENT

In certain monogenic disorders, such as epidermolysis bullosa (EB), RASopathies or disorders with tumor predisposition, cutaneous, as well as primary or secondary renal involvement may occur. In this section, we update the clinical and molecular features of the most relevant disorders of this vast group. In a large number of other genodermatoses and genetic syndromes, renal involvement may occur, but is not a defining feature. The clinical and molecular characteristics of these rare disorders are updated in **Tables 1** and **2**.

Epidermolysis Bullosa

Epidermolysis bullosa encompasses disorders defined by cutaneous and mucosal fragility. Classification into four major EB types, EB simplex, junctional EB, dystrophic EB, and the Kindler syndrome, is based on the ultrastructural level of skin cleavage (2, 3). Renal and urinary tract anomalies may occur in all EB types, in particular in junctional and dystrophic EB. In patients with severe dystrophic EB due to absence of collagen VII various renal pathologies may occur and lead to chronic renal failure. Hydronephrosis, poststreptococcal glomerulonephritis, IgA mesangial disease, or renal amyloidosis has been reported in dystrophic EB case series (4, 5). The mechanisms may include repetitive vesiculation within the lining epithelia of the urinary tract, and chronic systemic inflammation (6). Only EB types for which reno-urinary involvement is a primary feature will be described here.

Interstitial Lung Disease, Nephrotic Syndrome, and EB (ILNEB; MIM 614748)

Clinical Features

ILNEB is a rare autosomal recessive multiorgan disorder affecting the skin, kidneys and lungs. So far, 11 cases have been identified [reviewed in Ref. (5), and own unreported data], but the disease may be under recognized.

The clinical manifestations of ILNEB encompass the triad of early onset interstitial lung disease with respiratory distress, variable renal anomalies, and skin fragility. Since integrin α3 is widely expressed, clinical manifestations may occur in other organs, but are not characterized yet, because of the small number of cases and the early lethality. Skin involvement may include blistering, erosions or nail dystrophies, or may remain clinically unrecognized. The following renal anomalies were reported: congenital nephrotic syndrome, focal–segmental glomerulosclerosis, bilateral renal cysts, and a spectrum of CAKUT, including renal hypodysplasia, unilateral kidney hypoplasia, and ectopic conjoint kidney (7–12). Recently, two siblings of 13 and 9 years with viable ILNEB phenotypes presenting with growth retardation, severe pulmonary fibrosis, skin atrophy and erythema, scarce eyelashes/eyebrows, and nail anomalies (pachyonychia) but without renal features were described (13).

Genetics and Molecular Pathology

This disease is caused by mutations in the gene for integrin α3 (*ITGA3*) (7). Thus far, 10 *ITGA3* mutations have been reported: 2 frameshift, 2 splicing, and 6 missense mutations (5). Loss-of-function mutations were associated with lethality before the age of 2 years. The consequences of missense mutations cannot be easily predicted. Some of them were shown to disturb the post-translational modifications of integrin α3, which proved to be critical for the heterodimerization with integrin β1 and localization to the cell membrane (8, 9, 14).

Integrin α3 is the main integrin linking podocyte foot processes to the glomerular basement membrane [reviewed in Ref. (15, 16)]. In keratinocytes, it is located at cell–matrix adhesions, promoting epidermal adhesion primarily by maintaining the integrity of the basement membrane (17). The integrin α3 subunit is a widely expressed type I transmembrane protein consisting of a large extracellular region, a single transmembrane domain, and a short cytoplasmic tail (18). It forms obligate heterodimers with β1 integrin serving as a receptor for laminins, the major components of epithelial basement membranes (19). Integrin α3 is reduced or lost in several acquired conditions with glomerular disease, in which it is associated with reduction in podocyte adhesion to the glomerular basement membrane. For example, in podocytes of early-stage diabetic nephropathy integrin α3 expression was upregulated (20), while expression was suppressed with progression of the disease (21). In patients with primary focal segmental glomerulosclerosis, podocyte depletion was accompanied by reduced podocyte expression of α3β1 integrins (22). Moreover, integrin α3 is involved in podocyte foot process effacement during nephrotic syndrome (23).

Nephropathy with Pretibial EB and Deafness (MIM 609057)

Clinical Features

Two siblings with congenital nephrotic syndrome and pretibial EB were first described in 1988 (24). The disease-causing mutation in the gene for the tetraspanin CD151 was identified in 2004 (25), and very recently an additional case was reported (26). The first two cases had proteinuria in the nephrotic range and end-stage renal failure requiring hemodialysis or peritoneal dialysis from the age of 14 or 16 years on, respectively (24). The third case was a 33-year-old male with nephropathy manifesting with proteinuria below the nephrotic range, multiple episodes of pyelonephritis, and urinary incontinence, manifesting as a combination of overflow incontinence and intermittent urge incontinence (26). Additional manifestations included pretibial or extensive skin blistering, poikiloderma, nail dystrophy, hair loss, dystrophic teeth, involvement of the ocular, oral, gastrointestinal, and urogenital mucosal membranes (25, 26).

Genetics and Molecular Pathology

A homozygous single-nucleotide duplication in the *CD151* gene leading to frameshift and a premature stop codon was identified in the first two cases (25). Flow cytometry analysis demonstrated absence of reactivity for CD151, suggesting that the predicted truncated polypeptide was not functional. In the third case, a homozygous *CD151* splice site mutation, affecting a canonical donor splice site junction was found (26). Immunofluorescence staining and western blot analysis confirmed that the splice site mutation led to absence of CD151 in the cells of the patient (26).

TABLE 1 | Genodermatoses with reno-urinary involvement.

Disorder **MIM**	**Kidney involvement and its frequency (% of cases), if known**	**Skin involvement and its frequency (% of cases), if known**	**Affected gene and protein**	**Incidence**	**Onset of clinical manifestations**	**Inheritance**
Restrictive dermopathy 275210	Urethral duplication occasional	Skin is thin, translucent and forms a tight, rigid casing. Erosions and fissures occur mainly in folds 100	*ZMPSTE24* and *LAMNA* mutations, leading to abnormal function of lamin A	Approximately 60 cases reported	Prenatal/at birth	AR (*ZMPSTE24*) less frequently *de novo* dominant (*LMNA*)
Nephrosis with ichthyosis and adrenal insufficiency	Steroid-resistant nephrotic syndrome major feature	Ichthyosis Major feature	*SGPL1*, sphingosine-1-phosphate lyase	NA	Early adulthood	AR
Arthrogryposis-renal dysfunction-cholestasis (ARC) syndrome 208085	Renal tubular dysfunction with renal tubular acidosis, nephrogenic diabetes insipidus, glucosuria, aminoaciduria, and phosphaturia Major feature	Ichthyosis 50	*VPS33B*, Vacuolar protein sorting 33, yeast, homolog of, b	>80 cases reported	Birth	XLR or AR
Cockayne syndrome 216400	Proteinuria, renal failure 10	Photosensitive dermatitis (overlap with xeroderma pigmentosum); xerosis cutis; anhidrosis (occasional) 75	*ERCC6* and *ERCC8*	2.7:1,000,000 births	Infancy	AR
Ehlers–Danlos syndromes (EDS) 130000	Hypoplastic kidney, sporadic	Lax, smooth, hyperextensible skin, atrophic scars, bruises 100	*COL5A1* and *COL5A2* for classic EDS	1:5,000 for all types, classical type: 1:20,000–40,000	Childhood	AD
Cranio-ectodermal dysplasia (Sensenbrenner syndrome) 218330	Interstitial fibrosis of the kidneys: thickening of the tubular basement and tubular atrophy Common. renal failure is most common cause of death	Short nails, lax skin, fine sparse hair Common	*IFT122, WDR35, WDR19, IFT43;* their protein products constitute the intraflagellar transport complex A in cilia	>40 cases reported	Birth	AR
Ectrodactyly ectodermal dysplasia-clefting syndrome 129900	Renal agenesis and dysplasia, hydronephrosis, defects in urinary tract collection system 52	Fair pigmentation, thin skin, mild hyperkeratosis. Sparse, wiry hair common	*TP63* (homolog of tumor-suppressor gene p53), tp63	>200 patients described	Birth	AD
GAPO (growth deficiency, alopecia, pseudoanodontia, optic atrophy) 230740	Polycystic kidney Occasional	Mild skin laxity. Early alopecia Common	*ANTXR1, ANTXR1* appears necessary for actin assembly and thus cell adhesion	More than 30 patients reported	Infancy (6 months onward)	AR

TABLE 2 | Syndromes with cutaneous and reno-urinary involvement.

Disorder MIM	Kidney involvement and its frequency (% of cases)	Skin involvement and its frequency (% of cases)	Affected gene (locus) and protein	Incidence	Onset of clinical manifestations	Inheritance
Adams–Oliver syndrome 1 100300	Duplicated collecting system Occasional	Aplasia cutis congenita over posterior parietal region (common), on trunk and limbs (occasional); Cutis marmorata telangiectasia congenita; thin, hypopigmented skin (occasional) 20	Gain-of-function mutations in *ARHGAP31* (identified in some affected individuals); Cdc42/Rac1 GTPase regulator	Approximately 1 in 225,000 individuals, >100 cases reported	Intrauterine/birth	AD, in few cases AR inheritance suggested
Apert syndrome 101200	Polycystic kidneys, hydronephrosis 10	Hyperhidrosis and pronounced acne (including forearms) at adolescence Common	*FGFR2;* Fibroblast growth factor receptor 2	1:80,000	Infancy	AD
Beckwith–Wiedemann syndrome 130650	Large kidneys showing renal medullary dysplasia, renal cysts, anomalies in the urinary tract collection system and resulting hydronephrosis, nephrolithiasis. Natural history: Development of neuroblastoma and Wilms tumors. Tumor formation in approximately 7.5	Facial nevus flammeus, hemihypertrophy, unusual fissures and indentations in the external ear Common	Distal arm of 11p Imprinting disorder	1:13,700	Infancy/childhood	AD
Coffin–Siris syndrome 135900	Hydronephrosis, microureters with stenoses, ectopic kidneys Occasional	Hemangiomas, hypertrichosis, hirsutism Occasional	*ARIDIB (6q25) and SMARCB1;* encode subunits of switch/ sucrose non-fermenting complex, an epigenetic modifier	Approximately 140 cases reported	Birth/infancy	Probably AD
DiGeorge syndrome 188400	Congenital abnormalities of the kidney and urinary tract: single kidney, multicystic, dysplastic kidney/small kidneys, horseshoe kidney, duplicated collecting system 30	Severe acne 23%; seborrhea 35%	1.5- to 3.0-Mb hemizygous deletion of chromosome 22q11.2 including haploinsufficiency in the transcription factor gene TBX1, and CRKL which is a dosage-sensitive regulator of genitourinary development (1)	1 in 4,000	Birth/infancy	AD or sporadic resulting from *de novo* deletion
Early urethral obstruction sequence (Prune belly syndrome) 100100	Urethral obstruction (mostly due to urethral valves) leads to hydronephrosis and limits renal development 100	Excess and lax abdominal skin ("prune belly") if bladder ruptures during fetogenesis 100	Several genes identified: *ACTA2, CHRM3, HPSE2*	1 in 29,231	Prenatal	AR
Fabry disease 301500	Chronic kidney disease, glomerular sclerosis, vacuolization of glomerular and tubular epithelial cells, renal failure	Angiokeratomas, hypo- or anhidrosis	*GLA;* alpha-galactosidase A	1:1,500–1:3,100	Variable; males develop symptoms in childhood, females >50 years	XLR
Fanconi pancytopenia syndrome 227645 227646 227650 300514 600901 603467 609053 609054 610832 613390 613951 614082 614083 615272 616435 617243 617244 617247	Renal anomalies (hypoplasia or malformation) 34	Brownish pigmentation 64	15 genes identified	1:160,000	Childhood	AR

(Continued)

TABLE 2 | Continued

Disorder MIM	Kidney involvement and its frequency (% of cases)	Skin involvement and its frequency (% of cases)	Affected gene (locus) and protein	Incidence	Onset of clinical manifestations	Inheritance
Hajdu–Cheney syndrome 102500	Renal defects, especially cystic kidneys Occasional	Hirsutism Occasional	*NOTCH2*	NA	Childhood	AD
Nail-patella syndrome (hereditary osteo-onycho dyplasia) 161200	Glomerulonephritis, nephrotic syndrome, renal insufficiency 25	Triangular lunula, hypoplastic nails, webbing, absence of distal dorsal phalangeal skin creases Common	*LMX1B;* LIM homeobox transcription factor 1 B	1:50,000	Childhood	AD
Oral–facial–digital syndrome 311200	Polycystic kidney disease at adult age; glomerular cysts 50	Seborrheic skin, milia, alopecia Occasional	*OFD1*, involved in ciliary function	>160 cases reported	Birth	XLD
Pallister–Hall syndrome 146510	Renal ectopia or dysplasia Common	Midline facial hemangioma Common	*GLI3*	NA	Intrauterine/birth	AD
Roberts syndrome 268300	Polycystic or horseshoe kidney Occasional	Midfacial capillary hemangioma 78	*ESCO2* Essential in chromosomal alignment and adhesion in mitosis	Approximately 50 cases reported	Prenatal/at birth	AR
Robinow syndrome 268310	Renal anomalies 29	Nevus flammeus 23	*ROR2* and *WNT5A*	Sporadic cases	Prenatal	AR (*ROR2*) and AD (*WNT5A*)
Rubinstein–Taybi syndrome 180849	Renal anomalies 52	Hirsutism, capillary hemangioma, development of keloids 75, 25, and 22%, respectively	*CBP* (CREB-binding protein) and *EP300*	1:100,000–1:125,000	Infancy	AD
Russell–Silver syndrome 180860	Renal anomalies, occasional	Café-au-lait spots common	*ICR1* regulator of the expression of IGF-2, and others	1:30,000–1: 100,000	Infancy	Sporadic, genetically heterogeneous
Trichorhino Phalangeal syndrome (Langer–Giedion syndrome) 150230	Urethral reflux Occasional	Looseness or redundancy of skin in childhood, macularpapular nevi common	Deletion in 8q24.11–q24.13 (involving *TRPS1* and *EXT1*)	NA	Childhood	AD

CD151 (syn. Raph blood group, TSPAN24) is a member of the tetraspanin family of cell surface proteins and acts as a stabilizer of integrins (27). CD151 forms complexes with integrin α3β1 in cell culture and *in vivo* (28, 29). These complexes are assembled early during the integrin biosynthesis and precede the interaction of CD151 with other tetraspanins (30). CD151 also regulates glycosylation of α3β1 (31). CD151 is widely expressed in epithelia, endothelia, muscle cells, renal glomerular podocytes, Schwann and dendritic cells, in platelets and megakaryocytes. CD151 is involved in the formation and/or maintenance of the glomerular basement membrane (32).

Junctional EB with Pyloric Atresia (MIM 226730)

Clinical Features

Junctional EB with pyloric atresia manifests with aplasia cutis congenita (**Figure 1**), generalized skin blistering, and pyloric atresia. Several acquired complications of the reno-urinary system are reported, including pyelonephritis, hydronephrosis, urinary retention, development of bladder hypertrophy, and urethral meatal stenosis (4, 33, 34).

Genetics and Molecular Pathology

The disease is caused by mutations in the genes coding for the α6 or β4 integrin subunits, most mutations residing in *ITGB4*. Absence of α6β4 integrin is associated with a high rate of lethality in the first months of life, while missense and splicing mutations lead to moderate disease severity and reno-urinary manifestations.

Integrin α6β4 is a heterodimer composed of two type I transmembrane subunits localized in hemidesmosomes', which anchor keratin intermediate filaments to the cell membrane and extracellular matrix. The intracellular region of α6β4 consists of the short tail of α6 and a large β4 cytoplasmic domain, which interacts with plectin and collagen XVII in keratinocytes. The ligands of α6 integrin are CD151, collagen XVII and laminin 332. Integrin α6β4 has a major adhesive function and promotes polarization of the cells (35). α6β4 is expressed in the epithelial cells within the medulla of the kidney. In a mouse model, α6β4 was not required for morphogenesis of the urinary tract, but for maintaining the integrity of the kidney collecting system. Collecting duct anomalies appeared as the animals aged. α6-null collecting duct cells were not able to withstand mechanical stress and detached from the basement membrane (36, 37).

Junctional EB Generalized Severe (Formerly: Herlitz EB; MIM 226700)

Clinical Features

Junctional EB generalized severe is caused by complete lack of laminin 332, the major laminin expressed in the cutaneous basement membrane. Laminin 332 is a heterotrimeric glycoprotein consisting of three polypeptide chains: laminin α3, β3, and γ2, encoded by *LAMA3*, *LAMB3*, and *LAMC2*, respectively. The clinical picture is dominated by mucocutaneous blistering from birth onward. Extensive generalized blistering leads to loss of fluids and protein and failure to thrive. The most common complications are anemia, dyspnea, infections, and sepsis. Affected children show multiorgan involvement and commonly die before the age of 2 years (38). In an infant with *LAMB3* mutations, nephrotic syndrome with albuminuria due to failure of the glomerular filtration barrier, and high urinary *N*-acetylglucosaminidase levels, also indicating renal tubular involvement were reported (39).

Genetics and Molecular Pathology

Laminin 332 is the major laminin expressed by keratinocytes, but is also present in multiple epithelial basement membranes, including those of kidney. Like all laminins, it is a glycoprotein composed of three chains (α3, β3, and γ2) bound through disulfide bonds (5). In junctional EB generalized severe, mutations are found in one of the three genes encoding the laminin 332 chains. In the majority of cases, mutations are located in *LAMB3* and lead to premature termination codons, mRNA decay, and absence of laminin 332.

RASopathies

RASopathies represent an expanding common group of neurodevelopmental disorders caused by germline mutations in genes encoding components of the Ras/MAPK pathway (40). Collectively, they affect >1 in 1,000 individuals (41). The Ras/MAPK pathway is a conserved omnipresent intracellular signaling pathway that is critical in regulating cell cycle, differentiation, growth, apoptosis, and senescence (40). The group of RASopathies includes neurofibromatosis type 1 (NF1), Noonan syndrome (NS), NS with multiple lentigines, Legius syndrome, Costello syndrome, cardio-facio-cutaneous syndrome, capillary malformation-arteriovenous malformation, and autosomal dominant intellectual disability type 5. Because of the common

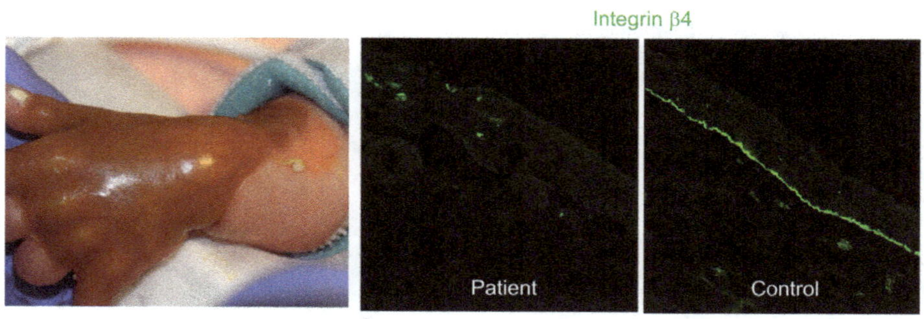

FIGURE 1 | Congenital absence of the skin, also known as aplasia cutis congenita, in a newborn with hydronephrosis and pyloric atresia due to integrin α6β4 deficiency (right panel) [clinical pictures, courtesy of Dr. P. Häusermann (Department of Dermatology Basel)].

molecular mechanisms, phenotypic features of these syndromes are overlapping.

NF1 (von Recklinghausen Disease, MIM 162200)

Clinical Features

With an incidence of 1:2,500–3,000 (42), NF1 is one of the most common disorders of this group. NF1 follows autosomal dominant inheritance, about half of all cases occur due to spontaneous mutations. Diagnosis of NF1 is established following a set of clinical diagnostic criteria established in 1988 [**Table 3**, diagnosis of NF1 is probable when more than two criteria are present (43)]. Most cases are diagnosed in childhood, but when the complete set of criteria is not yet evident, follow-up and re-evaluation are necessary. Cutaneous features include café-au-lait macules, cutaneous and internal neurofibromas, or plexiform neurofibromas and axillary freckling. Renal involvement occurs sporadically, manifestations include hypertension due to renal artery stenosis, renal neurofibromas, and renal metastases of malignant schwannomas. The cooccurrence of NF1 and Wilms' tumor has been reported in some cohorts (44, 45).

Individuals with NF1 have a high risk of developing malignancies, especially malignant peripheral nerve sheath tumors (46). Life expectancy has been found to be approximately 8 years lower than in the normal population (47).

The cutaneous features progress with age. Neurofibromas as the main cutaneous finding in NF1 can be itchy, lead to disfigurement, and cause psychological strain. They can be treated with excisions or laser ablation (Er:YAG or CO_2 laser) (48, 49), both with risk for hypertrophic scarring and recurrence (42).

In uncomplicated cases, clinical evaluation in childhood should be performed annually and include auxologic measurements, cardiovascular assessment, skin examination, and developmental progress (42). In childhood, visual assessment should be performed every 6–12 months for early detection of optical pathway glioma until the age of 7 years (42).

Genetics and Molecular Pathology

Monoallelic loss-of-function variants in *NF1* coding for neurofibromin 1 are disease-causing in NF1. Neurofibromin is a multifunctional tumor suppressive protein which functions as a GTPase-activating protein. Neurofibromin inhibits cell proliferation and growth by blocking RAS-mediated signal transduction and modulates cell motility and adhesion (50).

The mutational spectrum is highly heterogeneous including nonsense and missense mutations, splice site mutations (about 30% of cases), small insertion–deletions, whole-gene deletions (4–5%), and structural rearrangements (51). Penetrance is complete after childhood, but NF1 is characterized by extreme clinical variability which is poorly understood, as are genotype–phenotype correlations. Intra- and interfamilial evaluation of the NF1 phenotype suggests that genetic modifiers which are not linked to the *NF1* locus contribute to the variable expressivity of the disease (52, 53). Differently skewed expression of the *NF1* alleles as well as somatic "second hit" variants or loss of heterozygosity may account in part for the phenotypic variability (54, 55). In addition to NF1, atypical manifestations, such as familial spinal neurofibromatosis, multiple spinal ganglioneuromas, optic gliomas, or Lentigines, Electrocardiographic abnormalities, Ocular hypertelorism, Pulmonary stenosis, Abnormalities of genitalia, Retardation of growth and Deafness (LEOPARD) syndrome, have been associated with *NF1* mutations. Finally, incidental occurrence of *NF1* mutations together with mutations in other genes may account for atypical phenotypic associations.

TABLE 3 | Diagnostic criteria for neurofibromatosis 1 (NF1) (43).

- 6 or more café-au-lait macules (>0.5 cm in children or >1.5 cm in adults)
- 2 or more cutaneous/subcutaneous neurofibromas or one plexiform neurofibroma
- Axillary or groin freckling
- Optic pathway glioma
- 2 or more Lisch nodules (iris hamartomas seen on slit lamp examination)
- Bony dysplasia (sphenoid wing dysplasia, bowing of long bone ± pseudarthrosis)
- First degree relative with NF1

NS with Multiple Lentigines (syn. LEOPARD Syndrome, Multiple Lentigines Syndrome, Lentiginosis profusa and Progressive Cardiomyopathic Lentiginosis; MIM 151100)

Clinical Features

Noonan syndrome with multiple lentigines is a rare RASopathy that manifests in childhood. The incidence is unknown; so far, more than 200 cases were published. The characteristic cutaneous appearance is described well by the acronym LEOPARD: the skin appears spotted due to thousands of dark brown lentigines of 1–5 mm size which are distributed on the entire body (including sun-protected areas), cooccurring with café-au-lait macules (hence sometimes confused with NF1), hypomelanotic macules, and sometimes axillary freckling. Apart from LEOPARD are defining features (56). CAKUT, including horseshoe kidneys, occur in 11% of affected individuals (57). NS with multiple lentigines is sometimes difficult to distinguish from NF1 and the allelic NS (58), especially in early childhood when pigmentation anomalies are not yet pronounced (59). The prognosis is generally good, but can be limited by hypertrophic cardiomyopathy, arrhythmias, and sudden cardiac death. Annual cardiologic check-up should be performed life-long, and hearing assessment should be undertaken until adulthood. If auxologic follow-up indicates small statue, growth hormone therapy should be considered (56). Intense pulsed light has been used for cosmetic treatment of lentigines (60).

Genetics and Molecular Pathology

Noonan syndrome with multiple lentigines is allelic with NS and with the cardio-facio-cutaneous syndrome. The genetic basis of NS with multiple lentigines is heterogeneous including heterozygous pathogenic variants in one of four genes *PTPN11* (90% of cases), *RAF1* (less than 5% of cases), *BRAF* and *MAP2K1* (both in single cases) (61). One or more additional, as-yet undefined genes are probably associated with about 5% of cases in whom no pathogenic variant has been identified (61). Genotype–phenotype correlations are not well established (62).

All involved genes code for components of the Ras/MAPK pathway:

- *PTPN11* encodes the protein tyrosine phosphatase non-receptor type 11 that in its active form increases downstream Ras activity
- *RAF1* encodes a serine–threonine kinase that activates MEK1 and MEK2
- *BRAF* encodes the B-Raf proto-oncogene serine/threonine kinase that activates MEK1 and/or MEK2 by phosphorylation
- *MAP2K1* encodes the mitogen-activated protein kinase kinase 1 that activates ERK1 and/or ERK2 by phosphorylation (41).

Somatic mutations in all these genes are present in various types of cancers. Indeed, individuals with NS have a threefold increased risk of malignancies, such as juvenile myelomonocytic leukemia, acute lymphoblastic leukemia, rhabdomyosarcoma, and neuroblastoma (63, 64).

Genetic Tumor Predisposition Syndromes Affecting both Skin and Kidney

This is a large group of disorders characterized by both numerous hamartomas (benign tumors that can develop in basically all tissues) and premature development of malignant tumors during childhood. The molecular pathology of these conditions is highly heterogeneous. The most common conditions are described below or in **Table 4**. The tumors in these syndromes can occur in both cutaneous and extracutaneous locations, including the kidney (**Table 4**). Other tumor predisposition syndromes which usually manifest in adult age are only briefly mentioned.

Tuberous Sclerosis Complex (TSC, TSC1 and TSC2, syn. Bourneville Disease; MIM 191100)

Clinical Features

Tuberous sclerosis complex occurs with an estimated incidence of 1:5,800–1:10,000 (65). It is mostly diagnosed in infancy when it manifests with skin findings and seizures due to cerebral hamartomas and giant cell astrocytomas. The diagnosis of TSC is made according to clinical criteria (66) (**Table 5**, either two major features are required or, alternatively, one major and two or more minor features). Typical cutaneous features are hypopigmented macules (best seen in Wood's light), angiofibromas (mostly facial), periungual fibromas, and connective tissue nevi (shagreen patches). The frequency of cutaneous findings increases with age, but polygonal hypomelanotic macules, known as "ash-leaf spots," are the earliest manifestation and are invariably present at birth. Renal involvement is also common, with angiomyolipomas and cysts as the most frequent renal manifestations found in 17% of children with TSC by age 2 years and 65% of 14 years old children with TSC (67). Renal cell carcinoma is more common in TSC than in the overall population (68).

There is large variability in the clinical course, neurological development, and life expectancy in TSC, mostly depending on the number and location of hamartomas. While cutaneous features are crucial for clinical diagnosis, central nervous system tumors are the main cause of morbidity and mortality, while renal disease is the second leading cause of early death (69).

As TSC involves multiple organ systems, interdisciplinary care is necessary. Skin examinations should be performed annually. Diagnostic work-up of the kidney should include annual assessment of renal function and blood pressure and imaging (preferably with MRI) every 1–3 years (70). Since 2005, mTOR inhibitors have been evaluated for the use in TSC. Everolimus (Votubia®) is approved as a system therapeutic for use in children of 3 years and older with subependymal giant cell astrocytomas and for adults with complicated renal angiomyolipomas (71). Cutaneous lesions can be treated surgically, using laser (CO_2/Erbium:YAG/Dye laser combination, or CO_2, or Nd:YAG, or pulsed-dye laser) (72–74) and pharmacologically using topical mTOR inhibitors (75, 76). Surgical intervention can be considered as a therapeutic option for painful hemorrhagic renal angiomyolipomas and cerebral lesions.

TABLE 4 | Genetic tumor predisposition syndromes with cutaneous and reno-urinary involvement.

Disorder MIM	Kidney involvement and its frequency (% of cases, if known)	Skin involvement and its frequency (% of cases, if known)	Affected gene and protein	Incidence	Onset of symptoms	Inheritance
Cowden syndrome 158350	Renal cell carcinoma	Trichilemmomas, lipomas, acral keratoses, penile hyperpigmentation Main feature	*PTEN;* Phosphatase and tensin homolog	1:200,000–250,000	Adulthood	AD
Hereditary leiomyomatosis and renal cell cancer 150800	Renal cell carcinoma 10–20	Leiomyomas 76	*FH;* Fumarate hydratase	Unknown, approximately 100 families reported	>30 years onward	AD
Birt–Hogg–Dubé syndrome (syn: fibrofolliculomas with trichodoscomas and acrochordons) 135150	Renal tumors (both benign and malign) and cysts 27	Fibrofolliculomas, trichodiscomas and epidermoid cysts Common	*FLCN;* folliculin	>400 cases reported	Adulthood (>20 years), renal cancer at around 50 years	AD
Von Hippel–Lindau syndrome 193300	Renal clear cell carcinoma, renal cysts Variable	Capillary malformations, hemangioma, café-au-lait spots Variable	*VHL;* Von Hippel-Lindau tumor suppressor	1:36,000–1:45,000	Onset in adulthood	AD

TABLE 5 | Diagnostic criteria of tuberous sclerosis complex [adapted from Ref. (66)].

Major clinical features	Minor clinical features
• Hypomelanotic macules (≥3, at least 5 mm diameter) • Angiofibromas (≥3) or fibrous cephalic plaque • Ungual fibromas (≥2) • Shagreen patch • Retinal hamartomas (multiple) • Cortical dysplasia (≥3, including tubers and brain white matter radial migration lines) • Subependymal nodules • Subependymal giant cell astrocytoma • Cardiac rhabdomyoma • Lymphangioleiomyomatosis • Angiomyolipomas (≥2)	• "Confetti" lesions of the skin (hypomelanotic macules with 1–2 mm) • Dental enamel pits (≥3) • Intraoral fibromas (≥2) • Retinal achromic patch • Renal cysts (multiple) • Nonrenal hamartomas

Genetics and Molecular Pathology

Tuberous sclerosis complex is caused by monoallelic mutations in *TSC1* (about 20% of cases) or *TSC2* (about 70% of cases) (69) (Leiden open variation database). Two-thirds of TSC cases result from *de novo* pathogenic variants, and in about 10% no mutation can be detected (69). Large gene rearrangements, intronic pathogenic variants, and somatic or germ line mosaicism may explain the failure to detect mutations (77, 78). Specialized methods, such as targeted-deep sequencing of introns and exons and high-resolution SNP arrays improved the mutation detection rate to 94% (79). Genotype–phenotype correlations revealed that *TSC2* mutations lead to earlier onset and more severe phenotype, as compared with *TSC1* mutations (80). The occurrence of autosomal dominant polycystic kidney disease in TSC may be due to a contiguous deletion of *TSC2* and *PKD1* (81).

TSC1 and *TSC2* code for hamartin and tuberin which form heterodimers within the TSC protein complex. Loss-of-function mutations in either *TSC1* or *TSC2* lead to constitutive activation of the mammalian target of rapamycin complex 1 (mTORC1) that is uncoupled from inhibitory mechanisms. Thus tumor cells in TSC have increased activation of mTORC1 signaling, resulting in increased protein synthesis and cell growth, and reduced autophagy (82). In fact, somatic inactivation of normal alleles is expected to drive mTOR activation, but second hit mutations are not always observed. The pathogenesis of angiofibromas involves UV-induced mutations suggesting that sun exposure is the initiating event (83). In angiomyolipomas, about 70% of the second-hit events are loss-of-heterozygosity mutations (84). A recent study showed that in TSC, somatic mutation rates were lower than most malignant tumors, while whole or arm-level chromosome gains and losses were the most remarkable finding in over 10% of patients (79).

Basal Cell Nevus Syndrome (syn. Gorlin Syndrome, Gorlin–Goltz Syndrome, Nevoid Basal Cell Carcinoma Syndrome; MIM 109400)

Clinical Features

The basal cell nevus syndrome is a rare autosomal dominant condition, occurring with an estimated incidence of 1:30,000 (85). It formally belongs to the group of hamartoses, but is mainly ranked among the tumor predisposition syndromes. Its characteristic feature is the occurrence of multiple basal cell carcinomas from young adulthood onward. Development of basal cell carcinoma in infancy has also been described (86). Other skin manifestations include palmar and plantar punctate dyskeratotic pits and facial milia. Skeletal abnormalities (e.g., polydactily), jaw cysts, and medulloblastoma occurring in 5% of patients are early features that can hint toward the diagnosis of basal cell nevus syndrome. Renal anomalies, such as renal agenesis (87) or Wilms tumors (88, 89), were reported in single cases. Diagnosis can be difficult in childhood due to few or unspecific findings. In suspected basal cell nevus syndrome, a systematic work-up including examinations by a dermatologist, a radiologist, a dentist, a gynecologist, a cardiologist, and a geneticist is recommended (90). After the occurrence of the first basal cell carcinoma, dermatologic examinations should be performed every 6–12 months. A baseline cerebral MRI with yearly controls until the age of 8 years is recommended. Echocardiography should be performed at baseline to rule out cardiac fibromas. X-ray of the jaw should be repeated yearly until a first jaw cyst is detected, after that every 6 months or according to symptoms. For scoliosis detection, an X-ray at the age of 1 year or at time of diagnosis is recommended. If normal, it is only repeated in case of symptoms. If scoliosis is present, regular follow-ups are appointed. Other baseline evaluations include pelvic ultrasound and ophthalmologic assessments. Psychological evaluation and support is advisable (90).

For many years, excision of basal carcinoma was the main treatment option for this condition. Understanding of the molecular pathology has recently led to development and approval of vismodegib (Erivedge®) as an effective therapy. Vismodegib targets the sonic Hh pathway and leads to regression of existing and inhibits the development of new tumors (91). Radiation should be avoided as it will trigger the eruption of multiple new tumors (92).

Genetics and Molecular Pathology

The genetic basis of the basal cell nevus syndrome is heterogeneous. The main cause is represented by monoallelic germline pathogenic variants in *PTCH1* responsible for approximately 85% of the cases. *SUFU* pathogenic variants reside in about 5% of the cases (93). Rare causes are *PTCH2* and *SMO* mutations: a missense mutation in *PTCH2* was disclosed in a Chinese family (94), and a *SMO* mutation in a single case with a segmental basal cell nevus syndrome (95). In about 15–27% of cases, the genetic basis remains unclear (93). Low level of postzygotic mosaicism may explain some of the genetically unsolved cases (96). *PTCH1* pathogenic missense variants have also been associated with holoprosencephaly (97).

All these genes encode key players in the Hh signaling pathway, which is essential for development of vertebrates and drives proliferation, migration, and differentiation of progenitor cells (98):

- *PTCH1* encodes the patched homolog 1, the receptor for sonic Hh
- *SUFU* encodes the suppressor of fused homolog, a negative regulator of the Hh signaling pathway

- *PTCH2* encodes patched 2
- *SMO* encodes smoothened frizzled class receptor, a G protein-coupled receptor that interacts with the patched protein.

Activation of the Hh pathway is initiated by the Hh ligand binding and inhibition of the transmembrane receptor patched 1, allowing the signal transducer smoothened to activate Gli transcription factors and amplify the expression of Hh target genes (98). Somatic mutations that activate the Hh signaling pathway drive growth of various cancers including basal cell carcinomas, medulloblastomas, pancreatic, prostate, and small cell lung cancer, that account for up to 25% of all human cancer deaths (99).

Birt–Hogg–Dubé Syndrome

Clinical Features

The Birt–Hogg–Dubé syndrome is an autosomal dominant disorder which manifests with cutaneous lesions, pulmonary cysts and/or history of pneumothorax, and various types of renal tumors (100). Skin involvement occurs during the second, third, or fourth decade of life and progresses with age. It includes various benign tumors such as fibrofolliculomas, trichodiscomas/angiofibromas, perifollicular fibromas, and acrochordons. Fibrofolliculomas are the most common phenotypic features of the Birt–Hogg–Dubé syndrome, occurring in more than 85% of the patients over the age of 25 years (101). They appear as multiple, small, skin-colored papules disseminated on the face, neck, and upper trunk. Treatment by laser ablation results in temporary improvement, but relapse usually occurs.

Individuals with Birt–Hogg–Dubé syndrome have a sevenfold increased risk to develop renal tumors, that are typically bilateral and multifocal (102, 103). They are usually diagnosed in adults (median of diagnosis is 48 years, but have been described as early as 20 years of age) and have a slow progression (103). The histologic types of renal tumors found in individuals with Birt–Hogg–Dubé syndrome are: by far predominant are chromophobe renal cell carcinomas, followed by hybrid oncocytic tumors and oncocytomas, while clear cell renal cell carcinomas are uncommon. Yearly screening by renal MRI is indicated in individuals with Birt–Hogg–Dubé syndrome age 18 years or older. In some families, renal tumors and/or spontaneous pneumothorax occur without cutaneous manifestations.

Genetics and Molecular Pathology

The Birt–Hogg–Dubé syndrome is caused by monoallelic pathogenic variants in *FLCN,* encoding folliculin. Mutation analysis detects disease-causing variants in 88% of the affected families; the deletion or duplication of a cytosine at position c.1285 is a mutational hot spot. Partial- or whole-gene deletions account for 3–5% of the cases and must be identified with specific methods. About 7–9% of the cases remain genetically unsolved. The protein folliculin forms a complex with folliculin-interacting protein 1 or 2 and binds to the 5′ AMP-activated protein kinase suppressing tumorigenesis (104). Moreover, it plays a role in mTOR activation (105–107).

Hereditary Leiomyomatosis and Renal Cell Cancer (HLRCC)

Clinical Features

Hereditary leiomyomatosis and renal cell cancer is characterized by the occurrence of cutaneous and uterine leiomyomata, and/or a single, unilateral, and aggressive renal tumor (108). Cutaneous leiomyomata may be multiple or single, appear in adults (mean age of 25 years), and increase in size and number with age. They manifest as skin-colored papules or nodules, disseminated on the trunk, extremities, and face. The treatment consists of surgical or laser excision, or cryoablation. Renal tumors occur in about 10–16% of individuals with HLRCC at a median age of 44 years and cause hematuria and lower back pain. Histologically they are classically classified as type 2 papillary (108).

Genetics and Molecular Pathology

Hereditary leiomyomatosis and renal cell cancer is caused by monoallelic *FH* mutations that lead to reduced activity of the enzyme fumarate hydratase (109). In tumor tissue, somatic variants and loss of heterozygosity are found. No genotype–phenotype correlations are known, and there is significant intrafamilial variability. Biallelic mutations resulting in fumarase deficiency cause an inborn error of metabolism characterized by rapidly progressive neurologic impairment including hypotonia, seizures, and cerebral atrophy (110).

DISORDERS DUE TO POSTZYGOTIC MOSAICISM

The disorders in this group are caused by mutations that are mostly lethal if occurring as a germline mutation affecting all cells. However, if these mutations occur postzygotic in early embryogenesis, disorders with unilateral or segmental manifestations result, as proposed by Happle (111, 112). His hypothesis is supported by the elucidation of the molecular basis of several segmental disorders since the implementation of next-generation sequencing technologies.

Linear Sebaceous Nevus Sequence [Schimmelpenning–Feuerstein–Mims Syndrome, Nevus Sebaceous of Jadassohn; MIM 163200]

Clinical Features

This syndrome belongs to the group of epidermal nevus syndromes. More than 100 sporadic cases have been described, the incidence is not known. While solitary sebaceous nevi are a reasonably common finding in infants, the sebaceous nevi in this syndrome are associated with seizures, mental retardation, skeletal and ophthalmic anomalies, and asymmetric growth. At birth, one (or multiple) sebaceous nevi is/are found mostly in the mid-face. Involvement of the head/neck area is possible, as are locations on trunk or extremities. The sebaceous nevus shows a linear configuration along the lines of Blaschko. While it is mostly flat and wax-like in infancy, verrucous changes, hyperpigmentation, hyperkeratosis, and hypertrophy are seen toward puberty.

In adulthood, development of (mostly benign) tumors within the sebaceous nevus is noted. Skeletal, ophthalmic, and renal involvements occur occasionally, the latter comprising CAKUT, such as double urinary collecting system and horseshoe kidneys, and renal hamartoma and nephroblastoma.

Surgical treatment of sebaceous nevi can be offered for cosmetic or psychological reasons. Excision is generally not indicated because of cancer prophylaxis, as the risk for malignant tumors is very low (113). Therapeutic options include excision and laser ablation (114). Regarding the main complications, seizures, neurological retardation, and rickets, interdisciplinary care for children with linear sebaceous nevus sequence should be offered.

Genetics and Molecular Pathology

This syndrome can be considered a mosaic RASopathy because it is caused by postzygotic pathogenic variants in *HRAS* (HRas Proto-Oncogene, GTPase), *KRAS* (KRAS Proto-Oncogene, GTPase), or the *NRAS* (NRas Proto-Oncogene, GTPase) genes (115, 116). The recurrent activating mutations induce constitutive activation of the MAPK and PI3K/AKT signaling pathways. Somatic mutations in the *HRAS* and/or *KRAS* genes were also found in isolated sebaceous nevi. These mutations are only present in keratinocytes which give rise to the cutaneous lesions.

The proteins encoded by the Ras oncogene family have intrinsic GTPase activity and function in signal transduction pathways important for cell growth, proliferation, and survival. Defects in these genes are present in various cancers.

Neurocutaneous Melanocytosis (syn. Neurocutaneous Melanosis Sequence, Neuromelanosis; MIM 249400)

Clinical Features

The landmark lesion of this syndrome, a giant pigmented nevus, is seen at birth. It is usually located in the posterior head or trunk (117). Sometimes, three or more large congenital nevi are found rather than a single giant nevus. Numerous disseminated ("satellite") nevi can be present at birth and more will develop in the course of disease. The presence and proliferation of melanin-producing cells within cranium and spine leads to increased intracranial pressure, seizures, mental deterioration, and death in early childhood (117). Leptomeningeal and intracranial melanoma occur in a significant portion of patients. Occasional abnormalities found in neurocutaneous melanocytosis are cerebral malformations such as syringomyelia and Dandy–Walker malformation, CAKUT, and unilateral renal cysts. Other tumors occurring in the syndrome include rhabdomyosarcoma, liposarcoma, and malignant peripheral nerve sheath tumors.

There is a risk of development of cutaneous malignant melanoma within the congenital nevi. They develop in the depth of the lesion and can be felt earlier than they can be seen. This has been suggested to be as high as 15% (118) in giant congenital melanocytic nevi, although others have reported incidences of 0.7% (119). The amount of patients with the full picture of neurocutaneous melanocytosis developing malignant melanoma is not known, probably as most of these patients die before developing melanomas.

They clinical course is mostly determined by neurologic symptoms. If these occur, there is no effective therapeutic approach. If the child shows normal psychomotoric development, excision for the giant melanocytic nevi is recommended. Such surgical procedures may require several steps and the use of tissue expanders. Dermabrasio is not considered as a therapeutic option any more. To date, a causal therapy is not available, but a recent *in vitro* assessment of inhibitors of the NRAS-signaling pathway (drugs also successfully used in the therapy of malignant melanoma) showed promising results (120).

Genetics and Molecular Pathology

Somatic oncogenic missense mutations affecting codon 61 of the *NRAS* gene were identified in affected cutaneous (melanocytes) and nervous tissues from patients with congenital melanocytic nevus syndrome and/or neurocutaneous melanosis (118).

CHILD Syndrome (Congenital Hemidysplasia with Ichthyosiform Erythroderma and Limb Defects; MIM 308050)

Clinical Features

This epidermal nevus syndrome was coined with the acronyme "CHILD" by Happle and colleagues in 1980 (121) to sum up the main findings in children with this condition: a characteristic, mostly unilateral epidermal nevus in combination with ipsilateral congenital hemidysplasia of bones (affecting any part of the body, mainly limbs). The epidermal nevus is usually present at birth but can also develop in the first weeks of life. Spontaneous involution is sometimes witnessed (113). The CHILD nevus is red and scaly. It can show strict lateralization (right side more frequently than left side, 3:2) and midline demarcation, but it can also follow lines of Blaschko, and both patterns may be present in an affected individual (113) (**Figure 2**). Next to cardiovascular anomalies, renal findings comprise CAKUT, such as renal agenesis (122) or hypoplasia (123), to unilateral hydronephrosis, but their frequency is unknown (124).

Addressing the molecular pathology of CHILD, a therapeutic approach for treating the epidermal nevus combining simvastatin and cholesterol for topical use proved to be effective (125, 126) (**Figure 2**).

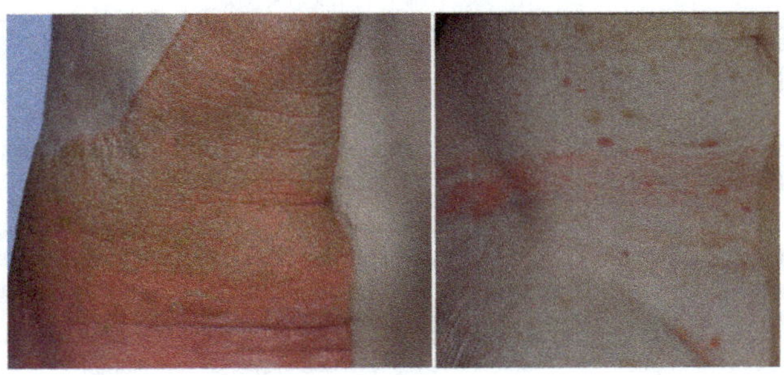

FIGURE 2 | Unilateral epidermal nevus in a patient with CHILD syndrome, before (left panel) and after 5 years topical application of a simvastatin/cholesterol cream (right panel).

Genetics, Molecular Pathology

CHILD syndrome is caused by monoallelic loss-of-function pathogenic variants in the *NSDHL* gene encoding the NAD(P) H steroid dehydrogenase-like protein, which is a C4 demethylase involved in postsqualene cholesterol biosynthesis (127). The enzyme is located within the membranes of the endoplasmic reticulum. Its deficiency leads to impaired cholesterol processing, causing abnormal sonic Hh signaling, which affects spatial patterning during embryogenesis (128). The cutaneous features may result from a dual mechanism: accumulation of cholesterol precursors and cholesterol deficiency (128).

This X-linked dominant disorder is lethal in male during gestation and thus predominantly affects females. The CK syndrome [initials of the original proband (129)] is an X-linked recessive disorder that affects males being also caused by pathogenic *NSDHL* variants (130). In CHILD syndrome, mosaicism results from inactivation of an X-chromosome in females. Interindividual differences in the pattern of X inactivation explain the phenotypic variations.

Focal Dermal Hypoplasia (Goltz syndrome; MIM 305600)

Clinical Features

Focal dermal hypoplasia is rare; more than 175 cases have been reported. The focal dermal hypoplasia is mostly encountered in females (90%), as its X-linked dominant inheritance leads to lethality in male fetuses. Affected males usually show a mosaic form of focal dermal hypoplasia. This syndrome is evident at birth, when skin and skeletal symptoms are predominant. Children with focal dermal hypoplasia show skin atrophy with Blaschko linear arrangement, appearing as depressed or slightly raised red macules. This finding explains the original name "focal dermal hypoplasia" (131). Over the course of disease, fatty tissue can herniate through gaps in the underdeveloped connective tissue forming lipomatous papules. Papillomas and angiofibroma occur on the face and in the urogenitoanal region (132). Additional findings are patchy alopecia and thin hair. Affected children show facial dysmorphies and asymmetric skeletal deformities (e.g., syndactyly, polydactyly, amelia, scoliosis). Renal anomalies occur occasionally and include horseshoes kidneys and hydronephrosis.

No specific therapy for focal dermal hypoplasia exists. Papillomas can be surgically removed, but may reoccur.

Genetics and Molecular Pathology

Focal dermal hypoplasia is an X-linked dominant disorder which reflects mosaicism resulting from inactivation of an X-chromosome in females. The pathogenic variants affect *PORCN* (133). *PORCN* is a gene of the porcupine family, which code for endoplasmic reticulum proteins with multiple transmembrane domains involved in the processing of Wnt (wingless and int homolog) proteins. Mutations in different players of the Wnt signaling pathway have been described before to cause CAKUT (134), explaining the pathogenesis of CAKUT in focal dermal hypoplasia. The disease is lethal in males; live-born affected males are rare and nearly always have somatic mosaicism for a *de novo* postzygotic pathogenic variant. Postzygotic mutations may also cause mild disease in females (135).

TABLE 6 | Chromosome anomalies with cutaneous and reno-urinary involvement.

Disorder MIM	Kidney involvement and its frequency (% of cases)	Skin involvement and its frequency (% of cases)	Affected gene and protein	Incidence	Onset of symptoms	Inheritance
Microdeletion 17q21 syndrome (Koolen–De Vries syndrome) 610443	Hydronephrosis, pyelectasis, renal dysplasia and duplex renal system 32	Altered pigmentation of hair and skin, hyperelastic skin, thickened skin in some areas, hyperpigmentation of nevi 55% (hair anomalies)	Microdeletion within chromosome 17 (17q21.31) involving *KANSL1, a* chromatin modifier gene	1:16,000	Birth	AD
Trisomy 18 (Edwards Syndrome)	Horseshoe kidneys, ectopic kidney, double ureter, hydronephrosis, polycystic kidneys. Wilms tumor 10–50% (Wilms tumor in <10%)	Redundant skin, cutis marmorata, hirsutism (especially at forehead) >50%	Trisomy 18	1–9/1,000 000	Birth	Random, mosaicism
Deletion 2q37 syndrome 600430	Kidney and urinary tract anomalies, Wilms tumors <5%	Eczema	Subtelomeric deletion in chromosome 2	>100 patients described	Variable	AD
Deletion 18q syndrome 601808	Horseshoe kidney, ureteral reflux occasional	Skin dimples (knuckles, shoulder), eczema occasional	Deletion of long arm of chromosome 18	1:40,000	Infancy	AD
Killian/Teschler–Nicola syndrome (=Pallister–Killian syndrome) 601803	Persistence of urogenital sinus/cloaca occasional	Streaky hypo- and hyperpigmentation, abnormal sweating occasional	Tissue-limited mosaicism with partial trisomy due to isochromosome of Chromosome 12p	5.1 per million live births	Neonatal period	Somatic mosaicism
Microdeletion 3q29 syndrome 609425	Horseshoe kidneys occasional	Abnormal skin pigmentation occasional	Microdeletion 3q29	>20 cases described	Usually onset in childhood	Unclear, only isolated cases described

AD, autosomal dominant; AR, autosomal recessive; NA, not available; XLD, X-linked dominant; XLR, X-linked recess.

CHROMOSOMAL ABERRATIONS

In case of chromosomal aberrations, e.g., deletions or trisomies, a large number of genes are affected by the defect. Therefore, the resulting clinical picture is broad and includes renal and cutaneous anomalies in some syndromes (**Table 6**). However, these are not defining for the clinical picture.

DIFFERENTIAL DIAGNOSIS IN NEWBORNS

Several acquired conditions affect both skin and kidney either pre- or postnatally. For example, maternal intake of valproate leads to fetal valproate syndrome commonly showing hemangiomas, altered pigmentation, and occasional renal malformations. Intake of phenytoin during pregnancy causes fetal hydantoin syndrome, in which hirsutism and coarse hair are common and renal malformations can occur. The oligohydramnios sequence (Potter syndrome) arises from lack of amniotic fluid. This anhydramnion or oligohydramnion can either be caused by primary renal problems such as agenesis, severe polycystic kidney deformation or obstruction of the urinary tract, or by chronic leakage from the amniotic sac. Fetal development, especially of the lungs, and life expectancy are severely limited.

CONCLUSION

Genetic disorders affecting the skin and the kidneys cover a broad range of phenotypes and molecular mechanisms, which have been largely uncovered in the last decades. Many of these conditions comprise involvement of multiple organs and systems. Although, in many cases, the cutaneous findings (e.g., café-au-lait spots, angiofibromas, nevi) have no significant impact on the prognosis they represent precious signs for the clinical diagnosis and should alert pediatricians to carefully evaluate the patients.

- Because of the clinical complexity these patients require an interdisciplinary care, comprising geneticists, dermatologists, nephrologists, cardiologists, etc., in which the pediatrician has a central coordinating role.
- The rarity of these disorders renders their diagnosis sometimes difficult, underrecognized and delayed. In addition, the cutaneous lesions have an esthetic impact (e.g., angiofibromas of the face, neurofibromas, nevi) and the tumors have an unpredictable, mostly progressive course. All these factors have a high psychological impact on the patients and their families, who require psychological aid and support from patients' organizations.
- Illumination of the molecular pathomechanisms of some rare disorders (e.g., Ras/MAPK, mTOR, cholesterol biosynthesis) opened new opportunities to repurpose known drugs and use them to slow down disease progression. Such evolving therapies, either in the clinical practice or in clinical trials, have been briefly outlined in this review.

AUTHOR CONTRIBUTIONS

AR wrote most of the clinical part (clinical features) and the tables. YH prepared the figures and reviewed the manuscript. CH drafted the manuscript, wrote the genetics and molecular part, and reviewed the entire manuscript.

FUNDING

CH was supported by the Deutsche Forschungsgemeinschaft (DFG) CRC/SFB 1140 and AR by the Berta-Ottenstein Programme of the Faculty of Medicine, University of Freiburg. YH was a fellow of the Else-Kröner-Fresenius Foundation.

REFERENCES

1. Haller M, Mo Q, Imamoto A, Lamb DJ. Murine model indicates 22q11.2 signaling adaptor CRKL is a dosage-sensitive regulator of genitourinary development. *Proc Natl Acad Sci U S A* (2017) 114:4981–6. doi:10.1073/pnas.1619523114
2. Has C, Bruckner-Tuderman L. The genetics of skin fragility. *Annu Rev Genomics Hum Genet* (2014) 15:245–68. doi:10.1146/annurev-genom-090413-025540
3. Fine J-D, Bruckner-Tuderman L, Eady RAJ, Bauer EA, Bauer JW, Has C, et al. Inherited epidermolysis bullosa: updated recommendations on diagnosis and classification. *J Am Acad Dermatol* (2014) 70:1103–26. doi:10.1016/j.jaad.2014.01.903
4. Fine JD, Johnson LB, Weiner M, Stein A, Cash S, DeLeoz J, et al. Genitourinary complications of inherited epidermolysis bullosa: experience of the national epidermylosis bullosa registry and review of the literature. *J Urol* (2004) 172:2040–4. doi:10.1097/01.ju.0000143200.86683.2c
5. Has C, He Y. Renal-skin syndromes. *Cell Tissue Res* (2017) 369:63–73. doi:10.1007/s00441-017-2523-y
6. Fine JD, Mellerio JE. Extracutaneous manifestations and complications of inherited epidermolysis bullosa: part I. Epithelial associated tissues. *J Am Acad Dermatol* (2009) 61:367–84. doi:10.1016/j.jaad.2009.03.052
7. Has C, Spartà G, Kiritsi D, Weibel L, Moeller A, Vega-Warner V, et al. Integrin α3 mutations with kidney, lung, and skin disease. *N Engl J Med* (2012) 366:1508–14. doi:10.1056/NEJMoa1110813
8. Nicolaou N, Margadant C, Kevelam SH, Lilien MR, Oosterveld MJ, Kreft M, et al. Gain of glycosylation in integrin alpha3 causes lung disease and nephrotic syndrome. *J Clin Invest* (2012) 122:4375–87. doi:10.1172/JCI64100
9. Yalcin EG, He Y, Orhan D, Pazzagli C, Emiralioglu N, Has C. Crucial role of posttranslational modifications of integrin α3 in interstitial lung disease and nephrotic syndrome. *Hum Mol Genet* (2015) 24:3679–88. doi:10.1093/hmg/ddv111
10. He Y, Balasubramanian M, Humphreys N, Waruiru C, Brauner M, Kohlhase J, et al. Intronic ITGA3 mutation impacts splicing regulation and causes interstitial lung disease, nephrotic syndrome, and epidermolysis bullosa. *J Invest Dermatol* (2016) 136:1056–9. doi:10.1016/j.jid.2015.11.031
11. Lovric S, Fang H, Vega-Warner V, Sadowski CE, Gee HY, Halbritter J, et al. Rapid detection of monogenic causes of childhood-onset steroid-resistant nephrotic syndrome. *Clin J Am Soc Nephrol* (2014) 9:1109–16. doi:10.2215/CJN.09010813
12. Shukrun R, Vivante A, Pleniceanu O, Vax E, Anikster Y, Dekel B, et al. A human integrin-alpha3 mutation confers major renal developmental defects. *PLoS One* (2014) 9:e90879. doi:10.1371/journal.pone.0090879
13. Colombo EA, Spaccini L, Volpi L, Negri G, Cittaro D, Lazarevic D, et al. Viable phenotype of ILNEB syndrome without nephrotic impairment in siblings heterozygous for unreported integrin alpha3 mutations. *Orphanet J Rare Dis* (2016) 11:136. doi:10.1186/s13023-016-0514-z
14. Yamada M, Sekiguchi K. Disease-associated single amino acid mutation in the calf-1 domain of integrin alpha3 leads to defects in its processing and

cell surface expression. *Biochem Biophys Res Commun* (2013) 441:988–93. doi:10.1016/j.bbrc.2013.11.003
15. Borza CM, Chen X, Zent R, Pozzi A. Cell receptor-basement membrane interactions in health and disease: a kidney-centric view. *Curr Top Membr* (2015) 76:231–53. doi:10.1016/bs.ctm.2015.07.003
16. Pozzi A, Zent R. Integrins in kidney disease. *J Am Soc Nephrol* (2013) 24:1034–9. doi:10.1681/ASN.2013010012
17. Longmate WM, Dipersio CM. Integrin regulation of epidermal functions in wounds. *Adv Wound Care* (2014) 3:229–46. doi:10.1089/wound.2013.0516
18. Campbell ID, Humphries MJ. Integrin structure, activation, and interactions. *Cold Spring Harb Perspect Biol* (2011) 3:a004994. doi:10.1101/cshperspect.a004994
19. Nishiuchi R, Takagi J, Hayashi M, Ido H, Yagi Y, Sanzen N, et al. Ligand-binding specificities of laminin-binding integrins: a comprehensive survey of laminin-integrin interactions using recombinant alpha3beta1, alpha6beta1, alpha7beta1 and alpha6beta4 integrins. *Matrix Biol* (2006) 25:189–97. doi:10.1016/j.matbio.2005.12.001
20. Sawada K, Toyoda M, Kaneyama N, Shiraiwa S, Moriya H, Miyatake H, et al. Upregulation of $\alpha3\beta1$-integrin in podocytes in early-stage diabetic nephropathy. *J Diabetes Res* (2016) 2016:9265074. doi:10.1155/2016/9265074
21. Chen HC, Chen CA, Guh JY, Chang JM, Shin SJ, Lai YH. Altering expression of alpha3beta1 integrin on podocytes of human and rats with diabetes. *Life Sci* (2000) 67:2345–53. doi:10.1016/S0024-3205(00)00815-8
22. Chen C-A, Hwang J-C, Guh J-Y, Chang J-M, Lai Y-H, Chen H-C. Reduced podocyte expression of alpha3beta1 integrins and podocyte depletion in patients with primary focal segmental glomerulosclerosis and chronic PAN-treated rats. *J Lab Clin Med* (2006) 147:74–82. doi:10.1016/j.lab.2005.08.011
23. Reiser J, Oh J, Shirato I, Asanuma K, Hug A, Mundel TM, et al. Podocyte migration during nephrotic syndrome requires a coordinated interplay between cathepsin L and alpha3 integrin. *J Biol Chem* (2004) 279:34827–32. doi:10.1074/jbc.M401973200
24. Kagan A, Feld S, Chemke J, Bar-Khayim Y. Occurrence of hereditary nephritis, pretibial epidermolysis bullosa and beta-thalassemia minor in two siblings with end-stage renal disease. *Nephron* (1988) 49:331–2. doi:10.1159/000185086
25. Karamatic Crew V, Burton N, Kagan A, Green CA, Levene C, Flinter F, et al. CD151, the first member of the tetraspanin (TM4) superfamily detected on erythrocytes, is essential for the correct assembly of human basement membranes in kidney and skin. *Blood* (2004) 104:2217–23. doi:10.1182/blood-2004-04-1512
26. Vahidnezhad H, Youssefian L, Saeidian AH, Mahmoudi HR, Touati A, Abiri M, et al. Recessive mutation in tetraspanin CD151 causes Kindler syndrome-like epidermolysis bullosa with multi-systemic manifestations including nephropathy. *Matrix Biol* (2017). doi:10.1016/j.matbio.2017.11.003
27. Zoller M. Tetraspanins: push and pull in suppressing and promoting metastasis. *Nat Rev Cancer* (2009) 9:40–55. doi:10.1038/nrc2543
28. Sterk LM, Geuijen CA, van den Berg JG, Claessen N, Weening JJ, Sonnenberg A. Association of the tetraspanin CD151 with the laminin-binding integrins alpha3beta1, alpha6beta1, alpha6beta4 and alpha7beta1 in cells in culture and in vivo. *J Cell Sci* (2002) 115:1161–73.
29. Serru V, Le Naour F, Billard M, Azorsa DO, Lanza F, Boucheix C, et al. Selective tetraspan-integrin complexes (CD81/alpha4beta1, CD151/alpha3beta1, CD151/alpha6beta1) under conditions disrupting tetraspan interactions. *Biochem J* (1999) 340(Pt 1):103–11. doi:10.1042/bj3400103
30. Berditchevski F, Gilbert E, Griffiths MR, Fitter S, Ashman L, Jenner SJ. Analysis of the CD151-alpha3beta1 integrin and CD151-tetraspanin interactions by mutagenesis. *J Biol Chem* (2001) 276:41165–74. doi:10.1074/jbc.M104041200
31. Baldwin G, Novitskaya V, Sadej R, Pochec E, Litynska A, Hartmann C, et al. Tetraspanin CD151 regulates glycosylation of (alpha)3(beta)1 integrin. *J Biol Chem* (2008) 283:35445–54. doi:10.1074/jbc.M806394200
32. Baleato RM, Guthrie PL, Gubler M-C, Ashman LK, Roselli S. Deletion of CD151 results in a strain-dependent glomerular disease due to severe alterations of the glomerular basement membrane. *Am J Pathol* (2008) 173:927–37. doi:10.2353/ajpath.2008.071149
33. Burgu B, Duffy PG, Wilcox DT. Single-centre experience of genitourinary complications of epidermolysis bullosa. *J Pediatr Urol* (2006) 2:583–6. doi:10.1016/j.jpurol.2006.01.007
34. Schumann H, Kiritsi D, Pigors M, Hausser I, Kohlhase J, Peters J, et al. Phenotypic spectrum of epidermolysis bullosa associated with alpha-6beta4 integrin mutations. *Br J Dermatol* (2013) 169:115–24. doi:10.1111/bjd.12317
35. Borza CM, Pozzi A. The role of cell-extracellular matrix interactions in glomerular injury. *Exp Cell Res* (2012) 318:1001–10. doi:10.1016/j.yexcr.2012.02.033
36. Yazlovitskaya EM, Tseng H-Y, Viquez O, Tu T, Mernaugh G, McKee KK, et al. Integrin $\alpha3\beta1$ regulates kidney collecting duct development via TRAF6-dependent K63-linked polyubiquitination of Akt. *Mol Biol Cell* (2015) 26:1857–74. doi:10.1091/mbc.E14-07-1203
37. Viquez OM, Yazlovitskaya EM, Tu T, Mernaugh G, Secades P, McKee KK, et al. Integrin alpha6 maintains the structural integrity of the kidney collecting system. *Matrix Biol* (2017) 57–58:244–57. doi:10.1016/j.matbio.2016.12.003
38. Hammersen J, Has C, Naumann-Bartsch N, Stachel D, Kiritsi D, Söder S, et al. Genotype, clinical course, and therapeutic decision making in 76 infants with severe generalized junctional epidermolysis bullosa. *J Invest Dermatol* (2016) 136:2150–7. doi:10.1016/j.jid.2016.06.609
39. Hata D, Miyazaki M, Seto S, Kadota E, Muso E, Takasu K, et al. Nephrotic syndrome and aberrant expression of laminin isoforms in glomerular basement membranes for an infant with Herlitz junctional epidermolysis bullosa. *Pediatrics* (2005) 116:e601–7. doi:10.1542/peds.2005-0160
40. Tidyman WE, Rauen KA. Expansion of the RASopathies. *Curr Genet Med Rep* (2016) 4:57–64. doi:10.1007/s40142-016-0100-7
41. Tidyman WE, Rauen KA. Pathogenetics of the RASopathies. *Hum Mol Genet* (2016) 25:R123–32. doi:10.1093/hmg/ddw191
42. Ferner RE, Huson SM, Thomas N, Moss C, Willshaw H, Evans DG, et al. Guidelines for the diagnosis and management of individuals with neurofibromatosis 1. *J Med Genet* (2007) 44:81–8. doi:10.1136/jmg.2006.045906
43. Neurofibromatosis. Conference statement. National Institutes of Health Consensus Development Conference. *Arch Neurol* (1988) 45:575–8.
44. Stay EJ, Vawter G. The relationship between nephroblastoma and neurofibromatosis (Von Recklinghausen's disease). *Cancer* (1977) 39:2550–5. doi:10.1002/1097-0142(197706)39:6<2550::AID-CNCR2820390636>3.0.CO;2-Y
45. Walden PA, Johnson AG, Bagshawe KD. Wilms's tumour and neurofibromatosis. *Br Med J* (1977) 1:813. doi:10.1136/bmj.1.6064.813
46. Korf BR. Malignancy in neurofibromatosis type 1. *Oncologist* (2000) 5:477–85. doi:10.1634/theoncologist.5-6-477
47. Evans DGR, O'Hara C, Wilding A, Ingham SL, Howard E, Dawson J, et al. Mortality in neurofibromatosis 1: in North West England: an assessment of actuarial survival in a region of the UK since 1989. *Eur J Hum Genet EJHG* (2011) 19:1187–91. doi:10.1038/ejhg.2011.113
48. Méni C, Sbidian E, Moreno JC, Lafaye S, Buffard V, Goldzal S, et al. Treatment of neurofibromas with a carbon dioxide laser: a retrospective cross-sectional study of 106 patients. *Dermatol Basel Switz* (2015) 230:263–8. doi:10.1159/000368078
49. Kriechbaumer LK, Susani M, Kircher SG, Distelmaier K, Happak W. Comparative study of CO_2- and Er:YAG laser ablation of multiple cutaneous neurofibromas in von Recklinghausen's disease. *Lasers Med Sci* (2014) 29:1083–91. doi:10.1007/s10103-013-1469-0
50. Rad E, Tee AR. Neurofibromatosis type 1: fundamental insights into cell signalling and cancer. *Semin Cell Dev Biol* (2016) 52:39–46. doi:10.1016/j.semcdb.2016.02.007
51. Friedman JM. Neurofibromatosis 1. In: Adam MP, Ardinger HH, Pagon RA, Wallace SE, Bean LJ, Mefford HC, Stephens K, Amemiya A, Ledbetter N, editors. *GeneReviews(®)*. Seattle, WA: University of Washington, Seattle (2017). Available from: http://www.ncbi.nlm.nih.gov/books/NBK1109/
52. Sabbagh A, Pasmant E, Laurendeau I, Parfait B, Barbarot S, Guillot B, et al. Unravelling the genetic basis of variable clinical expression in neurofibromatosis 1. *Hum Mol Genet* (2009) 18:2768–78. doi:10.1093/hmg/ddp212
53. Sabbagh A, Pasmant E, Imbard A, Luscan A, Soares M, Blanché H, et al. NF1 molecular characterization and neurofibromatosis type I genotype-phenotype correlation: the French experience. *Hum Mutat* (2013) 34:1510–8. doi:10.1002/humu.22392
54. Jentarra GM, Rice SG, Olfers S, Rajan C, Saffen DM, Narayanan V. Skewed allele-specific expression of the NF1 gene in normal subjects: a possible

mechanism for phenotypic variability in neurofibromatosis type 1. *J Child Neurol* (2012) 27:695–702. doi:10.1177/0883073811423439
55. Upadhyaya M, Spurlock G, Kluwe L, Chuzhanova N, Bennett E, Thomas N, et al. The spectrum of somatic and germline NF1 mutations in NF1 patients with spinal neurofibromas. *Neurogenetics* (2009) 10:251–63. doi:10.1007/s10048-009-0178-0
56. Sarkozy A, Digilio MC, Dallapiccola B. LEOPARD syndrome. *Orphanet J Rare Dis* (2008) 3:13. doi:10.1186/1750-1172-3-13
57. George CD, Patton MA, el Sawi M, Sharland M, Adam EJ. Abdominal ultrasound in Noonan syndrome: a study of 44 patients. *Pediatr Radiol* (1993) 23:316–8. doi:10.1007/BF02010926
58. Santoro C, Pacileo G, Limongelli G, Scianguetta S, Giugliano T, Piluso G, et al. LEOPARD syndrome: clinical dilemmas in differential diagnosis of RASopathies. *BMC Med Genet* (2014) 15:44. doi:10.1186/1471-2350-15-44
59. Digilio MC, Sarkozy A, de Zorzi A, Pacileo G, Limongelli G, Mingarelli R, et al. LEOPARD syndrome: clinical diagnosis in the first year of life. *Am J Med Genet A* (2006) 140:740–6. doi:10.1002/ajmg.a.31156
60. Kontoes PP, Vlachos SP, Marayiannis KV. Intense pulsed light for the treatment of lentigines in LEOPARD syndrome. *Br J Plast Surg* (2003) 56:607–10. doi:10.1016/S0007-1226(03)00218-2
61. Gelb BD, Tartaglia M. Noonan syndrome with multiple lentigines. In: Adam MP, Ardinger HH, Pagon RA, Wallace SE, Bean LJ, Mefford HC, Stephens K, Amemiya A, Ledbetter N, editors. *GeneReviews(®)*. Seattle, WA: University of Washington, Seattle (2017). Available from: http://www.ncbi.nlm.nih.gov/books/NBK1383/
62. Pandit B, Sarkozy A, Pennacchio LA, Carta C, Oishi K, Martinelli S, et al. Gain-of-function RAF1 mutations cause Noonan and LEOPARD syndromes with hypertrophic cardiomyopathy. *Nat Genet* (2007) 39:1007–12. doi:10.1038/ng2073
63. Jongmans MCJ, van der Burgt I, Hoogerbrugge PM, Noordam K, Yntema HG, Nillesen WM, et al. Cancer risk in patients with Noonan syndrome carrying a PTPN11 mutation. *Eur J Hum Genet EJHG* (2011) 19:870–4. doi:10.1038/ejhg.2011.37
64. Denayer E, Devriendt K, de Ravel T, Van Buggenhout G, Smeets E, Francois I, et al. Tumor spectrum in children with Noonan syndrome and SOS1 or RAF1 mutations. *Genes Chromosomes Cancer* (2010) 49:242–52. doi:10.1002/gcc.20735
65. Jones K, Jones MC, del Campo M. *Smith's Recognizable Patterns of Human Malformation: Expert Consult – Online and Print, 7e*. Philadelphia: Saunders (2013).
66. Northrup H, Krueger DA; International Tuberous Sclerosis Complex Consensus Group. Tuberous sclerosis complex diagnostic criteria update: recommendations of the 2012 Iinternational Tuberous Sclerosis Complex Consensus Conference. *Pediatr Neurol* (2013) 49:243–54. doi:10.1016/j.pediatrneurol.2013.08.001
67. Józwiak S, Schwartz RA, Janniger CK, Bielicka-Cymerman J. Usefulness of diagnostic criteria of tuberous sclerosis complex in pediatric patients. *J Child Neurol* (2000) 15:652–9. doi:10.1177/088307380001501003
68. Bjornsson J, Short MP, Kwiatkowski DJ, Henske EP. Tuberous sclerosis-associated renal cell carcinoma. Clinical, pathological, and genetic features. *Am J Pathol* (1996) 149:1201–8.
69. Northrup H, Koenig MK, Pearson DA, Au K-S. Tuberous sclerosis complex. In: Adam MP, Ardinger HH, Pagon RA, Wallace SE, Bean LJ, Mefford HC, Stephens K, Amemiya A, Ledbetter N, editors. *GeneReviews(®)*. Seattle, WA: University of Washington, Seattle (2017). Available from: http://www.ncbi.nlm.nih.gov/books/NBK1220/
70. Krueger DA, Northrup H; International Tuberous Sclerosis Complex Consensus Group. Tuberous sclerosis complex surveillance and management: recommendations of the 2012 International Tuberous Sclerosis Complex Consensus Conference. *Pediatr Neurol* (2013) 49:255–65. doi:10.1016/j.pediatrneurol.2013.08.002
71. Palavra F, Robalo C, Reis F. Recent advances and challenges of mTOR inhibitors use in the treatment of patients with tuberous sclerosis complex. *Oxid Med Cell Longev* (2017) 2017:9820181. doi:10.1155/2017/9820181
72. Fioramonti P, De Santo L, Ruggieri M, Carella S, Federico LT, Onesti MG, et al. Co_2/Erbium:YAG/Dye laser combination: an effective and successful treatment for angiofibromas in tuberous sclerosis. *Aesthetic Plast Surg* (2014) 38:192–8. doi:10.1007/s00266-013-0252-8
73. Ma G, Wu P, Lin X, Chen H, Li W, Hu X, et al. Nd:YAG laser for "fractional" treatment of angiofibromas. *Int J Dermatol* (2014) 53:638–42. doi:10.1111/ijd.12384
74. Weiss ET, Geronemus RG. New technique using combined pulsed dye laser and fractional resurfacing for treating facial angiofibromas in tuberous sclerosis. *Lasers Surg Med* (2010) 42:357–60. doi:10.1002/lsm.20939
75. Cardis MA, DeKlotz CMC. Cutaneous manifestations of tuberous sclerosis complex and the paediatrician's role. *Arch Dis Child* (2017) 102:858–63. doi:10.1136/archdischild-2016-312001
76. Jóźwiak S, Sadowski K, Kotulska K, Schwartz RA. Topical use of mammalian target of rapamycin (mTOR) inhibitors in tuberous sclerosis complex – a comprehensive review of the literature. *Pediatr Neurol* (2016) 61:21–7. doi:10.1016/j.pediatrneurol.2016.04.003
77. Rosset C, Netto CBO, Ashton-Prolla P. TSC1 and TSC2 gene mutations and their implications for treatment in tuberous sclerosis complex: a review. *Genet Mol Biol* (2017) 40:69–79. doi:10.1590/1678-4685-GMB-2015-0321
78. Tyburczy ME, Dies KA, Glass J, Camposano S, Chekaluk Y, Thorner AR, et al. Mosaic and intronic mutations in TSC1/TSC2 explain the majority of TSC patients with no mutation identified by conventional testing. *PLoS Genet* (2015) 11:e1005637. doi:10.1371/journal.pgen.1005637
79. Martin KR, Zhou W, Bowman MJ, Shih J, Au KS, Dittenhafer-Reed KE, et al. The genomic landscape of tuberous sclerosis complex. *Nat Commun* (2017) 8:15816. doi:10.1038/ncomms15816
80. Kothare SV, Singh K, Chalifoux JR, Staley BA, Weiner HL, Menzer K, et al. Severity of manifestations in tuberous sclerosis complex in relation to genotype. *Epilepsia* (2014) 55:1025–9. doi:10.1111/epi.12680
81. Boronat S, Caruso P, Auladell M, Van Eeghen A, Thiele EA. Arachnoid cysts in tuberous sclerosis complex. *Brain Dev* (2014) 36:801–6. doi:10.1016/j.braindev.2013.11.003
82. Lam HC, Nijmeh J, Henske EP. New developments in the genetics and pathogenesis of tumours in tuberous sclerosis complex. *J Pathol* (2017) 241:219–25. doi:10.1002/path.4827
83. Tyburczy ME, Wang J-A, Li S, Thangapazham R, Chekaluk Y, Moss J, et al. Sun exposure causes somatic second-hit mutations and angiofibroma development in tuberous sclerosis complex. *Hum Mol Genet* (2014) 23:2023–9. doi:10.1093/hmg/ddt597
84. Henske EP, Wessner LL, Golden J, Scheithauer BW, Vortmeyer AO, Zhuang Z, et al. Loss of tuberin in both subependymal giant cell astrocytomas and angiomyolipomas supports a two-hit model for the pathogenesis of tuberous sclerosis tumors. *Am J Pathol* (1997) 151:1639–47.
85. Evans DG, Howard E, Giblin C, Clancy T, Spencer H, Huson SM, et al. Birth incidence and prevalence of tumor-prone syndromes: estimates from a UK family genetic register service. *Am J Med Genet A* (2010) 152A:327–32. doi:10.1002/ajmg.a.33139
86. Mendes-Bastos P, Vale-Fernandes P, Brás S, Carvalho R, João A, Amaro C. Acral basal cell carcinomas in an infant with Gorlin syndrome: expanding the phenotype? *J Dtsch Dermatol Ges J Ger Soc Dermatol JDDG* (2017) 15:89–90. doi:10.1111/ddg.12934
87. Bacanli A, Ciftcioglu MA, Savas B, Alpsoy E. Nevoid basal cell carcinoma syndrome associated with unilateral renal agenesis: acceleration of basal cell carcinomas following radiotherapy. *J Eur Acad Dermatol Venereol JEADV* (2005) 19:510–1. doi:10.1111/j.1468-3083.2004.01169.x
88. Cajaiba MM, Bale AE, Alvarez-Franco M, McNamara J, Reyes-Múgica M. Rhabdomyosarcoma, Wilms tumor, and deletion of the patched gene in Gorlin syndrome. *Nat Clin Pract Oncol* (2006) 3:575–80. doi:10.1038/ncponc0608
89. Garavelli L, Piemontese MR, Cavazza A, Rosato S, Wischmeijer A, Gelmini C, et al. Multiple tumor types including leiomyoma and Wilms tumor in a patient with Gorlin syndrome due to 9q22.3 microdeletion encompassing the PTCH1 and FANC-C loci. *Am J Med Genet A* (2013) 161A:2894–901. doi:10.1002/ajmg.a.36259
90. Bree AF, Shah MR, BCNS Colloquium Group. Consensus statement from the first international colloquium on basal cell nevus syndrome (BCNS). *Am J Med Genet A* (2011) 155A:2091–7. doi:10.1002/ajmg.a.34128
91. Bakshi A, Chaudhary SC, Rana M, Elmets CA, Athar M. Basal cell carcinoma pathogenesis and therapy involving hedgehog signaling and beyond. *Mol Carcinog* (2017) 56(12):2543–57. doi:10.1002/mc.22690
92. Solis DC, Kwon GP, Ransohoff KJ, Li S, Chahal HS, Ally MS, et al. Risk factors for basal cell carcinoma among patients with basal cell nevus syndrome:

development of a basal cell nevus syndrome patient registry. *JAMA Dermatol* (2016). doi:10.1001/jamadermatol.2016.4347

93. Evans DG, Farndon PA. Nevoid basal cell carcinoma syndrome. In: Adam MP, Ardinger HH, Pagon RA, Wallace SE, Bean LJ, Mefford HC, Stephens K, Amemiya A, Ledbetter N, editors. *GeneReviews(®)*. Seattle, WA: University of Washington, Seattle (2017). Available from: http://www.ncbi.nlm.nih.gov/books/NBK1151/
94. Fan Z, Li J, Du J, Zhang H, Shen Y, Wang C-Y, et al. A missense mutation in PTCH2 underlies dominantly inherited NBCCS in a Chinese family. *J Med Genet* (2008) 45:303–8. doi:10.1136/jmg.2007.055343
95. Khamaysi Z, Bochner R, Indelman M, Magal L, Avitan-Hersh E, Sarig O, et al. Segmental basal cell naevus syndrome caused by an activating mutation in smoothened. *Br J Dermatol* (2016) 175:178–81. doi:10.1111/bjd.14425
96. Reinders MGHC, Boersma HJ, Leter EM, Vreeburg M, Paulussen ADC, Arits AHMM, et al. Postzygotic mosaicism in basal cell naevus syndrome. *Br J Dermatol* (2017) 177:249–52. doi:10.1111/bjd.15082
97. Ribeiro LA, Murray JC, Richieri-Costa A. PTCH mutations in four Brazilian patients with holoprosencephaly and in one with holoprosencephaly-like features and normal MRI. *Am J Med Genet A* (2006) 140:2584–6. doi:10.1002/ajmg.a.31369
98. Atwood SX, Chang ALS, Oro AE. Hedgehog pathway inhibition and the race against tumor evolution. *J Cell Biol* (2012) 199:193–7. doi:10.1083/jcb.201207140
99. Epstein EH. Basal cell carcinomas: attack of the hedgehog. *Nat Rev Cancer* (2008) 8:743–54. doi:10.1038/nrc2503
100. Toro JR. Birt-Hogg-Dubé syndrome. In: Adam MP, Ardinger HH, Pagon RA, Wallace SE, Bean LJ, Mefford HC, Stephens K, Amemiya A, Ledbetter N, editors. *GeneReviews®*. Seattle, WA: University of Washington, Seattle (2017). Available from: http://www.ncbi.nlm.nih.gov/books/NBK1522/
101. Schmidt LS, Linehan WM. Molecular genetics and clinical features of Birt-Hogg-Dubé syndrome. *Nat Rev Urol* (2015) 12:558–69. doi:10.1038/nrurol.2015.206
102. Zbar B, Alvord WG, Glenn G, Turner M, Pavlovich CP, Schmidt L, et al. Risk of renal and colonic neoplasms and spontaneous pneumothorax in the Birt-Hogg-Dubé syndrome. *Cancer Epidemiol Biomark Prev* (2002) 11:393–400.
103. Schmidt LS, Nickerson ML, Warren MB, Glenn GM, Toro JR. Germline BHD-mutation spectrum and phenotype analysis of a large cohort of families with Birt-Hogg-Dubé syndrome. *Am J Hum Genet* (2005) 76(6):1023–33. doi:10.1086/430842
104. Yan M, Gingras MC, Dunlop EA, Nouet Y, Dupuy F, Jalali Z, et al. The tumor suppressor folliculin regulates AMPK-dependent metabolic transformation. *J Clin Invest* (2014) 124:2640–50. doi:10.1172/JCI71749
105. Baba M, Hong S-B, Sharma N, Warren MB, Nickerson ML, Iwamatsu A, et al. Folliculin encoded by the BHD gene interacts with a binding protein, FNIP1, and AMPK, and is involved in AMPK and mTOR signaling. *Proc Natl Acad Sci U S A* (2006) 103:15552–7. doi:10.1073/pnas.0603781103
106. Hasumi H, Baba M, Hong S-B, Hasumi Y, Huang Y, Yao M, et al. Identification and characterization of a novel folliculin-interacting protein FNIP2. *Gene* (2008) 415:60–7. doi:10.1016/j.gene.2008.02.022
107. Takagi Y, Kobayashi T, Shiono M, Wang L, Piao X, Sun G, et al. Interaction of folliculin (Birt-Hogg-Dubé gene product) with a novel Fnip1-like (FnipL/Fnip2) protein. *Oncogene* (2008) 27:5339–47. doi:10.1038/onc.2008.261
108. Pithukpakorn M, Toro JR. Hereditary leiomyomatosis and renal cell cancer. In: Adam MP, Ardinger HH, Pagon RA, Wallace SE, Bean LJ, Mefford HC, Stephens K, Amemiya A, Ledbetter N, editors. *GeneReviews®*. Seattle, WA: University of Washington, Seattle (2017). Available from: http://www.ncbi.nlm.nih.gov/books/NBK1252/
109. Tomlinson IPM, Alam NA, Rowan AJ, Barclay E, Jaeger EEM, Kelsell D, et al. Germline mutations in FH predispose to dominantly inherited uterine fibroids, skin leiomyomata and papillary renal cell cancer. *Nat Genet* (2002) 30:406–10. doi:10.1038/ng849
110. Coughlin EM, Christensen E, Kunz PL, Krishnamoorthy KS, Walker V, Dennis NR, et al. Molecular analysis and prenatal diagnosis of human fumarase deficiency. *Mol Genet Metab* (1998) 63:254–62. doi:10.1006/mgme.1998.2684
111. Happle R. Cutaneous manifestation of lethal genes. *Hum Genet* (1986) 72:280. doi:10.1007/BF00291899
112. Happle R. Lethal genes surviving by mosaicism: a possible explanation for sporadic birth defects involving the skin. *J Am Acad Dermatol* (1987) 16:899–906. doi:10.1016/S0190-9622(87)80249-9
113. Happle R. The group of epidermal nevus syndromes Part I. Well defined phenotypes. *J Am Acad Dermatol* (2010) 63:1–22–24. doi:10.1016/j.jaad.2010.01.017
114. Kiedrowicz M, Kacalak-Rzepka A, Królicki A, Maleszka R, Bielecka-Grzela S. Therapeutic effects of CO_2 laser therapy of linear nevus sebaceous in the course of the Schimmelpenning-Feuerstein-Mims syndrome. *Postepy Dermatol Alergol* (2013) 30:320–3. doi:10.5114/pdia.2013.38363
115. Groesser L, Herschberger E, Ruetten A, Ruivenkamp C, Lopriore E, Zutt M, et al. Postzygotic HRAS and KRAS mutations cause nevus sebaceous and Schimmelpenning syndrome. *Nat Genet* (2012) 44:783–7. doi:10.1038/ng.2316
116. Sun BK, Saggini A, Sarin KY, Kim J, Benjamin L, LeBoit PE, et al. Mosaic activating RAS mutations in nevus sebaceous and nevus sebaceus syndrome. *J Invest Dermatol* (2013) 133:824–7. doi:10.1038/jid.2012.377
117. DeDavid M, Orlow SJ, Provost N, Marghoob AA, Rao BK, Wasti Q, et al. Neurocutaneous melanosis: clinical features of large congenital melanocytic nevi in patients with manifest central nervous system melanosis. *J Am Acad Dermatol* (1996) 35:529–38. doi:10.1016/S0190-9622(96)90674-X
118. Kinsler VA, Thomas AC, Ishida M, Bulstrode NW, Loughlin S, Hing S, et al. Multiple congenital melanocytic nevi and neurocutaneous melanosis are caused by postzygotic mutations in codon 61 of NRAS. *J Invest Dermatol* (2013) 133:2229–36. doi:10.1038/jid.2013.70
119. Krengel S, Hauschild A, Schäfer T. Melanoma risk in congenital melanocytic naevi: a systematic review. *Br J Dermatol* (2006) 155:1–8. doi:10.1111/j.1365-2133.2006.07218.x
120. Basu D, Salgado CM, Bauer BS, Johnson D, Rundell V, Nikiforova M, et al. Nevospheres from neurocutaneous melanocytosis cells show reduced viability when treated with specific inhibitors of NRAS signaling pathway. *Neuro Oncol* (2016) 18:528–37. doi:10.1093/neuonc/nov184
121. Happle R, Koch H, Lenz W. The CHILD syndrome. Congenital hemidysplasia with ichthyosiform erythroderma and limb defects. *Eur J Pediatr* (1980) 134:27–33. doi:10.1007/BF00442399
122. Happle R, Karlić D, Steijlen PM. [CHILD syndrome in a mother and daughter]. *Hautarzt Z Dermatol Venerol Verwandte Geb* (1990) 41:105–8.
123. Schmidt-Sidor B, Obersztyn E, Szymańska K, Wychowski J, Mierzewska H, Wierzba-Bobrowicz T, et al. Brain and cerebellar hemidysplasia in a case with ipsilateral body dysplasia and suspicion of CHILD syndrome. *Folia Neuropathol* (2008) 46:232–7.
124. du Souich C, Raymond FL, Grzeschik K-H, Boerkoel CF. NSDHL-related disorders. In: Adam MP, Ardinger HH, Pagon RA, Wallace SE, Bean LJ, Mefford HC, Stephens K, Amemiya A, Ledbetter N, editors. *GeneReviews(®)*. Seattle, WA: University of Washington, Seattle (2017). Available from: http://www.ncbi.nlm.nih.gov/books/NBK51754/
125. Kiritsi D, Schauer F, Wolfle U, Valari M, Bruckner-Tuderman L, Has C, et al. Targeting epidermal lipids for treatment of Mendelian disorders of cornification. *Orphanet J Rare Dis* (2014) 9:33. doi:10.1186/1750-1172-9-33
126. Paller AS, van Steensel MAM, Rodriguez-Martín M, Sorrell J, Heath C, Crumrine D, et al. Pathogenesis-based therapy reverses cutaneous abnormalities in an inherited disorder of distal cholesterol metabolism. *J Invest Dermatol* (2011) 131:2242–8. doi:10.1038/jid.2011.189
127. König A, Happle R, Bornholdt D, Engel H, Grzeschik KH. Mutations in the NSDHL gene, encoding a 3beta-hydroxysteroid dehydrogenase, cause CHILD syndrome. *Am J Med Genet* (2000) 90:339–46. doi:10.1002/(SICI)1096-8628(20000214)90:4<339::AID-AJMG15>3.0.CO;2-5
128. Seeger MA, Paller AS. The role of abnormalities in the distal pathway of cholesterol synthesis in the Congenital Hemidysplasia with Ichthyosiform erythroderma and Limb Defects (CHILD) syndrome. *Biochim Biophys Acta* (2014) 1841:345–52. doi:10.1016/j.bbalip.2013.09.006
129. du Souich C, Chou A, Yin J, Oh T, Nelson TN, Hurlburt J, et al. Characterization of a new X-linked mental retardation syndrome with microcephaly, cortical malformation, and thin habitus. *Am J Med Genet A* (2009) 149A:2469–78. doi:10.1002/ajmg.a.33071
130. McLarren KW, Severson TM, du Souich C, Stockton DW, Kratz LE, Cunningham D, et al. Hypomorphic temperature-sensitive alleles of NSDHL

cause CK syndrome. *Am J Hum Genet* (2010) 87:905–14. doi:10.1016/j.ajhg.2010.11.004

131. Goltz RW, Peterson WC, Gorlin RJ, Ravits HG. Focal dermal hypoplasia. *Arch Dermatol* (1962) 86:708–17. doi:10.1001/archderm.1962.01590120006002
132. Bree AF, Grange DK, Hicks MJ, Goltz RW. Dermatologic findings of focal dermal hypoplasia (Goltz syndrome). *Am J Med Genet C Semin Med Genet* (2016) 172C:44–51. doi:10.1002/ajmg.c.31472
133. Grzeschik K-H, Bornholdt D, Oeffner F, König A, del Carmen Boente M, Enders H, et al. Deficiency of PORCN, a regulator of Wnt signaling, is associated with focal dermal hypoplasia. *Nat Genet* (2007) 39:833–5. doi:10.1038/ng2052
134. Sanna-Cherchi S, Westland R, Ghiggeri GM, Gharavi AG. Genetic basis of human congenital anomalies of the kidney and urinary tract. *J Clin Invest* (2018) 128:4–15. doi:10.1172/JCI95300
135. Sheu J, Divito SJ, Hoffman EP, Frank NY, Merola JF. Mosaic focal dermal hypoplasia caused by a novel somatic mutation in PORCN detected in affected skin. *Br J Dermatol* (2015) 173:568–70. doi:10.1111/bjd.13649

22

Developmental Programming of Renal Function and Re-Programming Approaches

Eva Nüsken, Jörg Dötsch, Lutz T. Weber and Kai-Dietrich Nüsken*

Pediatric Nephrology, Department of Pediatrics, Medical Faculty, University of Cologne, Cologne, Germany

Correspondence:
Kai-Dietrich Nüsken
kai-dietrich.nuesken@uk-koeln.de

Chronic kidney disease affects more than 10% of the population. Programming studies have examined the interrelationship between environmental factors in early life and differences in morbidity and mortality between individuals. A number of important principles has been identified, namely permanent structural modifications of organs and cells, long-lasting adjustments of endocrine regulatory circuits, as well as altered gene transcription. Risk factors include intrauterine deficiencies by disturbed placental function or maternal malnutrition, prematurity, intrauterine and postnatal stress, intrauterine and postnatal overnutrition, as well as dietary dysbalances in postnatal life. This mini-review discusses critical developmental periods and long-term sequelae of renal programming in humans and presents studies examining the underlying mechanisms as well as interventional approaches to "re-program" renal susceptibility toward disease. Clinical manifestations of programmed kidney disease include arterial hypertension, proteinuria, aggravation of inflammatory glomerular disease, and loss of kidney function. Nephron number, regulation of the renin–angiotensin–aldosterone system, renal sodium transport, vasomotor and endothelial function, myogenic response, and tubuloglomerular feedback have been identified as being vulnerable to environmental factors. Oxidative stress levels, metabolic pathways, including insulin, leptin, steroids, and arachidonic acid, DNA methylation, and histone configuration may be significantly altered by adverse environmental conditions. Studies on re-programming interventions focused on dietary or anti-oxidative approaches so far. Further studies that broaden our understanding of renal programming mechanisms are needed to ultimately develop preventive strategies. Targeted re-programming interventions in animal models focusing on known mechanisms will contribute to new concepts which finally will have to be translated to human application. Early nutritional concepts with specific modifications in macro- or micronutrients are among the most promising approaches to improve future renal health.

Keywords: kidney development, nephron number, renin–angiotensin–aldosterone system, renal sodium transport, blood pressure, early nutrition, re-programming intervention

INTRODUCTION

Prevention of chronic kidney disease is a major public health challenge (1). Although diabetes mellitus is the most common cause of chronic kidney disease worldwide (2), developmental programming processes that have been reviewed by us (3, 4) and others (5–7) before substantially contribute to differences in morbidity and mortality between individuals. The normal development of the kidney can be disturbed by multiple environmental factors, including intrauterine deficiencies by disturbed placental function or maternal malnutrition, prematurity, intrauterine and postnatal stress, intrauterine and postnatal overnutrition, as well as dietary dysbalances of macro- and micronutrients. Since developmental steps take place during unique developmental periods, timing, and duration of an adverse environment specifically impact on developmental programming. Adverse kidney programming increases the incidence of severe renal and cardiovascular sequels later in life. This includes arterial hypertension and associated end organ damage, the aggravation of inflammatory glomerular disease and the occurrence of end-stage renal disease. Specific "re-programming" interventions may mitigate or even prevent programmed disease. Consequently, our mini-review will address the following topics:

(1) Which developmental stages are especially vulnerable?
(2) What are the long-term sequelae of adverse renal programming?
(3) Which environmental factors may have impact on kidney development and what are potential mechanisms of developmental kidney programming?
(4) What are potential therapeutic "re-programming" interventions?

CRITICAL DEVELOPMENTAL PERIODS OF RENAL PROGRAMMING IN HUMANS

In humans the pronephros begins to form around day 22, urine production starts after 10 weeks (8), and maximum renal growth occurs between 26 and 34 weeks of gestation (9). Around week 36, nephrogenesis is completed and the number of nephrons is determined (8, 10). In preterm infants, adaptation to extra-uterine conditions impairs nephrogenesis, and the children end up with fewer nephrons and a higher percentage of morphologically abnormal glomeruli (5, 6, 11, 12). In small for gestational age (SGA) fetuses, intrauterine renal growth is reduced compared to appropriate for gestational age controls (9). In both term and preterm infants, glomerular and tubular functions undergo further maturational changes during the first months of life (8, 13). In these vulnerable periods, babies are often exposed to nephrotoxic medication, such as non-steroidal anti-inflammatory drugs (14), antibiotics, or diuretics, during neonatal intensive care unit treatment (15, 16).

LONG-TERM SEQUELAE OF RENAL PROGRAMMING IN HUMANS

Blood Pressure and Loss of Kidney Function

Hypertension is the most important risk factor for cardiovascular events and mortality worldwide (17). Elevated blood pressure contributes to progression of renal insufficiency (18) and is a strong independent risk factor for end-stage renal disease (19). *Vice versa*, decreased renal function is associated with increased blood pressure and cardiovascular morbidity (20). Early detection of blood pressure elevation plays a major role in the prevention of end organ damage (21). Many studies, including a systematic meta-analysis of studies tracking blood pressure during life course, demonstrated that childhood blood pressure predicts blood pressure (22–24) and vascular end organ damage in adulthood (25). Abnormal birth weight, either low or high, increases the risk for blood pressure elevation and loss of renal function in a U-shaped manner (26–31). In SGA individuals, some studies demonstrated elevated blood pressure in childhood (32) or adulthood (33, 34) especially when rapid postnatal catch-up growth and later adiposity were present (35). Further risk factors include high maternal BMI (36) or elevated protein/carbohydrate ratios in maternal diet during pregnancy (37, 38), rapid postnatal weight gain (39), or being born large for gestational age (36, 40, 41).

Proteinuria and Loss of Kidney Function

Several risk factors during early life predispose toward proteinuria and related decline of renal function. Accordingly, the prevalence of microalbuminuria among adults whose mothers had been exposed to the Dutch Hunger Winter 1944/45 was elevated (42). Chinese women born in the famine years 1959–1961 had a higher risk to develop more severe stages of proteinuria in their forties (43). Low birthweight itself is associated with elevated risks for albuminuria (OR, 1.81; 95% CI, 1.19–2.77), end-stage renal disease (OR, 1.58; 95% CI, 1.33–1.88), or low estimated glomerular filtration rate (GFR) (29, 44, 45). A birthweight-dependent decline in GFR may already be seen in childhood (29, 46, 47).

Glomerular Disease and Inflammation

Furthermore, a number of studies have evaluated the association between perinatal risk factors and later glomerular disease. Thus, SGA individuals have a higher risk to experience steroid resistance and a more severe course in nephrotic syndrome (48, 49). In IgA-nephropathy, they develop arterial hypertension and glomerulosclerosis more often (50).

MECHANISMS OF RENAL PROGRAMMING

In human studies, it is difficult to establish mechanistic links in the field of developmental programming since there usually is a large delay between an adverse event and the related clinical phenotype. This makes it very challenging to distinguish the underlying causes from multiple modifying factors. Thus, animal models providing the possibility of equalized postnatal conditions and specific interventions are especially valuable. In rodents, kidney development during the early postnatal period corresponds to the third trimester in humans (10). For an overview of mechanisms see **Figure 1**.

Nephron Number

Nephron number in humans ranges from ~200,000 to >2.5 million nephrons per kidney (51). The well-known hypothesis of Brenner et al. linked decreased glomerular number with increased glomerular size, hyperfiltration, hypertension, and progressive glomerular injury (7, 52). Nephron number positively correlates with birth weight (53, 54) and is reduced after low-protein (LP) diet throughout pregnancy (55–59), utero-placental insufficiency

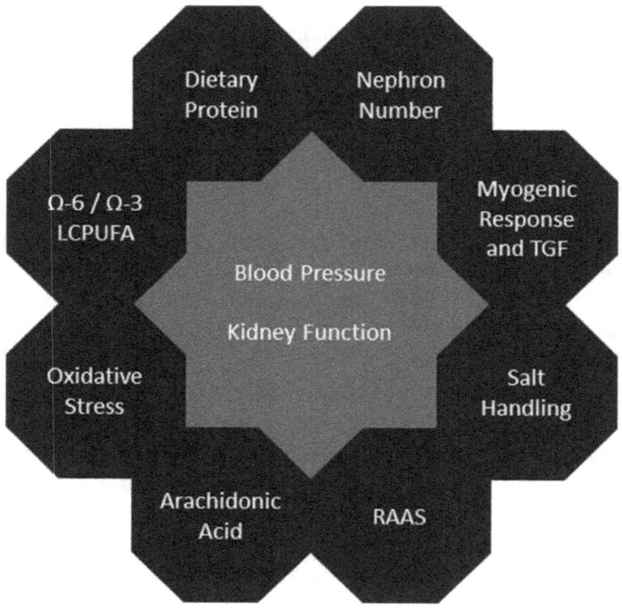

FIGURE 1 | Programming mechanisms affecting blood pressure and kidney function.

(60–62), intrauterine glucocorticoid exposure (63), preterm birth (11, 64), and oxidative stress (65). In addition, a diet deficient in vitamin A (58, 66), zinc (67), or iron (68) is associated with low nephron count. Finally, nephrons get lost with age (69). Interestingly, low nephron number in young individuals is not necessarily associated with hypertension (70, 71). Thus, modulating factors such as early hyperalimentation and aging processes certainly have an impact on renal outcome in individuals with low nephron count (71, 72).

Renin–Angiotensin–Aldosterone System (RAAS)

Dysregulation of all or single components of the RAAS system may severely impair renal development (73, 74). Both activating and deactivating effects on the RAAS can induce a vicious circle of persisting hormonal dysbalances which may finally contribute to the development of arterial hypertension and renal failure.

In the fetal and perinatal period, downregulation of the RAAS has been identified as a relevant mechanism. In neonatal rats after LP diet during gestation, renal renin and angiotensin II levels (75) as well as angiotensin II receptors type 1 (AT1R) and 2 (AT2R) protein expressions (76) were reduced. Similarly, renal AT2R gene and protein expressions were reduced in fetal rats after prenatal caffeine exposure (77). Fetal angiotensin II levels in plasma were decreased after maternal high-salt diet in sheep (78).

Later in life, most environmental influences during early childhood end up with a RAAS activation. Adult rat offspring from the LP diet model showed elevated blood pressure (59), increased AT1R expression (79, 80) and elevated plasma angiotensin-converting enzyme (ACE) activity going along with slightly elevated angiotensin II levels (81). When challenged with angiotensin II infusion, adult LP offspring reacted with a greater decline in GFR than controls (80). In another LP study, there were more angiotensin II-positive cells in the cortical tubulointerstitium of adult offspring (82). Offspring from diabetic mothers had marked upregulation of angiotensinogen (AGT) and AT1R gene expression as well as increased ACE:ACE2 mRNA ratio (83). Some environmental influences induce RAAS activation already in fetal life. Thus, ovine offspring exposed to high salt during gestation presented with increased gene expression of AGT, ACE, AT1R, and increased ACE:ACE2 and AT1R:AT2R mRNA ratio (78). In the human situation, plasma renin concentrations were elevated in umbilical veins of SGA infants, and birth weight was inversely associated with circulating aldosterone concentrations (84). Treatment of human proximal tubule epithelial cells with palmitic acid demonstrated susceptibility to nutritional factors, as it induced intracellular endoplasmic reticulum (ER) stress and increased angiotensin II concentrations in cell medium. Co-treatment with AT1R-blocker or renin-inhibitor prevented ER stress (85).

Renal Sodium Transport

In rats, LP nutrition or dexamethasone treatment during gestation both resulted in an upregulation of the bumetanide-sensitive Na-K-2Cl cotransporter and of the thiazide-sensitive Na-Cl cotransporter in the offspring (86, 87). Adult offspring exposed to LP nutrition during gestation and lactation presented with a reduced diuretic response after a single dose of furosemide (88). After prenatal dexamethasone treatment, proximal tubule Na/H exchanger protein expression was increased, going along with an increase in proximal tubule sodium and volume reabsorption (86, 89). Sodium uptake in renal proximal tubule cells from adult male sheep was enhanced after prenatal betamethasone exposure (90). In rat offspring exposed to experimental utero-placental insufficiency (91) or maternal diabetes (92), sodium-dependent hypertension was observed.

Vasomotor and Endothelial Function

Another interesting aspect is the maturation of vascular smooth muscle function and small artery resistance regulation. Sympathectomy suppresses maturation of the gene program involved in small artery resistance regulation (93). Intrauterine and perinatal stress could, therefore, have a major impact on vascular tone regulation. In addition, vasomotor function can be impaired by perinatal hyperoxia (65) and LP diet (94). Endothelial dysfunction has also been described after intrauterine deficiency and may add to hypertension and glomerular damage (95).

Myogenic Response and Tubuloglomerular Feedback (TGF)

An impaired myogenic response as well as a disturbed TGF are important contributors to glomerular damage in diabetic and hypertensive nephropathy (96). An altered myogenic response has been described in intrauterine growth-restricted (IUGR) neonates, which may be beneficial postnatally, but harmful in the long run (97). The TGF mechanism matures during fetal life and could, therefore, be susceptible to programming *in utero* (98).

However, no study has examined the specific consequences of disturbed intrauterine environment for TGF function.

Epigenetic Mechanisms

The molecular details of kidney development have been extensively studied (99, 100). Altered DNA methylation, histone modification, and other mechanisms modifying the renal transcriptome may significantly impair renal organogenesis and predispose toward renal disease which has lately been reviewed in detail (101). In this context, it is important to separate epigenetic changes during kidney disease (102) from epigenetic changes during early life leading to "programmed" disease. So far, there is little evidence that single, kidney-specific epigenetic alterations during early life might actually cause renal disease later on. Candidate genes would be all genes which are activated during specific developmental windows. Pax-2, for example, is essential for kidney development, ontogenetically regulated and can be reactivated in repair processes after acute kidney injury (103, 104). Global alterations of methylation associated with hypertension were observed after significant periconceptional deficiency of B vitamins and methionine (105). Thus, nutritional modifications may induce temporary or permanent epigenetic alterations that certainly have the potential to modulate kidney disease.

Oxidative Stress

Oxidative stress and inflammation are major contributors to vascular remodeling and hypertension (106). In LP (94, 107) and maternal smoking models (108), it was shown that oxidative stress during critical developmental steps may significantly contribute to renal susceptibility toward disease. In addition, both IUGR offspring after global undernutrition of the dam (109) and after high-fat died during gestation and lactation (110) showed increased oxidative stress and elevated blood pressure later in life. Reduction of oxidative stress during early life can prevent programmed hypertension and renal damage (94, 107, 108).

Metabolism

Rapid postnatal weight gain and early life obesity have been associated with adverse renal outcome (111, 112). Interplay between adiposity, leptin, and insulin resistance with RAAS regulation and sympathetic activity has been described (113, 114). Early postnatal overfeeding in rats by litter size reduction induced increased early postnatal weight gain and was associated with increased blood pressure, glomerulosclerosis, and proteinuria in adulthood (71). In a similar study, postnatal overfeeding resulted in decreased GFR, increased proteinuria and increased deposition of collagens. On the molecular level, intrinsic renal leptin resistance could be demonstrated (115). Dysregulation of renal leptin and Akt/AMPKα signaling associated with increased renal matrix deposition could also be shown in overweight offspring from mothers fed a high-fat diet during gestation and lactation (116). Maternal LP nutrition during rat gestation persistently decreased the expression of renal 11β-hydroxysteroid dehydrogenase type 2 (11β-HSD2) (117, 118) and increased the expression of the renal glucocorticoid receptor in the offspring (118). The same was shown for sheep offspring exposed to temporary maternal calorie restriction (119).

Arachidonic Acid Metabolism Pathway

Finally, there is evidence that the arachidonic acid metabolism pathway could be involved in the development of programmed hypertension (120, 121). 20-hydroxyeicosatetraenoic acid (20-HETE), a metabolite of arachidonic acid, contributes to the normal myogenic pressure response. Physiologically, arachidonic acid is released from cell membranes by phospholipase A2, converted to 20-HETE, which then adds to vasoconstriction of the afferent arteriole (96, 122). However, 20-HETE has also been linked to systemic hypertension and endothelial dysfunction in rats (123). Further arachidonic acid metabolites like Cox-2 derived prostaglandins contribute to counter regulatory vasodilation of the afferent arteriole after TGF-mediated vasoconstriction (124) and oxidative stress in the kidney (125), and therefore modulate intraglomerular pressure and GFR as well as renal inflammation (82). Thus, nutritional intake of arachidonic acid may significantly affect blood pressure, kidney function, and kidney survival.

POTENTIAL THERAPEUTIC "RE-PROGRAMMING" INTERVENTIONS

The ultimate goal of all research on programmed disease is to develop preventive strategies. So far, the number of studies on re-programming interventions is still limited and mainly restricted to dietary or anti-oxidative approaches.

Early Dietary Interventions

Data on nutritional interventions are available from both animal and human studies. A meta-analysis showed slightly, but significantly lower blood pressure in infants, children, and adolescents who were breast fed during infancy compared to those being formula fed (126). Micronutrient (127), calcium (128), vitamin A (129, 130), and iron (131) supplementation during pregnancy as well as long-chain polyunsaturated fatty acid (LCPUFA) supplementation in infant formula (132) may be beneficial to renal outcome.

In detail, children of women receiving a multiple micronutrient supplementation during the second and third trimesters of pregnancy were heavier and had lower systolic blood pressure during infancy (127). Calcium supplementation from the 20th gestational week until delivery lowered systolic blood pressure in children aged 7 years, with a stronger effect when children were overweight (128). Supplementation of iron and folate until the end of pregnancy in rural Bangladesh caused a slightly decreased diastolic blood pressure and a slightly increased GFR in infants at the age of 4.5 years when started at the ninth, but not when started at the 20th gestational week (131). Another dietary intervention with micronutrient supplementation in malnourished pregnant Nepalese women until 3 months postpartum showed that folic acid or the combination of folic acid, iron, and zinc reduced the risk of microalbuminuria, but not blood pressure in the children aged 6–8 years (133). The effects of retinoic acid have mainly been studied in animals. Decreased availability of retinoic acid induced by down-regulated vitamin A metabolism after previous overexposure to vitamin A strongly impairs metanephric kidney development, which can be restored by adequate retinoic acid supplementation (129). In rat offspring exposed to LP diet of the dam during pregnancy, a single injection of retinoic acid to the dam at midgestation increased postnatal nephron number at 4 weeks of age (130). Postnatal administration of retinoic acid in preterm baboons, however, did not alter kidney growth or nephron number, presumably because the timing of the intervention was chosen too late (134).

Long-chain polyunsaturated fatty acid supplementation with arachidonic acid and docosahexaenoic acid (ratio 2:1) in infant milk formula (IF) during the first 4 months of life lowered blood pressure at 6 years of age compared to IF without LCPUFAs. Blood pressure of children fed LCPUFA-IF was similar compared to breast fed children (132). A diet sufficient in ω-3 PUFAs reduced blood pressure levels compared to a diet almost free of ω-3 PUFAs in TGR(mRen-2)27 rats which have high angiotensin II levels (135). Finally, the importance of the amino acid composition was demonstrated. Addition of glycine to maternal LP diet throughout gestation normalized body weight and blood pressure at 4 weeks of age in rat offspring, whereas alanine or urea had no effect (136).

Anti-Oxidative Substances

Re-programming interventions with anti-oxidative substances have only been performed in animals. Supplementation of maternal LP diet with anti-oxidative (ACH09)-derived polyphenols extracted from grape skins reduced signs of renal oxidative stress in the offspring on the first postnatal day and attenuated the adverse effects of maternal LP diet on glomerular number and maturity (107). Administration of a lipid peroxidation inhibitor along with LP diet in gestation reduced prenatal oxidative stress and prevented programming of elevated blood pressure, enhanced vasoconstriction after angiotensin II administration and reduced vasodilation after sodium nitroprusside administration in adult animals (94). Similarly, treatment of previously malnourished dams with α-tocopherol during lactation prevented the development of hypertension in the offspring. In addition, upregulated angiotensin II levels and down-regulated Cox-2 expression in the tubulointersititum were brought back to control levels and oxidative stress as well as macrophage infiltration was prevented. However, treatment of control dams with α-tocopherol resulted in arterial hypertension of the offspring (82).

CONCLUSION AND FUTURE DIRECTIONS

The concept of "developmental origins of health and disease" highlights the interrelationship between environmental factors throughout life and differences in morbidity and mortality between individuals. Chronic kidney disease affects more than 10% of the population (1). High blood pressure, childhood underweight, and suboptimal breastfeeding are among the top risk factors contributing to global burden of disease (137). Prematurity, IUGR, overweight in early life, and other conditions have been associated with the development of arterial hypertension, proteinuria, and decline of renal function. Around 11% of all live-born infants worldwide are born preterm (138). IUGR is seen in 3–7% of all pregnancies (139). During childhood, 5–6% of girls and 7–8% of boys become overweight (140). Thus, renal programming is not a rare phenomenon but affects large parts of the population. Further studies that broaden our understanding of renal programming mechanisms are needed to ultimately develop preventive strategies. Targeted re-programming interventions in animal models focusing on known mechanisms will contribute to new concepts which finally will have to be translated to human application. Early nutritional concepts with specific modifications in macro- or micronutrients are among the most promising approaches to improve future renal health.

AUTHOR CONTRIBUTIONS

EN performed the majority of literature research, and designed and wrote the review. K-DN contributed to literature research, and designed and wrote the review. JD and LW contributed to literature research and writing. All authors revised and approved the review.

REFERENCES

1. Eckardt KU, Coresh J, Devuyst O, Johnson RJ, Köttgen A, Levey AS, et al. Evolving importance of kidney disease: from subspecialty to global health burden. *Lancet* (2013) 382(9887):158–69. doi:10.1016/S0140-6736(13)60439-0
2. Jha V, Garcia-Garcia G, Iseki K, Li Z, Naicker S, Plattner B, et al. Chronic kidney disease: global dimension and perspectives. *Lancet* (2013) 382(9888):260–72. doi:10.1016/S0140-6736(13)60687-X
3. Nüsken E, Nüsken K-D, Dötsch J. Diet and epigenetic alteration of renal function. In: Patel V, Preedy V, editors. *Handbook of Nutrition, Diet, and Epigenetics*. Cham: Springer International Publishing (2017). p. 1–20.
4. Dötsch J, Alejandre-Alcazar M, Janoschek R, Nüsken E, Weber LT, Nüsken KD. Perinatal programming of renal function. *Curr Opin Pediatr* (2016) 28(2):188–94. doi:10.1097/MOP.0000000000000312
5. Stritzke A, Thomas S, Amin H, Fusch C, Lodha A. Renal consequences of preterm birth. *Mol Cell Pediatr* (2017) 4(1):2. doi:10.1186/s40348-016-0068-0
6. Luyckx VA. Preterm birth and its impact on renal health. *Semin Nephrol* (2017) 37(4):311–9. doi:10.1016/j.semnephrol.2017.05.002
7. Luyckx VA, Brenner BM. Low birth weight, nephron number, and kidney disease. *Kidney Int Suppl* (2005) 97:S68–77. doi:10.1111/j.1523-1755.2005.09712.x
8. Quigley R. Developmental changes in renal function. *Curr Opin Pediatr* (2012) 24(2):184–90. doi:10.1097/MOP.0b013e32834fe863
9. Konje JC, Bell SC, Morton JJ, de Chazal R, Taylor DJ. Human fetal kidney morphometry during gestation and the relationship between weight, kidney morphometry and plasma active renin concentration at birth. *Clin Sci (Lond)* (1996) 91(2):169–75. doi:10.1042/cs0910169
10. Seely JC. A brief review of kidney development, maturation, developmental abnormalities, and drug toxicity: juvenile animal relevancy. *J Toxicol Pathol* (2017) 30(2):125–33. doi:10.1293/tox.2017-0006
11. Rodríguez MM, Gómez AH, Abitbol CL, Chandar JJ, Duara S, Zilleruelo GE. Histomorphometric analysis of postnatal glomerulogenesis in extremely preterm infants. *Pediatr Dev Pathol* (2004) 7(1):17–25. doi:10.1007/s10024-003-3029-2
12. Sutherland MR, Gubhaju L, Moore L, Kent AL, Dahlstrom JE, Horne RS, et al. Accelerated maturation and abnormal morphology in the preterm neonatal kidney. *J Am Soc Nephrol* (2011) 22(7):1365–74. doi:10.1681/ASN.2010121266
13. Aperia A, Broberger O, Herin P, Thodenius K, Zetterström R. Postnatal control of water and electrolyte homeostasis in pre-term and full-term infants. *Acta Paediatr Scand Suppl* (1983) 305:61–5. doi:10.1111/j.1651-2227.1983.tb09861.x

14. Giniger RP, Buffat C, Millet V, Simeoni U. Renal effects of ibuprofen for the treatment of patent ductus arteriosus in premature infants. *J Matern Fetal Neonatal Med* (2007) 20(4):275–83. doi:10.1080/14767050701227950
15. Rhone ET, Carmody JB, Swanson JR, Charlton JR. Nephrotoxic medication exposure in very low birth weight infants. *J Matern Fetal Neonatal Med* (2014) 27(14):1485–90. doi:10.3109/14767058.2013.860522
16. Girardi A, Raschi E, Galletti S, Poluzzi E, Faldella G, Allegaert K, et al. Drug-induced renal damage in preterm neonates: state of the art and methods for early detection. *Drug Saf* (2015) 38(6):535–51. doi:10.1007/s40264-015-0288-6
17. Lopez AD, Mathers CD, Ezzati M, Jamison DT, Murray CJ. Global and regional burden of disease and risk factors, 2001: systematic analysis of population health data. *Lancet* (2006) 367(9524):1747–57. doi:10.1016/S0140-6736(06)68770-9
18. Wingen AM, Fabian-Bach C, Schaefer F, Mehls O. Randomised multicentre study of a low-protein diet on the progression of chronic renal failure in children. European Study Group of Nutritional Treatment of Chronic Renal Failure in Childhood. *Lancet* (1997) 349(9059):1117–23. doi:10.1016/S0140-6736(96)09260-4
19. Klag MJ, Whelton PK, Randall BL, Neaton JD, Brancati FL, Ford CE, et al. Blood pressure and end-stage renal disease in men. *N Engl J Med* (1996) 334(1):13–8. doi:10.1056/NEJM199601043340103
20. Vanholder R, Massy Z, Argiles A, Spasovski G, Verbeke F, Lameire N, et al. Chronic kidney disease as cause of cardiovascular morbidity and mortality. *Nephrol Dial Transplant* (2005) 20(6):1048–56. doi:10.1093/ndt/gfh813
21. Schmieder RE. End organ damage in hypertension. *Dtsch Arztebl Int* (2010) 107(49):866–73. doi:10.3238/arztebl.2010.0866
22. Chen X, Wang Y. Tracking of blood pressure from childhood to adulthood: a systematic review and meta-regression analysis. *Circulation* (2008) 117(25):3171–80. doi:10.1161/CIRCULATIONAHA.107.730366
23. Bao W, Threefoot SA, Srinivasan SR, Berenson GS. Essential hypertension predicted by tracking of elevated blood pressure from childhood to adulthood: the Bogalusa Heart Study. *Am J Hypertens* (1995) 8(7):657–65. doi:10.1016/0895-7061(95)97901-3
24. Dekkers JC, Snieder H, Van Den Oord EJ, Treiber FA. Moderators of blood pressure development from childhood to adulthood: a 10-year longitudinal study. *J Pediatr* (2002) 141(6):770–9. doi:10.1067/mpd.2002.128113
25. Erlingsdottir A, Indridason OS, Thorvaldsson O, Edvardsson VO. Blood pressure in children and target-organ damage later in life. *Pediatr Nephrol* (2010) 25(2):323–8. doi:10.1007/s00467-009-1350-3
26. Edvardsson VO, Steinthorsdottir SD, Eliasdottir SB, Indridason OS, Palsson R. Birth weight and childhood blood pressure. *Curr Hypertens Rep* (2012) 14(6):596–602. doi:10.1007/s11906-012-0311-6
27. Lackland DT, Bendall HE, Osmond C, Egan BM, Barker DJ. Low birth weights contribute to high rates of early-onset chronic renal failure in the Southeastern United States. *Arch Intern Med* (2000) 160(10):1472–6. doi:10.1001/archinte.160.10.1472
28. Luyckx VA, Brenner BM. Birth weight, malnutrition and kidney-associated outcomes – a global concern. *Nat Rev Nephrol* (2015) 11(3):135–49. doi:10.1038/nrneph.2014.251
29. Vikse BE, Irgens LM, Leivestad T, Hallan S, Iversen BM. Low birth weight increases risk for end-stage renal disease. *J Am Soc Nephrol* (2008) 19(1):151–7. doi:10.1681/ASN.2007020252
30. Hallan S, Euser AM, Irgens LM, Finken MJ, Holmen J, Dekker FW. Effect of intrauterine growth restriction on kidney function at young adult age: the Nord Trondelag Health (HUNT 2) study. *Am J Kidney Dis* (2008) 51(1):10–20. doi:10.1053/j.ajkd.2007.09.013
31. Low Birth Weight and Nephron Number Working Group. The impact of kidney development on the life course: a consensus document for action. *Nephron* (2017) 136(1):3–49. doi:10.1159/000457967
32. Primatesta P, Falaschetti E, Poulter NR. Birth weight and blood pressure in childhood: results from the Health Survey for England. *Hypertension* (2005) 45(1):75–9. doi:10.1161/01.HYP.0000150037.98835.10
33. Barker DJ, Osmond C. Low birth weight and hypertension. *BMJ* (1988) 297(6641):134–5. doi:10.1136/bmj.297.6641.134-b
34. Spence D, Stewart MC, Alderdice FA, Patterson CC, Halliday HL. Intrauterine growth restriction and increased risk of hypertension in adult life: a follow-up study of 50-year-olds. *Public Health* (2012) 126(7):561–5. doi:10.1016/j.puhe.2012.03.010
35. Eriksson JG, Forsén TJ, Kajantie E, Osmond C, Barker DJ. Childhood growth and hypertension in later life. *Hypertension* (2007) 49(6):1415–21. doi:10.1161/HYPERTENSIONAHA.106.085597
36. Perng W, Gillman MW, Mantzoros CS, Oken E. A prospective study of maternal prenatal weight and offspring cardiometabolic health in midchildhood. *Ann Epidemiol* (2014) 24(11):793–800.e1. doi:10.1016/j.annepidem.2014.08.002
37. Hrolfsdottir L, Halldorsson TI, Rytter D, Bech BH, Birgisdottir BE, Gunnarsdottir I, et al. Maternal macronutrient intake and offspring blood pressure 20 years later. *J Am Heart Assoc* (2017) 6(4):e005808. doi:10.1161/JAHA.117.005808
38. Campbell DM, Hall MH, Barker DJ, Cross J, Shiell AW, Godfrey KM. Diet in pregnancy and the offspring's blood pressure 40 years later. *Br J Obstet Gynaecol* (1996) 103(3):273–80. doi:10.1111/j.1471-0528.1996.tb09718.x
39. Ben-Shlomo Y, McCarthy A, Hughes R, Tilling K, Davies D, Smith GD. Immediate postnatal growth is associated with blood pressure in young adulthood: the Barry Caerphilly Growth study. *Hypertension* (2008) 52(4):638–44. doi:10.1161/HYPERTENSIONAHA.108.114256
40. Filler G, Yasin A, Kesarwani P, Garg AX, Lindsay R, Sharma AP. Big mother or small baby: which predicts hypertension? *J Clin Hypertens (Greenwich)* (2011) 13(1):35–41. doi:10.1111/j.1751-7176.2010.00366.x
41. Bowers K, Liu G, Wang P, Ye T, Tian Z, Liu E, et al. Birth weight, postnatal weight change, and risk for high blood pressure among Chinese children. *Pediatrics* (2011) 127(5):e1272–9. doi:10.1542/peds.2010-2213
42. Painter RC, Roseboom TJ, van Montfrans GA, Bossuyt PM, Krediet RT, Osmond C, et al. Microalbuminuria in adults after prenatal exposure to the Dutch famine. *J Am Soc Nephrol* (2005) 16(1):189–94. doi:10.1681/ASN.2004060474
43. Huang C, Guo C, Nichols C, Chen S, Martorell R. Elevated levels of protein in urine in adulthood after exposure to the Chinese famine of 1959–61 during gestation and the early postnatal period. *Int J Epidemiol* (2014) 43(6):1806–14. doi:10.1093/ije/dyu193
44. White SL, Perkovic V, Cass A, Chang CL, Poulter NR, Spector T, et al. Is low birth weight an antecedent of CKD in later life? A systematic review of observational studies. *Am J Kidney Dis* (2009) 54(2):248–61. doi:10.1053/j.ajkd.2008.12.042
45. Ruggajo P, Skrunes R, Svarstad E, Skjærven R, Reisæther AV, Vikse BE. Familial factors, low birth weight, and development of ESRD: a nationwide registry study. *Am J Kidney Dis* (2016) 67(4):601–8. doi:10.1053/j.ajkd.2015.11.015
46. López-Bermejo A, Sitjar C, Cabacas A, Vázquez-Ruíz M, García-González MM, Mora C, et al. Prenatal programming of renal function: the estimated glomerular filtration rate is influenced by size at birth in apparently healthy children. *Pediatr Res* (2008) 64(1):97–9. doi:10.1203/PDR.0b013e31817282db
47. Franco MC, Nishida SK, Sesso R. GFR estimated from cystatin C versus creatinine in children born small for gestational age. *Am J Kidney Dis* (2008) 51(6):925–32. doi:10.1053/j.ajkd.2008.02.305
48. Sheu JN, Chen JH. Minimal change nephrotic syndrome in children with intrauterine growth retardation. *Am J Kidney Dis* (2001) 37(5):909–14. doi:10.1016/S0272-6386(05)80005-8
49. Zidar N, Avgustin Cavić M, Kenda RB, Ferluga D. Unfavorable course of minimal change nephrotic syndrome in children with intrauterine growth retardation. *Kidney Int* (1998) 54(4):1320–3. doi:10.1046/j.1523-1755.1998.00121.x
50. Zidar N, Cavić MA, Kenda RB, Koselj M, Ferluga D. Effect of intrauterine growth retardation on the clinical course and prognosis of IgA glomerulonephritis in children. *Nephron* (1998) 79(1):28–32. doi:10.1159/000044987
51. Bertram JF, Douglas-Denton RN, Diouf B, Hughson MD, Hoy WE. Human nephron number: implications for health and disease. *Pediatr Nephrol* (2011) 26(9):1529–33. doi:10.1007/s00467-011-1843-8
52. Brenner BM, Lawler EV, Mackenzie HS. The hyperfiltration theory: a paradigm shift in nephrology. *Kidney Int* (1996) 49(6):1774–7. doi:10.1038/ki.1996.265
53. Hughson M, Farris AB III, Douglas-Denton R, Hoy WE, Bertram JF. Glomerular number and size in autopsy kidneys: the relationship to birth weight. *Kidney Int* (2003) 63(6):2113–22. doi:10.1046/j.1523-1755.2003.00018.x
54. Hinchliffe SA, Lynch MR, Sargent PH, Howard CV, Van Velzen D. The effect of intrauterine growth retardation on the development of renal nephrons. *Br J Obstet Gynaecol* (1992) 99(4):296–301. doi:10.1111/j.1471-0528.1992.tb13726.x

55. Langley-Evans SC, Welham SJ, Jackson AA. Fetal exposure to a maternal low protein diet impairs nephrogenesis and promotes hypertension in the rat. *Life Sci* (1999) 64(11):965–74. doi:10.1016/S0024-3205(99)00022-3
56. Jones SE, Bilous RW, Flyvbjerg A, Marshall SM. Intra-uterine environment influences glomerular number and the acute renal adaptation to experimental diabetes. *Diabetologia* (2001) 44(6):721–8. doi:10.1007/s001250051681
57. Woods LL, Weeks DA, Rasch R. Programming of adult blood pressure by maternal protein restriction: role of nephrogenesis. *Kidney Int* (2004) 65(4):1339–48. doi:10.1111/j.1523-1755.2004.00511.x
58. Sampogna RV, Schneider L, Al-Awqati Q. Developmental programming of branching morphogenesis in the kidney. *J Am Soc Nephrol* (2015) 26(10):2414–22. doi:10.1681/ASN.2014090886
59. Vehaskari VM, Aviles DH, Manning J. Prenatal programming of adult hypertension in the rat. *Kidney Int* (2001) 59(1):238–45. doi:10.1046/j.1523-1755.2001.00484.x
60. Merlet-Bénichou C, Gilbert T, Muffat-Joly M, Lelièvre-Pégorier M, Leroy B. Intrauterine growth retardation leads to a permanent nephron deficit in the rat. *Pediatr Nephrol* (1994) 8(2):175–80. doi:10.1007/BF00865473
61. Schreuder MF, Nyengaard JR, Fodor M, van Wijk JA, Delemarre-van de Waal HA. Glomerular number and function are influenced by spontaneous and induced low birth weight in rats. *J Am Soc Nephrol* (2005) 16(10):2913–9. doi:10.1681/ASN.2004100875
62. Sanders MW, Fazzi GE, Janssen GM, de Leeuw PW, Blanco CE, De Mey JG. Reduced uteroplacental blood flow alters renal arterial reactivity and glomerular properties in the rat offspring. *Hypertension* (2004) 43(6):1283–9. doi:10.1161/01.HYP.0000127787.85259.1f
63. Dickinson H, Walker DW, Wintour EM, Moritz K. Maternal dexamethasone treatment at midgestation reduces nephron number and alters renal gene expression in the fetal spiny mouse. *Am J Physiol Regul Integr Comp Physiol* (2007) 292(1):R453–61. doi:10.1152/ajpregu.00481.2006
64. Stelloh C, Allen KP, Mattson DL, Lerch-Gaggl A, Reddy S, El-Meanawy A. Prematurity in mice leads to reduction in nephron number, hypertension, and proteinuria. *Transl Res* (2012) 159(2):80–9. doi:10.1016/j.trsl.2011.10.004
65. Yzydorczyk C, Comte B, Cambonie G, Lavoie JC, Germain N, Ting Shun Y, et al. Neonatal oxygen exposure in rats leads to cardiovascular and renal alterations in adulthood. *Hypertension* (2008) 52(5):889–95. doi:10.1161/HYPERTENSIONAHA.108.116251
66. Lelièvre-Pégorier M, Vilar J, Ferrier ML, Moreau E, Freund N, Gilbert T, et al. Mild vitamin A deficiency leads to inborn nephron deficit in the rat. *Kidney Int* (1998) 54(5):1455–62. doi:10.1046/j.1523-1755.1998.00151.x
67. Tomat AL, Inserra F, Veiras L, Vallone MC, Balaszczuk AM, Costa MA, et al. Moderate zinc restriction during fetal and postnatal growth of rats: effects on adult arterial blood pressure and kidney. *Am J Physiol Regul Integr Comp Physiol* (2008) 295(2):R543–9. doi:10.1152/ajpregu.00050.2008
68. Lisle SJ, Lewis RM, Petry CJ, Ozanne SE, Hales CN, Forhead AJ. Effect of maternal iron restriction during pregnancy on renal morphology in the adult rat offspring. *Br J Nutr* (2003) 90(1):33–9. doi:10.1079/BJN2003881
69. Tan JC, Workeneh B, Busque S, Blouch K, Derby G, Myers BD. Glomerular function, structure, and number in renal allografts from older deceased donors. *J Am Soc Nephrol* (2009) 20(1):181–8. doi:10.1681/ASN.2008030306
70. Mühle A, Mühle C, Amann K, Dötsch J, Nüsken KD, Boltze J, et al. No juvenile arterial hypertension in sheep multiples despite reduced nephron numbers. *Pediatr Nephrol* (2010) 25(9):1653–61. doi:10.1007/s00467-010-1512-3
71. Boubred F, Daniel L, Buffat C, Feuerstein JM, Tsimaratos M, Oliver C, et al. Early postnatal overfeeding induces early chronic renal dysfunction in adult male rats. *Am J Physiol Renal Physiol* (2009) 297(4):F943–51. doi:10.1152/ajprenal.90704.2008
72. Boubred F, Daniel L, Buffat C, Tsimaratos M, Oliver C, Lelièvre-Pégorier M, et al. The magnitude of nephron number reduction mediates intrauterine growth-restriction-induced long term chronic renal disease in the rat. A comparative study in two experimental models. *J Transl Med* (2016) 14(1):331. doi:10.1186/s12967-016-1086-3
73. Guron G, Friberg P. An intact renin-angiotensin system is a prerequisite for normal renal development. *J Hypertens* (2000) 18(2):123–37. doi:10.1097/00004872-200018020-00001
74. Terada T, Urushihara M, Saijo T, Nakagawa R, Kagami S. (Pro)renin and (pro)renin receptor expression during kidney development in neonates. *Eur J Pediatr* (2017) 176(2):183–9. doi:10.1007/s00431-016-2820-9
75. Woods LL, Ingelfinger JR, Nyengaard JR, Rasch R. Maternal protein restriction suppresses the newborn renin-angiotensin system and programs adult hypertension in rats. *Pediatr Res* (2001) 49(4):460–7. doi:10.1203/00006450-200104000-00005
76. Alwasel SH, Kaleem I, Sahajpal V, Ashton N. Maternal protein restriction reduces angiotensin II AT(1) and AT(2) receptor expression in the fetal rat kidney. *Kidney Blood Press Res* (2010) 33(4):251–9. doi:10.1159/000317739
77. Ao Y, Sun Z, Hu S, Zuo N, Li B, Yang S, et al. Low functional programming of renal AT2R mediates the developmental origin of glomerulosclerosis in adult offspring induced by prenatal caffeine exposure. *Toxicol Appl Pharmacol* (2015) 287(2):128–38. doi:10.1016/j.taap.2015.05.007
78. Mao C, Liu R, Bo L, Chen N, Li S, Xia S, et al. High-salt diets during pregnancy affected fetal and offspring renal renin-angiotensin system. *J Endocrinol* (2013) 218(1):61–73. doi:10.1530/JOE-13-0139
79. Luzardo R, Silva PA, Einicker-Lamas M, Ortiz-Costa S, do Carmo Mda G, Vieira-Filho LD, et al. Metabolic programming during lactation stimulates renal Na+ transport in the adult offspring due to an early impact on local angiotensin II pathways. *PLoS One* (2011) 6(7):e21232. doi:10.1371/journal.pone.0021232
80. Sahajpal V, Ashton N. Renal function and angiotensin AT1 receptor expression in young rats following intrauterine exposure to a maternal low-protein diet. *Clin Sci (Lond)* (2003) 104(6):607–14. doi:10.1042/CS20020355
81. Langley-Evans SC, Jackson AA. Captopril normalises systolic blood pressure in rats with hypertension induced by fetal exposure to maternal low protein diets. *Comp Biochem Physiol A Physiol* (1995) 110(3):223–8. doi:10.1016/0300-9629(94)00177-U
82. Vieira-Filho LD, Cabral EV, Farias JS, Silva PA, Muzi-Filho H, Vieyra A, et al. Renal molecular mechanisms underlying altered Na+ handling and genesis of hypertension during adulthood in prenatally undernourished rats. *Br J Nutr* (2014) 111(11):1932–44. doi:10.1017/S0007114513004236
83. Chen YW, Chenier I, Tran S, Scotcher M, Chang SY, Zhang SL. Maternal diabetes programs hypertension and kidney injury in offspring. *Pediatr Nephrol* (2010) 25(7):1319–29. doi:10.1007/s00467-010-1506-1
84. Martinez-Aguayo A, Aglony M, Bancalari R, Avalos C, Bolte L, Garcia H, et al. Birth weight is inversely associated with blood pressure and serum aldosterone and cortisol levels in children. *Clin Endocrinol (Oxf)* (2012) 76(5):713–8. doi:10.1111/j.1365-2265.2011.04308.x
85. Li C, Lin Y, Luo R, Chen S, Wang F, Zheng P, et al. Intrarenal renin-angiotensin system mediates fatty acid-induced ER stress in the kidney. *Am J Physiol Renal Physiol* (2016) 310(5):F351–63. doi:10.1152/ajprenal.00223.2015
86. Dagan A, Kwon HM, Dwarakanath V, Baum M. Effect of renal denervation on prenatal programming of hypertension and renal tubular transporter abundance. *Am J Physiol Renal Physiol* (2008) 295(1):F29–34. doi:10.1152/ajprenal.00123.2008
87. Manning J, Beutler K, Knepper MA, Vehaskari VM. Upregulation of renal BSC1 and TSC in prenatally programmed hypertension. *Am J Physiol Renal Physiol* (2002) 283(1):F202–6. doi:10.1152/ajprenal.00358.2001
88. DuBois BN, Pearson J, Mahmood T, Nguyen D, Thornburg K, Cherala G. Perinatal growth restriction decreases diuretic action of furosemide in adult rats. *Eur J Pharmacol* (2014) 728:39–47. doi:10.1016/j.ejphar.2014.01.056
89. Dagan A, Gattineni J, Cook V, Baum M. Prenatal programming of rat proximal tubule Na+/H+ exchanger by dexamethasone. *Am J Physiol Regul Integr Comp Physiol* (2007) 292(3):R1230–5. doi:10.1152/ajpregu.00669.2006
90. Su Y, Bi J, Pulgar VM, Figueroa J, Chappell M, Rose JC. Antenatal glucocorticoid treatment alters Na+ uptake in renal proximal tubule cells from adult offspring in a sex-specific manner. *Am J Physiol Renal Physiol* (2015) 308(11):F1268–75. doi:10.1152/ajprenal.00047.2015
91. Sanders MW, Fazzi GE, Janssen GM, Blanco CE, De Mey JG. High sodium intake increases blood pressure and alters renal function in intrauterine growth-retarded rats. *Hypertension* (2005) 46(1):71–5. doi:10.1161/01.HYP.0000171475.40259.d1
92. Nehiri T, Duong Van Huyen JP, Viltard M, Fassot C, Heudes D, Freund N, et al. Exposure to maternal diabetes induces salt-sensitive hypertension and impairs renal function in adult rat offspring. *Diabetes* (2008) 57(8):2167–75. doi:10.2337/db07-0780
93. Reho JJ, Zheng X, Benjamin JE, Fisher SA. Neural programming of mesenteric and renal arteries. *Am J Physiol Heart Circ Physiol* (2014) 307(4):H563–73. doi:10.1152/ajpheart.00250.2014

94. Cambonie G, Comte B, Yzydorczyk C, Ntimbane T, Germain N, Lê NL, et al. Antenatal antioxidant prevents adult hypertension, vascular dysfunction, and microvascular rarefaction associated with in utero exposure to a low-protein diet. *Am J Physiol Regul Integr Comp Physiol* (2007) 292(3):R1236–45. doi:10.1152/ajpregu.00227.2006

95. Yzydorczyk C, Armengaud JB, Peyter AC, Chehade H, Cachat F, Juvet C, et al. Endothelial dysfunction in individuals born after fetal growth restriction: cardiovascular and renal consequences and preventive approaches. *J Dev Orig Health Dis* (2017) 8(4):448–64. doi:10.1017/S2040174417000265

96. Burke M, Pabbidi MR, Farley J, Roman RJ. Molecular mechanisms of renal blood flow autoregulation. *Curr Vasc Pharmacol* (2014) 12(6):845–58. doi:10.2174/15701611113116660149

97. Bauer R, Walter B, Brust P, Füchtner F, Zwiener U. Impact of asymmetric intrauterine growth restriction on organ function in newborn piglets. *Eur J Obstet Gynecol Reprod Biol* (2003) 110(Suppl 1):S40–9. doi:10.1016/S0301-2115(03)00171-4

98. Brown RD, Turner AJ, Carlström M, Persson AE, Gibson KJ. Tubuloglomerular feedback response in the prenatal and postnatal ovine kidney. *Am J Physiol Renal Physiol* (2011) 300(6):F1368–74. doi:10.1152/ajprenal.00019.2011

99. Rumballe B, Georgas K, Wilkinson L, Little M. Molecular anatomy of the kidney: what have we learned from gene expression and functional genomics? *Pediatr Nephrol* (2010) 25(6):1005–16. doi:10.1007/s00467-009-1392-6

100. Kuure S, Vuolteenaho R, Vainio S. Kidney morphogenesis: cellular and molecular regulation. *Mech Dev* (2000) 92(1):31–45. doi:10.1016/S0925-4773(99)00323-8

101. Dressler GR, Patel SR. Epigenetics in kidney development and renal disease. *Transl Res* (2015) 165(1):166–76. doi:10.1016/j.trsl.2014.04.007

102. Reddy MA, Natarajan R. Recent developments in epigenetics of acute and chronic kidney diseases. *Kidney Int* (2015) 88(2):250–61. doi:10.1038/ki.2015.148

103. Soofi A, Levitan I, Dressler GR. Two novel EGFP insertion alleles reveal unique aspects of Pax2 function in embryonic and adult kidneys. *Dev Biol* (2012) 365(1):241–50. doi:10.1016/j.ydbio.2012.02.032

104. Imgrund M, Gröne E, Gröne HJ, Kretzler M, Holzman L, Schlöndorff D, et al. Re-expression of the developmental gene Pax-2 during experimental acute tubular necrosis in mice 1. *Kidney Int* (1999) 56(4):1423–31. doi:10.1046/j.1523-1755.1999.00663.x

105. Sinclair KD, Allegrucci C, Singh R, Gardner DS, Sebastian S, Bispham J, et al. DNA methylation, insulin resistance, and blood pressure in offspring determined by maternal periconceptional B vitamin and methionine status. *Proc Natl Acad Sci U S A* (2007) 104(49):19351–6. doi:10.1073/pnas.0707258104

106. Guzik TJ, Touyz RM. Oxidative stress, inflammation, and vascular aging in hypertension. *Hypertension* (2017) 70(4):660–7. doi:10.1161/HYPERTENSIONAHA.117.07802

107. Costa MR, Pires KM, Nalbones-Barbosa MN, Dos Santos Valença S, Resende ÂC, de Moura RS. Grape skin extract-derived polyphenols modify programming-induced renal endowment in prenatal protein-restricted male mouse offspring. *Eur J Nutr* (2016) 55(4):1455–64. doi:10.1007/s00394-015-0963-5

108. Stangenberg S, Nguyen LT, Chen H, Al-Odat I, Killingsworth MC, Gosnell ME, et al. Oxidative stress, mitochondrial perturbations and fetal programming of renal disease induced by maternal smoking. *Int J Biochem Cell Biol* (2015) 64:81–90. doi:10.1016/j.biocel.2015.03.017

109. Rodríguez-Rodríguez P, de Pablo AL, Condezo-Hoyos L, Martín-Cabrejas MA, Aguilera Y, Ruiz-Hurtado G, et al. Fetal undernutrition is associated with perinatal sex-dependent alterations in oxidative status. *J Nutr Biochem* (2015) 26(12):1650–9. doi:10.1016/j.jnutbio.2015.08.004

110. Tain YL, Lin YJ, Sheen JM, Yu HR, Tiao MM, Chen CC, et al. High fat diets sex-specifically affect the renal transcriptome and program obesity, kidney injury, and hypertension in the offspring. *Nutrients* (2017) 9(4):E357. doi:10.3390/nu9040357

111. Yim HE, Yoo KH. Early life obesity and chronic kidney disease in later life. *Pediatr Nephrol* (2015) 30(8):1255–63. doi:10.1007/s00467-014-2922-4

112. Wang Y, Chen X, Klag MJ, Caballero B. Epidemic of childhood obesity: implications for kidney disease. *Adv Chronic Kidney Dis* (2006) 13(4):336–51. doi:10.1053/j.ackd.2006.07.016

113. Manrique C, Lastra G, Gardner M, Sowers JR. The renin angiotensin aldosterone system in hypertension: roles of insulin resistance and oxidative stress. *Med Clin North Am* (2009) 93(3):569–82. doi:10.1016/j.mcna.2009.02.014

114. Ramalingam L, Menikdiwela K, LeMieux M, Dufour JM, Kaur G, Kalupahana N, et al. The renin angiotensin system, oxidative stress and mitochondrial function in obesity and insulin resistance. *Biochim Biophys Acta* (2017) 1863(5):1106–14. doi:10.1016/j.bbadis.2016.07.019

115. Alcazar MA, Boehler E, Rother E, Amann K, Vohlen C, von Hörsten S, et al. Early postnatal hyperalimentation impairs renal function via SOCS-3 mediated renal postreceptor leptin resistance. *Endocrinology* (2012) 153(3):1397–410. doi:10.1210/en.2011-1670

116. Kasper P, Vohlen C, Dinger K, Mohr J, Hucklenbruch-Rother E, Janoschek R, et al. Renal metabolic programming is linked to the dynamic regulation of a Leptin-Klf15 axis and Akt/AMPKalpha signaling in male offspring of obese dams. *Endocrinology* (2017) 158(10):3399–415. doi:10.1210/en.2017-00489

117. Ostreicher I, Almeida JR, Campean V, Rauh M, Plank C, Amann K, et al. Changes in 11beta-hydroxysteroid dehydrogenase type 2 expression in a low-protein rat model of intrauterine growth restriction. *Nephrol Dial Transplant* (2010) 25(10):3195–203. doi:10.1093/ndt/gfq354

118. Bertram C, Trowern AR, Copin N, Jackson AA, Whorwood CB. The maternal diet during pregnancy programs altered expression of the glucocorticoid receptor and type 2 11beta-hydroxysteroid dehydrogenase: potential molecular mechanisms underlying the programming of hypertension in utero. *Endocrinology* (2001) 142(7):2841–53. doi:10.1210/endo.142.7.8238

119. Whorwood CB, Firth KM, Budge H, Symonds ME. Maternal undernutrition during early to midgestation programs tissue-specific alterations in the expression of the glucocorticoid receptor, 11beta-hydroxysteroid dehydrogenase isoforms, and type 1 angiotensin ii receptor in neonatal sheep. *Endocrinology* (2001) 142(7):2854–64. doi:10.1210/endo.142.7.8264

120. Sheen JM, Yu HR, Tiao MM, Chen CC, Huang LT, Chang HY, et al. Prenatal dexamethasone-induced programmed hypertension and renal programming. *Life Sci* (2015) 132:41–8. doi:10.1016/j.lfs.2015.04.005

121. Tain YL, Wu KL, Lee WC, Leu S, Chan JY. Maternal fructose-intake-induced renal programming in adult male offspring. *J Nutr Biochem* (2015) 26(6):642–50. doi:10.1016/j.jnutbio.2014.12.017

122. Imig JD, Zou AP, Stec DE, Harder DR, Falck JR, Roman RJ. Formation and actions of 20-hydroxyeicosatetraenoic acid in rat renal arterioles. *Am J Physiol* (1996) 270(1 Pt 2):R217–27.

123. Cheng J, Ou JS, Singh H, Falck JR, Narsimhaswamy D, Pritchard KA Jr, et al. 20-hydroxyeicosatetraenoic acid causes endothelial dysfunction via eNOS uncoupling. *Am J Physiol Heart Circ Physiol* (2008) 294(2):H1018–26. doi:10.1152/ajpheart.01172.2007

124. Ichihara A, Imig JD, Inscho EW, Navar LG. Cyclooxygenase-2 participates in tubular flow-dependent afferent arteriolar tone: interaction with neuronal NOS. *Am J Physiol* (1998) 275(4 Pt 2):F605–12.

125. Vaziri ND, Bai Y, Ni Z, Quiroz Y, Pandian R, Rodriguez-Iturbe B. Intra-renal angiotensin II/AT1 receptor, oxidative stress, inflammation, and progressive injury in renal mass reduction. *J Pharmacol Exp Ther* (2007) 323(1):85–93. doi:10.1124/jpet.107.123638

126. Owen CG, Whincup PH, Gilg JA, Cook DG. Effect of breast feeding in infancy on blood pressure in later life: systematic review and meta-analysis. *BMJ* (2003) 327(7425):1189–95. doi:10.1136/bmj.327.7425.1189

127. Vaidya A, Saville N, Shrestha BP, Costello AM, Manandhar DS, Osrin D. Effects of antenatal multiple micronutrient supplementation on children's weight and size at 2 years of age in Nepal: follow-up of a double-blind randomised controlled trial. *Lancet* (2008) 371(9611):492–9. doi:10.1016/S0140-6736(08)60172-5

128. Belizán JM, Villar J, Bergel E, del Pino A, Di Fulvio S, Galliano SV, et al. Long-term effect of calcium supplementation during pregnancy on the blood pressure of offspring: follow up of a randomised controlled trial. *BMJ* (1997) 315(7103):281–5. doi:10.1136/bmj.315.7103.281

129. Lee LM, Leung CY, Tang WW, Choi HL, Leung YC, McCaffery PJ, et al. A paradoxical teratogenic mechanism for retinoic acid. *Proc Natl Acad Sci U S A* (2012) 109(34):13668–73. doi:10.1073/pnas.1200872109

130. Makrakis J, Zimanyi MA, Black MJ. Retinoic acid enhances nephron endowment in rats exposed to maternal protein restriction. *Pediatr Nephrol* (2007) 22(11):1861–7. doi:10.1007/s00467-007-0572-5

131. Hawkesworth S, Wagatsuma Y, Kahn AI, Hawlader MD, Fulford AJ, Arifeen SE, et al. Combined food and micronutrient supplements during pregnancy have limited impact on child blood pressure and kidney function in rural Bangladesh. *J Nutr* (2013) 143(5):728–34. doi:10.3945/jn.112.168518

132. Forsyth JS, Willatts P, Agostoni C, Bissenden J, Casaer P, Boehm G. Long chain polyunsaturated fatty acid supplementation in infant formula and blood pressure in later childhood: follow up of a randomised controlled trial. *BMJ* (2003) 326(7396):953. doi:10.1136/bmj.326.7396.953
133. Stewart CP, Christian P, Schulze KJ, Leclerq SC, West KP Jr, Khatry SK. Antenatal micronutrient supplementation reduces metabolic syndrome in 6- to 8-year-old children in rural Nepal. *J Nutr* (2009) 139(8):1575–81. doi:10.3945/jn.109.106666
134. Sutherland MR, Gubhaju L, Yoder BA, Stahlman MT, Black MJ. The effects of postnatal retinoic acid administration on nephron endowment in the preterm baboon kidney. *Pediatr Res* (2009) 65(4):397–402. doi:10.1203/PDR.0b013e3181975f52
135. Jayasooriya AP, Begg DP, Chen N, Mathai ML, Sinclair AJ, Wilkinson-Berka J, et al. Omega-3 polyunsaturated fatty acid supplementation reduces hypertension in TGR(mRen-2)27 rats. *Prostaglandins Leukot Essent Fatty Acids* (2008) 78(1):67–72. doi:10.1016/j.plefa.2007.11.001
136. Jackson AA, Dunn RL, Marchand MC, Langley-Evans SC. Increased systolic blood pressure in rats induced by a maternal low-protein diet is reversed by dietary supplementation with glycine. *Clin Sci (Lond)* (2002) 103(6):633–9. doi:10.1042/cs1030633
137. Lim SS, Vos T, Flaxman AD, Danaei G, Shibuya K, Adair-Rohani H, et al. A comparative risk assessment of burden of disease and injury attributable to 67 risk factors and risk factor clusters in 21 regions, 1990–2010: a systematic analysis for the Global Burden of Disease study 2010. *Lancet* (2012) 380(9859):2224–60. doi:10.1016/S0140-6736(12)61766-8
138. Blencowe H, Cousens S, Oestergaard MZ, Chou D, Moller AB, Narwal R, et al. National, regional, and worldwide estimates of preterm birth rates in the year 2010 with time trends since 1990 for selected countries: a systematic analysis and implications. *Lancet* (2012) 379(9832):2162–72. doi:10.1016/S0140-6736(12)60820-4
139. Romo A, Carceller R, Tobajas J. Intrauterine growth retardation (IUGR): epidemiology and etiology. *Pediatr Endocrinol Rev* (2009) 6(Suppl 3):332–6.
140. NCD Risk Factor Collaboration (NCD-RisC). Worldwide trends in body-mass index, underweight, overweight, and obesity from 1975 to 2016: a pooled analysis of 2416 population-based measurement studies in 128.9 million children, adolescents, and adults. *Lancet* (2017) 390(10113):2627–42. doi:10.1016/S0140-6736(17)32129-3

23

Heterozygous *COL4A3* Variants in Histologically Diagnosed Focal Segmental Glomerulosclerosis

*Matthias C. Braunisch[1,2], Maike Büttner-Herold[3], Roman Günthner[1,2], Robin Satanovskij[1,2], Korbinian M. Riedhammer[1,2], Pierre-Maurice Herr[2], Hanns-Georg Klein[4], Dagmar Wahl[4], Claudius Küchle[1], Lutz Renders[1], Uwe Heemann[1], Christoph Schmaderer[1] and Julia Hoefele[2]**

[1] Department of Nephrology, Klinikum Rechts der Isar, Technical University of Munich, Munich, Germany, [2] Institute of Human Genetics, Klinikum Rechts der Isar, Technical University of Munich, Munich, Germany, [3] Department of Nephropathology, Institute of Pathology, Friedrich-Alexander-University, Erlangen, Germany, [4] Center for Human Genetics and Laboratory Diagnostics Dr. Klein, Dr. Rost and Colleagues, Martinsried, Germany

***Correspondence:**
Julia Hoefele
julia.hoefele@tum.de

Introduction: Steroid-resistant nephrotic syndrome (SRNS) is one of the most frequent causes for chronic kidney disease in childhood. In ~30% of these cases a genetic cause can be identified. The histological finding in SRNS is often focal segmental glomerulosclerosis (FSGS). In rare cases, however, pathogenic variants in genes associated with Alport syndrome can be identified in patients with the histological finding of FSGS.

Materials and Methods: Clinical information was collected out of clinical reports and medical history. Focused molecular genetic analysis included sequencing of *COL4A5* and *COL4A3* in the index patient. Segregation analysis of identified variants was performed in the parents and children of the index patient.

Results: The female index patient developed mild proteinuria and microscopic hematuria in childhood (12 years of age). The histological examination of the kidney biopsies performed at the age of 21, 28, and 32 years showed findings partly compatible with FSGS. However, immunosuppressive treatment of the index patient did not lead to a sufficient reduction of in part nephrotic-range proteinuria. After the patient developed hearing impairment at the age of 34 years and her daughter was diagnosed with microscopic hematuria at the age of 6 years, re-examination of the index's kidney biopsies by electron microscopy revealed textural changes of glomerular basement membrane compatible with Alport syndrome. Molecular genetic analysis identified two missense variants in *COL4A3* in a compound heterozygous state with maternal and paternal inheritance. One of them is a novel variant that was also found in the 6 year old daughter of the index patient who presented with microscopic hematuria.

Discussion: We were able to show that a novel variant combined with a previously described variant in compound heterozygous state resulted in a phenotype that was histologically associated with FSGS. Molecular genetic analysis therefore can be essential to solve difficult cases that show an unusual appearance and therefore improve diagnostic accuracy. Additionally, unnecessary and inefficient treatment with multiple side effects can be avoided.

Keywords: Alport syndrome, *COL4A3*, focal segmental glomerulosclerosis, FSGS, nephrotic syndrome, hearing impairment

INTRODUCTION

Steroid-resistant nephrotic syndrome (SRNS) is one of the most frequent causes for chronic kidney disease especially in young adulthood (1, 2). In around 30% of cases a monogenetic cause can be identified (3). Histological findings in SRNS largely present as focal segmental glomerulosclerosis (FSGS) with progressive glomerular scarring (4). To date, more than 30 genes associated with SRNS have been identified placing the podocyte into the center of attention regarding the pathogenesis of SRNS and FSGS (5). Immunosuppressive treatment of proteinuria in hereditary FSGS often cannot induce remission and is also poorly tolerated (6, 7).

In rare cases, FSGS can be caused by variants in *COL4A3* and *COL4A4,* both genes associated with Alport syndrome (AS) (8). AS typically occurs with the leading symptoms of progressive renal failure, sometimes associated with the extrarenal manifestations of hearing impairment (sensorineural deafness) and/or ocular abnormalities (anterior lenticonus, cataract) (9). In AS the first sign is microscopic hematuria in early childhood. Proteinuria increases as disease progresses. However, proteinuria commonly does not reach nephrotic range in contrast to FSGS or SRNS (10).

Variants in *COL4A5* are the most frequent causes involved in the pathogenesis of AS and account for about 85% of cases (9). Due to the X-linked inheritance of *COL4A5* mostly men are affected. In fewer cases, variants in *COL4A3* and *COL4A4* located at the long arm of chromosome 2 account for an autosomal recessive (14% of cases) or autosomal dominant (1% of cases) AS (11, 12). Male and female patients are equally affected.

Due to mainly economic reasons, genetic testing is often reluctantly used in clinical routine. Molecular genetic diagnosis can improve accuracy of disease classification, especially in phenotypes with multiple symptoms and unusual appearance and help to create personalized treatment options.

Here we report one novel *COL4A3* variant in a compound heterozygous state in a 34 year old woman with hematuria and proteinuria who presented initially with histological findings compatible with FSGS. Only after hearing impairment occurred later in life, genetic testing of AS associated genes was initiated and the correct diagnosis was made.

Abbreviations: ACE, angiotensin-converting enzyme; AS, Alport syndrome; ESRD, end-stage renal disease; FSGS, focal segmental glomerulosclerosis; GBM, glomerular basement membrane; MMF, mycophenolate mofetil; NC1, C-terminal globular non-collagenous domain; SRNS, steroid-resistant nephrotic syndrome; TBMN, thin basement membrane nephropathy.

MATERIALS AND METHODS

Clinical Case Information

The study was approved by the local Ethics Committee of the Technical University of Munich and performed according to the standard of the Helsinki Declaration of 1975. Written informed consent was obtained from the index patient and their relatives for publication. Clinical and phenotype information was gathered out of clinical reports and medical history.

Histology

Histological examinations of the kidney biopsies at the age of 28 and 32 years were performed with light microscopy of sections stained with Periodic acid-Schiff (PAS) reaction and hematoxylin and eosin staining, immunohistochemistry and electron microscopy. Immunohistochemistry of the latest biopsy was performed with antibodies specific for IgA, IgG, IgM, C1q, and C3c (all polyclonal rabbit antibodies, Dako; Dilution and Code No. IgA 1:200000, A0262, IgG 1:150000, A0423, IgM 1:100000, A0425, C1q 1:100000, A0136, C3c 1:100000, A0062) after digestion with PronaseE for 45 min. For detection Envision Kit (Dako) was applied and DAB was used as a chromogen. For electron microscopy fixed renal biopsies were dehydrated and embedded in Epon. Semithin and ultrathin sections were prepared and stained with methylene blue or uranyl acetate/lead citrate, respectively. Ultrathin sections were then analyzed with a Zeiss electron microscope LEO EM 910 or LEO EM 912 (Zeiss, Oberkochen, Germany) at various magnifications. Histological and electron microscopic images were only available from the latest kidney biopsy.

Genetics

Blood samples were collected after written informed consent. Genomic DNA was extracted from peripheral blood of the index patient, her parents, and her children using the Gentra Puregene Blood Kit (Qiagen, Hilden, Germany) according to manufacturer's instructions. In the index patient exon 1 to 51 of *COL4A5* were examined followed by exon 1 to 52 of *COL4A3* using direct DNA sequencing on both strands applying the dideoxy chain termination method on an ABI capillary sequencer 3730 (Applied Biosystems, Foster City, USA). Primers were designed by Primer3 program (http://frodo.wi.mit.edu/primer3/input.htm). For segregation analysis, subsequent targeted sequencing was performed in both parents and children of the index patient in exon 26 and 52 of the *COL4A3* gene. DNA alignment and sequence variant analysis were carried out using the Sequence Pilot^{CE} software (JSI Medical Systems GmbH, Kippenheim, Germany) and compared to EMBL (European

Molecular Biology Laboratory) and GenBank databases as well as our in-house database. All variants were validated in a second independent DNA sample. Scaled gene structure was created with the Gene Structure Display Server version 2.0 (13).

RESULTS

Clinical Phenotype

Index Patient

A 34 year old Caucasian woman of German ancestry presented in our department (**Figure 1A**, II-2). At the age of 12 years, mild proteinuria and microscopic hematuria was detected. This finding was, however, not followed.

At the age of 21 years, the index patient had, for the first-time, increased proteinuria (>1 g per day) and mild hypertension. The histology of a kidney biopsy showed, besides minimal mesangial cell proliferation, uncharacteristic findings. Therefore, no specific therapy was initiated. Unfortunately, no detailed report of the first kidney biopsy was available.

In the presence of persistent proteinuria of >1 g/d and a decrease of creatinine clearance from 83 to 65 mL/min/1.73 m^2 re-biopsy of the kidney was performed at the age of 28 years. The diagnosis at that time was chronic kidney disease due to FSGS with secondary hypertension and proteinuria. The clinical presentation was normal, besides a slightly increased weight (body mass index 24.7 kg/m^2) possibly due to the discrete lower leg edema. Especially, there was no report of hearing impairment. Further laboratory work-up is shown in **Table 1**. Ultrasound examination showed morphologically normal kidneys. The histology of the kidney biopsy revealed focal global glomerulosclerosis with mild chronic tubulo-interstitial damage. Electron microscopy showed one scarred glomerulus and one glomerulus with clumsy podocyte foot processes with effacement compatible with the diagnosis of primary FSGS. Due to a gross proteinuria and the progressive decline of kidney function an angiotensin-converting enzyme (ACE) inhibitor and immunosuppressive therapy with cyclosporine for 7 months and prednisolone were initiated.

Four years later, at the age of 32 years, the patient experienced nephrotic range proteinuria (4.5 g per day). In the beginning, the patient responded well to immunosuppressive treatment with prednisolone (starting dose 60 mg, tapered to 7.5 mg once daily) and mycophenolate mofetil (MMF) (250 mg twice daily) with a reduction of the proteinuria to 1.7 g per day. To further reduce the proteinuria, MMF was increased to 500 mg twice daily. Nonetheless, proteinuria increased again to 4.3 g/d. Therefore, MMF was discontinued and the patient was admitted to our hospital for a kidney biopsy. Clinical presentation at that time was age-appropriate, besides discrete lower leg edema. Abnormal laboratory values are shown in **Table 1**.

Light microscopy of the third kidney biopsy revealed renal parenchyma with 11 glomeruli of which four were obliterated (**Figure 2A**). In one obliterated glomerulus fibrous thickening of the Bowman's capsule was present, indicating fibrous synechia (**Figure 2C**). Crescents were not identified. The remaining glomeruli were unremarkable (**Figure 2D**). No segmental sclerosis, extra- or intracapillary proliferation was seen. Patchy tubular atrophy and interstitial fibrosis was present in ~15% (**Figures 2E,F**) and was accompanied by a mild lymphoplasmacytic interstitial infiltrate. Additionally, multiple foam cell nests were present in the interstitium (**Figure 2B**). Arterial vessel walls showed mild thickening (**Figure 2G**) and moderate arteriolar hyalinosis (**Figure 2H**). In immunohistochemical stainings with antisera against IgA, IgG, IgM, C1q, and C3c only mild mesangial staining for IgM was seen (**Figure 3**). Furthermore, electron microscopy showed that the GBM (glomerular basement membrane) was moderately thinned with extensive foot process effacement and microvillous transformation of podocytes going in line with the former report of primary FSGS (**Figure 4**). After an in-patient stay, an increase of MMF to 750 mg/d was recommended. Hypertension and proteinuria were treated with an ACE inhibitor and candesartan.

Two years later, at the age of 34 years, the patient developed moderate inner ear hearing impairment. Additionally, the 6 year old daughter of the index patient was diagnosed with microscopic hematuria. This new clinical symptomatology combined with a conspicuous family history led to a re-examination of electron microscopy of the kidney biopsy performed at the age of 32 years. In further electron microscopic analyses, segments with thinning and thickening of the GBM (170–700 nm) were found. Moreover, changes in the texture of the GBM were seen in some segments with mild lamellation and basket-woven texture. Moderate effacement of the foot processes was present (**Figure 4**). The re-evaluation of the ultra-thin sections revealed the beforehand described podocyte abnormalities in addition to structural changes of the GBM. Therefore, the changes in GBM structure in the context of the clinical findings and family history were suspicious of hereditary kidney disease and prompted a molecular genetic examination of genes involved in the pathogenesis of AS.

Relatives

The daughter of the index patient presented with microscopic hematuria at the age of 6 years as already mentioned above. So far, the son of the index patient does not show any clinical symptoms of a kidney disease at the age of 9 years. Neither the mother nor the father of the index patient developed (chronic) kidney disease until the age of 54 and 58 years, respectively.

Genetic Analysis

Pathogenic variants in *COL4A5* could not be identified. The sequencing of *COL4A3* (NM_000091.4) revealed two missense variants in a compound heterozygous state in the index patient: c.1892G>T, p.Gly631Val (paternally inherited) and c.4981C>T, p.Arg1661Cys (maternally inherited) (**Figure 1A**, I-1 and I-2). The variants are located in exon 26 and 52, respectively (**Figures 1B,D**). Each parent is a heterozygous carrier for one variant (**Figure 1B**). The amino acid at position 631 is highly conserved in evolution (**Figure 1C**). It is located in the triple helical collagenous domain of the type IV collagen alpha-3 chain (**Figure 1D**). The variant has not been described in the literature before. The second variant, p.Arg1661Cys, has been described previously and is mostly associated to early development of end-stage renal disease (ESRD) (8, 12, 14). The encoded amino

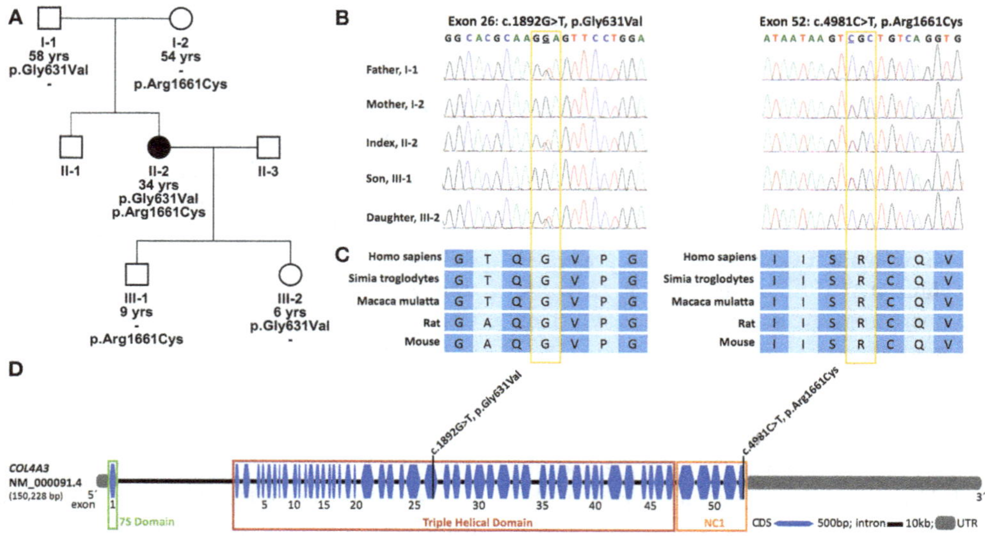

FIGURE 1 | Pedigree of the family, conservations and location of identified variants. **(A)** Pedigree of the family; solid symbols, affected individuals; circles, females; squares, males; yrs, years. **(B)** Partial nucleotide sequence of exon 26 and 52 of *COL4A3* of the patient, her parents and her children. **(C)** Conservation of the affected amino acid over five different species; A, Alanine; C, Cysteine; G, Glycine; I, Isoleucine; P, Proline; Q, Glutamine; R, Arginine; S, Serine; T, Threonine; V, Valine. **(D)** Exon-intron structure of *COL4A3* (NM_000091.4) with the localization of the two identified variants. The variant p.Gly631Val lies in the central triple helical domain, whereas the variant p.Arg1661Cys lies in the C-terminal cysteine-rich non-collagenous domain (NC1) which is together with the 7S domain at the N-terminal a cross-linking domain. bp, base pairs; CDS, coding sequence; kb, kilo base pairs; UTR, untranslated region.

acid is located in the cross-linking C-terminal globular non-collagenous domain (NC1) (14) (**Figure 1D**). The daughter of the index patient carries the newly discovered variant p.Gly631Val (**Figure 1A**, III-2). This variant was also present in the father of the index patient (**Figure 1A**, I-1). The son of the index patient carries the variant p.Arg1661Cys (**Figure 1A**, III-1).

DISCUSSION

We identified a novel variant in *COL4A3* combined with a previously described variant in a compound heterozygous state. In the context of the progressive proteinuria and the young age of the index patient the initial diagnosis was erroneously considered to be hereditary FSGS as it was the most probable differential diagnosis. The present study highlights the importance of including AS in the differential diagnosis of FSGS, especially when disease onset is early in life (<25 years of age). In these cases, it would be helpful to start a molecular genetic analysis promptly (i.e., already if mild proteinuria is present).

Several reports have linked variants in *COL4A3* and *COL4A4* to patients with nephrotic-range proteinuria and the histological findings of FSGS (8, 15).

In these cases, FSGS most likely occurs secondary to GBM pathology and therefore represents an independent entity different from primary FSGS with podocytopathy. Histologic diagnosis of FSGS depends on the size of the kidney biopsy as FSGS due to its local nature is prone to sampling error.

Using molecular diagnostics, we identified a novel missense variant in *COL4A3*. The variant p.Gly631Val is assumed to be disease-causing as it segregates within the family and since glycine is important for the spatial organization of the collagen triple helix as it resides at every third position of the collagen type IV chain. Using PolyPhen-2 (http://genetics.bwh.harvard.edu/pph/) and MutationTaster (http://www.mutationtaster.org) to predict possible functional effects, the variant was classified as probably damaging (PolyPhen-2) and disease-causing (MutationTaster). The variant was not found in our in-house database and in the genome Aggregation Database (gnomAD).

The daughter of the index patient, who is a heterozygous carrier of the variant, already demonstrated microscopic hematuria in early childhood (6 years of age). This can be a first sign of thin basement membrane nephropathy (TBMN). However, the father of the index patient, who also carried this variant, showed no signs of (chronic) kidney disease going in line with the wide range of clinical phenotypes reported in individuals with single heterozygous variants (8, 12, 16).

The second variant, p.Arg1661Cys, has been identified both in a heterozygous and compound-heterozygous state in patients with autosomal recessive AS mostly at an early age at diagnosis of 10–18 years (in one case 44 years of age). In one case ESRD was reached at 19 years of age (8, 12). Previous cases presented with nephrotic range proteinuria (2–5 g/d), thickened GBM and foot process effacement. Hearing loss was reported in one of six cases. No ocular disease was reported (8, 12). However, so far, the variant was only reported in heterozygous form to be associated with ESRD (8) (family DUK6585, individual 1). Elsewhere, the variant was reported in a compound-heterozygous state, however, age of renal failure was not indicated (12).

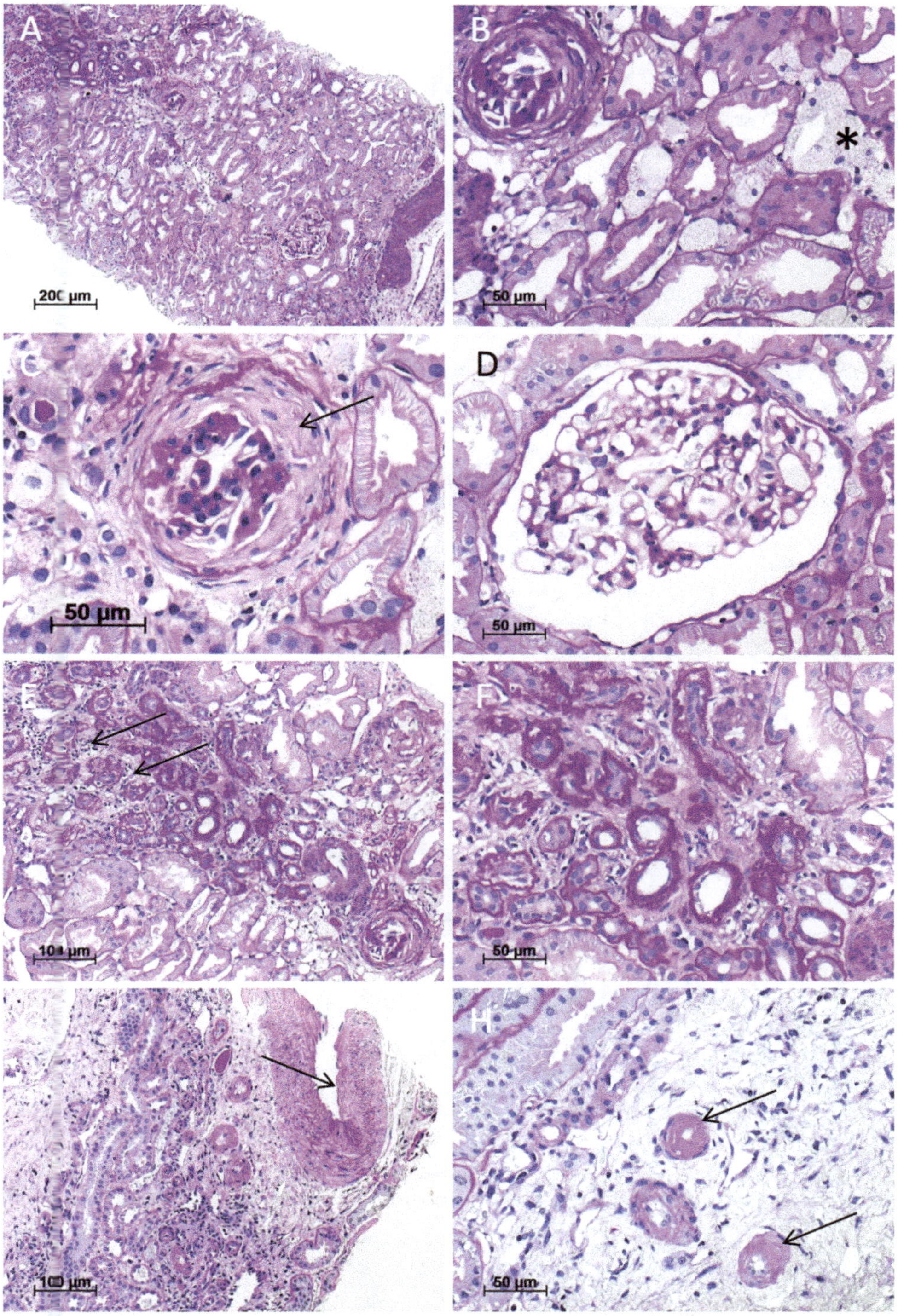

FIGURE 2 | Light microscopy of the kidney biopsy. **(A)** Renal biopsy performed at the age of 32 years with patchy tubular atrophy and interstitial fibrosis (upper left; magnification x100). **(B)** Multiple interstitial foam cell nests (asterisk) and an obliterated glomerulus (upper left; magnification x400), which shows in **(C)** residues of fibrous synechia (arrow; magnification x400). **(D)** One unremarkable glomerulus (magnification x400). **(E,F)** Interstitial fibrosis and tubular atrophy with mild lymphoplasmacytic interstitial infiltrate (arrows) (**E**; magnification x200; **F**; magnification x400). **(G)** Arterial vessel walls showed mild thickening (arrow) and moderate arteriolar hyalinosis **(H)**. All images were taken from sections stained with Periodic acid-Schiff (PAS) reaction.

TABLE 1 | Abnormal blood and urine laboratory values.

	Reference range	Values	
		28 years of age	32 years of age
BLOOD			
Blood urea nitrogen	7–18 md/dL	19.6	39
Creatinine	0.5–1.1 mg/dL	1.2	1.1–1.4
Phosphate	2.5–4.5 mg/dL	–	4.7
GFR (MDRD)	>60 mL/min/1.73 m^2	–	>60
Uric acid	3–7 mg/dL	8.1	–
Total serum protein	6.0–8.0 g/dL	5.6	5.7
Lactate dehydrogenase	<244 U/L	284	353–433
Anti-nuclear antibodies	<1: 120	1:120	–
SERUM ELECTROPHORESIS			
Alpha-1	1.5–4.0%	4.2	–
Alpha-2	5.0–9.0%	11.5	–
ß-globulin	7.0–12.0%	12.9	–
URINE			
Proteinuria	<150 mg/g creatinine	1465	316
Albuminuria	<20 mg/g creatinine	1384	–
Alpha-1-microglobulinuria	<14 mg/g creatinine	14.1	–
Leukocyturia	0–3 per visual field	–	4–10
Erythrocyturia	0–3 per visual field	-	4–10

GFR, glomerular filtration rate; MDRD, Modification of Diet in Renal Disease.

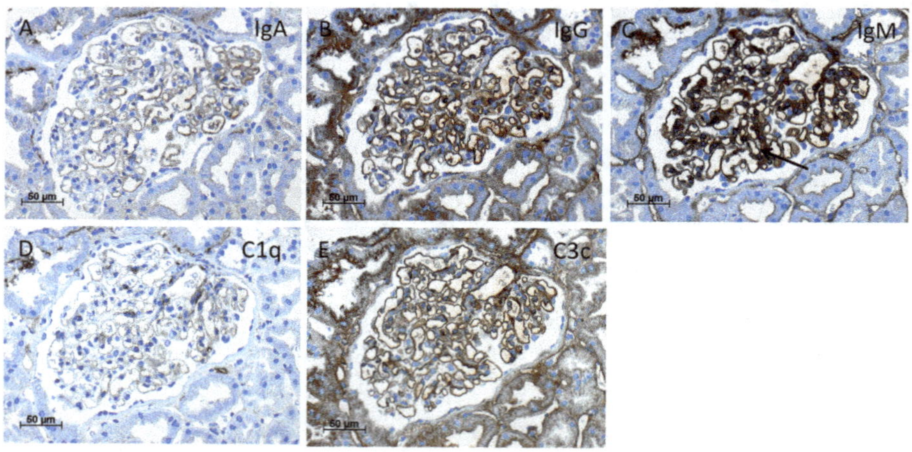

FIGURE 3 | Immunohistochemistry of the kidney biopsy. Immunohistochemistry stainings (magnification x400) with antisera against IgA **(A)**, IgG **(B)**, IgM with mild mesangial staining (**C**, arrow), C1q **(D)**, and C3c **(E)** showed only mild background staining at the endothelial aspect of the capillary loops without deposits suspicious of immune-complex glomerulonephritis.

This exemplifies the wide range of clinical manifestation of heterozygous variants reaching from familial benign hematuria to AS with development of ESRD. The healthy son and the mother of the index patient carry the same variant and did not develop (chronic) kidney disease so far.

Because both parents and children of the index patient carry a heterozygous variant they should be monitored closely by a (pediatric) nephrologist if hypertension, proteinuria, or renal impairment is present (17). In this case, an ACE inhibitor therapy should be evaluated. Otherwise, in the absence of these symptoms regular examination every 1–2 years should be performed by a primary care physician (17). In patients with TBMN and isolated microscopic hematuria chronic renal failure is rare (16). However, if TBMN is accompanied by proteinuria, it has been associated with an increased risk to late onset FSGS with nephrotic syndrome (18, 19). Furthermore, in clinically

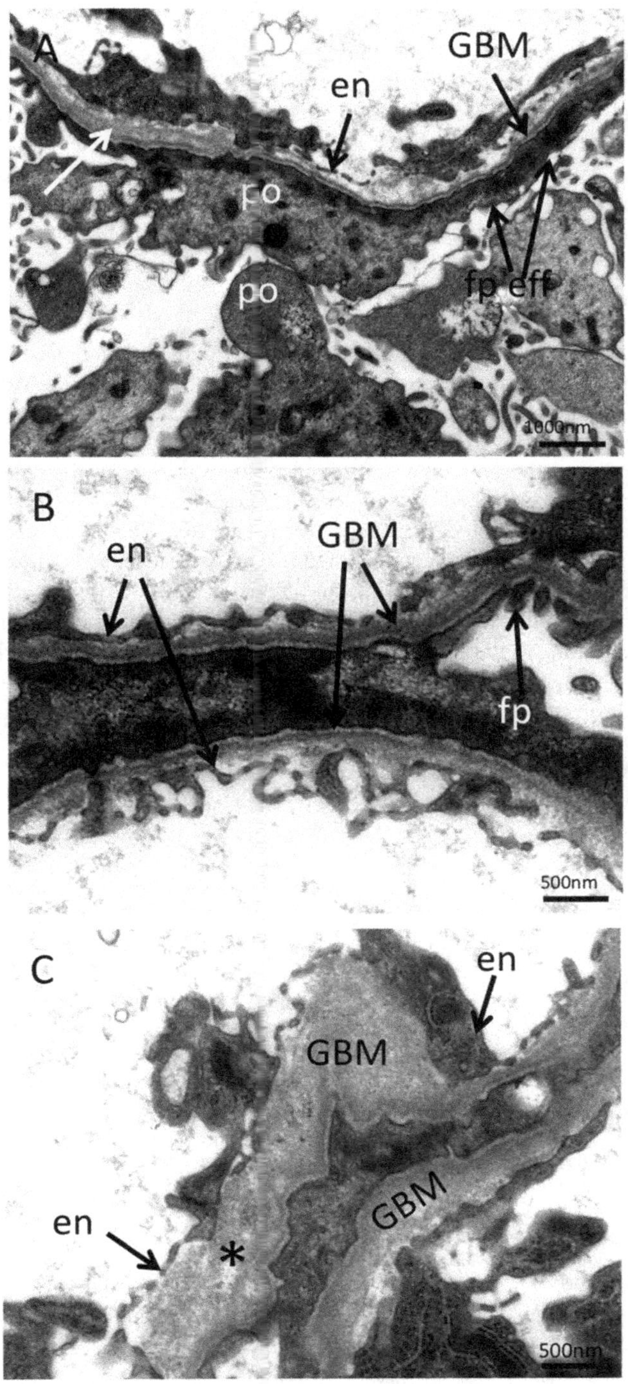

FIGURE 4 | Electron microscopy of the kidney biopsy. **(A)** In the ultrastructural analysis performed at the age of 32, podocytes showed strong foot process effacement with microvillous transformation and thinned glomerular basement membrane (GBM) with mild lamellation (white arrow) compatible with the preexisting diagnosis of primary FSGS (magnification x10,000). In additional ultrastructural analyses performed at the age of 34, segments with thinning and thickening of the GBM (**B**; magnification x16,000) with disrupted basket-woven texture (**C**, asterisk; magnification x16,000) were found. en, endothelium; po, podocyte; fp, foot process; fp eff, podocyte food process effacement.

affected patients with heterozygous variants in *COL4A3, COL4A4* an increased risk of progression to chronic renal failure was observed in up to 38% and a progression to ESRD was observed in up to 20% (15). Age of ESRD onset was significantly earlier in untreated patients with heterozygous variants in *COL4A3, COL4A4,* and *COL4A5* compared to those treated with blockade of the renin aldosterone system (20). Patients that progress to chronic renal failure and ESRD could have variants in hitherto unknown modifier genes.

The rapid course of disease in one family (DUK6696) with compound heterozygous variants in *COL4A3* (p.Glu131fs*151 and p.Gln936*) and nephrotic range proteinuria and hematuria with ESRD at 8 to 12 years of age described by Malone et al. is comparable to our family (8). However, the severity and the more rapid course to ESRD in the previous report could be explained by the presence of two loss of function variants whereas our index patient has compound heterozygous missense variants. This is in line with a genotype-phenotype correlation postulated for *COL4A3* as nonsense or larger rearrangement variants lead to a shortening of the protein and are associated with a younger age at renal failure (<20 years) (15, 21). The unusual appearance of AS with nephrotic range proteinuria in our index patient and the cases described by Malone et al. could be additionally modified by variants in FSGS genes that alter the podocyte in collagen IV-related kidney disease and therefore, could explain the high clinical variability. However, Malone et al. was not able to identify variants in genes associated with FSGS in his cohort (8).

Our index patient developed hearing impairment at the age of 34 years. In general, hearing loss seems to occur more often in cases with variants in *COL4A3* as compared to *COL4A4* (8, 12), but is not mandatory. In the study of Malone et al., hearing impairment was only diagnosed in all 8 of 15 individuals with variants in *COL4A3* after genetic testing had already been done (8). Accordingly, in our case otologic examination was not performed at earlier age probably due to the absence of (severe) symptoms.

Several points may have led to the misdiagnosis of hereditary FSGS in our index patient. First, the quality of the kidney biopsy was low. The histological definition of FSGS comprises a broad spectrum of different pathologies together. So far it is not possible to definitely differentiate between subgroups of FSGS based on the morphology. To improve diagnostic accuracy ultrastructural analysis including measurements of the GBM in ultra-thin slices could be helpful to identify GBM defects. In most cases genetic testing has no therapeutic consequence except for the omission of immunosuppressive therapy and therefore avoidance of adverse side effects. Next generation sequencing would allow a much faster and more accurate diagnosis in clinically and genetically heterogeneous cases. Second, nephrotic proteinuria is unusual for AS (10). Third, classical AS symptoms (e.g., hearing impairment) occurred late in the medical history. Fourth, variants in *COL4A3* show a highly variable clinical phenotype. Fifth, as classically men are affected by X-linked inherited AS female patients may be overseen.

Genetic implications are different for patients with autosomal recessive AS and could highlight caution in case of a kidney transplantation. The mode of inheritance is different compared to X-linked AS. A heterozygous (autosomal dominant) affection with microscopic hematuria and TBMN warrants a restrained selection as kidney donor. This is especially important if blood pressure is high or proteinuria is present (17). Therefore, the newly discovered p.Gly631Val variant with the clinical presentation of microscopic hematuria in the daughter indicates caution for selection as kidney donor.

In patients with AS and TBMN ACE inhibitors are recommended by the expert guidelines for the treatment of hypertension and proteinuria especially in individuals with genetic variants (17). Angiotensin-receptor blockers and aldosterone inhibitors could show additional effects on the reduction of proteinuria (22). To date, new insights for the treatment of AS are expected from the EARLY PRO-TECT Alport trail that is evaluating the effect of renin-angiotensin blockade on proteinuria and renal failure progression (23).

Some limitations of the present study have to be stated. We performed only targeted sequencing of *COL4A3* and *COL4A5* as this study was already performed several years ago. Examination of disease modifiers for collagen IV that could explain the high variability of phenotypes described before were not performed (8). Today panel diagnostics, whole exome or whole genome sequencing would be done in such a case. Also, we did not examine other genes or modifiers related to FSGS, which should be included in further studies to improve the understanding of the high variability of the clinical phenotype. Due to the absence of cryopreserved tissue of the kidney biopsies, it was not possible to perform immunofluorescence analysis with antibodies specific for alpha-3,4,5 subunits of collagen IV complex in the GBM and therefore directly document collagen dysfunction. Unfortunately, electron microscopic images for a re-examination were only available from the last kidney biopsy.

CONCLUSION

We were able to show that a novel variant combined with a previously described variant in *COL4A3* in compound heterozygous state can lead to a phenotype that was erroneously associated with hereditary FSGS. Finally, our study exemplifies the importance of molecular examination in the diagnosis of the renal phenotype to improve diagnostic accuracy and avoid unnecessary inefficient treatment with immunosuppression.

AUTHOR CONTRIBUTIONS

MB and JH, analyzed and interpreted the patient data regarding the genetic and clinical findings and wrote the manuscript. MB-H conducted the histological examination of the third kidney biopsy, compiled histological, and electron microscopy figures and contributed to the writing of the manuscript. H-GK, DW, and JH performed the molecular diagnostics. CK, LR, UH, and CS conducted in-patient treatment. RG, RS, KR, P-MH, CK, LR, UH, and CS contributed important intellectual content during manuscript drafting and revision. All authors accept accountability for the overall work by ensuring that questions pertaining to the accuracy or integrity of any portion of the work are appropriately investigated and resolved. Text revision was performed by all authors. All authors read and approved the final manuscript.

ACKNOWLEDGEMENTS

We thank the index patient and her family for their participation in the study. This work was supported by the German Research Foundation (DFG) and the Technical University of Munich (TUM) in the framework of the Open Access Publishing Program.

REFERENCES

1. Benoit G, Machuca E, Antignac C. Hereditary nephrotic syndrome: a systematic approach for genetic testing and a review of associated podocyte gene mutations. *Pediatr Nephrol.* (2010) 25:1621–32. doi: 10.1007/s00467-010-1495-0
2. Caridi G, Trivelli A, Sanna-Cherchi S, Perfumo F, Ghiggeri GM. Familial forms of nephrotic syndrome. *Pediatr Nephrol.* (2010) 25:241–52. doi: 10.1007/s00467-008-1051-3
3. Sadowski CE, Lovric S, Ashraf S, Pabst WL, Gee HY, Kohl S, et al. A single-gene cause in 29.5% of cases of steroid-resistant nephrotic syndrome. *J Am Soc Nephrol.* (2015) 26:1279–89. doi: 10.1681/ASN.2014050489
4. D'agati VD, Kaskel FJ, Falk RJ. Focal segmental glomerulosclerosis. *N Engl J Med.* (2011) 365:2398–411. doi: 10.1056/NEJMra1106556
5. Warejko JK, Tan W, Daga A, Schapiro D, Lawson JA, Shril S, et al. (2018). Whole exome sequencing of patients with steroid-resistant nephrotic syndrome. *Clin J Am Soc Nephrol.* 13:53–62. doi: 10.2215/CJN.04120417
6. Korbet SM. Treatment of primary FSGS in adults. *J Am Soc Nephrol.* (2012) 23:1769–76. doi: 10.1681/ASN.2012040389
7. Ponticelli C, Graziani G. Current and emerging treatments for idiopathic focal and segmental glomerulosclerosis in adults. *Expert Rev Clin Immunol.* (2013) 9:251–61. doi: 10.1586/eci.12.109
8. Malone AF, Phelan PJ, Hall G, Cetincelik U, Homstad A, Alonso AS, et al. Rare hereditary COL4A3/COL4A4 variants may be mistaken for familial focal segmental glomerulosclerosis. *Kidney Int.* (2014) 86:1253–9. doi: 10.1038/ki.2014.305
9. Kashtan CE. Alport syndrome. An inherited disorder of renal, ocular, and cochlear basement membranes. *Medicine* (1999) 78:338–60. doi: 10.1097/00005792-199909000-00005
10. Hebert LA, Parikh S, Prosek J, Nadasdy T, Rovin BH. Differential diagnosis of glomerular disease: a systematic and inclusive approach. *Am J Nephrol.* (2013) 38:253–66. doi: 10.1159/0003 54390
11. Pescucci C, Mari F, Longo I, Vogiatzi P, Caselli R, Scala E, et al. Autosomal-dominant Alport syndrome: natural history of a disease due to COL4A3 or COL4A4 gene. *Kidney Int.* (2004) 65:1598–603. doi: 10.1111/j.1523-1755.2004.00560.x
12. Storey H, Savige J, Sivakumar V, Abbs S, Flinter FA. COL4A3/COL4A4 mutations and features in individuals with autosomal recessive Alport syndrome. *J Am Soc Nephrol.* (2013) 24:1945–54. doi: 10.1681/ASN.2012100985
13. Hu B, Jin J, Guo AY, Zhang H, Luo J, Gao G. GSDS 2.0: an upgraded gene feature visualization server. *Bioinformatics* (2015) 31:1296–7. doi: 10.1093/bioinformatics/btu817

14. Heidet L, Arrondel C, Forestier L, Cohen-Solal L, Mollet G, Gutierrez B, et al. Structure of the human type IV collagen gene COL4A3 and mutations in autosomal Alport syndrome. *J Am Soc Nephrol.* (2001) 12:97–106.
15. Voskarides K, Damianou L, Neocleous V, Zouvani I, Christodoulidou S, Hadjiconstantinou V, et al. COL4A3/COL4A4 mutations producing focal segmental glomerulosclerosis and renal failure in thin basement membrane nephropathy. *J Am Soc Nephrol.* (2007) 18:3004–16. doi: 10.1681/ASN.2007040444
16. Savige J, Rana K, Tonna S, Buzza M, Dagher H, Wang YY. Thin basement membrane nephropathy. *Kidney Int.* (2003) 64:1169–78. doi: 10.1046/j.1523-1755.2003.00234.x
17. Savige J, Gregory M, Gross O, Kashtan C, Ding J, Flinter F. Expert guidelines for the management of Alport syndrome and thin basement membrane nephropathy. *J Am Soc Nephrol.* (2013) 24:364–75. doi: 10.1681/ASN.2012020148
18. Van Paassen P, Van Breda Vriesman PJ, Van Rie H, Tervaert JW. Signs and symptoms of thin basement membrane nephropathy: a prospective regional study on primary glomerular disease-The Limburg Renal Registry. *Kidney Int.* (2004) 66:909–13.doi: 10.1111/j.1523-1755.2004.00835.x
19. Deltas C. Thin basement membrane nephropathy: is there genetic predisposition to more severe disease? *Pediatr Nephrol.* (2009) 24:877–9. doi: 10.1007/s00467-008-1042-4
20. Temme J, Peters F, Lange K, Pirson Y, Heidet L, Torra R, et al. Incidence of renal failure and nephroprotection by RAAS inhibition in heterozygous carriers of X-chromosomal and autosomal recessive Alport mutations. *Kidney Int.* (2012) 81:779–83. doi: 10.1038/ki.2011.452
21. Savige J, Storey H, Il Cheong H, Gyung Kang H, Park E, Hilbert P, et al. X-Linked and autosomal recessive alport syndrome: pathogenic variant features and further genotype-phenotype correlations. *PLoS ONE* (2016) 11:e0161802. doi: 10.1371/journal.pone.0161802
22. Kaito H, Nozu K, Iijima K, Nakanishi K, Yoshiya K, Kanda K, et al. The effect of aldosterone blockade in patients with alport syndrome. *Pediatr Nephrol.* (2006) 21:1824–9. doi: 10.1007/s00467-006-0270-8
23. Gross O, Friede T, Hilgers R, Gorlitz A, Gavenis K, Ahmed R, et al. Safety and efficacy of the ACE-inhibitor ramipril in Alport syndrome: the double-blind, randomized, placebo-controlled, multicenter phase III Early Pro-Tect Alport trial in pediatric patients. *ISRN Pediatr.* (2012) 2012:436046. doi: 10.5402/2012/436046

24

Network for Early Onset Cystic Kidney Diseases—A Comprehensive Multidisciplinary Approach to Hereditary Cystic Kidney Diseases in Childhood

Jens Christian König, Andrea Titieni, Martin Konrad and The NEOCYST Consortium*

Department of General Pediatrics, University Children's Hospital Münster, Münster, Germany

Correspondence:
Jens Christian König
jens.koenig@ukmuenster.de

Hereditary cystic kidney diseases comprise a complex group of genetic disorders representing one of the most common causes of end-stage renal failure in childhood. The main representatives are autosomal recessive polycystic kidney disease, nephronophthisis, Bardet–Biedl syndrome, and hepatocyte nuclear factor-1beta nephropathy. Within the last years, genetic efforts have brought tremendous progress for the molecular understanding of hereditary cystic kidney diseases identifying more than 70 genes. Yet, genetic heterogeneity, phenotypic variability, a lack of reliable genotype–phenotype correlations and the absence of disease-specific biomarkers remain major challenges for physicians treating children with cystic kidney diseases. To tackle these challenges comprehensive scientific approaches are urgently needed that match the ongoing "revolution" in genetics and molecular biology with an improved efficacy of clinical data collection. Network for early onset cystic kidney diseases (NEOCYST) is a multidisciplinary, multicenter collaborative combining a detailed collection of clinical data with translational scientific approaches addressing the genetic, molecular, and functional background of hereditary cystic kidney diseases. Consisting of seven work packages, including an international registry as well as a biobank, NEOCYST is not only dedicated to current scientific questions, but also provides a platform for longitudinal clinical surveillance and provides precious sources for high-quality research projects and future clinical trials. Funded by the German Federal Government, the NEOCYST collaborative started in February 2016. Here, we would like to introduce the rationale, design, and objectives of the network followed by a short overview on the current state of progress.

Keywords: hereditary cystic kidney diseases, ciliopathy, nephronophthisis, autosomal recessive polycystic kidney disease, Bardet–Biedl syndrome, hepatocyte nuclear factor-1beta nephropathy

BACKGROUND

Hereditary cystic kidney diseases comprise a group of slowly progressive, chronically debilitating disorders with a high level of complexity. Despite rare individually, as a group they represent one of the most common causes of end-stage renal failure in childhood and, therefore, have an enormous socioeconomic impact. The main representatives of this group of diseases are autosomal recessive polycystic kidney disease (ARPKD), nephronophthisis and nephronophthisis-related ciliopathies (NPH/NPH-RC), Bardet–Biedl syndrome (BBS), and hepatocyte nuclear factor-1beta (HNF1B) nephropathy (1). The incidence ranges from 1:5,000 to 1:100,000 and the estimated overall prevalence is about 300–450 children in Germany (2–7).

Most early onset cystic kidney diseases are inherited as an autosomal recessive trait. One important exception is the HNF1B nephropathy, which follows autosomal dominant inheritance (6). Within the past 20 years scientific efforts have brought tremendous progress for the molecular understanding of hereditary cystic kidney diseases. To date, mutations in more than 70 individual genes have been identified (**Table 1**)

TABLE 1 | Update on genes identified to cause early onset cystic kidney diseases (2, 10, 19–25).

Nephronophthisis (NPH) (~63% rate of genetic proof)	**Genes accounting for more than 1% of cases**	**Genes accounting for less than 1% of cases**
	• NPHP1 (NPHP1/SLS1/JBTS4) (20–39%) • INVS (NPHP2) • NPHP3 (NPHP3/MKS7) • NPHP4 (NPHP4/SLS4) • IQCB1 (NPHP5) • CEP290 [NPHP6/SLS6/JBTS5/MKS4/Bardet–Biedl syndrome (BBS)14] • TMEM67 (NPHP11/JBTS6/MKS3/COACH)	• GLIS2 (NPHP7) • RPGRIP1L (NPHP8/JBTS7/MKS5/COACH) • NEK8 (NPHP9) • SDCCAG8 (NPHP10/SLS7/BBS16) • TTC21B (NPHP12/JBTS11/SRTD4) • WDR19 (NPHP13/SLS8/SRTD5) • ZNF423 (NPHP14/JBTS19) • CEP164 (NPHP15) • ANKS6 (NPHP16) • IFT172 (NPHP17/SRTD10) • CEP83 (NPHP18) • DCDC2 (NPHP19) • MAPKBP1 (NPHP20)
Joubert Syndrome (62–94% rate of genetic proof)	**Genes accounting for more than 1% of cases**	**Genes accounting for less than 1% of cases**
	• INPP5E (JBTS1) • TMEM216 (JBTS2/MKS2) • AHI1 (JBTS3) • NPHP1 (JBTS4/NPHP1/SLS1) • CEP290 (JBTS5/NPHP6/SLS6/MKS4/BBS14) • TMEM67 (JBTS6/NPHP11/MKS3/COACH) • RPGRIP1L (JBTS7/NPHP8/MKS5/COACH) • CC2D2A (JBTS9/MKS6) • C5orf42 (JBTS17/OFD6) • CSPP1 (JBTS21) • KIAA0586 (JBTS23/SRTD14) • TCTN2 (JBTS24/MKS8) • MKS1 (JBTS28/BBS13/MKS1)	• ARL13B (JBTS8) • OFD1 (JBTS10) • TTC21B (JBTS11/NPHP12/SRTD4) • KIF7 (JBTS12) • TCTN1 (JBTS13) • TMEM237 (JBTS14) • CEP41 (JBTS15) • TMEM138 (JBTS16) • TCTN3 (JBTS18/OFD4) • ZNF423 (JBTS19/NPHP14) • TMEM231 (JBTS20/MKS11/OFD3) • PDE6D (JBTS22) • CEP104 (JBTS25) • KIAA0556/KATNIP (JBTS26) • B9D1 (JBTS27/MKS9) • TMEM107 (JBTS29/MKS13) • ARMC9 (JBTS30) • CEP120 (JBTS31/SRTD13) • SUFU (JBTS32) • PIBF1 (JBTS33) • B9D2 (JBTS34/MKS10)
Bardet–Biedl syndrome (70–80% rate of genetic proof)	**Most common genes**	**Less common genes**
	• BBS1 (20–30%) • BBS2 (15%) • BBS7 (15%) • BBS4 (8%) • PTHB1 (BBS9) (8%) • BBS10 (20–30%)	• ARL6 (BBS3) • BBS5 • MKKS (BBS6) • TTC8 (BBS8) • TRIM32 (BBS11) • BBS12 (BBS12) • MKS1 (BBS13/JBTS28/MKS1) • CEP290 (BBS14/NPHP6/SLS6/JBTS5/MKS4) • WDPCP (BBS15) • SDCCAG8 (BBS16/NPHP10/SLS7) • LZTFL1 (BBS17) • BBIP1 (BBS18) • IFT27 (BBS19) • IFT74 (BBS20) • C8orf37 (BBS21)

(Continued)

TABLE 1 | Continued

	Most common genes	Less common genes
Meckel–Gruber Syndrome (60% rate of genetic proof)	• MKS1 (MKS1/JBTS28/BBS13) (~7%) • TMEM67 (~16–50%) (MKS3/NPHP11/JBTS6/COACH) • CEP290 (MKS4/NPHP6/SLS6/JBTS5/BBS14) • RPGRIP1L (MKS5/JBTS7/NPHP8/COACH)	• TMEM216 (MKS2/JBTS2) • CC2D2A (MKS6/JBTS9/COACH) • NPHP3 (MKS7/NPHP3) • TCTN2 (MKS8/JBTS24) • B9D1 (MKS9/JBTS27) • B9D2 (MKS10/JBTS34) • TMEM231 (MKS11/JBTS20/OFD3) • KIF14 (MKS12) • TMEM107 (MKS13/JBTS29)
Short rib thoracic dysplasia with or without polydactyly	• IFT80 (SRTD2) • DYNC2H1 (SRTD3) • TTC21B/IFT139 (SRTD4/JBTS11/NPHP12) • WDR19/IFT144 (SRTD5/NPHP13/SLS8) • NEK1 (SRTD6) • WDR35 (SRTD7) • WDR60 (SRTD8) • IFT140 (SRTD9) • IFT172 (SRTD10/NPHP17) • WDR34 (SRTD11) • CEP120 (SRTD13/JBTS31) • KIAA0586 (SRTD14/JBTS23)	

(8). Yet, genetic heterogeneity is a major problem since, there is a significant amount of genetic as well as phenotypic overlap and reliable data on genotype–phenotype correlations are still lacking (9). Moreover, the phenotypic spectrum covered by cystic kidney diseases is highly complex and extremely variable. Although all disease entities are characterized by the development of renal cysts as a common characteristic, clinical courses as well as the onset of chronic renal failure differ significantly. Furthermore, most phenotypes are not limited to the kidneys, but comprise extrarenal organ manifestations (10, 11).

- ARPKD: the clinical presentation of ARPKD is determined by grossly enlarged polycystic kidneys usually diagnosed before birth. Depending on prenatal kidney function, an early oligohydramnion may lead to pulmonary hypoplasia resulting in a perinatal mortality of about 20% in ARPKD. Children surviving the first months of life usually present a preserved renal function for several years. There is obligate hepatic involvement and the clinical presentation of some patients is dominated by a hepatic phenotype rather than by chronic kidney disease (2, 3, 12–14).
- NPH: reduced urinary concentrating capacity, polyuria/polydipsia, and a slowly progressive loss of renal function are the clinical hallmarks of NPH. Urine analysis is typically unremarkable (4). In contrast to ARPKD, kidney volumes are small or normal, and renal cysts have no obligatory feature (15). NPH can be limited to the kidneys, but extrarenal manifestations are found in 20–40% of patients depending on the underlying genetic defect (10). Moreover, many complex syndromes encompass the renal phenotype with NPH, including Senior–Løken syndrome, Joubert-like syndromes, and other NPH-related ciliopathies (16, 17).
- BBS: Bardet–Biedl syndrome is a complex genetic disorder clinically characterized by progressive visual impairment, obesity, developmental delay, postaxial hexadactyly, hypogonadism, and slowly progressive CKD. The clinical presentation is highly variable and can be accompanied by further organ involvement (5). The renal phenotype usually resembles NPH, including polyuria and small- to normal-sized kidneys showing cystic lesions at the corticomedullary junction. However, renal involvement is not mandatory and reported in only 31–42% of BBS (18).
- HNF1B nephropathy: HNF1B is a transcription factor playing a central role in the tissue-specific regulation of gene expression in various organs, such as kidney, liver, biliary duct, pancreas, and genital organs. Initially, mutations in the *HNF1B* gene were described in association with maturity onset diabetes of the young (MODY type 5). Subsequently, it was shown that in patients with congenital cystic renal dysplasia *HNF1B* mutations could frequently be identified (renal cysts and diabetes syndrome, RCAD). In contrast to the NPH spectrum, renal cysts may already be detected prenatally, but renal ultrasound presentation is variable including unilateral and bilateral renal dysplasia with different numbers and sizes of cysts. Depending on the extent of renal dysplasia some patients develop renal failure in early childhood while others preserve normal renal function for their whole life (6). Beyond the renal involvement, the clinical spectrum comprises elevated liver enzymes, hyperuricemia, genital tract malformations, and electrolyte disturbances, such as hypomagnesemia and hypokalemia (11).

GENETIC AND PHENOTYPIC HETEROGENEITY

Although the clinical characteristics of the different hereditary cystic kidney diseases appear quite discriminative, there is significantly genetic as well as phenotypic overlap that hampers an early diagnosis and an individual clinical management (**Figure 1**) (1). The tremendous progress that has been achieved within the genetic field had major impact on the classification of cystic kidney diseases. However, the newly generated insights seem to further complicate the clinical situation for physicians dealing with affected individuals: it has become increasingly evident that so far well-defined clinical entities can be caused by mutations in multiple genes. Even in ARPKD, which for a long time has been assumed to be a single gene disease, modern NGS-based sequencing techniques just recently were able to identify a new genetic cause encoding a ciliary transition zone protein (26). Also, mutations in the same gene can cause very different phenotypes that range from lethal early embryonic multivisceral manifestations to single organ involvement starting in adolescence (**Figure 1**) (1, 27). Thus, recent advances in genomics challenged the classical Mendelian conditions and highlighted the genetic complexity of hereditary cystic kidney diseases and related ciliopathies (28). This complexity has been attributed to allelic heterogeneity, locus heterogeneity, reduced penetrance, variable expressivity, modifier genes, and/or environmental factors (29).

Based on these newly generated insights it has become clear that the "diagnostic odyssey" experienced by patients does not end with the identification of a disease-causing genotype (30). Neither does the traditional approach using textbook signs nor symptoms to guide diagnosis and management seem to be sufficient any longer (31). Rather a systematic and deep phenotyping approach supplementary to careful genotyping is critical in order to discover nonobvious phenotypes and to determine a precise diagnosis. Thus, physicians addressing hereditary cystic kidney diseases should combine both—detailed, multisystemic phenotyping and careful assessment of genotype pathogenicity—in order to capture all facets of the underlying disease (30). Against this background, it will be important to overcome the financial restraints associated with modern NGS-based sequencing currently hampering a comprehensive genetic characterization.

MOLECULAR UNDERSTANDING

The genetic discoveries revolutionized our molecular understanding of cystic kidney diseases. The observation that most genes that have been identified so far encode proteins that co-localize in primary cilia and even interact as functional ciliary clusters suggested the existence of a common pathophysiological pathway and lead to the so-called ciliary hypothesis (**Figure 2**) (32, 33). However, different molecular mechanisms have been described to be altered in renal cyst formation, including cell-proliferation, apoptosis, DNA repair, fluid secretion into the cyst lumen, altered

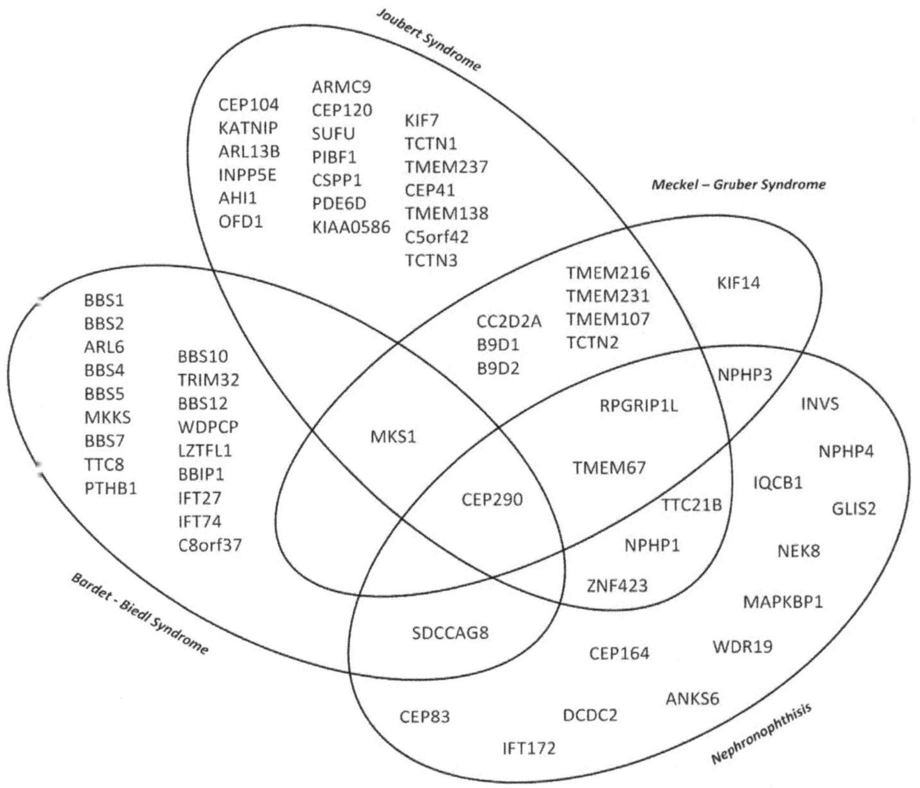

FIGURE 1 | Venn diagram illustrating the major genetic and phenotypic overlap in hereditary ciliopathies featuring cystic kidney disease. So far well-defined clinical entities can be caused by mutations in multiple genes, whereas at the same time mutations in the same gene can cause very different phenotypes depending on the type of mutation ranging from isolated nephronophthisis (NPH) to lethal early embryonic multivisceral manifestations like Meckel–Gruber syndrome.

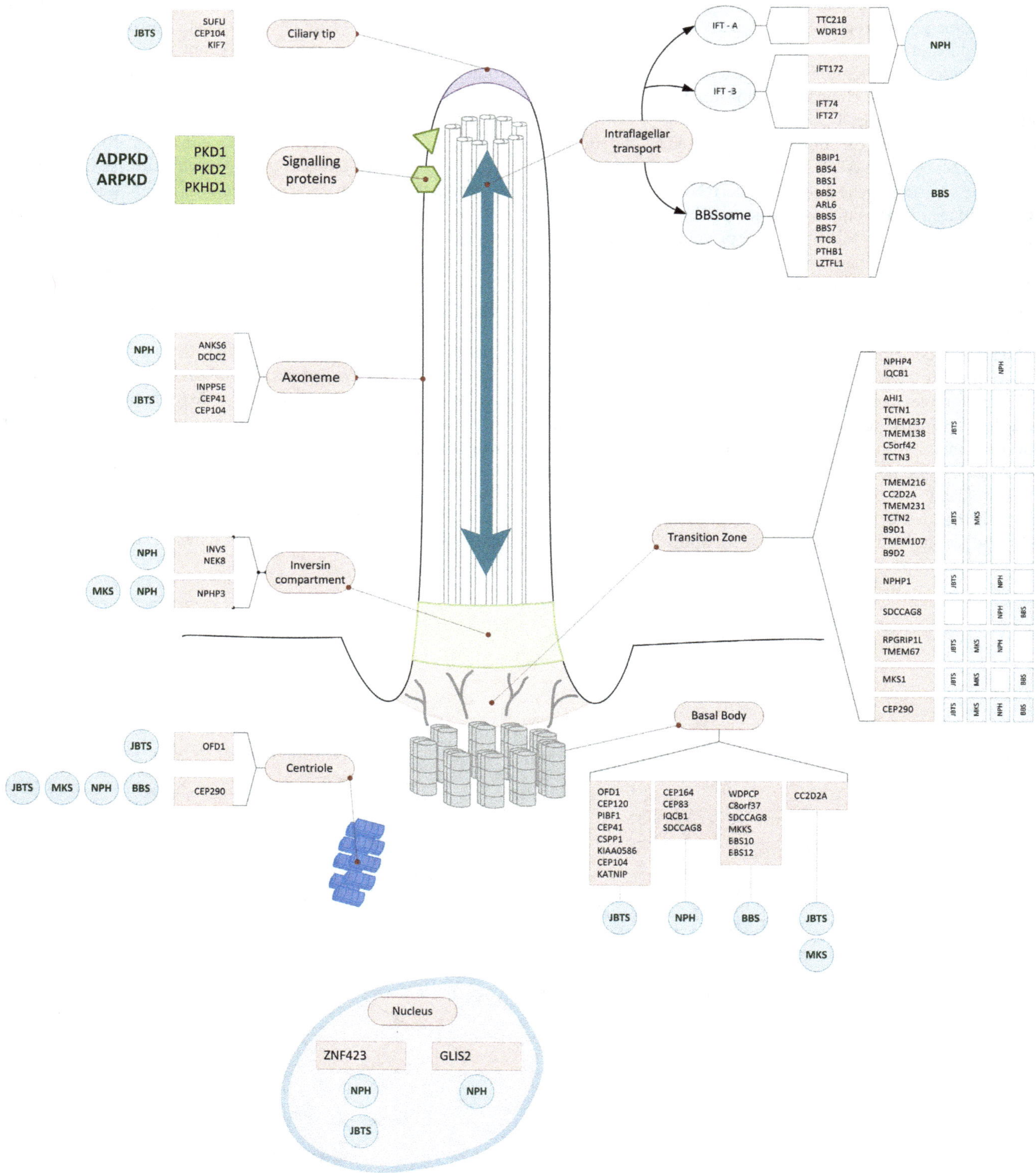

FIGURE 2 | Ciliary localization of the proteins encoded by genes causing early onset cystic kidney diseases. Almost all gene products mutated in hereditary cystic kidney diseases are located at the primary cilium, the ciliary base, or the basal body. Some of the proteins form functional units (Polycystin1/2; BBSom; Nephrocystin-4,5) and are found at characteristic parts of the cilium (e.g., ciliary base). While for some of the gene mutations there is a clear impact on regular ciliary function (e.g., disrupting intraflagellar transport), for most others the exact pathophysiological mechanisms still remain to be unraveled. Abbreviations: NPH, nephronophthisis; JBTS, Joubert syndrome; BBS, Bardet–Biedl syndrome; MKS, Meckel–Gruber syndrome; ARPKD, autosomal recessive polycystic kidney disease; ADPKD, autosomal dominant polycystic kidney disease.

apico-basal cell polarity, directional cell migration, cell–cell adhesion, interaction with the extracellular matrix and ciliary function. Additionally, various intracellular signaling pathways were identified to be activated in epithelia developing cystic lesion, such as intracellular calcium signaling, cAMP triggered fluid secretion, the wnt-, hedgehog, mTOR-, notch-, YAP-hippo-, and other pathways. Whether or not these observations are related to each other and how the mentioned mechanisms could be connected with an altered ciliary function remains poorly understood and is the topic of ongoing research. Details on these topics are beyond the scope of this perspective. However, this has been excellently reviewed by Ong et al. recently (34–36).

NETWORK FOR EARLY ONSET CYSTIC KIDNEY DISEASES (NEOCYST)—A COMPREHENSIVE APPROACH ON HEREDITARY CYSTIC KIDNEY DISEASES

Despite all the achievements mentioned above, enormous challenges remain to be solved: the complex phenotypic spectrum, genetic heterogeneity, a lack of reliable genotype–phenotype correlations, a limited molecular understanding and the absence of disease-specific biomarkers still hamper an early diagnosis and individual counseling. Data from international registry studies like the NEPHREG or the ARegPKD registry will certainly help to define robust genotype–phenotype associations by increasing sample sizes and following individual disease courses in a longitudinal fashion (10, 37). However, in order to achieve a deeper clinical as well as molecular understanding, international collaborative efforts comprising various subspecialists will be necessary to move knowledge forward especially in the context of rare diseases. A detailed molecular understanding will be fundamental in order to identify new therapeutic targets and develop disease specific treatment approaches. Therefore, future research activities should go one step further and try to verify the hypotheses gained from cell culture experiments in specimen harvested from actual patients.

To address all these questions, the NEOCYST was initiated in 2016 in order to match the ongoing "revolution" in genetics and molecular biology with an improved efficacy of clinical data collection. Here, we would like to introduce the structure, the goals, and the individual work-packages of the NEOCYST collaborative accompanied by a short overview on the current state of progress.

DESIGN

Network for early onset cystic kidney diseases is a multidisciplinary, multicenter observational study of hereditary cystic kidney diseases in childhood. It combines a detailed and comprehensive clinical data collection with translational scientific approaches covering the genetic, molecular, and functional background.

AIMS

The primary goal of the NEOCYST consortium is to improve the clinical situation and the management of children with hereditary cystic kidney diseases. In order to reach this goal a multimodal approach was chosen including:

- A detailed and comprehensive longitudinal characterization of different hereditary cystic kidney diseases in childhood.
- The establishment of reliable genotype–phenotype correlations.
- The identification of new cystic disease genes.
- An improved molecular understanding.
- The identification of disease-specific marker proteins.
- A standardized clinical management based on standard-of-care-guidelines.
- The implementation of a national biobank generating a platform for future research projects.

STUDY COHORT

Eligible are patients with the diagnosis of ARPKD, isolated NPH or NPH-related ciliopathies, BBS, and HNF1B-nephropathy. While for the first four study, inclusion is justified either by clinical or genetic criteria, HNF1B-nephropathy has to be confirmed genetically in order to avoid phenotypic overlap with other urinary tract malformations. For the clinical diagnosis of NPH at least two of the following criteria have to be met: (i) characteristic clinical course with polyuria/polydipsia; (ii) chronic kidney disease; (iii) kidney ultrasound or biopsy suggestive of NPH (24); (iv) pedigree compatible with autosomal recessive inheritance. The clinical diagnosis of BBS is based on the diagnostic criteria according to Beales et al. (38). Phenotypes reassembling a NPH-related ciliopathy are classified by the clinical criteria published by Bergmann (1).

Exclusion criteria encompass the definite genetic or clinical diagnosis of other cystic kidney diseases, in particular autosomal dominant polycystic kidney disease (ADPKD) which is addressed by other clinical registry studies.

Patient inclusion is preceded by a written informed consent and an approval by the local ethics committee of each contributing center, guaranteeing accordance with the principles of the Declaration of Helsinki and Good Clinical Practice guidelines.

WORK PACKAGES

To address the goals mentioned above the NEOCYST consortium comprises seven work packages (**Figure 3**). Subsequently, we will outline the main topics covered by these work-packages:

- Clinical registry study: the web-based NEOCYST registry is a newly created retro- and prospective clinical registry providing a detailed genetic and phenotypic characterization of all hereditary cystic kidney diseases in one common database collecting cross-sectional as well as longitudinal data. Three pre-existing registries on NPH-RC,[1] BBS, and HNF1B were merged to build the fundaments of this new database. Additionally, technical bridgehead components

[1] www.nephreg.de.

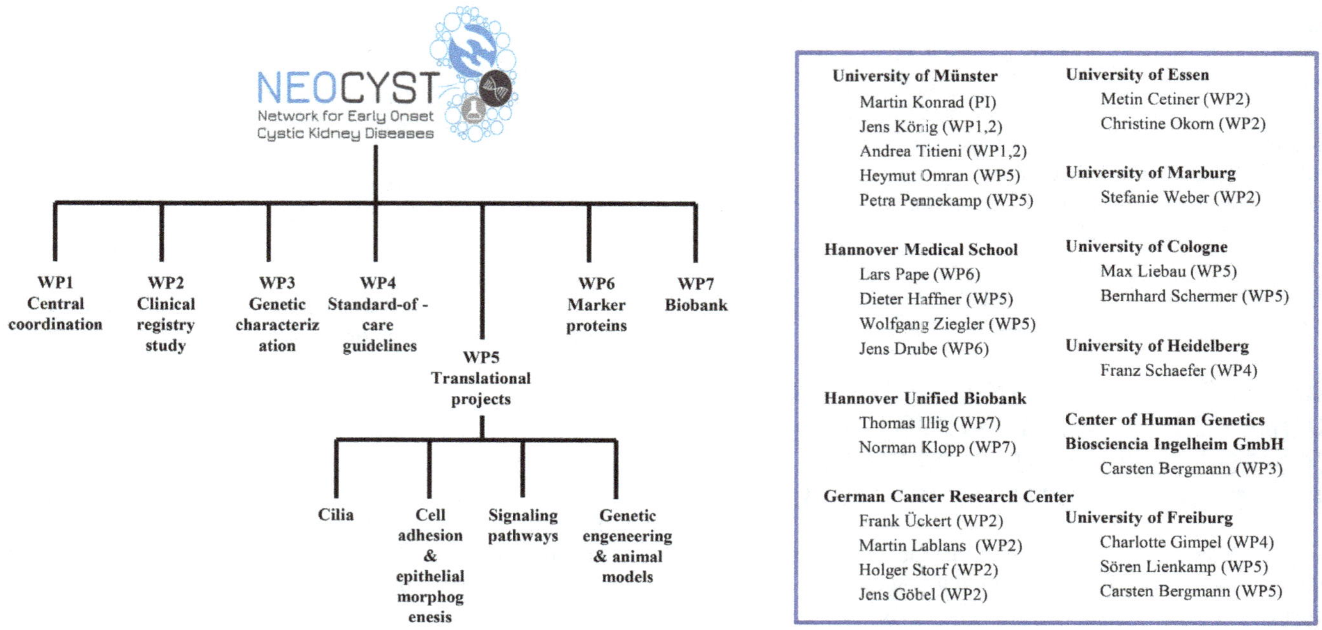

FIGURE 3 | Organizational structure of the network for early onset cystic kidney diseases (NEOCYST) collaborative.

have been implemented that allow a direct comparative data analysis with the international ARPKD registry[2] (37). Thereby, NEOCYST is the first registry study providing a comprehensive approach to early onset hereditary cystic kidney diseases and allowing back-to-back analyses on similarities and differences of the individual disease entities. At the same time, the database supplies technical features that enable external international cooperation and provide a platform for further research projects and future clinical trials throughout Europe.

- Genetic characterization: as the majority of NPH/NPH-RC patients as well as some ARPKD and BBS patients are still genetically unsolved, the NEOCYST network has set out to genetically characterize as many patients as possible, including potential genetic modifiers. The genetic approach applied consists of NGS-based panel diagnostics covering more than 100 ciliary genes followed by whole exome sequencing for those patients in whom no convincing mutations can be identified.
- Molecular biology: the molecular focus of the NEOCYST collaborative is on the characterization of an altered ciliary structure and function, intracellular signaling pathways as well as cell programming and cell adhesion processes. These topics get addressed by internationally acknowledged experts in the field of hereditary cystic kidney diseases (for details see NEOCYST consortium section below). Using conventional cell cultures as well as urine-derived renal epithelial cells (UREC) from patients carrying different mutations, modern techniques, such as proteomics, 3D spheroid models, cell (re)programming, and genomic engineering are applied to analyze different signaling pathways and their impact on cystogenesis *in vivo* and *in vitro*. Additionally, in order to characterize altered ciliary processes in hereditary cystic kidney diseases, nasal brushes from affected patients are generated and techniques like high-frequency video microscopy, freeze-fracture analysis, and immunohistological staining are applied to motile as well as immotile cilia. Finally, it is a goal to identify disease-specific proteome marker profiles from patients' spot urine using a blinded prospective approach based on capillary electrophoresis coupled with mass spectrometry.
- Biobank: due to the paucity of patients characterized by an early onset renal failure, biological samples of such patients are highly precious. Thus, to ensure current as well as future research projects, the NEOCYST collaborative includes a biobank for storing urine, blood, and respiratory epithelial cells. All samples get stored at the Hannover Unified Biobank, one of the most modern biobanks in Europe. It is characterized by a high degree of automation and state-of-the-art biobank infrastructure according to standard operating procedures with data safety concepts, pseudonymization tools, sample identification *via* 2D bar codes and integrated IT systems that enable high quality and safety standards.
- Standard-of-care guidelines: so far, the clinical management of patients with hereditary cystic kidney diseases is mainly based on local physician's experience and differs quite considerably between different centers. Due to the limited number of patients, the experience of most clinical centers is based on only a few single cases and clinical guidelines on the

[2]www.aregpkd.org.

management of hereditary cystic kidney diseases are scarcely available. Thus, NEOCYST has set itself the task to develop and elaborate recommendations on different topics concerning hereditary cystic kidney diseases based on the given evidence in the literature as well as experts' opinions.

CURRENT STATUS

The NEOCYST project started in February 2016 after initiation and approval of funding by the Federal Ministry of Education and Research (BMBF). After 24 months crucial milestones have been reached.

First of all, a homepage[3] has been installed addressing patients, clinicians, and researchers to the same extent. Valuable information on the NEOCYST collaborative, the study goals as well as the medical background is provided in German and English language. A download domain contains all necessary study documents.

Furthermore, in September 2017 the technical implementation of the new online NEOCYST database has been completed merging three pre-existing clinical registries. Up-to-date 344 patients have been included comprising 194 patients with NPH and related ciliopathies, 88 patients with BBS, and 62 patients with HNF1B nephropathy. Especially, regarding HNF1B a rapid increase of participants has been observed ever since HNF1B became a part of the regular genetic screening in patients with hereditary cystic kidney diseases. However, we still assume a high number of unreported cases anticipating a further expansion of the study cohort within the next few years. The database is accessible *via* the NEOCYST-homepage (see text footnote 3).

Major success has been achieved by the genetic workgroup in identifying *DZIP1L* as a new cause for early onset cystic kidney diseases. *DZIP1L* encodes a protein located at the ciliary-transition-zone leading to a phenotype mimicking ARPKD when mutated (26). Additionally, mutations in *MKS1* so far only associated with lethal Meckel–Gruber syndrome were found also to be responsible for a milder phenotype resembling Joubert syndrome accompanied by agenesis of the corpus callosum (39).

The number of biological samples stored in the biobank is continuously growing and substantial progress has been achieved by the projects attended to the molecular biology of cystic kidney diseases. Methods that have been established in another context were successfully transferred to the scientific issues addressed by the NEOCYST project. Detailed imaging and structural analyses of primary and motile cilia have been elaborated and brought to a new scale. First results suggest that structural abnormalities and differences in ciliary protein composition specific for the underlying genetic defect. Furthermore, urine-derived renal epithelial cells, URECs have been established as a valid model on studying cell polarity and epithelial morphogenesis in cystic kidney diseases producing distinguishable patterns of cell clusters. Most results are still preliminary and part of an ongoing research process that will be the subject of future publications.

So far, 19 manuscripts from the NEOCYST cohort have been published or accepted for publication—including a positional paper on the "perinatal management of early onset cystic kidney diseases" (40). Two further positional papers on "imaging of early onset cystic kidney diseases" and "management of early onset ADPKD" have been finalized and are about to be published.

[3]www.neocyst.de.

CONCLUSION

Since initiation in February 2016, the NEOCYST collaborative has made substantial progress in addressing clinical, genetic, and molecular questions related to hereditary cystic kidney diseases. However, the mentioned achievements just represent the first steps of an ongoing process and further scientific initiatives and funding as well as international cooperation will be needed in order to answer these questions. Thus, any participation by international centers is warmly welcome. By setting up the infrastructure of an international clinical registry accompanied by several biological projects and the longtime storage of biomaterial, NEOCYST provides a platform that guarantees a detailed collection of precious longitudinal clinical data going along with further high-quality research approaches and enabling future clinical trials.

NEOCYST CONSORTIUM

C. Bergmann, Ingelheim, Germany; **M. Cetiner**, Essen, Germany; **J. Drube**, Hannover, Germany; **C. Gimpel**, Freiburg, Germany; **J. Göbel**, Frankfurt, Germany; **D. Haffner**, Hannover, Germany; **T. Illig**, Hannover, Germany; **N. Klopp**, Hannover, Germany; **J. König**, Münster, Germany; **M. Konrad**, Münster, Germany; **M. Lablans**, Heidelberg, Germany; **M. C. Liebau**, Cologne, Germany; **S. Lienkamp**, Freiburg, Germany; **C. Okorn**, Essen, Germany; **H. Omran**, Münster, Germany; **L. Pape**, Hannover, Germany; **P. Pennekamp**, Münster, Germany; **F. Schaefer**, Heidelberg, Germany; **B. Schermer**, Cologne, Germany; **H. Storf**, Frankfurt, Germany; **A. Titieni**, Münster, Germany; **F. Ückert**, Heidelberg, Germany; **S. Weber**, Marburg, Germany; **W. Ziegler**, Hannover, Germany.

AUTHOR CONTRIBUTIONS

JK, AT, and MK drafted the manuscript. MK is the principle investigator and JK the central coordinator of the described consortium.

FUNDING

The authors thank GPN for their support. The NEOCYST consortium is funded by the German Federal Ministry of Research and Education (BMBF, grant 01GM1515).

REFERENCES

1. Bergmann C. Educational paper: ciliopathies. *Eur J Pediatr* (2012) 171(9):1285–300. doi:10.1007/s00431-011-1553-z
2. Igarashi P, Somlo S. Genetics and pathogenesis of polycystic kidney disease. *J Am Soc Nephrol* (2002) 13:2384–98. doi:10.1097/01.ASN.0000028643.17901.42
3. Bergmann C, Zerres K. Early manifestations of polycystic kidney disease. *Lancet* (2007) 369(9580):2157. doi:10.1016/S0140-6736(07)61005-8
4. Hildebrandt F, Attanasio M, Otto E. Nephronophthisis: disease mechanisms of a ciliopathy. *J Am Soc Nephrol* (2009) 20(1):23–35. doi:10.1681/ASN.2008050456
5. Forsythe E, Beales PL. Bardet-Biedl syndrome. *Eur J Hum Genet* (2013) 21(1):8–13. doi:10.1038/ejhg.2012.115
6. Ulinski T, Lescure S, Beaufils S, Guigonis V, Decramer S, Morin D, et al. Renal phenotypes related to hepatocyte nuclear factor-1beta (TCF2) mutations in a pediatric cohort. *J Am Soc Nephrol* (2006) 17(2):497–503. doi:10.1681/ASN.2005101040
7. Weber S, Moriniere V, Knüppel T, Charbit M, Dusek J, Ghiggeri GM, et al. Prevalence of mutations in renal developmental genes in children with renal hypodysplasia: results of the ESCAPE study. *J Am Soc Nephrol* (2006) 17(10):2864–70. doi:10.1681/ASN.2006030277
8. Arts HH, Knoers NV. Current insights into renal ciliopathies: what can genetics teach us? *Pediatr Nephrol* (2013) 28(6):863–74. doi:10.1007/s00467-012-2259-9
9. Waters AM, Beales PL. Ciliopathies: an expanding disease spectrum. *Pediatr Nephrol* (2011) 26(7):1039–56. doi:10.1007/s00467-010-1731-7
10. König J, Kranz B, König S, Schlingmann KP, Titieni A, Tönshoff B, et al. Phenotypic spectrum of children with nephronophthisis and related ciliopathies. *Clin J Am Soc Nephrol* (2017) 12(12):1974–83. doi:10.2215/CJN.01280217
11. Bockenhauer D, Jaureguiberry G. HNF1B-associated clinical phenotypers: the kidney and beyond. *Pediatr Nephrol* (2016) 31(5):707–14. doi:10.1007/s00467-015-3142-2
12. Dell KM. The spectrum of polycystic kidney disease in children. *Adv Chronic Kidney Dis* (2011) 18(5):339–47. doi:10.1053/j.ackd.2011.05.001
13. Sweeney WE Jr, Avner ED. Diagnosis and management of childhood polycystic kidney disease. *Pediatr Nephrol* (2011) 26:675–92. doi:10.1007/s00467-010-1656-1
14. Büscher R, Büscher AK, Weber S, Mohr J, Hegen B, Vester U, et al. Clinical manifestations of autosomal recessive polycystic kidney disease (ARPKD): kidney-related and non-kidney-related phenotypes. *Pediatr Nephrol* (2014) 29(10):1915–25. doi:10.1007/s00467-013-2634-1
15. Blowey DL, Querfeld U, Geary D, Warady BA, Alon U. Ultrasound findings in juvenile nephronophthisis. *Pediatr Nephrol* (1996) 10:22–4. doi:10.1007/BF00863431
16. Hildebrandt F, Zhou W. Nephronophthisis-associated ciliopathies. *J Am Soc Nephrol* (2007) 18(6):1855–71. doi:10.1681/ASN.2006121344
17. Wolf M. Nephronophthisis and related syndromes. *Curr Opin Pediatr* (2015) 27(2):201–11. doi:10.1097/MOP.0000000000000194
18. Forsythe E, Sparks K, Best S, Borrows S, Hoskins B, Sabir A, et al. Risk factors for severe renal disease in Bardet-Biedl Syndrome. *J Am Soc Nephrol* (2017) 28(3):963–70. doi:10.1681/ASN.2015091029
19. Parisi M, Glass I. Joubert syndrome. In: Adam MP, Ardinger HH, Pagon RA, Wallace SE, Bean LJH, Mefford HC, Stephens K, Amemiya A, Ledbetter N, editors. *GeneReviews®*. Seattle, WA: University of Washington, Seattle (2003). p. 1993–2017.
20. Ece Solmaz A, Onay H, Atik T, Aykut A, Cerrah Gunes M, Ozalp Yuregir O, et al. Targeted multi-gene panel testing for the diagnosis of Bardet Biedl syndrome: identification of nine novel mutations across BBS1, BBS2, BBS4, BBS7, BBS9, BBS10 genes. *Eur J Med Genet* (2015) 58(12):689–94. doi:10.1016/j.ejmg.2015.10.011
21. Hartill V, Szymanska K, Sharif SM, Wheway G, Johnson CA. Meckel-Gruber syndrome: an update on diagnosis, clinical management, and research advances. *Front Pediatr* (2017) 5:244. doi:10.3389/fped.2017.00244
22. Szymanska K, Berry I, Logan CV, Cousins SR, Lindsay H, Jafri H, et al. Foundermutations and genotype-phenotype correlations in Meckel-Gruber syndrome and associated ciliopathies. *Cilia* (2012) 1(1):18. doi:10.1186/2046-2530-1-18
23. Braun DA, Hildebrandt F. Ciliopathies. *Cold Spring Harb Perspect Biol* (2017) 9(3):a028191. doi:10.1101/cshperspect.a028191
24. König J, Ermisch-Omran B, Omran H. Nephronophthisis and autosomal dominant interstitial kidney disease (ADIKD). In: Geary DF, Schaefer F, editors. *Pediatric Kidney Diseases*. Berlin: Springer Verlag (2016):369–88.
25. Stokman M, Lilien M, Knoers N. Nephronophthisis. In: Adam MP, Ardinger HH, Pagon RA, Wallace SE, Bean LJH, Mefford HC, Stephens K, Amemiya A, Ledbetter N, editors. *GeneReviews®*. Seattle, WA: University of Washington, Seattle (2016). p. 1993–2017.
26. Lu H, Galeano MCR, Ott E, Kaeslin G, Kausalya PJ, Kramer C, et al. Mutations in DZIP1L, which encodes a ciliary-transition-zone protein, cause autosomal recessive polycystic kidney disease. *Nat Genet* (2017) 49(7):1025–34. doi:10.1038/ng.3871
27. Ware SM, Gunay-Aygun M, Hildebrandt F. Spectrum of clinical diseases caused by disorders of primary cilia. *Proc Am Thorac Soc* (2011) 8(5):444–50. doi:10.1513/pats.201103-025SD
28. Gilissen C, Hoischen A, Brunner HG, Veltman JA. Unlocking Mendelian disease using exome sequencing. *Genome Biol* (2014) 12:228. doi:10.1186/gb-2011-12-9-228
29. Lemaire M, Parekh RS. A perspective on inherited kidney disease: lessons for practicing nephrologists. *Clin J Am Soc Nephrol* (2017) 12(12):1914–6. doi:10.2215/CJN.11751017
30. Sawyer SL, Hartley T, Dyment DA, Beaulieu CL, Schwartzentruber J, Smith A, et al. Utility of whole-exome sequencing for those near the end of the diagnostic odyssey: time to address gaps in care. *Clin Genet* (2016) 89:275–84. doi:10.1111/cge.12654
31. Joly D, Beroud C, Grünfeld JP. Rare inherited disorders with renal involvement-approach to the patient. *Kidney Int* (2015) 87:901–8. doi:10.1038/ki.2014.432
32. Fliegauf M, Horvath J, von Schnakenburg C, Olbrich H, Müller D, Thumfart J, et al. Nephrocystin specifically localizes to the transition zone of renal and respiratory cilia and photoreceptor connecting cilia. *J Am Soc Nephrol* (2006) 17:2424–33. doi:10.1681/ASN.2005121351
33. Hildebrandt F, Benzing T, Katsanis N. Ciliopathies. *N Engl J Med* (2011) 364(16):1533–43. doi:10.1056/NEJMra1010172
34. Ong AC, Devuyst O, Knebelmann B, Walz G; ERA-EDTA Working Group for Inherited Kidney Diseases. Autosomal dominant polycystic kidney disease: the changing face of clinical management. *Lancet* (2015) 385(9981):1993–2002. doi:10.1016/S0140-6736(15)60907-2
35. Loftus H, Ong AC. Cystic kidney diseases: many ways to form a cyst. *Pediatr Nephrol* (2013) 28(1):33–49. doi:10.1007/s00467-012-2221-x
36. Ong AC, Harris PC. A polycystin-centric view of cyst formation and disease: the polycystins revisited. *Kidney Int* (2015) 88(4):699–710. doi:10.1038/ki.2015.207
37. Ebner K, Feldkoetter M, Ariceta G, Bergmann C, Buettner R, Doyon A, et al. Rationale, design and objectives of ARegPKD, a European ARPKD registry study. *BMC Nephrol* (2015) 18(16):22. doi:10.1186/s12882-015-0002-z
38. Beales PL, Elcioglu N, Woolf AS, Parker D, Flinter FA. New criteria for improved diagnosis of Bardet-Biedl syndrome: results of a population survey. *J Med Genet* (1999) 36(6):437–46.
39. Bader I, Decker E, Mayr JA, Lunzer V, Koch J, Boltshauser E, et al. MKS1 mutations cause Joubert syndrome with agenesis of the corpus callosum. *Eur J Med Genet* (2016) 59(8):386–91. doi:10.1016/j.ejmg.2016.06.007
40. Gimpel C, Avni FE, Bergmann C, Cetiner M, Habbig S, Haffner D, et al. Perinatal diagnosis, management, and follow-up of cystic renal diseases: a clinical practice recommendation with systematic literature reviews. *JAMA Pediatr* (2018) 172(1):74–86. doi:10.1001/jamapediatrics.2017.3938

25

Is it Ethical to Test Apparently "Healthy" Children for Autosomal Dominant Polycystic Kidney Disease and Risk Medicalizing Thousands?

*Tess Harris**

PKD International, Geneva, Switzerland

***Correspondence:**
Tess Harris
tess.harris@pkdinternational.org

Keywords: autosomal dominant polycystic kidney disease, genetic test, presymptomatic testing, genetic counseling, medicalization, next-generation sequencing

INTRODUCTION

A frequent question asked by parents of children at risk of inheriting autosomal dominant polycystic kidney disease (ADPKD) is: "should my child be tested?" Until recently, most doctors answered "no." They regarded ADPKD as an "adult" condition and advised families to wait until their children were grown up and not to worry them during childhood. But is this an ethical response today given growing evidence of manifestation in children already diagnosed with ADPKD and the prospect of a treatment (1).

BACKGROUND

Autosomal dominant polycystic kidney disease is the most common inherited renal disease worldwide, affecting 1–2 in 1,000 people (2), an estimated 12.5 million individuals across all ethnic groups. Mutations in three genes (*PKD1*, *PKD2*, and *GANAB*) cause multiple fluid-filled cysts to develop in both kidneys and other organs. The kidney cysts grow and expand throughout life causing complications, such as chronic and acute pain, infections, hematuria, stones, hernia, and disfiguring abdominal swelling. Over time, the cysts overwhelm and destroy healthy tissue resulting in kidney failure. ADPKD also causes cysts to form in the liver (polycystic liver disease or PLD), with some patients experiencing massive liver growth, infection, and pain. Brain aneurysms are four times as common in ADPKD as the general population and patients are at risk of cardiovascular disease from high blood pressure. Other, rarer manifestations can occur, such as cysts in the pancreas, brain, and seminal vesicles (**Figure 1**).

Autosomal dominant polycystic kidney disease accounts for one in 10 patients in end-stage renal disease (ESRD) requiring renal replacement therapy (dialysis or kidney transplant) and is a major health-care burden. Across Europe, ESRD in ADPKD is estimated to cost €1.5 billion/year (3). Those with severe PLD may require life-saving liver transplantation due to comorbidities from liver enlargement. Perversely, cystic livers remain functional and patients with PLD can spend years on transplant waiting lists owing to low Model for End-Stage Liver Disease score.

Pre-ESRD, ADPKD patients often experience significant diminution in quality of life. This is due not only to the clinical burden, but also to the impact that this chronic, progressive incurable, genetic disease has on personal and family life. Anxiety, depression, shock, fear of the future, and genetic guilt have been observed in patients (4). Average ESRD age in ADPKD is mid to late 50s (5). Kidney failure at an age when many people are economically productive can result in lost jobs and income—with consequent socio-economic burden.

There are no proven treatments that will stop cyst development. Management is focused on treating the symptoms: anti-hypertensive medication, antibiotics, pain relief, and then dialysis or transplantation. In 2015, the first-ever drug to treat ADPKD in adults was approved by regulators

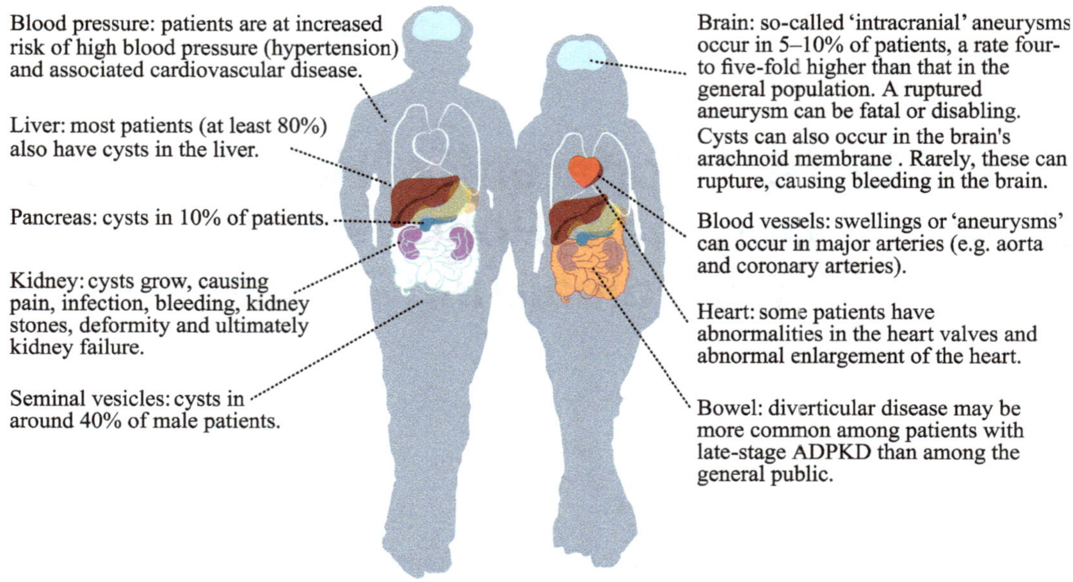

FIGURE 1 | Parts of the body that may be affected by autosomal dominant polycystic kidney disease (ADPKD). The author kindly acknowledges the European ADPKD Forum Report: Translating science into policy to improve ADPKD care in Europe. (2015). Available from: http://www.pkdinternational.org/eaf_adpkd_forum_policy_report_2015/.

in Japan, Canada, and the EU. In a trial, tolvaptan (a vasopressin V2 receptor antagonist) was shown to help slow ADPKD progression by reducing the rate at which kidneys become enlarged by cysts and helping slow the speed of kidney function decline (6). Tolvaptan does not alter liver cyst growth. In the EU, only adult ADPKD patients with CKD stage 1–3 and evidence of rapidly progressing disease are eligible for this therapy.

ADPKD IN CHILDREN

Autosomal dominant polycystic kidney disease is present from conception but symptoms are primarily adult-onset and rare during childhood. Being an autosomal dominant condition, ADPKD carries an inheritance risk of 1 in 2 (50%) from an affected parent. However, *de novo* mutations have been found in 1 in 10–13 people (7). Despite continuous, silent cyst growth, kidney function is typically normal during childhood owing to compensatory hyperfiltration in the nephrons. Many people are not diagnosed until adulthood (even with family histories) when symptoms, such as hypertension, chronic back pain or blood in the urine trigger an investigation for ADPKD. Some patients are diagnosed incidentally, e.g., during scans for kidney stones or pregnancy (unpublished data from PKD Charity UK survey 2015).

Diagnosis is usually by ultrasound. However, cysts in children are not always detected and there is a chance of cyst development in later life. Genetic testing is uncommon owing to cost and genetic complexity. Rarely, genetic testing is used where diagnosis by imaging is inconclusive or to distinguish ADPKD from other cystic kidney diseases such as autosomal recessive polycystic kidney disease and ciliopathies which can "mimic" PKD (8).

There is wide variability in ADPKD progression, even in families with the same mutation. Individuals with ADPKD caused by *PKD1* mutations typically have a more severe progression than those with *PKD2* mutations. ESRD, for instance, can be up to 20 years earlier in patients with *PKD1* mutations (9). Clinical features do overlap, however, and clinicians do not differentiate in practice. Monitoring and treatment are indicated by kidney function progression and comorbidities.

Molecular mechanisms that may explain the variability are starting to be understood. It is suggested that stochastic, epistatic and environmental events may influence ADPKD expression in individuals (10). Advances in next-generation sequencing should provide more knowledge and insights but this technique is not widely available or affordable.

Unless a child has a diagnosis of ADPKD, they probably will not need treatment until later in life. Symptom rarity, perception of ADPKD being an "adult" condition, and lack of licensed treatments for children to slow disease progression, mean that historically doctors and parents felt safe to wait until the child was old enough to decide about testing for themselves.

Presymptomatic testing was discussed at the ADPKD Kidney Disease: Improving Global Outcomes (KDIGO) Consensus Conference (2014). The conference included patients and parents, and at that time there was agreement that minors should not be offered presymptomatic testing (11). Three approaches were proposed for parents considering screening or testing at-risk but undiagnosed children: "screen children as young as possible and disclose the results to the entire family; screen and disclose results only to the parents; do not screen." Parents would in all cases have the final decision regarding screening.

The KDIGO report's authors felt that negative outcomes of a positive diagnosis in a child outweighed positives (11). When anyone is diagnosed with ADPKD (or any other potentially life-changing, incurable genetic condition), there are long-term consequences. Career choices may be limited, e.g., patients may be unable to join the armed forces or pursue vigorous contact sports such as rugby or martial arts. Insurance policies for life, critical illness, and private health may be impossible to obtain; other types of insurance will incur higher premiums. A diagnosis has implications for family planning and may negatively influence a patient's perspective of their future (unpublished data from PKD Charity UK survey 2015).

Undiagnosed at-risk children may appear "healthy" on the outside. However, there is evidence of early symptoms that may be overlooked in the undiagnosed ADPKD population. In a meta-analysis, Marlais et al. estimated that at least one in five children with ADPKD have hypertension (12); in some centers one in three children are affected. Left ventricular hypertrophy is seen. Cyst and kidney growth is evident, sometimes accompanied by pain. Some children have hematuria and urinary tract infections. Early interventions such as anti-hypertensive medication are inexpensive to prescribe and provide long-term positive outcomes with minimal side-effects. Children can be advised about kidney protection during sports.

There is evidence of changing attitudes among clinicians. In a survey, European geneticists, pediatric and adult nephrologists generally agreed that at-risk minors be clinically tested for ADPKD but did not agree about genetic testing (13). The authors called for a consensus, in particular to clarify the sometimes "conflicting information given to families."

Autosomal dominant polycystic kidney disease was historically called an "adult" condition. The term "adult PKD" is still in use in the SNOMED CT International Codes (14). But it is clearly not just a disease of adulthood, so why are doctors—and parents—reluctant to test children for ADPKD?

ETHICS OF PRESYMPTOMATIC TESTING IN CHILDREN

Although genetic testing is rarely used to diagnose ADPKD, declining costs mean this may become cost-effective and more available. Moreover, the author anticipates there will a rise in parents asking about screening with the potential of access to a licensed therapy (tolvaptan) at 18, as well as growth in clinicians' awareness of manifestations in children. In the author's opinion, international recommendations on presymptomatic testing—to encompass both imaging and genetic testing—should be developed as a priority to guide ADPKD screening/testing in children.

It is instructive to examine current recommendations for presymptomatic genetic testing in children and consider customizing them for ADPKD to include imaging. The prevailing view is that children should not be offered genetic tests for inherited conditions that develop in adult life and are currently untreatable. If a test is being considered, parents and doctors need to ask if the test is in the child's "best interests," i.e., will it do more harm than good to have a diagnosis or should it wait until the child is sufficiently mature and emotionally competent to decide for themselves?

The European Society of Human Genetics (ESHG) recommends (15) that children (minors) can decide for themselves about genetic testing when they are "well informed, have an adequate understanding of the test and its potential consequences, have the capacity to make this decision, are not exposed to external pressure, and have had appropriate counseling."

These are laudable recommendations but the author knows from personal family history of ADPKD and 10-year experience moderating a large ADPKD support group (PKD Charity UK) that information and counseling provided to families and individuals undergoing genetic tests are not offered to those considering an ultrasound test. Indeed, many families are given referrals for ultrasound tests without the opportunity to discuss pros and cons. This standard of care is unlikely to change in the short-term as the routine commissioning of genetic services for ADPKD is not expected for many years.

The ESHG recommendations state that presymptomatic testing can be done if preventive interventions can start in childhood. At present, unfortunately, there are no guidelines for the care of children with or at risk of ADPKD and thus no motivation or incentive for physicians to suggest presymptomatic testing (genetic or imaging).

WHAT ARE THE MEDICALIZATION IMPLICATIONS OF PRESYMPTOMATIC TESTING OF CHILDREN AT RISK OF ADPKD?

It is estimated that 12,000 children (under 18 years) in the UK have ADPKD, of whom about 500 are seen in specialist clinics (unpublished survey of UK nephrologists 2015). The actual undiagnosed population is unknown but presumed to be many thousands. Most children will not have symptoms until adulthood. Many doctors and parents feel that medicalizing children, labeling them with a "disease" while asymptomatic, is inappropriate. Over 90% of parents of these children will also be dealing with the impact of ADPKD on one of them (and possibly other family members). Burdening them with caring for a diagnosed child could add unnecessary anxiety and stress. Moreover, medicalization incurs intervention costs, even if these are limited to hypertensive monitoring and low cost drug prescribing.

Medicalization can have benefits, however (16). Getting a diagnosis can be enabling and empowering. Early anti-hypertensive intervention may reduce cardiovascular risk (and consequent costs) in later life and can help families prepare their children for adulthood. These benefits need to be weighed against the costs to society; there is no immediate solution to this dilemma.

OPINION

In the author' opinion, it is ethical to test apparently "healthy" children at risk of ADPKD, but only when there is a specific framework in place for presymptomatic ADPKD testing accompanied by approved international recommendations for follow-up management and long-term care. The framework should set quality standards which ensure: (i) that parents have the opportunity to discuss the implications in advance of referrals for imaging and/or genetic testing; (ii) that testing by ultrasound for ADPKD is considered equivalent to genetic testing and accompanied by access to appropriate counseling; (iii) that the child is involved in the decision-making if they are sufficiently mature and well informed; (iv) that parents are enabled to discuss the diagnostic implications of ADPKD with children and supported by appropriate services and information; and (v) that genetic testing is considered and provided where feasible and cost effective.

AUTHOR CONTRIBUTIONS

TH contributed the content of the article, which expresses the personal opinion of TH and not necessarily the official views of the PKD Charity UK and PKD International.

ACKNOWLEDGMENTS

The author acknowledges the inputs from families and individuals affected by ADPKD. TH is also a patient with ADPKD with several affected siblings and relatives.

REFERENCES

1. Clinical Trial. *Safety, Pharmacokinetics, Tolerability and Efficacy of Tolvaptan in Children and Adolescents with ADPKD (Autosomal Dominant Polycystic Kidney Disease)*. (2016). Available from: https://clinicaltrials.gov/ct2/show/NCT02964273.
2. Torres VE, Harris PC, Pirson Y. Autosomal dominant polycystic kidney disease. *Lancet* (2007) 369(9569):1287–301. doi:10.1016/S0140-6736(07)60601-1
3. Spithoven EM, Kramer A, Meijer E, Orskov B, Wanner C, Abad JM, et al. Renal replacement therapy for autosomal dominant polycystic kidney disease (ADPKD) in Europe: prevalence and survival – an analysis of data from the ERA-EDTA Registry. *Nephrol Dial Transplant* (2014) 29(Suppl 4):iv15–25. doi:10.1093/ndt/gfu017
4. Simms RJ, Thong KM, Dworschak GC, Ong AC. Increased psychosocial risk, depression and reduced quality of life living with autosomal dominant polycystic kidney disease. *Nephrol Dial Transplant* (2016) 31(7):1130–40. doi:10.1093/ndt/gfv299
5. Shaw C, Simms RJ, Pitcher D, Sandford R. Epidemiology of patients in England and Wales with autosomal dominant polycystic kidney disease and end-stage renal failure. *Nephrol Dial Transplant* (2014) 29(10):1910–8. doi:10.1093/ndt/gfu087
6. Torres VE, Chapman AB, Devuyst O, Gansevoort RT, Grantham JJ, Higashihara E, et al. Tolvaptan in patients with autosomal dominant polycystic kidney disease. *N Engl J Med* (2012) 367(25):2407–18. doi:10.1056/NEJMoa1205511
7. Reed B, McFann K, Kimberling WJ, Pei Y, Gabow PA, Christopher K, et al. Presence of de novo mutations in autosomal dominant polycystic kidney disease patients without family history. *Am J Kidney Dis* (2008) 52(6):1042–50. doi:10.1053/j.ajkd.2008.05.015
8. Bergmann C. ARPKD and early manifestations of ADPKD: the original polycystic kidney disease and phenocopies. *Pediatr Nephrol* (2015) 30:15–30. doi:10.1007/s00467-013-2706-2
9. Cornec-Le Gall E, Audrézet M-P, Chen J-M, Hourmant M, Morin M-P, Perrichot R, et al. Type of PKD1 mutation influences renal outcome in ADPKD. *J Am Soc Nephrol* (2013) 24(6):1006–13. doi:10.1681/ASN.2012070650
10. Bergmann C, von Bothmer J, Ortiz Brüchle N, Venghaus A, Frank V, Fehrenbach H, et al. Mutations in multiple PKD genes may explain early and severe polycystic kidney disease. *J Am Soc Nephrol* (2011) 22(11):2047–56. doi:10.1681/ASN.2010101080
11. Chapman AB, Devuyst O, Eckardt K-U, Gansevoort RT, Harris T, Horie S, et al. Autosomal-dominant polycystic kidney disease (ADPKD): executive summary from a kidney disease: improving global outcomes (KDIGO) Controversies Conference. *Kidney Int* (2015) 88(1):17–27. doi:10.1038/ki.2015.59
12. Marlais M, Cuthell O, Langan D, Dudley J, Sinha MD, Winyard PJ. Hypertension in autosomal dominant polycystic kidney disease: a meta-analysis. *Arch Dis Child* (2016) 101(12):1142–7. doi:10.1136/archdischild-2015-310221
13. De Rechter S, Kringen J, Janssens P, Liebau MC, Devriendt K, Levtchenko E, et al. Clinicians' attitude towards family planning and timing of diagnosis in autosomal dominant polycystic kidney disease. *PLoS One* (2017) 12(9):e0185779. doi:10.1371/journal
14. Snomed CT. (2017). Available from: http://browser.ihtsdotools.org/?perspective=full&conceptId1=28728008&edition=en-edition&release=v20170731&server=http://browser.ihtsdotools.org/api/v1/snomed&langRefset=900000000000509007
15. European Society of Human Genetics. Genetic testing in asymptomatic minors: recommendations of the European Society of Human Genetics. *Eur J Hum Genet* (2009) 17:720–1. doi:10.1038/ejhg.2009.26
16. van Dijk W, Faber M, Tanke M, Jeurissen P, Westert G. Medicalisation and overdiagnosis: what society does to medicine. *Int J Health Policy Manag* (2016) 5(11):619–22. doi:10.15171/ijhpm.2016.121

Permissions

All chapters in this book were first published by Frontiers; hereby published with permission under the Creative Commons Attribution License or equivalent. Every chapter published in this book has been scrutinized by our experts. Their significance has been extensively debated. The topics covered herein carry significant findings which will fuel the growth of the discipline. They may even be implemented as practical applications or may be referred to as a beginning point for another development.

The contributors of this book come from diverse backgrounds, making this book a truly international effort. This book will bring forth new frontiers with its revolutionizing research information and detailed analysis of the nascent developments around the world.

We would like to thank all the contributing authors for lending their expertise to make the book truly unique. They have played a crucial role in the development of this book. Without their invaluable contributions this book wouldn't have been possible. They have made vital efforts to compile up to date information on the varied aspects of this subject to make this book a valuable addition to the collection of many professionals and students.

This book was conceptualized with the vision of imparting up-to-date information and advanced data in this field. To ensure the same, a matchless editorial board was set up. Every individual on the board went through rigorous rounds of assessment to prove their worth. After which they invested a large part of their time researching and compiling the most relevant data for our readers.

The editorial board has been involved in producing this book since its inception. They have spent rigorous hours researching and exploring the diverse topics which have resulted in the successful publishing of this book. They have passed on their knowledge of decades through this book. To expedite this challenging task, the publisher supported the team at every step. A small team of assistant editors was also appointed to further simplify the editing procedure and attain best results for the readers.

Apart from the editorial board, the designing team has also invested a significant amount of their time in understanding the subject and creating the most relevant covers. They scrutinized every image to scout for the most suitable representation of the subject and create an appropriate cover for the book.

The publishing team has been an ardent support to the editorial, designing and production team. Their endless efforts to recruit the best for this project, has resulted in the accomplishment of this book. They are a veteran in the field of academics and their pool of knowledge is as vast as their experience in printing. Their expertise and guidance has proved useful at every step. Their uncompromising quality standards have made this book an exceptional effort. Their encouragement from time to time has been an inspiration for everyone.

The publisher and the editorial board hope that this book will prove to be a valuable piece of knowledge for researchers, students, practitioners and scholars across the globe.

List of Contributors

Verity Hartill
Department of Clinical Genetics, Yorkshire Regional Genetics Service, Leeds Teaching Hospitals NHS Trust, Leeds, United Kingdom
Leeds Institute of Biomedical and Clinical Sciences, University of Leeds, Leeds, United Kingdom

Katarzyna Szymanska and Colin A. Johnson
Leeds Institute of Biomedical and Clinical Sciences, University of Leeds, Leeds, United Kingdom

Saghira Malik Sharif
Department of Clinical Genetics, Yorkshire Regional Genetics Service, Leeds Teaching Hospitals NHS Trust, Leeds, United Kingdom

Gabrielle Wheway
Faculty of Health and Applied Sciences, Department of Applied Sciences, UWE Bristol, Bristol, United Kingdom

Stéphanie De Rechter and Djalila Mekahli
PKD Lab, Department of Development and Regeneration, KU Leuven, Leuven, Belgium
Department of Pediatric Nephrology, University Hospitals Leuven, Leuven, Belgium

Luc Breysem
Department of Radiology, University Hospitals Leuven, Leuven, Belgium

Kirsten Y. Renkema and Nine V. A. M. Knoers
Department of Genetics, Center for Molecular Medicine, University Medical Center Utrecht, Utrecht University, Utrecht, Netherlands

Rachel H. Giles
Department of Nephrology and Hypertension, University Medical Center Utrecht, Utrecht University, Utrecht, Netherlands

Marc R. Lilien
Department of Pediatric Nephrology, Wilhelmina Children's Hospital, University Medical Center Utrecht, Utrecht University, Utrecht, Netherlands

Philip L. Beales
UCL Great Ormond Street Institute of Child Health, London, United Kingdom

Ronald Roepman and Machteld M. Oud
Department of Genetics, Radboud University Medical Center, Nijmegen, Netherlands

Heleen H. Arts
Department of Pathology and Molecular Medicine, McMaster University, Hamilton, ON, Canada

Roman-Ulrich Müller and Thomas Benzing
Department II of Internal Medicine and Center for Molecular Medicine Cologne, University of Cologne, Cologne, Germany

Adrián Cordido, Lara Besada-Cerecedo and Miguel A. García-González
Grupo de Genética y Biología del Desarrollo de las Enfermedades Renales, Laboratorio de Nefrología (n.° 11), Instituto de Investigación Sanitaria (IDIS), Complexo Hospitalario de Santiago de Compostela (CHUS), Santiago de Compostela, Spain

Shalabh Srivastava
Institute of Genetic Medicine, Newcastle University, Newcastle upon Tyne, United Kingdom
Renal Unit, City Hospitals Sunderland and South Tyneside NHS Foundation Trust, Sunderland, United Kingdom

Elisa Molinari
Institute of Genetic Medicine, Newcastle University, Newcastle upon Tyne, United Kingdom

Shreya Raman
Department of Histopathology, Newcastle upon Tyne Hospitals NHS Foundation Trust, Newcastle upon Tyne, United Kingdom

John A. Sayer
Institute of Genetic Medicine, Newcastle University, Newcastle upon Tyne, United Kingdom
Renal Services, Newcastle upon Tyne Hospitals NHS Foundation Trust, Newcastle upon Tyne, United Kingdom

Xuejun Yang, Gaofu Zhang, Mo Wang, Haiping Yang and Qiu Li
Department of Nephrology, Children's Hospital of Chongqing Medical University, Chongqing, China

Jochen Gehrig
Acquifer is a Division of Ditabis, Digital Biomedical Imaging Systems AG, Pforzheim, Germany

Jens H. Westhoff
Department of Pediatrics I, University Children's Hospital Heidelberg, Heidelberg, Germany

Gunjan Pandey
Acquifer is a Division of Ditabis, Digital Biomedical Imaging Systems AG, Pforzheim, Germany
Department of Pediatrics I, University Children's Hospital Heidelberg, Heidelberg, Germany

Sören Bäumner and Lutz T. Weber
Pediatric Nephrology, Children's and Adolescents' Hospital, University Hospital Cologne, Cologne, Germany

George C. Gabriel and Cecilia W. Lo
Department of Developmental Biology, University of Pittsburgh School of Medicine, Pittsburgh, PA, United States

Gregory J. Pazour
Program in Molecular Medicine, University of Massachusetts Medical School, Worcester, MA, United States

Martin Helmstädter and Tobias Hermle
Renal Division, University Medical Center Freiburg, Freiburg, Germany
Faculty of Medicine, University of Freiburg, Freiburg, Germany

Tobias B. Huber
III. Department of Medicine, University Medical Center Hamburg-Eppendorf, Hamburg, Germany

Paula Giménez-Mascarell and Luis Alfonso Martínez-Cruz
CIC bioGUNE, Bizkaia Science and Technology Park, Derio, Spain

Carlotta Else Schirrmacher and Dominik Müller
Department of Pediatric Gastroenterology, Nephrology and Metabolism, Charité - Universitätsmedizin Berlin, Berlin, Germany

Elizabeth Forsythe, Joanna Kenny, Chiara Bacchelli and Philip L. Beales
Genetics and Genomic Medicine Programme, UCL Great Ormond Street Institute of Child Health, University College London, London, United Kingdom

Henning Hagmann and Paul T. Brinkkoetter
Department II of Internal Medicine, Center for Molecular Medicine Cologne, University of Cologne, Cologne, Germany

Jan Halbritter, Anna Seidel, Luise Müller and Ria Schönauer
Division of Nephrology, Department of Internal Medicine, University of Leipzig, Leipzig, Germany

Bernd Hoppe
Division of Pediatric Nephrology, University Children's Hospital, Bonn, Germany

Emily Kim
Department of Radiation Oncology, Faculty of Medicine, Albert Ludwigs University of Freiburg, Freiburg, Germany
German Cancer Consortium (DKTK), Partner Site Freiburg, Freiburg, Germany

Stefan Zschiedrich
Renal Division, Department of Medicine IV, Faculty of Medicine, Albert Ludwigs University of Freiburg, Freiburg, Germany

Markus J. Kemper
AK Nord Heidberg, Asklepios Medical School GmbH, Hamburg, Germany

Anja Lemke
Universitätsklinikum Hamburg-Eppendorf, Hamburg, Germany

Korbinian Maria Riedhammer
Department of Nephrology, Klinikum rechts der Isar, Technical University of Munich, Munich, Germany
Institute of Human Genetics, Klinikum rechts der Isar, Technical University of Munich, Munich, Germany

Corinna Siegel, Bader Alhaddad, Reka Kovacs-Nagy, Pierre-Maurice Herr and Julia Hoefele
Institute of Human Genetics, Klinikum rechts der Isar, Technical University of Munich, Munich, Germany

Carmen Montoya
KfH Center of Pediatric Nephrology, Children's Hospital Munich Schwabing, Munich, Germany

Matias Wagner
Institute of Human Genetics, Klinikum rechts der Isar, Technical University of Munich, Munich, Germany
Institute of Human Genetics, Helmholtz Zentrum Munich, Neuherberg, Germany
Institute of Neurogenomics, Helmholtz Zentrum Munich, Neuherberg, Germany

Thomas Meitinger
Institute of Human Genetics, Klinikum rechts der Isar, Technical University of Munich, Munich, Germany
Institute of Human Genetics, Helmholtz Zentrum Munich, Neuherberg, Germany

Kathrin Burgmaier, Joy Brandt, Lutz T. Weber and Jörg Dötsch
Department of Pediatrics, University Hospital of Cologne, Cologne, Germany

Rukshana Shroff
Great Ormond Street Hospital for Children NHS Foundation Trust, London, United Kingdom

Peter Witters
Department of Pediatric Gastroenterology and Hepatology, University Hospitals Leuven, Leuven, Belgium

Djalila Mekahli
Department of Pediatric Nephrology, University Hospitals Leuven, Leuven, Belgium
PKD Research Group, Department of Development and Regeneration, KU Leuven, University of Leuven, Leuven, Belgium

Max C. Liebau
Department of Pediatrics, University Hospital of Cologne, Cologne, Germany
Center for Molecular Medicine, University Hospital of Cologne, Cologne, Germany

Agnes Trautmann and Franz Schaefer
Division of Pediatric Nephrology, University Center for Pediatrics and Adolescent Medicine, Heidelberg, Germany

Eva Nüsken, Jörg Dötsch, Lutz T. Weber and Kai-Dietrich Nüsken
Pediatric Nephrology, Department of Pediatrics, Medical Faculty, University of Cologne, Cologne, Germany

Matthias C. Braunisch, Roman Günthner, Robin Satanovskij and Korbinian M. Riedhammer
Department of Nephrology, Klinikum Rechts der Isar, Technical University of Munich, Munich, Germany
Institute of Human Genetics, Klinikum Rechts der Isar, Technical University of Munich, Munich, Germany

Maike Büttner-Herold
Department of Nephropathology, Institute of Pathology, Friedrich-Alexander-University, Erlangen, Germany

Hanns-Georg Klein and Dagmar Wahl
Center for Human Genetics and Laboratory Diagnostics Dr. Klein, Dr. Rost and Colleagues, Martinsried, Germany

Claudius Küchle, Lutz Renders, Uwe Heemann and Christoph Schmaderer
Department of Nephrology, Klinikum Rechts der Isar, Technical University of Munich, Munich, Germany

Beata S. Lipska-Ziętkiewicz
Clinical Genetics Unit, Department of Biology and Medical Genetics, Medical University of Gdańsk, Gdańsk, Poland

Jens Christian König, Andrea Titieni and Martin Konrad
Department of General Pediatrics, University Children's Hospital Münster, Münster, Germany

Tess Harris
PKD International, Geneva, Switzerland

Index